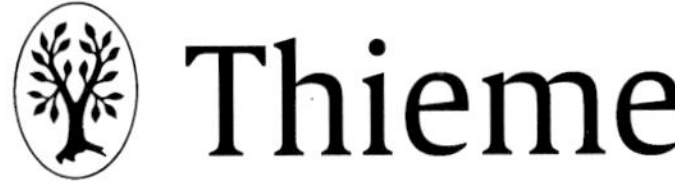
Thieme

Dedicated in gratitude
to my wife Barbara

Surgery of the Auricle

Tumors · Trauma · Defects · Abnormalities

Hilko Weerda, MD, DMD
Professor and Former Head
Department of Otorhinolaryngology
University Hospital Schleswig-Holstein
Campus Lübeck
Lübeck, Germany

With contributions by

F.X. Brunner, G. Burg, S. Gottschalk, I. Greiner, A. Haisch, A.A. Hartmann, A. Hasse, D. Hoehmann, R.A. Jahrsdoerfer, R. Katzbach, J.H.N. Kim, S. Klaiber, M. Landthaler, D. Petersen, R. Schoenweiler, R. Siegert, H. Sommer, H. Weerda, M.B. Wimmershoff

1340 illustrations
33 tables

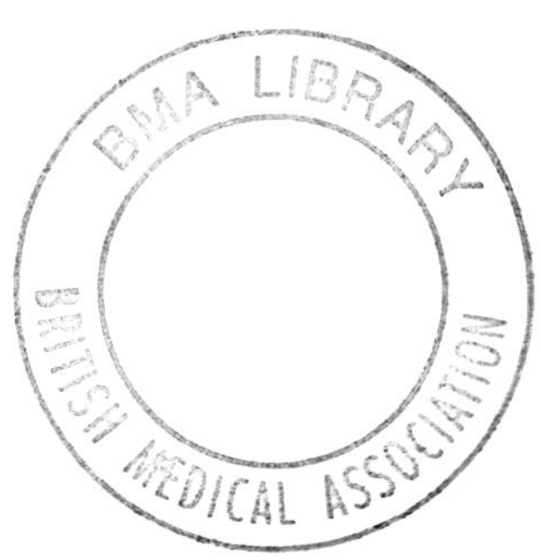

Thieme
Stuttgart · New York

Library of Congress Cataloging-in-Publication Data is available from the publisher.

Important note: Medicine is an ever-changing science undergoing continual development. Research and clinical experience are continually expanding our knowledge, in particular our knowledge of proper treatment and drug therapy. Insofar as this book mentions any dosage or application, readers may rest assured that the authors, editors, and publishers have made every effort to ensure that such references are in accordance with **the state of knowledge at the time of production of the book.**

Nevertheless, this does not involve, imply, or express any guarantee or responsibility on the part of the publishers in respect to any dosage instructions and forms of applications stated in the book. **Every user is requested to examine carefully** the manufacturers' leaflets accompanying each drug and to check, if necessary in consultation with a physician or specialist, whether the dosage schedules mentioned therein or the contraindications stated by the manufacturers differ from the statements made in the present book. Such examination is particularly important with drugs that are either rarely used or have been newly released on the market. Every dosage schedule or every form of application used is entirely at the user's own risk and responsibility. The authors and publishers request every user to report to the publishers any discrepancies or inaccuracies noticed. If errors in this work are found after publication, errata will be posted at www.thieme.com on the product description page.

This book is an authorized and revised translation of the German edition published and copyrighted 2004 by Georg Thieme Verlag, Stuttgart, Germany. Title of the German edition: Chirurgie der Ohrmuschel

Translator: Grahame Larkin, MD, Wimborne, UK

Illustrator: Katharina Schumacher, Munich, Germany

Rüdigerstrasse 14, 70469 Stuttgart, Germany
http://www.thieme.de
Thieme New York, 333 Seventh Avenue,
New York, NY 10001, USA
http://www.thieme.com

Typesetting by Primustype Hurler, Notzingen
Printed in Germany by Druckhaus Götz, Ludwigsburg

ISBN 978-3-13-139411-8 (TPS, Rest of World)
ISBN 978-1-58890-359-4 (TPN, The Americas) 1 2 3 4 5 6

Forewords

Surgical creation of the outer ear with autogenous tissues is a unique blend of art and science. The result will be influenced by the surgeon's adherence to the basic principles of plastic surgery, but his or her sculpture and design skills will ultimately determine the final outcome.

Over the years numerous surgeons have visited me in the operating room, but only a handful have blossomed into auricular artists. Dr Hilko Weerda is one of these gifted few.

I have been honored not only to watch Dr Weerda perform ear surgery, but also to be the recipient of a number of his wonderful self-made Christmas card paintings over the years. During my visit to Lübeck, I was most impressed with his artistic flair and the lovely paintings that he had created both for his home and office.

Both the art and the surgical world are privileged to have Dr Weerda's presence, for the impact he has made on both is outstanding.

His book on ear reconstruction will certainly be another wonderful contribution of artistic and scientific endeavor.

Professor Burton Brent, MD
El Camino Hospital,
Woodside, CA, USA

My acquaintance with Professor Hilko Weerda of the Lübeck University School of Medicine in Germany began in May 1995 at the 11th International Congress of Plastic, Reconstructive, and Aesthetic Surgery (IPRAS) in Yokohama, Japan. Professor Weerda's concern for the treatment of auricular and middle ear defects led to the organization of the 3rd International Symposium on Auricular and Middle Ear Malformation, Ear Defects and Their Reconstructions in Lübeck, Germany, September 1997. At this meeting, Professor Weerda was able to invite prominent surgeons from throughout the world to present lectures and perform demonstration surgeries: this was indeed one of the most educational and scientific meetings concerned with problems related to the auricle to take place in the twentieth century.

Auricular reconstruction is still considered to be one of the most difficult reconstructive surgeries for a plastic reconstructive surgeon to perform. This is due to the fact that anatomical and morphological knowledge is required prior to being able to reconstruct an auricle in the proper anatomical location with all the detailed morphological features of the auricle. In addition, there is the problem of insufficient skin surface area to cover the fabricated three-dimensional costal cartilage framework (3-D frame), and its associated complications like low hairline and craniofacial skeletal defects. The Nagata method described in this textbook by Professor Weerda is a two-stage method for total auricular reconstruction, where anatomical and morphological problems have been solved; and with Professor Weerda's expertise, the problem of middle ear malformation (auditory function) is in the midst of being solved for the attainment of the ultimate goal, the reconstruction of a functional auricle of normal appearance.

It is an honor for me to write a foreword for Professor Weerda's textbook. I would like to recommend this textbook to all surgeons involved in, and/or considering a clinical practice in, reconstructive surgery for auricular and middle ear defects.

Professor Satoru Nagata, MD, PhD
Department of Reconstructive Plastic Surgery
AKIBA-Hospital, Saitama, Japan

Preface

When I began my work as a physician at the Hospital for Oral and Maxillofacial Surgery in Erlangen in 1965, the thalidomide disaster was just emerging and we had to make external prostheses for a great many children with auricular malformations. Because I had studied sculpture at an art academy before attending medical school, I was called upon to fabricate the prostheses. The relatively poor psychological rehabilitation of these children moved me deeply and prompted me to seek more satisfactory methods of reconstruction.

I have maintained a keen interest in this area during more than 30 years' practice as a plastic and reconstructive surgeon, working first at the Department of Otolaryngology at Freiburg University Hospital under Fritz Zöllner and Chlodwig Beck and later at the Department of Otolaryngology of Lübeck Medical University.

Particularly in Lübeck, I was able to pursue my work in this field along with a number of colleagues and doctoral candidates, some of whom have kindly contributed their results to this volume.

I also wish to acknowledge all the specialists who enriched this book with their contributions.

I extend special thanks to our photographer, Mrs Ellen Liegmann, who was responsible for years of difficult image documentation and effectively illustrated essential diseases and operations. I also thank Mrs Bettina Villmann, who worked tirelessly to put my partially handwritten notes into an intelligible form.

I am grateful to Thieme Publishing and its dedicated staff, particularly Ms. Elisabeth Kurz, Ms. Stefanie Langner, and Mr. Stephan Konnry. I appreciate the high quality of the illustrations prepared from my sketches by Mrs K. Schumacher and her patience in implementing my suggested changes.

For didactic reasons, the majority of conditions and procedures have been illustrated for the right ear.

I hope that this book will encourage my colleagues to explore auricular reconstruction and to advance both the theory and practice of this challenging field.

Hilko Weerda

Contributors

Franz Xaver Brunner, MD
Professor and Director
Department of Otorhinolaryngology
Augsburg Central Hospital
Augsburg, Germany

Guenter Burg, MD
Professor
Department of Dermatology
University Hospital of Zürich
Zürich, Switzerland

Stefan Gottschalk, MD
Institute of Neuroradiology
University Hospital Schleswig-Holstein
Campus Lübeck
Lübeck, Germany

Ingo Greiner
Greiner Epithesen GmbH
Kiel, Germany

Andreas Haisch, MD
Department of Otorhinolaryngology
Charité—University Medicine Berlin
Campus Benjamin Franklin
Berlin, Germany

Albert A. Hartmann, MD
Professor
Dermatology, Allergology
Aachen, Germany

Andreas Hasse, MD
Schlosspark-Klinik
Department of Oral-Maxillofacial Surgery
Berlin, Germany

Dirk Hoehmann, MD
Associate Professor
Private Practice Clinic
Otorhinolaryngology, Plastic Surgery, Allergology
Nuremberg, Germany

Robert A. Jahrsdoerfer, MD
Professor of Clinical Otolaryngology—Head and Neck Surgery
University of Virginia Medical Center
Department of Otolaryngology—Head and Neck Surgery
Division of Otolgy, Neurotology
Charlottesville, VA, USA

R. Katzbach, MD
Department of Otorhinolaryngology
University Hospital Schleswig-Holstein
Campus Lübeck
Lübeck, Germany

Jeffrey Hung N. Kim, MD
Assistant Professor
Georgetown University Medical Center
Department of Otolaryngology—Head and Neck Surgery
Washington, DC, USA

Susanne Klaiber, MD
Department of Otorhinolaryngology
University Hospital Schleswig-Holstein
Campus Lübeck
Lübeck, Germany

Michael Landthaler, MD
Professor
Clinic and Polyclinic for Dermatology
University of Regensburg
Regensburg, Germany

Dirk Petersen, MD
Professor
Institute of Neuroradiology
University Hospital Schleswig-Holstein
Campus Lübeck
Lübeck, Germany

Rainer Schoenweiler, MD
Professor
Department of Otorhinolaryngology
Division of Phoniatrics
University Hospital Schleswig-Holstein
Campus Lübeck
Lübeck, Germany

Ralf Siegert, MD
Professor
Department of Otorhinolaryngology
Prosper Hospital
Recklinghausen, Germany

Hilke Sommer, MD
Department of Otorhinolaryngology
Klinikum Oldenburg
Oldenburg, Germany

Hilko Weerda, MD, DMD
Professor and Former Head
Department of Otorhinolaryngology
University Hospital Schleswig-Holstein
Campus Lübeck
Lübeck, Germany

Monika Wimmershoff, MD
Dermatologist and Venereologist
Private Practice
Ulm, Germany

Table of Contents

1 Basic Principles

1.1 Anatomy of the External Ear

H. Weerda

The external ear (*auris externa*) comprises the **auricle** (Fig. 1.1 **a**, **b**) and the **auditory canal**.

The **anterior surface** of the ear is referred to as the **anteroauricular** (lateral, anterior auricular) surface, the **posterior surface** of the ear as the **postauricular** (medial, cranial, posterior auricular) surface (Rogers 1974).

The auricle consists of a skin envelope about 0.8–1.2 mm thick, which is firmly attached to the perichondrium (Fig. 1.2). The posterior surface bears an additional layer of fat between the skin and perichondrium, which, unlike the anterior surface, allows good mobility of the skin (1.2–3.0 mm) on the posterior surface (Smahel and Converse 1980).

The **framework** of the auricle (Fig. 1.3 **a**, **b**) consists of a convoluted elastic cartilage, 1.0–3.0 mm thick.

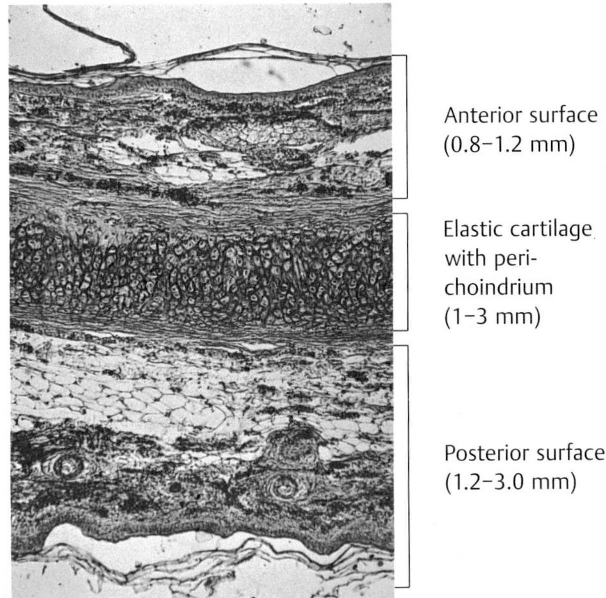

Fig. 1.2 **Histological structure of the auricle.**

Anterior auricular surface (Fig. 1.1 **a**). The anterior relief of the auricle is characterized by its typical convolutions: the helix in the marginal region, the shell-like concha in the middle of the ear merging into the antihelix, which divides into an upper and lower crus. Between these lies the triangular fossa. The antihelix blends inferiorly into the antitragus, and between the tragus and antitragus lies the inter-

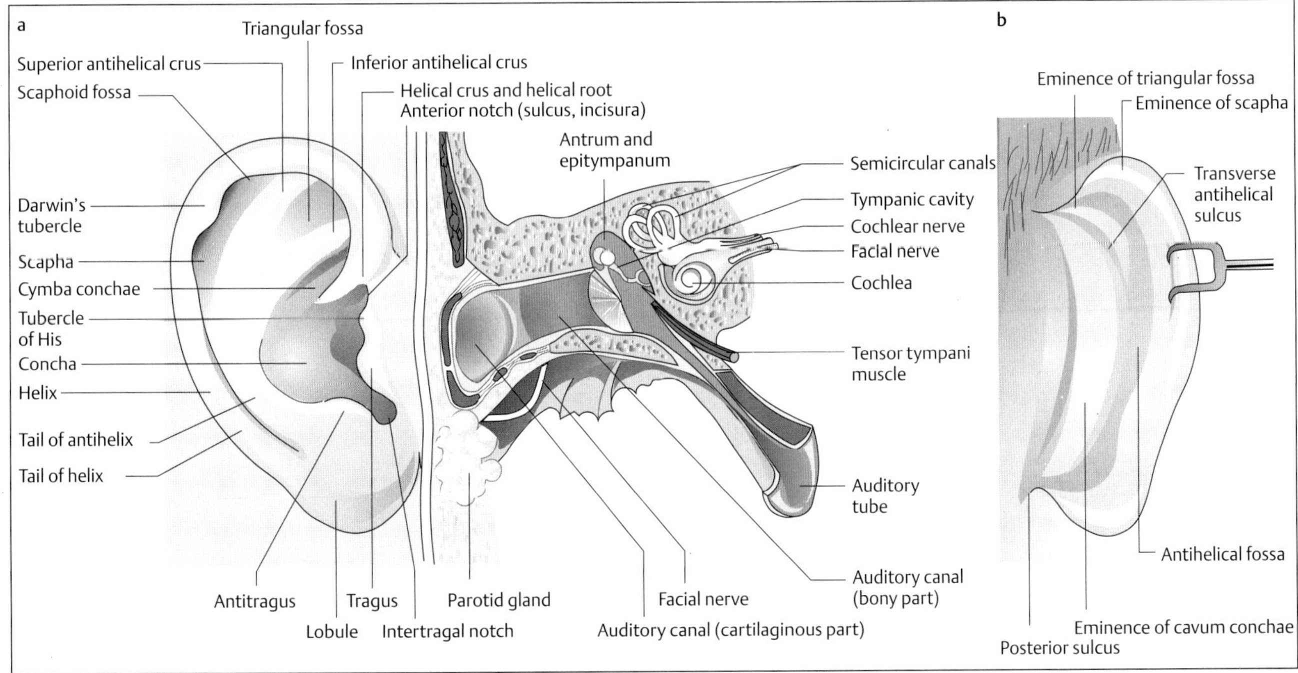

Fig. 1.1 **External ear and adjacent structures (after Weerda 1994 d).**
a Anterior auricular surface. **b** Posterior auricular surface.

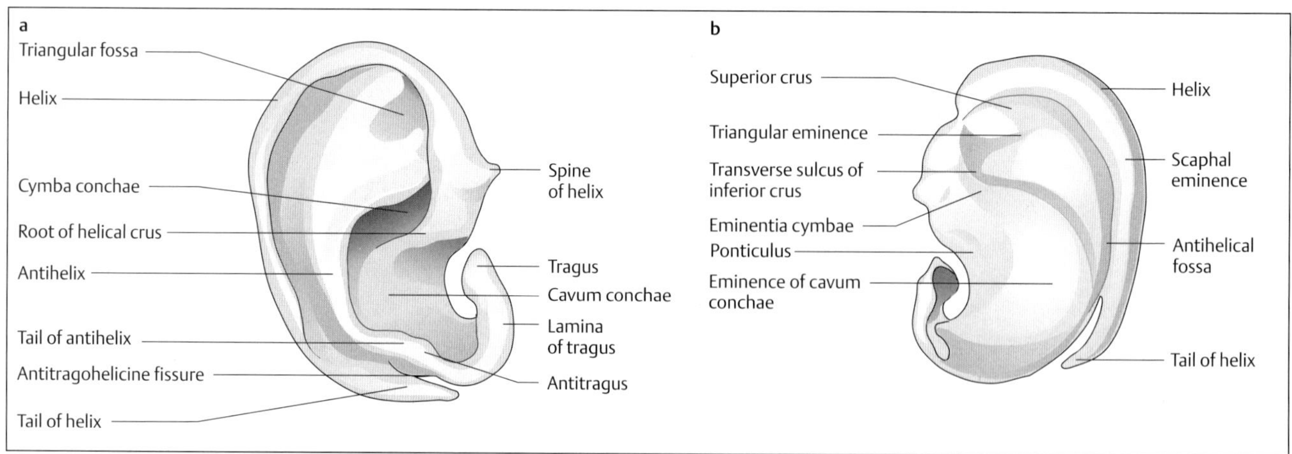

Fig. 1.3 **Anterior view (a) and posterior view (b) of the elastic auricular cartilage (after Feneis 1982; Weerda 1985 a; Quatela and Cheney 1995).**

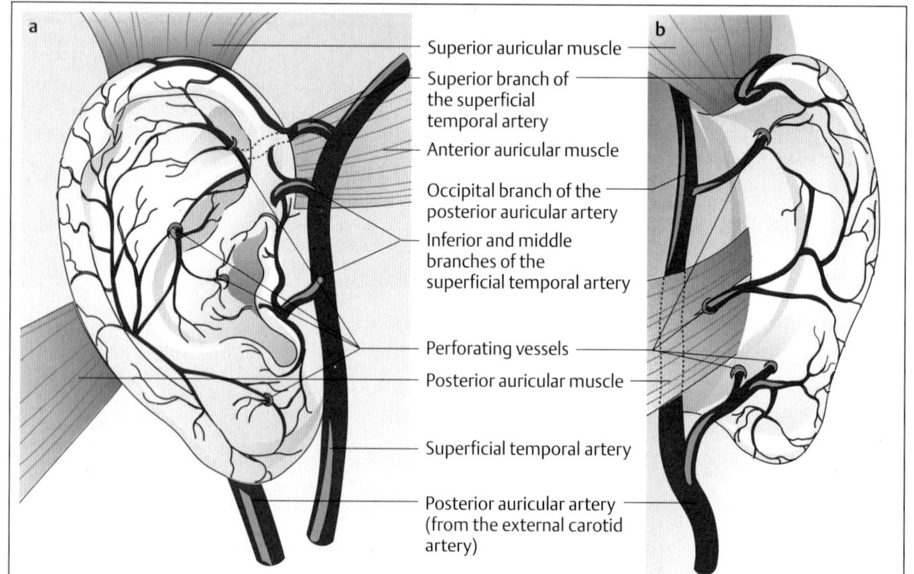

Fig. 1.4 **Arterial supply of the anterior (a) and posterior (b) auricular surface (after Weerda 1985 a).**

tragal notch. For evolutionary reasons, there may be a small duplication above the tragus, which is referred to as the tubercle of His. Darwin's tubercle can be found in the superior portion of the helix, towards the scapha. The concha gives rise to the cartilaginous part of the external auditory canal.

The cartilaginous auditory canal extends into the bony part of the auditory canal, is about 3.5 cm long in all, and ends with the tympanic membrane. Note its proximity to the parotid gland anteriorly, as well as to the facial nerve, which courses in a lateral direction after emerging from the stylomastoid foramen and divides within the parotid (Davis 1987; Weerda 1994 d; see Figs. 1.1 **a**; 1.**15**).

Posterior auricular surface. The posterior auricular surface (see Fig. 1.1 **b**) is characterized by the eminences of the scapha, the triangular fossa, and the concha, between which are found the antihelical sulcus and fossa (see Fig. 1.1 **b**).

Auricular cartilage. The cartilaginous relief of the anterior (see Fig. 1.3 **a**) and the posterior surfaces (see Fig. 1.3 **b**) corresponds to the structure of the anterior and posterior auricular surfaces. The earlobe lacks any elastic cartilage.

Vascular supply. Knowledge of the vascular supply of the external ear and the surrounding area is essential for auricular reconstruction (Rauber-Kopsch 1987; Park et al. 1992). The supply of the ear is based on two arteries: the superficial temporal and the posterior auricular (Fig. 1.**4 a, b**). The anterior surface is supplied by numerous perforating vessels; the branches of the superficial temporal artery are most variable. The arteries have a diameter of between 0.4 and 0.7 mm, the veins between 0.3 and 2.0 mm.

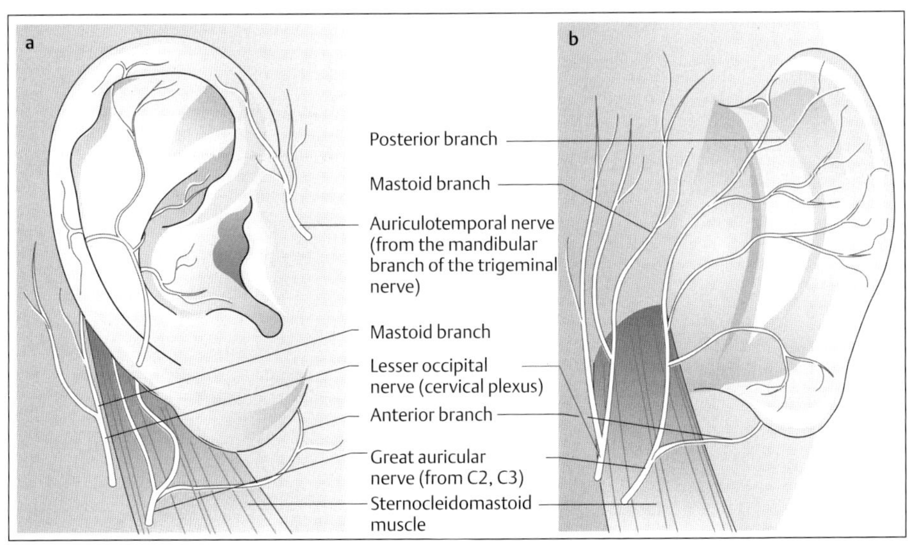

Fig. 1.5 **Sensory supply of the anterior auricular surface (a) and the posterior auricular surface (b; Quatela and Cheney 1995).**

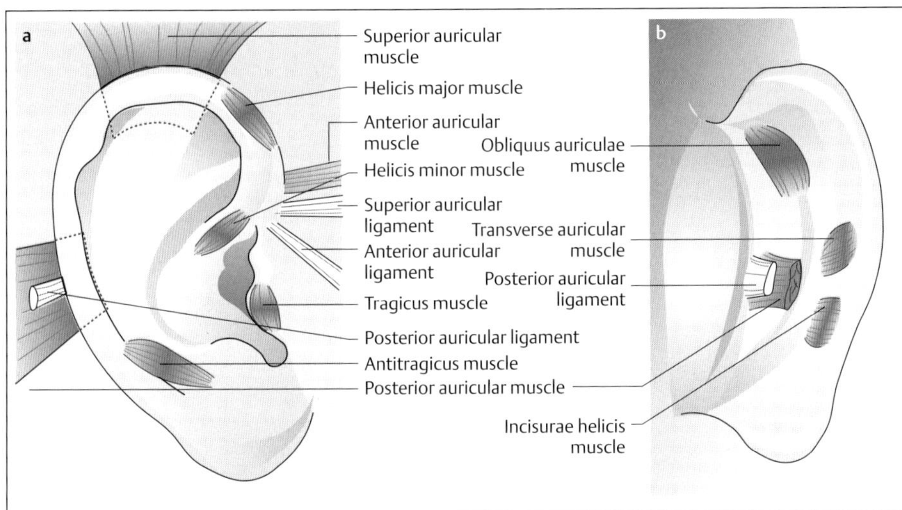

Fig. 1.6 **Muscles and ligaments of the anterior (a) and posterior (b) auricular surface (after Davis 1987).**

Sensory supply. The sensory supply of the **anterior surface** is via the auriculotemporal and great auricular nerves (Fig. 1.5 **a**), the **posterior surface** by the great auricular nerve and the mastoid branch of the lesser occipital nerve (Fig. 1.5 **b**; Quatela and Cheney 1995).

Muscles and ligaments. Although the muscles and ligaments play only a minor role for the human ear, the position of the large muscles, particularly the posterior auricular muscle and its corresponding artery, as well as the superior auricular muscle, should be known (Fig. 1.6 **a**, **b**; Davis 1987).

Lymphatic drainage system. The draining basin of the external ear lies both superficially in the preauricular region in the parotid and in the submandibular region (Fig. 1.7 **a**, lymph node groups 1, 2, 5, and 6) as well as in the postauricular and mastoid region (Fig. 1.7 **a**, lymph node groups 3 and 4).

In the peripheral region, drainage is into the superficial lymph node groups and the deep cervical lymph node groups 7–11 (Fig. 1.7 **a**, **b**).

Position. The position of the external ear plays an extremely important role in auricular reconstruction. The determination of its position, axis, etc. is discussed in the section on anthropometry (see p. 4), in the section on basic aesthetic principles (see p. 6) and in the section "Fabrication of a template" (see pp. 64, 202, 203).

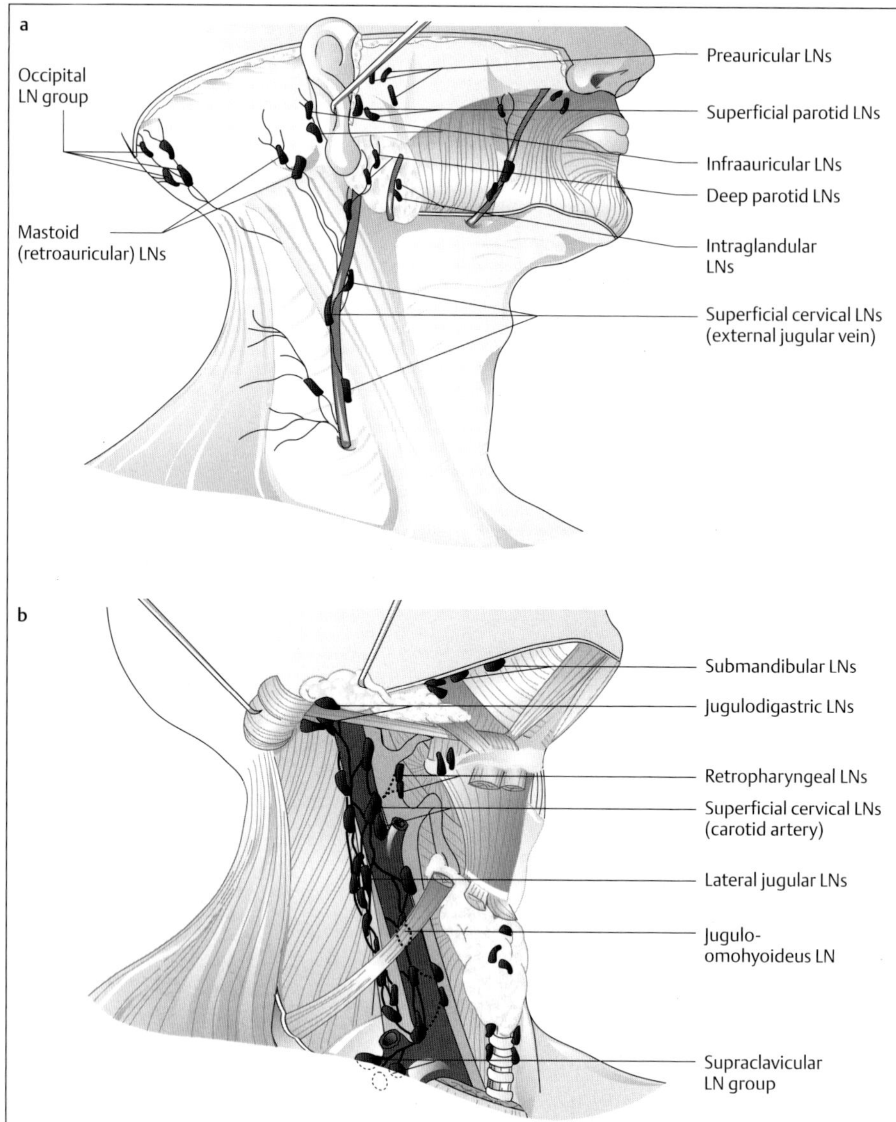

Fig. 1.7 **Superficial (a) and deep (b) lymph nodes (LNs) of the auricular region and the neck (after Feneis 1982; Richter and Feyerabend 1991).**

Lymph node groups (see p. 3):

1 Preauricular LNs
2 Superficial parotid LNs
3 Infraauricular LNs
4 Occipital LN group
5 Mastoid (retroauricular) LNs
6 Deep parotid LNs
7 Intraglandular LNs
8 Superficial cervical LNs (external jugular vein)
9 Jugulodigastric LNs
10 Submandibular LNs
11 Retropharyngeal LNs
12 Superficial cervical LNs (carotid artery)
13 Lateral jugular LNs
14 Jugulomohyoideus LN
15 Supraclavicular LN group

1.2 Anthropometry of the Auricle

R. Siegert

1.2.1 Introduction

Reconstructive and corrective surgery of the external ear requires exact knowledge of the normal auricular anatomy. This includes the position of the external ear with respect to the head and the relative positions of the various structures of its relief. These data, relative to the age, height, and sex of the patient, are required for individual surgical planning.

Classic **cephalometry** (measurement of the dimensions of the head) gained importance from the middle to the end of the last century. Farkas in the USA concerned herself with the specific anthropometry of the ear. In her classic work, she compiled a wealth of measurements gathered manually from volunteers and patients (Farkas 1981). We conducted our own study which, with the aid of a computer, digitalized and evaluated in detail standardized photographs of over 1000 normal and malformed ears (Kaesemann 1991; Siegert et al. 1998 b). In this chapter, the clinically most important standard anthropometric values (Tables **1.1** and **1.2**), and sometimes their relationship to age and height, are presented as a basis for operative planning.

1.2.2 Variables Relative to Age and Height

The following variables are relative to age and, in particular, to height. The positions of important parameters will be described below.

When reconstructing the external ears of children and adolescents who are not yet fully grown, the expected body height should first be estimated. This can be calculated from the relative height in comparison with peers and from the height of the parents. A more exact method, which is not usually necessary for surgery of the external ear, is the analysis of growth using radiographs of the carpal bones.

Horizontal position of the ear. The horizontal position of the external ear increases almost linearly with height and is therefore related to head size. The symmetry of the head should also be taken into consideration in the clinical assessment of malformations. There may be considerable differences between the left and right side in combined malformations of the ear and lower jaw, so that the position of the ear cannot be determined strictly according to standard values, but will always be a compromise between the norm and individual asymmetry. For this purpose, the position of the readily palpable mandibular joint should be taken into consideration, situated as it is immediately in front of the tragus (see Fig. 1.11, p. 7).

Length of the auricle. The length of the external ear (Fig. 1.8 a–c, Table 1.3) is closely related both to height and to age. Between the 5th year of life and adulthood it increases from 53 mm by at least 10 mm. Growth of the auricle continues until the 20th year of life. By the 6th year of life, it has on average reached 85% of its final length, by the 9th year 90% and by the 15th year 95%. Smaller changes occur

Table 1.1 Reference lines

Line	Definition
Facial profile line	Line connecting glabella and most protruded point of upper lip (see Fig. 1.8 a)
Pupil line	Line connecting both pupils

Table 1.2 Landmarks

Points	Definition
Glabella	The most prominent point in the median sagittal plane between the eyebrows
Vertex	The highest point of the head in the median sagittal plane
Occipital point	The most prominent posterior point, with the head in profile, usually located in the median sagittal plane
Upper lip	Border between the red and white portions of the lip
Nasion	Landmark where the nasofrontal suture meets the median sagittal plane, projected onto the soft-tissue contour (most dorsal point of the root of the nose)
Tragion	Superior margin of the tragus. This point usually corresponds to the lowest notch between tragus and helix
Supraaurale	Highest point of the auricle
Subaurale	Lowest point of the earlobe
Postaurale	The most posterior point on the posterior helical rim
Otobasion superius	The highest point of attachment of the external ear to the scalp
Otobasion inferius	The lowest point of attachment of the external ear to the scalp

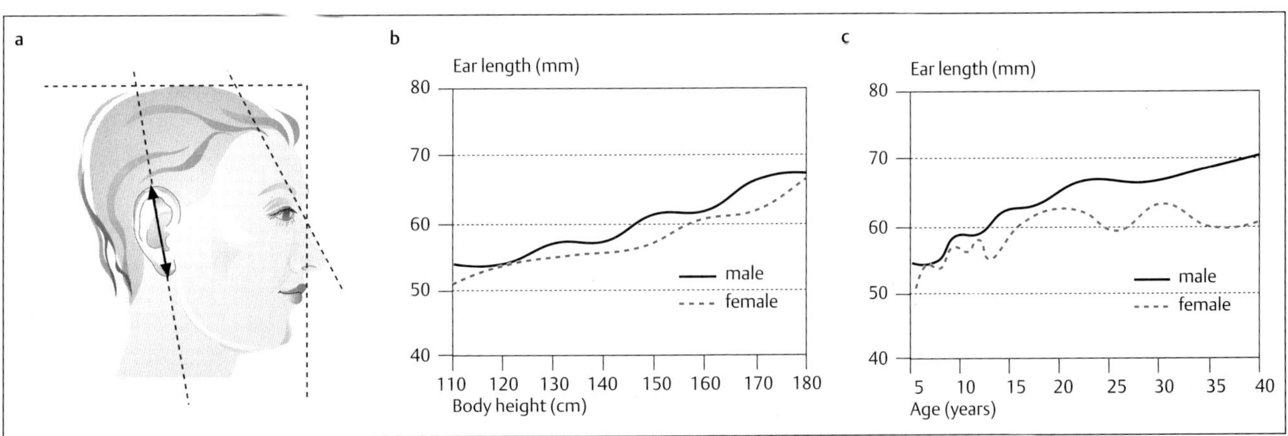

Fig. 1.8 **Ear length.**
a Measurement line.
b Mean values relative to body height.
c Mean values relative to age.

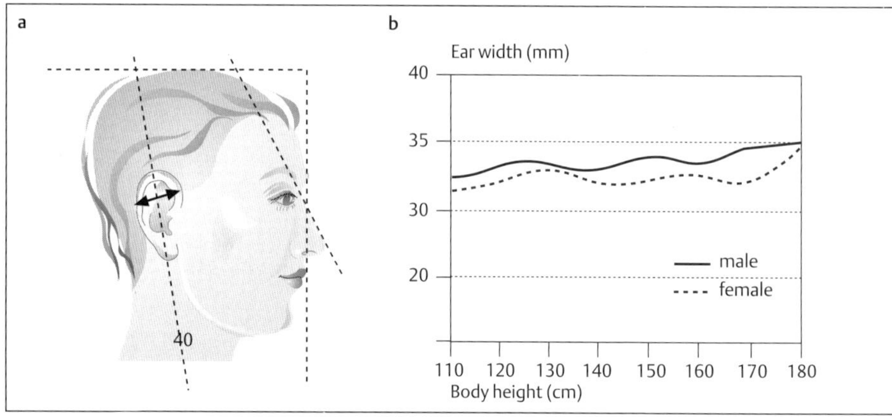

Fig. 1.9 **Ear width.**
a Measurement line.
b Mean values relative to body height.

Table 1.3 Ear length

Height (cm)	x̄ (mm)
<120	53
120–130	54
130–140	56
140–150	57
150–160	58
160–170	60
170–180	64
> 180	66

Table 1.4 Ear width (lateral view)

Height (cm)	x̄ (mm)
<120	32
120–130	32
130–140	33
140–150	32
150–160	33
160–170	34
170–180	34
> 180	> 35

throughout later life, particularly soft-tissue alterations of the lower third, which has no cartilaginous support.

The length of the auricle can be calculated with the aid of growth charts. Surgically constructed external ears do not demonstrate any significant increase in size, so the size of the auricle for children and adolescents should be calculated in relation to their prospective body height when fully grown.

Width of the auricle. The width of the auricle (lateral view; Fig. 1.9 a, b, Table 1.4) with reference to its long axis is also related to both age and height, but here the relationship is much less pronounced. Its increase between the 5th year of life and adulthood is only about 2 mm. By the 6th year of life, the auricle has reached 95% of its final width.

1.2.3 Summary

Exact planning of the size and position of the new auricle is a prerequisite for successful corrective, constructive, and reconstructive surgery of the external ear. Furthermore, prospective growth has to be considered when dealing with children.

1.3 Aesthetic Principles of Auricular Reconstruction

H. Weerda

The external ear is paired and lies at an angle of less than 30° to the mastoid plane. Any changes or asymmetries, such as scars, differences of contour, abnormalities, differences in height, changes in size, are easily noticed (Fig. 1.10 a, b). Apart from an exact reconstruction modeled on the contralateral healthy ear, **skin color**, **skin texture**, and **thickness of the skin** are just as important as the **same size**, **same length**, and **same position** (Pierce 1930; Broadbent and Mathews 1957; Gorney et al. 1971).

The following landmarks should be observed during reconstruction (Suracie 1944; Broadbent and Mathews 1957; Gorney et al. 1971; Farkas 1974; Brent 1977; Song et al. 1982; Tolleth 1978; Nagata 1994 a–c; Weerda 1985 a, 1994 a; Goedecke 1995):

- The long axis of the ear, which extends from the highest point on the superior helix to the anterior border of the earlobe, should be roughly parallel to the nasal bridge. The angle amounts to about 10–25° (Fig. 1.11, 1).

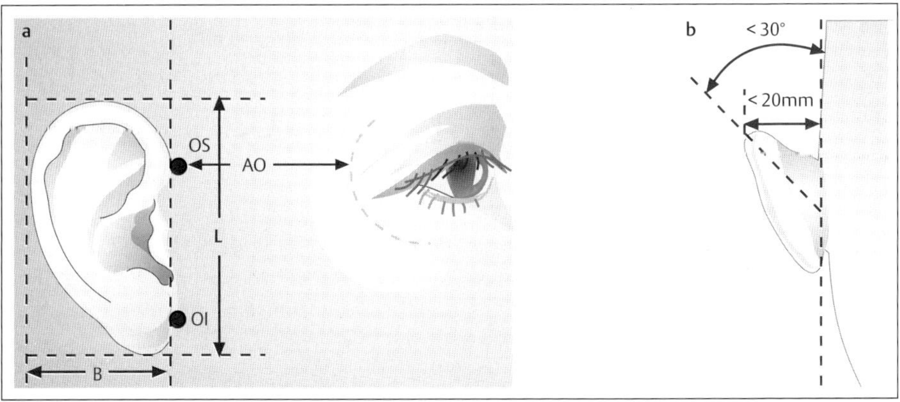

Fig. 1.**10** **Measurements of the auricle (see Chapter 5, pp. 64, 202, 203; after Farkas 1974).**

a Measurements of the lateral auricle; L: length is the distance between the lowest point on the free margin of the earlobe and the highest point on the free margin of the helix; W: width is the distance between the otobasion line and the parallel line on the outermost point of the posterior helical rim; OS: otobasion superius; OI: otobasion inferius; AO: auriculo-orbital distance (see Fig. 1.**11**).

- The connection between the attachments of the anterior helix and the earlobe (otobasion) forms the extension of the posterior margin of the mandibular ramus (line PF).
- The earlobe lies roughly at the same level as the tip of the nose (Fig. 1.**11**, 2).
- The attachment of the helix to the head (otobasion superior = OS) lies roughly on the same level as the lateral canthus.
- The distance between helix attachment and the lateral orbital margin amounts approximately to the length of the ear (the distance from attachment of the ear and lateral bony orbital margin amounts to about 65–70 mm; Fig. 1.**11**, 4).
- The highest point of the superior helix lies approximately at the same height as the arch of the eyebrow (Fig. 1.**11**, 3).
- The external auditory canal lies on same level as the midpoint between the eyebrow and the tip of the nose.
- The two ears should be the same size.
- The contours of both ears should be the same.
- The protrusion of both ears should be the same (see Fig. 1.**10 b**).
- The auricular height should be the same on each side.
- The form of the ear should not appreciably change after surgery.
- Suitable tissue should be selected for fabricating the framework and for coverage.
- The skin of both auricles should be of appropriate color, i. e., the tissue covering the auricular framework must come from the vicinity of the auricle.

The posterior margin of the ascending mandibular ramus and the position of the temperomandibular joint are also important for determining the position of the ear (see Fig. 1.**11**), provided there is only slight dysplasia of the mandibular head. The line of the otobasion lies directly on the

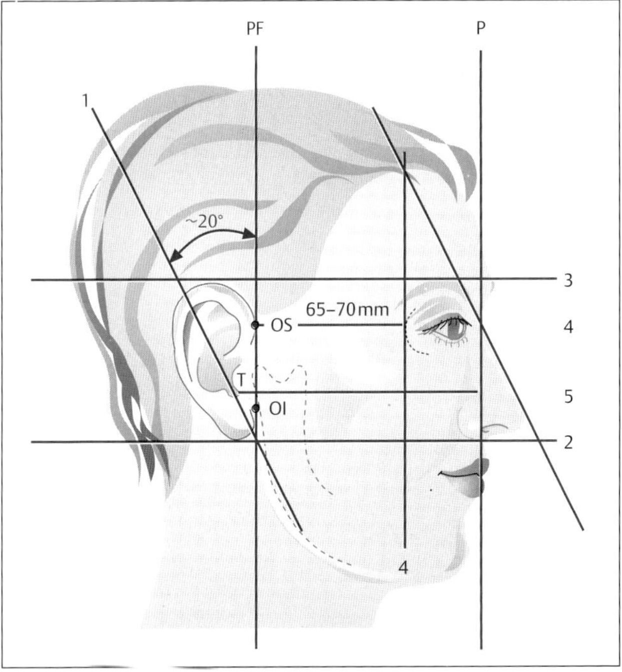

Fig. 1.**11** **Anatomically aesthetic relationships of the auricle to landmarks of the face.**

Ear inclination: The angle between line PF (parallel to facial profile line P) and the medial longitudinal axis (1) of the auricle is 10–25°. The otobasion line (OS–OI) lies immediately behind the posterior margin of the ascending mandibular ramus; OS: otobasion superius (helical attachment to the head); OI: otobasion inferius (attachment of the earlobe).

Lower border of the auricle:
Line 2, earlobe margin–base of nose.

Upper border of the auricle:
Line 3, upper helical margin–eyebrow height.

Distance from the lateral orbital margin to the otobasion AO (line 4):
approximately one ear length = 65–70 mm.
Tragus (T): positioned behind the mandibular head.

extension of the ascending mandibular ramus, the tragus lies directly behind the mandibular head (see also p. 202).

Given that 90% of all malformations of the auricle are unilateral, the position of the normal ear can be projected onto the contralateral side (see pp. 202, 203; see Figs. 5.**154** and 5.**155**).

1.4 Basic Principles of Plastic Surgery

H. Weerda

1.4.1 Instruments and Auxiliary Equipment

We generally use loupes with 2- to 2.5-fold magnification for the operation and for suturing. High-quality instruments are also required, including size 11, 15, and 19 scalpels (Fig. 1.**12 a**) and a somewhat stronger needle holder for atraumatic needles (Fig. 1.**12 b**). In addition, fine surgical forceps, e.g., Adson's forceps, and nontoothed forceps (Fig. 1.**12 c**) are required, as well as fine, angled bipolar forceps for the coagulation of vessels, 2–3 haemostats, mucosal clamps, and assorted sharp-pointed scissors and paper scissors (Fig. 1.**12 d**). The instrument set also includes single- and double-pronged skin hooks (Fig. 1.**12 e**) to hold and manipulate flaps. A good alternative is the hooked forceps after Weerda (Fig. 1.**13**). The margins of the skin flaps should not be crushed with the forceps. A ruler and a caliper (Fig. 1.**12 f**), sterile colored marker pens, wooden marker sticks and methylene blue, 5–0, 6–0, and 7–0 monofilament suture material and 5–0 absorbable material, braided, and monofilament sutures (see Appendix 2 for a list of suture materials) are also required. For carving the cartilaginous framework of the ear, we use a variety of tools (Fig. 1.**12 g**).

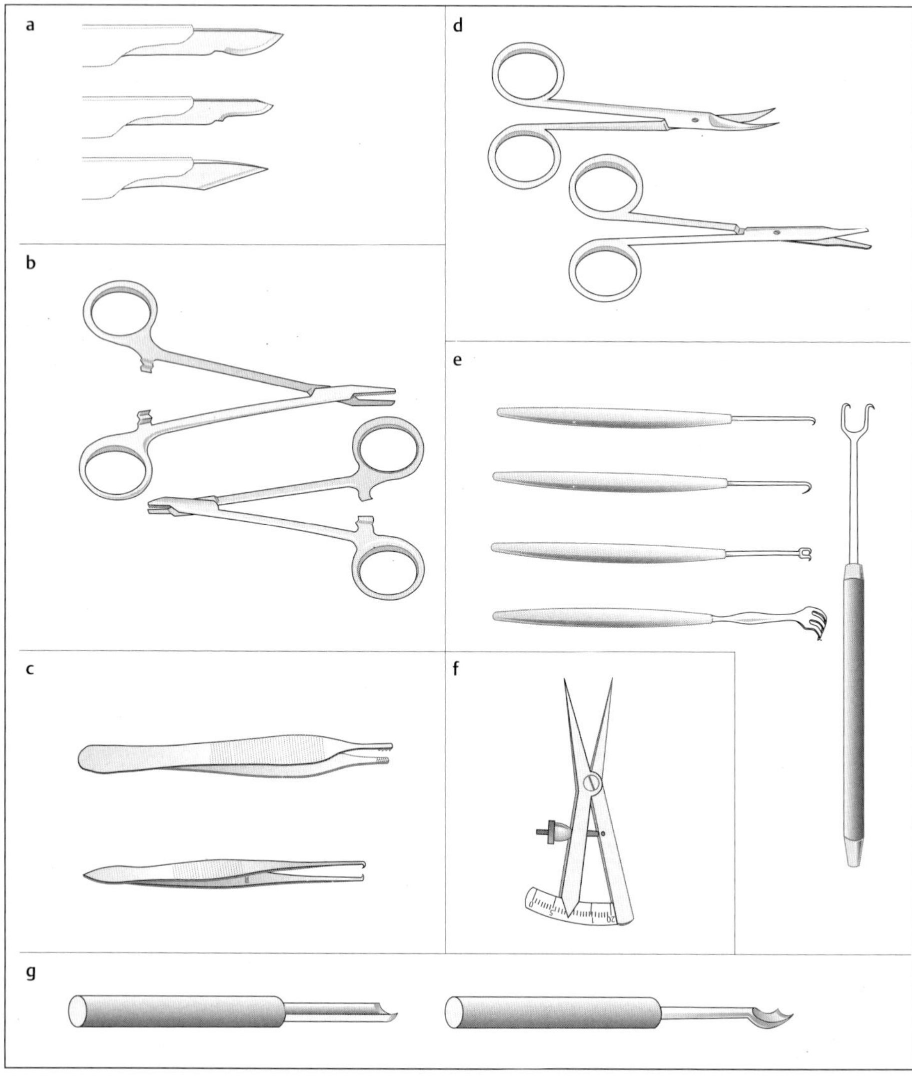

Fig. 1.**12** **a–g Instruments for surgery of the external ear (see text; K. Storz, Inc., Tuttlingen).**

We also use adhesive tapes of various lengths for dressings, as well as nonaqueous ointments, usually containing petroleum jelly. Finally, we attach suction drains and mini suction drains, using the vacuum to suction off wound secretions and to improve adaptation of the skin to the wound bed (see also Weerda 1999 a).

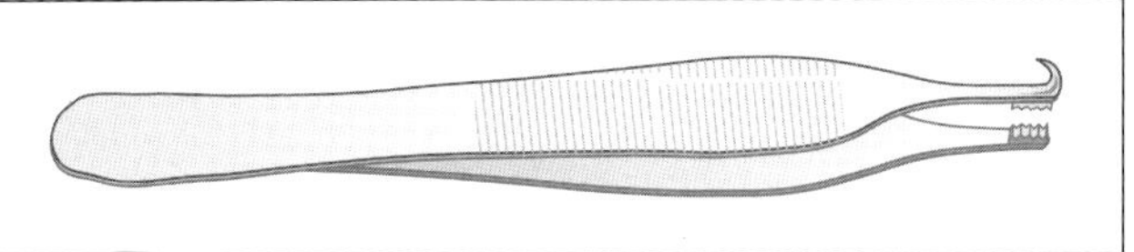

Fig. 1.13 **Weerda's hooked forceps (K. Storz, Inc., Tuttlingen).**

1.4.2 Wound Management, Care of Small Defects, and Scar Revision

Knowledge of the vascular supply of the face (Fig. 1.14) as well as of the course of the facial nerve (Fig. 1.15), is essential.

Operations can be performed under local anesthesia for up to 2.5 hours. Longer operations, larger scar revisions, and time-consuming procedures are done under general anesthesia. Care should be taken not to distort the face by plaster fixation of the endotracheal tube. The face should not be covered up during operations in the region of the facial nerve. We use transparent foils to drape the face, allowing the function of the facial nerve to be monitored.

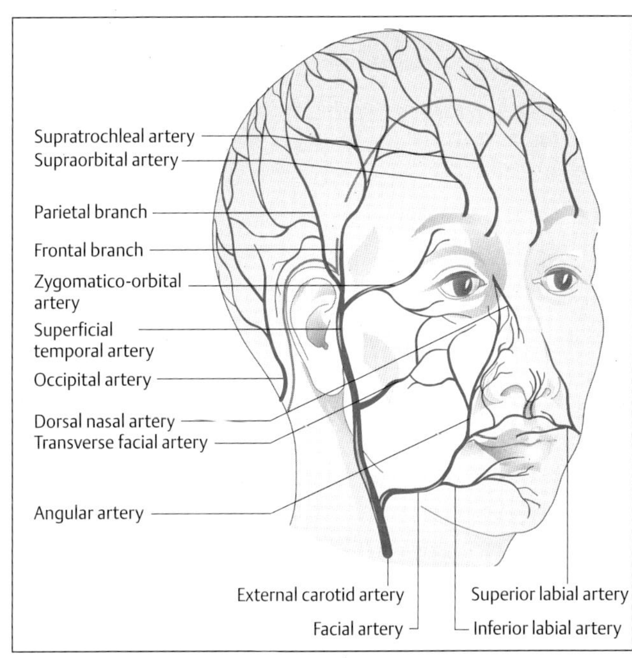

Fig. 1.14 **Arterial blood supply of the face is derived from the external carotid artery and anastomotic regions.**

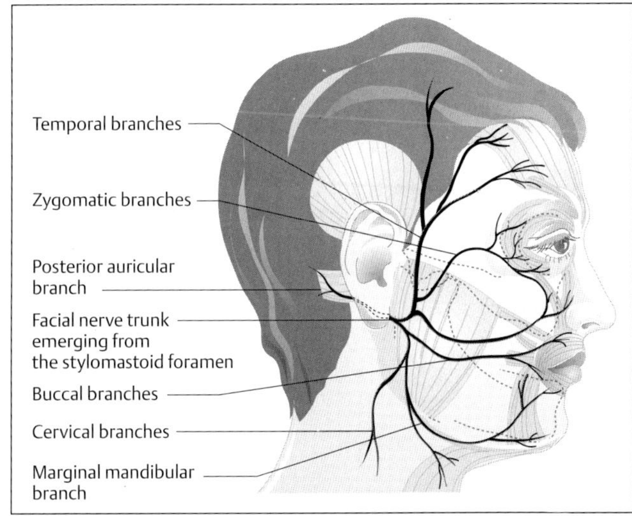

Fig. 1.15 **The facial nerve and its distribution on the face.** Buccal, marginal mandibular, and cervical branches from the cervicofacial branch; zygomatic branches and temporal branches from the temporofacial branch.

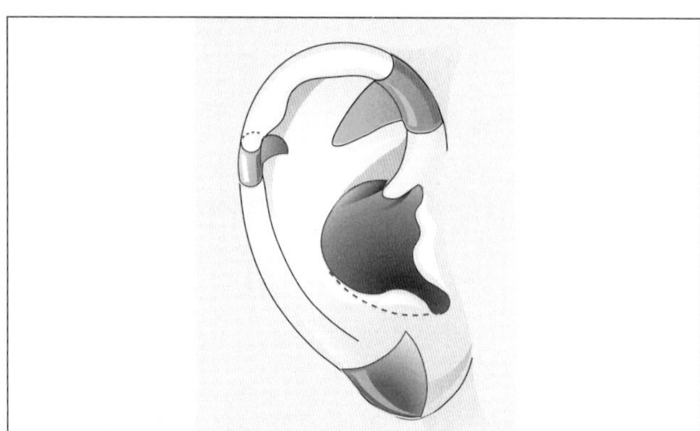

Fig. 1.**16** **Options for harvesting two- and three-layered composite grafts with primary closure of the defects.** Fat–skin graft in the region of the earlobe (for defect closure see pp. 53, 63, 166, 167).

1.4.3 Composite Grafts

Composite grafts, usually skin–cartilage transplants (two-layered composite grafts) or skin–cartilage–skin transplants (three-layered composite grafts) are normally harvested from the auricle (Fig. 1.**16**). They are generally used for the reconstruction of the nose, but can also be used for the auricle itself. Because the skin shrinks a little, it should be excised slightly larger than the defect and also larger than the harvested cartilage. We use templates of the defects cut from aluminum foil (the suture packaging) or from glove paper. The skin of the anterior surface is more firmly adherent to the perichondrium and cartilage than the skin on the posterior surface.

If the skin of the posterior surface is also harvested, it should be fixed to the cartilage with a few interrupted sutures because otherwise it easily becomes detached.

The wound margins of the composite graft should not be crushed with forceps, and the sutures should not be placed too close together. Dusky discoloration of the graft during the first few days is no cause for alarm, given that 20% of these transplants do not survive. It is also essential that the inset composite graft is kept as **immobile** as possible in a dressing for 6–7 days to prevent tearing of the small, freshly sprouting vessels.

1.4.4 Graft and Implant Terminology

- **Autogenic (autologous).** Donor and recipient are identical (**autograft**).
- **Syngenic (isogenic).** Donor and recipient are genetically identical (e. g., identical twins, animals of the same inbred strain; **isograft**).
- **Allogenic.** Donor and recipient are of the same species (human–human, dog–dog; **allograft**).
- **Xenogenic.** Donor and recipient are of different species (**xenograft**, bovine cartilage).
- **Alloplastic.** Synthetic materials such as metal, plastic, ceramic (**alloplasts, alloplastic implants**).

2 Tumors of the External Ear

H. Weerda, A.A. Hartmann, F.X. Brunner, G. Burg, and D. Hoehmann

2.1 Introduction

Benign and malignant lesions of the ear can derive from all types of tissue found in this region: the skin and its appendages, vessels, nerves, cartilage and, in the external auditory canal, bone. The lesions can occur primarily and solitarily; they can also initially appear in the adjacent skin and encroach on the ear. The ear can also be involved in generalized neoplastic changes, such as mycosis fungoides and Kaposi sarcoma. Tumorous alterations associated with metabolic diseases, e. g., gout tophi, or secondary to inflammatory alterations, such as relapsing polychondritis, chondrodermatitis nodularis chronica helicis, or of hamartoma-like origin, are only briefly mentioned here.

About 85% of malignant skin lesions are localized in the region of the head and neck. Over 70% are so-called light-induced (actinic or solar) lesions (Hertig 1978; Koplin and Zarem 1980; Hartmann et al. 1994; Weerda 1994 b; Lee et al. 1996).

Precancerous lesions. The common element of precancerous lesions is that they can give rise to malignant, metastatic tumors (Müller and Petres 1984). Their proportion of all skin changes in the region of the head and neck is reported to be about 20–25%. The number of precancerous lesions of the external ear is cited at 17% (Koplin et al. 1980; Müller and Petres 1984; Weerda 1994 b, 1999 a).

Here we discuss in detail only basal cell carcinoma, squamous cell carcinoma, and melanoma (see Hartmann et al. 1994).

2.2 Basal Cell Carcinoma and Squamous Cell Carcinoma

The proportion of lesions in the region of the external ear, including precancerous lesions, is considerable. In collective statistics of 6121 basal cell carcinomas of the face and neck region we found basal cell carcinomas of the external ear in 8.6% of cases, while in further collective statistics of 1796 skin carcinomas in the face and neck region there were 16.3% on the external ear. In these total statistics of 8187 malignant lesions of the face and neck region, **10.6%** of the cases were malignant tumors in the region of the external ear (Müller and Petres 1984; Weerda 1994 b).

The distribution of the lesions on the external ear has been reported in only a few studies (Table 2.1). In collective statistics from 13 authors, we were able to ascertain the distribution of 1438 tumors, without however differentiating between basal cell and squamous cell carcinomas. In all, approximately **70%** of the lesions were located on the anterior surface and **30%** on the posterior surface of the external ear. The distribution on the external ear (Fig. 2.1) shows that the largest number (40%) are found on the helix, almost 12% on the antihelix, and 11% in the region of the concha. The remainder are distributed on the tragus, antitragus, and lobulus (see Fig. 2.1, Table 2.1; Ledermann 1965; Blake and Wilson 1974; Schiffmann 1975; Avila et al. 1977; Ceilley et al. 1979; Baillin et al. 1980; Alvares Cruz et al. 1981; Freedlander and Chung 1983; Draf 1984; Schrader et al. 1988; Lee et al. 1996; Levin et al. 1996).

2.2.1 Basal Cell Carcinoma

Synonyms: epithelioma basocellulare, basalioma.

Definition

Basal cell carcinoma (Figs. 2.2–2.4) is a tumor originating from the cells of the basal layer of the epidermis, the sebaceous glands and hair follicles. Its growth is locally destructive, so under certain circumstances its course can be fatal, although it metastasizes extremely rarely. Together with squamous cell carcinoma, it is one of the most common malignant neoplasms of the skin (Garbe 1995).

Pathogenesis

Although basal cell carcinoma sometimes arises for no obvious reason, it often appears in individuals with sun-reactive skin type I (red hair, freckles, and skin that sunburns easily) and after longer sun exposure. The effect of sun exposure is evident in patients with xeroderma pigmentosum, in whom basal cell carcinoma and spinal cell carcinoma occur with increased frequency. In certain syndromes there is also a genetic predisposition. The incidence rates have risen considerably in the last 20 years, from 53 : 100 000 to 171 : 100 000 inhabitants in 1992 (figures from the cancer register of Saarland, Germany). In Australia the incidence rate is over 1000 : 100 000 inhabitants per year.

Table 2.1 Distribution of malignant tumors of the external ear

Author	Helix and scapha	Antihelix	Concha	Tragus and antitragus	Earlobe	Postauricular, retroauricular, and sulcus	Total
Lederman 1965	60	23	12	19	4	46	164
Blake and Wilson et al. 1974	59	16	8	4	–	42	129
Schiffmann 1975	27	9	3	–	2	42	52
Avila et al. 1977	39	13	3	4	7	22	88
Ceilley et al. 1979	12	6	13	3	3	6	43
Bailin et al. 1980	29	11	4	7	1	22	74
Alvarez Cruz et al. 1981	31	17	20	4	4	27	103
Freedlander and Chung 1983	95	15	7	–	1	29	147
Draf 1984	11	1	10	–	1	10	33
Schrader et al. 1988	35	15	14	–	–	39	103
Niparko et al. 1990	84	15	41	3	3	115	261
Lee et al. 1996	37	19	8	–	7	32	103
Levin et al. 1996	51	18	14	16	9	30	138
n	**570**	**178**	**157**	**60**	**42**	**431**	**1438** **Anterior: 1007** **Posterior: 431**
% of total no.	39.6	12.4	10.9	4.2	2.9	30	100 Anterior: 70 Posterior: 30
% of anterior tumors	56.6	17.7	15.6	6.0	4.1	–	–

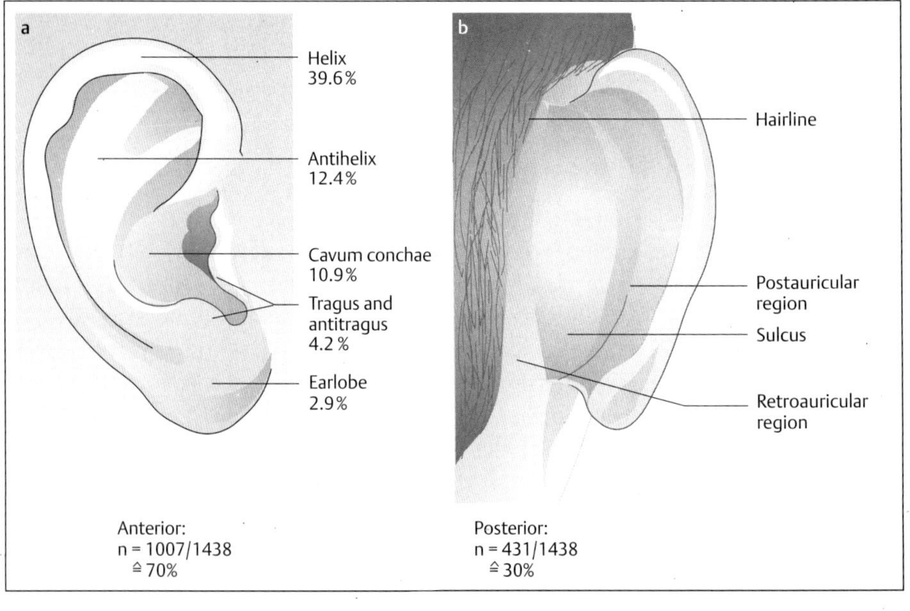

Fig. 2.1 **Distribution of malignant tumors of the external ear (n = 1438).**
Almost 57% of anterior malignant tumors are found on the helix, almost 18% on the antihelix, c. 16% in the concha (see Table 2.1; after Weerda 1994b).

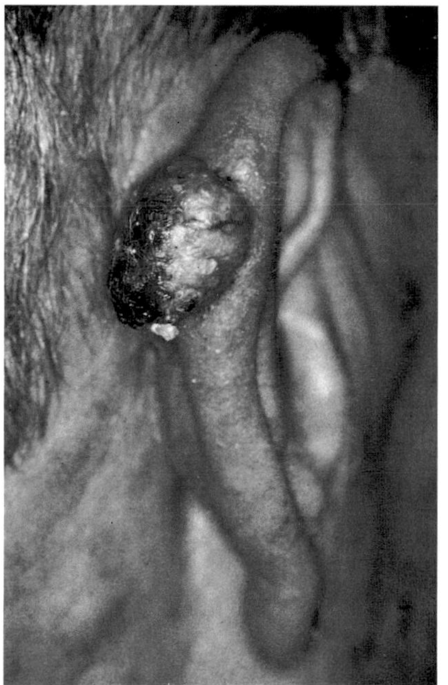

Fig. 2.**2** **Nodular ulcerative basal cell carcinoma (Type I).**

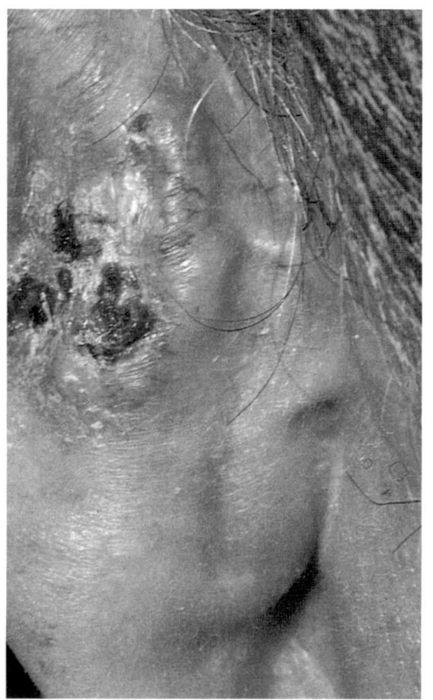

Fig. 2.**3** **Metatypical basal cell carcinoma (Type IV).**

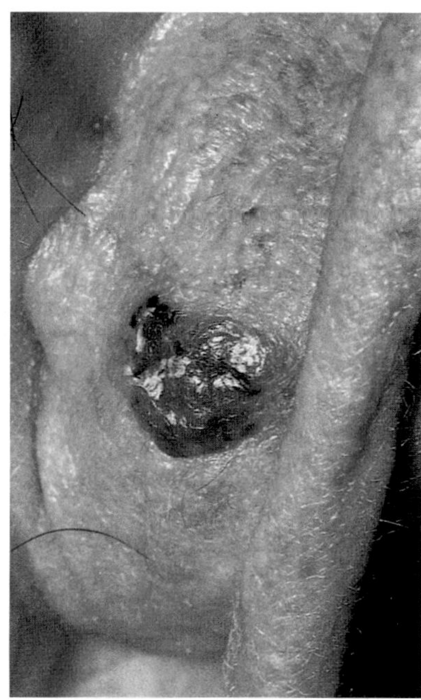

Fig. 2.**4** **Pigmented basal cell carcinoma.**

Differential Diagnosis

Keratoacanthoma (see Fig. 2.7), spinal cell carcinoma (see Fig. 2.**8**), Bowen's disease (see Fig. 2.**9**).

Clinical Presentation

Because of differences in growth behavior, a distinction is made between various types of basal cell carcinoma (Table 2.2).

Type I

Nodular ulcerative solid basal cell carcinomas (see Fig. 2.**2**) have the macroscopic appearance of a pearly shiny nodule, often with a crater-like central depression. Sometimes cystic or ulcerative changes are seen. Pigmented basal cell carcinomas with medium-brown to dirty-brown pigmentation also belong to this group (see Fig. 2.**4**). Other forms are extremely rare on the ear.

Type II

The morphea-type, fibrosing, sclerodermiform basal cell carcinoma often demonstrates a yellowish, wax-like alteration, sometimes with telangiectasias.

Differential diagnosis. Circumscribed scleroderma, malignant melanoma, exophytic seborrhoeic keratosis, pigmented histiocytoma.

Table 2.**2** Differentiation of basal cell carcinomas (after Bukal et al. 1982)

Type	Differentiation
Type I	Clinical presentation: nodular ulcerative form (see Fig. 2.**2**) Histological picture: solid basal cell carcinoma
Type II	Clinical presentation: morphea-like basal cell carcinoma (sclerodermiform basal cell carcinoma) Histological picture: fibrosing basal cell carcinoma
Type III	Clinical presentation: basal cell carcinoma of trunk skin Histological picture: superficial multicentric basal cell carcinoma
Type IV	Metatypical (basosquamous) basal cell carcinoma (see Fig. 2.**3**; wildly growing solid basal cell carcinoma)

Basalioma Exulcerans

Synonym: rodent ulcer.

Destructive, invasive, ulcerative basal cell carcinoma, often uncontrolled, untreated basal cell carcinoma which preferentially grows deeply between the earlobe and the mastoid (Fig. 2.**5**). A metatypical alteration is possible.

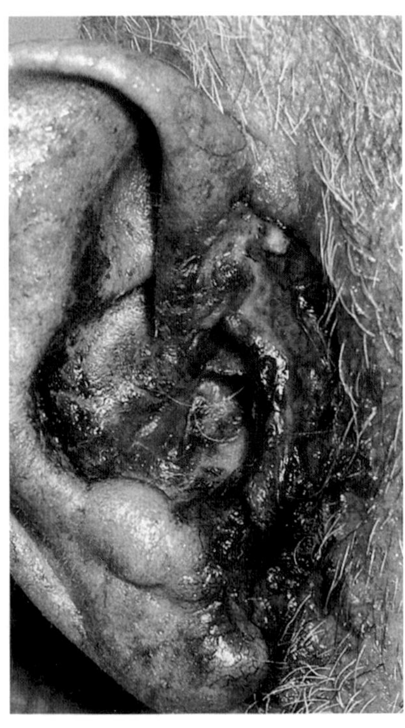

Fig. 2.**5** **Basalioma exulcerans.**

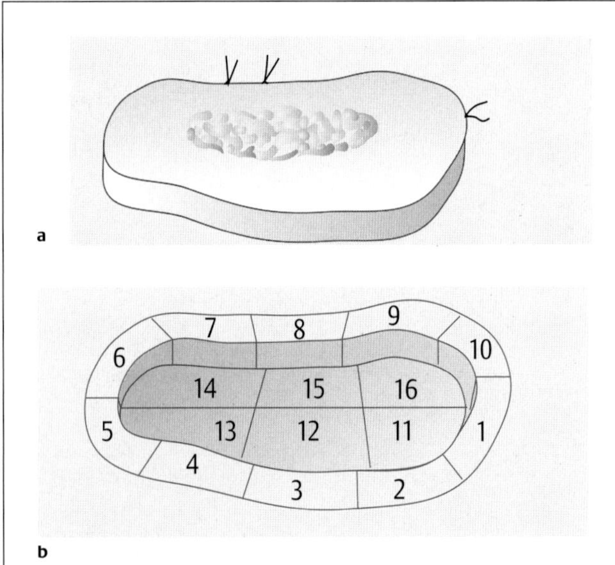

Fig. 2.**6** **Microscopically controlled tumor excision** (from Weerda 1999 a).

a Tumor excision "orientated" on a cork using various sutures or needles or differently colored cannulae.

b Additional samples from the margins and tumor base for the purpose of histological (microscopically controlled) confirmation of freedom from tumor.

Differential diagnosis. Spinal cell carcinoma (see Fig. 2.**8**).

Surgical Treatment

Surgical excision of tumors of the external ear depends on type, size, and degree of invasion and metastatic spread. Excision should be achieved with an adequate safety margin on all sides, depending on the type of carcinoma. In the region of the face, including the region of the ear, we prefer a modified form of **microscopically controlled surgery** to minimize the recurrence rate (see Fig. 2.**6**).

The purpose of any form of tumor surgery is the **radical removal of the tumor**. The following method of simplified, histologically controlled tumor excision has proven reliable in our hands (Mohs 1941, 1988; Haas 1982; Weerda 1984 b, 1994 b, 1999 a):

- With increasing size and increasing malignity, a larger safety margin from the main tumor is selected.
- The exact location of the tumor is indicated to the pathologist by a marker stitch (Fig. 2.**6 a**) and an illustration. The pathologist cuts the main tumor into slices and carefully examines both the defined excision margins and the underside of the excised lesion for freedom of tumor.
- In addition, we remove multiple, small excision samples from the margins and from the base of the tumor in a clockwise fashion (Fig. 2.**6 b**), and these are sent separately for examination.

If primary coverage of the defect is intended, these samples are examined immediately as **frozen sections**. This readily allows primary reconstruction after excision of small carcinomas and nodular basal cell carcinomas with an adequate safety margin. **Recurrences and all other tumors are subject to secondary reconstruction. This means that the defect is only covered after knowledge of the histopathology result and, in particular, after confirmation of clear surgical margins.**

Where the tumor has penetrated the cartilage, or if there is invasion in the direction of the facial nerve, radical surgery is indicated; if necessary with dissection and resection of the nerve followed by reconstruction and, in severe cases, removal of the entire petrous bone (see pp. 102–104).

Solid nodular basal cell carcinomas (see Fig. 2.**2**) are excised with a surgical margin of 3 mm. Small recurrent lesions, or tumors extending more than 2 cm, the clinical margins of which are uncertain and which have histological evidence of sclerodermiform growth, are excised with a margin of 8–10 mm or more. Attention should be paid to an adequate depth of excision. If the pathologist reports marginal involvement, then histologically controlled excisions are performed in this area until the margins are free of tumor tissue (Koplin and Zarem 1980). Only then is any final coverage done.

The paramount objective is excision with adequate lateral surgical margins, depending on the type of lesion (see prognosis) (see Fig. 2.**6**).

Mohs' micrographic surgical technique (MGS) (1947) is recommended for recurrent tumors, i. e., histological inspection of the lateral and deep surgical margins, with re-excision if necessary, until all cut surfaces are free of tumor.

This often requires temporary coverage with some type of skin replacement. Coverage of the defect can then be undertaken as a secondary procedure after histological confirmation of complete excision.

Although basal cell carcinoma responds well to radiotherapy (total dose about 40–60 Gy), this should not be used on the ear because it will damage the underlying cartilage. The stroma-rich sclerodermiform basal cell carcinoma is less suitable for therapeutic irradiation and is associated with a recurrence rate of about 30%.

Prognosis

The prognosis of basal cell carcinoma is good, given its very low rate of metastatic spread (0.0028%) and its usually slow rate of growth (Paver et al. 1977). The vertically and destructively growing basalioma terebrans (ulcus terebrans), however, can rapidly lead to death through the destruction of vital structures. The growth pattern of many basal cell carcinomas—deeper and wider than they may at first appear, like icebergs—demands a somewhat more generous excision in width as well as in depth. Assessment of the complete excision of this flat growing, multicentric carcinoma is clinically and histologically uncertain, because the surgical margins may be free of tumor although further cancerous foci may still be present in the non-excised skin.

2.2.2 Keratoacanthoma

Definition

A rapidly growing spinocellular tumor, not infrequently located on the helix, with a tendency to spontaneous resolution within 6–12 months (Fig. 2.7).

Pathogenesis

The pathogenesis of keratoacanthoma is still uncertain. The identification of HPV type 40 virus in the tumor is pathogenetically not proof, although spontaneous involution, as is also known of verruca vulgaris, and the formation of microabscesses in acanthomas point in that direction.

Differential Diagnosis

Spinal cell carcinoma, giant molluscum contagiosum, nodular ulcerative basal cell carcinoma.

Therapy

If you do not want to wait for spontaneous involution, the tumour should be excised with histological confirmation of free surgical margins.

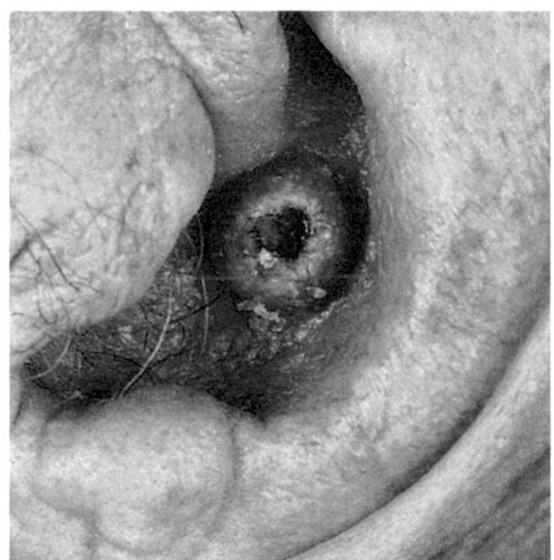

Fig. 2.7 **Keratoacanthoma.**

Table 2.3 Histopathological grading of invasive squamous cell carcinomas (after Broders; UICC 1998)

UICC	Differentiation	Broders' grade	Percentage of undifferentiated tumor cells (%)
GX	Grade of differentiation cannot be determined	–	–
G1	Highly differentiated	Grade I	< 25
G2	Moderately differentiated	Grade II	< 50
G3	Poorly differentiated	Grade III	< 75
G4	Undifferentiated	Grade IV	> 75

2.2.3 Spinal Cell Carcinoma

Synonyms: spinalioma, keratinizing squamous cell carcinoma, carcinoma spinocellulare.

Definition

This malignant tumor originates from the cells of the stratum spinosum (spinous or prickle-cell layer). Its formations spread via the epidermis into the dermis (Fig. 2.8; Brauer et al. 1977; Chen and Dehner 1978).

Of the malignant lesions of the external ear, spinal cell carcinomas are found about twice as frequently as basal cell carcinomas (Bauer et al. 1977; Chen and Dehner 1978; Müller and Petres 1984; Weerda 1994b).

The degree of differentiation is described by four histopathologic grades according to the UICC (1998) (see Table 2.3).

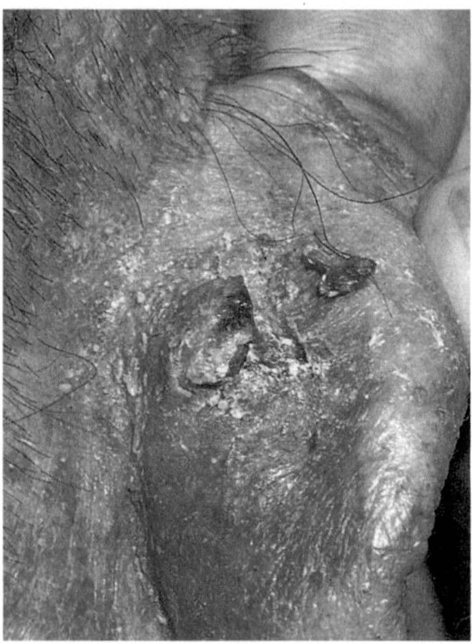

Fig. 2.8 **Spinal cell carcinoma.**

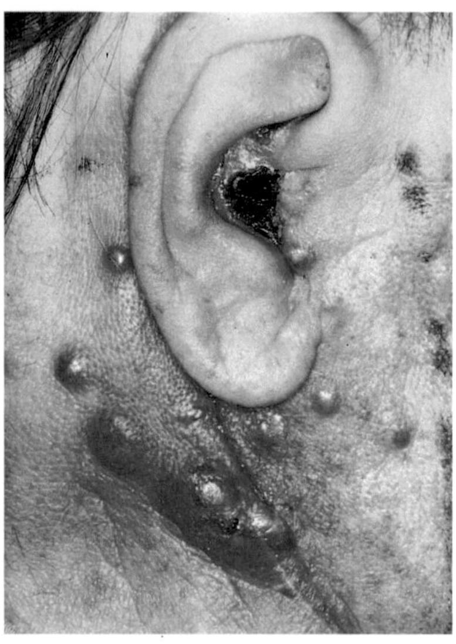

Fig. 2.9 **Metastatic spinal cell carcinoma of the concha.**

Pathogenesis

A number of pathogenetic factors have been suggested, primarily sunlight, coal tar in road construction workers, x-rays, and arsenic (Fowler's solution, etc.). Skin damaged by sunlight with actinic keratoses often forms the basis for spinal cell carcinoma. Consequently, older individuals (50–80 years old) are most commonly affected. The tumors are preferentially found on the rim of the helix and on the antihelix (see p. 12; see Fig. 2.1, see Table 2.1).

Clinical Presentation

The initial impression is that of a 0.5–1 cm solid, flat, skin-colored to gray papule with a firmly attached hyperkeratosis. This hard papule displays an exophytic and endophytic destructive form of growth through the cartilage or bone and gives rise to initially lymphogenic, and later hematogenic, metastatic spread. The affected lymph nodes are hard and may be adherent to each other and to the overlying skin. The rate of **metastatic spread** (Fig. 2.9) for spinal cell carcinomas varies considerably: between 0.1 and 4%, depending on the degree of differentiation and type of tumor.

Histomorphology

This is a squamous cell carcinoma of the epidermis; the degree of differentiation is classified after Broders (Lever and Schaumburg-Lever 1999; Table 2.3).

Therapy

The considerations are the same as in the treatment of basal cell carcinoma (see p. 14). Small spinal cell carcinomas are excised with a surgical margin of 3–6 mm. In tumors that penetrate the ear in an anterior or posterior direction, the extent of excision of healthy tissue is decided according to the rules of radical tumor surgery (Hauben et al. 1982; Weerda 1994 b, 1999 a). The rule for positive excision margins applies here, too: a histologically controlled excision is repeated until the margins are pathohistologically free (see Fig. 2.6). Chapter 4 deals in more detail with the classification of the resulting defects and defect surgery.

Surgical treatment consists of excision of the primary lesion with a margin of healthy tissue, e. g., by wedge excision and, when detected, removal of regional metastases (parotidectomy, neck dissection). Defect coverage is by primary or secondary wound closure, flap coverage, transplantation of a composite graft from the contralateral ear, split-skin graft, or full-thickness graft. The options for defect coverage using plastic surgery are manifold, and the cosmetic result usually quite acceptable. Depending on the patient's age and the prognosis of the tumor, facial prostheses with their cosmetically and functionally good results are recommended for older patients, rather than the use of plastic reconstruction (see pp. 101–104; see Chapter 6.6, p. 270, Fig. 6.52; Schuchardt 1967; Tolsdorf and Walter 1974; Converse 1977; Kastenbauer 1977; Weerda 1978; Manktelow 1986; Kaufmann and Landes 1987; Schulz 1988; Haas 1991).

Metastases. Estimates of the incidence of regional lymph node metastasis vary widely (Weerda 1984 c). Freelander and Chung (1983) discovered that 50% of metastatic tumors were larger than 3 cm. Afzelius et al. (1980) found an incidence of metastasis of over 17% in 65 patients with an average age of 77 years. They saw a relationship to mode of invasion, depth of growth, and size (Lundt and Greensborough 1965; Hedington 1974; Byers 1983; Freelander and Chung 1983; Afzelius and Nordgreen 1984; Schrader et al. 1988). In contrast, Byers (1983) saw no correlation between size and incidence of metastasis. Lee et al. (1996) report metastatic lymph node involvement in 9.6% (14 of 147 patients). They also saw a relationship to location, with almost **80%** of the metastatic tumors being found **in the preauricular region** and only **2% of the auricular tumors displaying metastases** (see Fig. 2.**9**). Of peri-auricular tumors, Hertig (1978) finds only 3% in the preauricular region.

If metastatic spread occurs, the regional lymph nodes of the parotid, the deep cervical lymph nodes, or even both regions may be involved, independent of whether the site of the tumor is pre-, post- or retroauricular (Fig. 1.7). Apart from ultrasound, CT or MRI is used to establish the diagnosis.

Ultrasound controlled fine needle aspiration biopsy and cytologic (bioptic) examination are recommended to confirm the diagnosis when suspicious lymph nodes are discovered (Russ 1978, Lee et al. 1985; Weerda and Gehrking 2000). The status of the lymph node can be assessed with a high degree of certainty by needle biopsy under ultrasound control (Weerda and Gehrking 2000). We reject selective neck dissection without proof of metastatic lymph node involvement (Garbe 1995). If involvement is confirmed, selective, and at times even radical, neck dissection is undertaken.

Radiotherapy. We prefer excisional biopsy. Once the cartilage has been invaded, however, the prospects of cure are lower, with the 5-year cure rate being reported as below 50% (Ledermann 1965; Hansen et al. 1968). In tumors where surgical cure is no longer feasible because the invasion is too deep, or that are inoperable for other reasons, combination therapy should be considered, involving palliative surgical measures (laser surgery or cryosurgery) and subsequent irradiation, or a combination of chemotherapy and radiotherapy.

Photodynamic laser tumor therapy may be an alterative, although its value cannot yet be judged with certainty.

2.3 Malignant Melanoma

Definition

Malignant melanoma is one of the most malignant tumors of the skin and mucous membrane, displaying lymphogenic and hematogenic metastatic spread. There are few data on the frequency of malignant melanoma of the ear, but the frequency of malignant melanoma in the head and neck region is reported to be 10% in men and 9.8% in women (Weidner and Tonak, no year given). Of the total number of malignant melanomas in the head and neck region, the proportion on the ear is reported to be 12.6–18.6% (Sylven and Hamberger 1950; Fitzpatrick 1972; Conley and Pack 1974).

Pathogenesis

Genetic predisposition, UV exposure, and chronic irritation play important roles in the development of malignant melanoma (Schwartz 1980; Kaufmann et al. 1989; Garbe and Orfanos 1991; Jung 1991).

Clinical Presentation

When there is justifiable suspicion of malignant melanoma, incisional biopsy is ruled out because of the possibility of initiating metastatic spread (Blake and Wilson 1974; Altmeyer et al. 1991). However, unnecessarily large, disfiguring operations should not be performed, nor are cosmetically disturbing scars acceptable. Accordingly, if there is the slightest suspicion of malignant melanoma, the diagnosis should be clinically established or excluded before any surgical procedure.

An experienced dermatologist can differentiate a malignant melanoma clinically from other pigmented skin changes with a 95% level of certainty with the aid of history, clinical presentation, and, if necessary, light microscopy (Czarnetzki et al. 1992, 1993).

The ABCDE Rule

The so-called ABCDE rule was devised to clinically differentiate a melanoma from other skin changes of similar appearance:

- A = asymmetry
- B = border irregularity
- C = color variation
- D = diameter (> 6 mm)
- E = elevation

In situ melanomas often appear clinically as asymmetrical, irregularly bordered macules with a diameter of more than

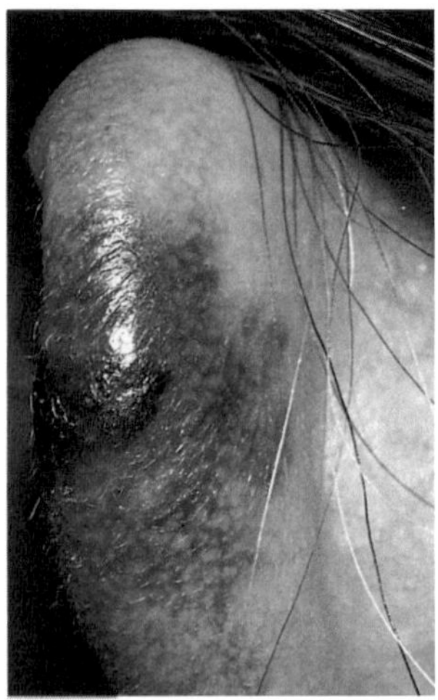

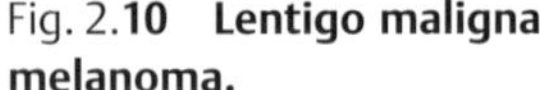

Fig. 2.10 **Lentigo maligna melanoma.**

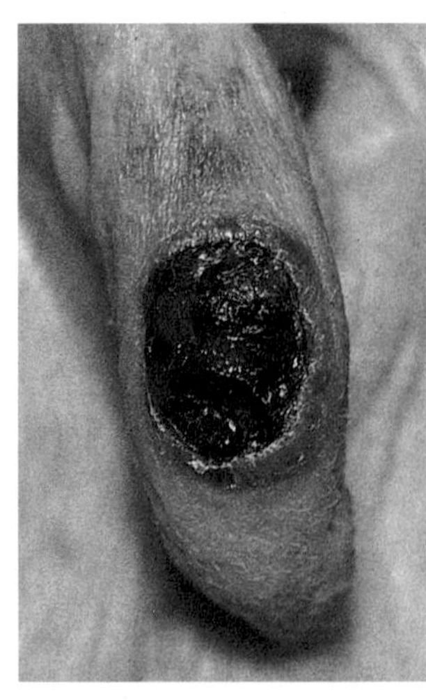

Fig. 2.11 **Ulcerative nodular melanoma.**

5 mm, indistinct marginal extensions, and irregular pigmentation, ranging from light to deep blackish-brown.

Suspicious signs, which are also found in other pigmented lesions, include pruritus, signs of regression, inflammatory margins, vertical growth, and possibly loss of hair, ulceration, and bleeding.

Types of Melanoma

A distinction is made between different types of melanoma:

- Lentigo maligna melanoma (c.15–20 % of all melanomas)
- Superficial spreading melanoma (c.60 %)
- Nodular melanoma (c.10 %)
- Acral lentiginous melanoma (c.5 %)
- Amelanotic melanoma (c.5 %)
- Non-classifiable melanoma (c.5 %)

Lentigo maligna melanoma (Fig. 2.**10**). This develops from a lentigo maligna after a latency period lasting years, sometimes even decades, and is characterized by the appearance of usually darkly pigmented, nodular areas and infiltrated foci within the lentigo maligna. The clinical picture is that of the lentigo maligna.

Superficial spreading melanoma. This often has a history of only a few years. It grows firstly in a radial, then a vertical, direction and morphologically displays a large degree of variation with foci of up to 3 cm in size, polycyclic, well defined, often with tongue-shaped extensions, inhomogeneously pigmented, light to dark brown, in part interspersed with bluish, light gray, reddish inflammatory amelanotic components; during regression it has leukodermic patches and secondary nodular components.

Nodular melanoma. The primary nodular melanoma, with a history of only months to a few years, usually develops de novo, less often on the basis of a pre-existing pigmented lesion. Its appearance is nodular, exophytic tumorous in with a homogeneous dark-brown coloring. It is rarely amelanotic, and not infrequently displays erosions or ulcerations and bleeding (Fig. 2.**11**).

Table 2.**4** presents the classification of malignant melanomas according to the **TNM system** (Sobin 2002).

Histomorphology

The histological diagnosis includes the **Clark level of invasion** (see also Table 2.**4**) and the **Breslow vertical tumor thickness.**

Invasion Level (Clark)

- Level I: intraepidermal malignant melanoma (surgically curable)
- Level II: invasion of the papillary dermis
- Level III: tumor cells have infiltrated the entire papillary dermis
- Level IV: invasion of the reticular dermis
- Level V: invasion of the subcutaneous tissue

Tumor Thickness (Breslow)

- Tumor thickness $<$ 0.5–0.75 mm—**low risk** of metastatic spread
- Tumor thickness 0.75–1.5 mm—**medium risk** of metastatic spread
- Tumor thickness $>$ 1.5 mm—**high risk** of metastatic spread

The **prognostic index** after Schmoeckel (in Braun-Falco et al. 1991) can be calculated from tumor thickness and tumor mitotic rate (number of mitoses/mm^2). A prognostic index of 13 represents a high risk.

Patterns of Metastatic Spread

The following distinctions are made:

- Local metastases: recurrence in the surgical scar and/or satellite metastases in the immediate vicinity of the primary lesion ($<$ 2 cm; Fig. 2.**12**; surgical therapy, see Figs. **4.52** to **4.55**)
- In-transit metastases: situated more that 2 cm from the primary side, between primary lesion and regional lymph nodes
- Regional lymph node metastases
- Distant metastases, including lymph nodes beyond the regional lymph nodes and all other metastases

Therapy

The only therapy for malignant melanoma that promises any degree of success, to the extent of even being curative in cases of Clark level I, is excision of the lesion within healthy tissue, attempting to achieve lateral surgical margins of up to 2 cm, depending on the assumed tumor thickness.

Standard surgical treatment. The following excisional margins should be observed:

- 1 cm margin of resection for pT1 (level II and/or < 0.75 mm)
- 2 cm margin of resection for pT2 (level III and/or > 0.75–1.5 mm)
- 2–3 cm margin of resection for pT3 (level IV–V and/or > 1.5 mm)

This approach cannot always be strictly adhered to during primary excision, especially with the ear, because of course the differentation between pT1 and pT2 can only be determined in the histological section. This may necessitate re-excision, which should be undertaken within 10 days to a maximum of 4 weeks after primary excision. The practical approach is set out in Table 2.5.

Surgery of metastases and neck dissection. All metastases amenable to surgery (cutis/subcutis, lung, CNS) should be approached surgically with the objective of reducing the total mass of the tumor.

There is still some controversy regarding the role of prophylactic functional neck dissection for melanomas in the auricular area (Wilmes et al. 1988). If the general condition of the patient or the prognosis justifies it, and depending on the degree of regional metastatic spread, a selective or radical neck dissection in combination with a lateral or total parotidectomy should be performed when metastases have been detected by palpation, cytological evidence, or imaging.

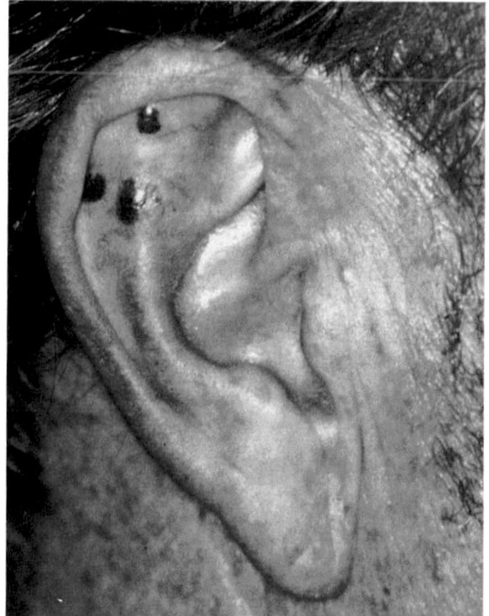

Fig. 2.**12** **Satellite metastases secondary to a malignant melanoma of the antithelix originally situated below these lesions (surgical therapy see p. 65).**

Table 2.**4** pTNM classification of malignant melanoma (Sobin 2002)

pT*: Primary Tumor (* The extent of the tumor is classified after excision.)	
pTX	Primary tumor cannot be assessed (includes shave biopsies and regressed melanomas)
pT0	No evidence of primary tumor
pTis	Melanoma in situ (Clark level I) (atypical melanocytic hyperplasia, severe melanocytic dysplasia, not an invasive malignant lesion)
pT1	Tumor 1 mm or less in thickness
pT1a	Clark level II or III, without ulceration
pT1b	Clark level IV or V, or with ulceration
pT2	Tumor more than 1 mm but not more than 2 mm in thickness
pT2a	Without ulceration
pT2b	With ulceration
pT3	Tumor more than 2 mm but not more than 4 mm in thickness
pT3a	Without ulceration
pT3b	With ulceration
pT4	Tumor more than 4 mm in thickness
pT4a	Without ulceration
pT4b	With ulceration
pN*: Regional Lymph Nodes (* The pN categories correspond to the N categories.)	
NX	Regional lymph nodes cannot be assessed
N0	No regional lymph node metastasis
N1	Metastasis in one regional lymph node
N1a	Only microscopic metastasis (clinically occult)
N1b	Macroscopic metastasis (clinically apparent)
N2	Metastasis in two or three regional lymph nodes or intralymphatic regional metastasis
N2a	Only microscopic nodal metastasis
N2b	Macroscopic nodal metastasis
N2c	Satellite or in-transit metastasis without regional nodal metastasis
N3	Metastasis in four or more regional lymph nodes, or matted metastatic regional lymph nodes, or satellite or in-transit metastasis with metastasis in regional lymph node(s)
pM*: Distant Metastasis (* The pM categories correspond to the M categories.)	
MX	Distant metastasis cannot be assessed
M0	No distant metastasis
M1	Distant metastasis
M1a	Skin, subcutaneous tissue, or lymph node(s) beyond the regional lymph nodes
M1b	Lung
M1c	Other sites, or any site with elevated serum lactic dehydrogenase (LDH)

Table 2.5 Practical approach to the standard therapy of malignant melanoma

Suspicion of malignant melanoma	Tumor elevation low (< 1 mm)	high (> 1 mm)
Low	1 cm margin, local anesthesia	1 cm margin, frozen section under general anesthesia (re-excision if necessary)
High	1 cm margin, frozen section under general anesthesia (re-excision if necessary)	3 cm margin under general anesthesia

Sentinel node biopsy. In order to map the lymph node basin more exactly, either vital blue dye or a radioactive tracer is injected around the primary tumor to identify the sentinel node from its increased blue staining or by using a gamma probe. After histological proof of nodal metastases, formal lymphadenectomy of the region is performed (Hausschild et al. 1998).

Adjuvant chemotherapy. Adjuvant forms of therapy are available to prevent recurrence or to eliminate micrometastases. The success of such treatment is inversely proportional to the size of the tumor. Adjuvant therapy should be initiated as soon as possible after surgery.

Cytostatic therapy. Systemic dacarbazine therapy demonstrates a response rate of 10–20% and can be used for inoperable metastases or after excision of metastases (Stadler and Orfanos 1991), if necessary in combination with immunomodulators (interferon).

Immunostimulation therapy. Immunostimulation therapy using bacillus Calmette–Guerin (BCG) has not produced the expected success. Various therapeutic protocols are currently being conducted using interleukin in combination with interferon alpha for high-risk melanomas.

Prognosis

The prognosis of malignant melanoma is difficult to predict in individual cases. Favorable prognostic factors that have been identified include female sex, location (face and leg), Clark level I, and tumor thickness <1.0 mm (Rassner et al. 1991).

Disease course curves for remission and survival of malignant melanomas stabilize only after about 8–10 years, although cases of late metastatic spread have been observed after more than 20 years (Tilgen and Kaufmann 1995).

Our melanoma patients are always treated in cooperation with the dermatology clinic.

2.4 Keloid

Definition

Benign, fibrous, elevated lesion which occurs after trauma (ear piercing, Fig. 2.**13**; otoplasty, Fig. 2.**14b**, **c**; surgery) and extends beyond the original scar to invade healthy tissue.

Pathogenesis

There are familial and racial predilections for keloid formation. It is more common in black people.

Clinical Presentation

Initially there is no distinction between keloids and hypertrophic scars; the appearance is that of a raised, red, hard, papulous efflorescence or scar with a smooth, shiny surface. However, after 1–2 years the hypertrophic scar regresses spontaneously, whereas the keloid persists and becomes progressively larger.

Differential Diagnosis

Hypertrophic scar, dermatofibrosarcoma protuberans (see Fig. 4.**89**, p. 83).

Histomorphology

Extensive collagen fiber bundles and pathological vessels arranged in whorls and bands.

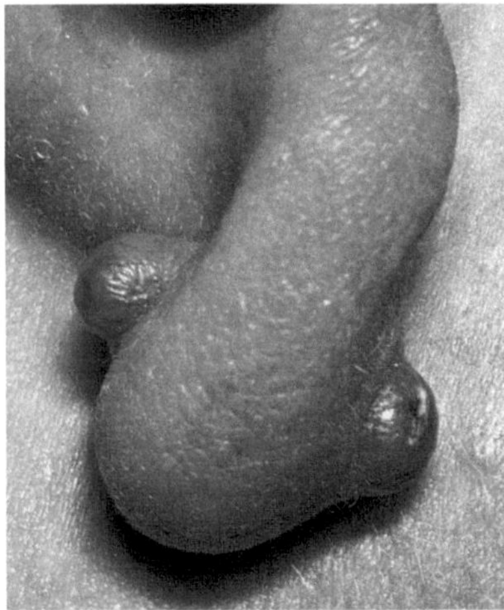

Fig. 2.**13** **Keloid formation after earlobe piercing** (see Fig. 4.**89**, p. 85).

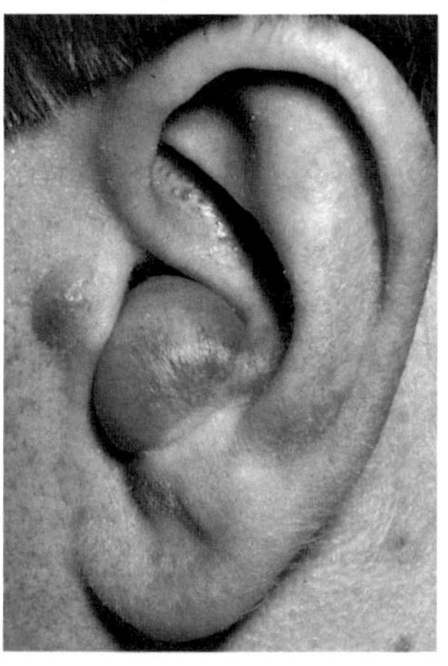
a

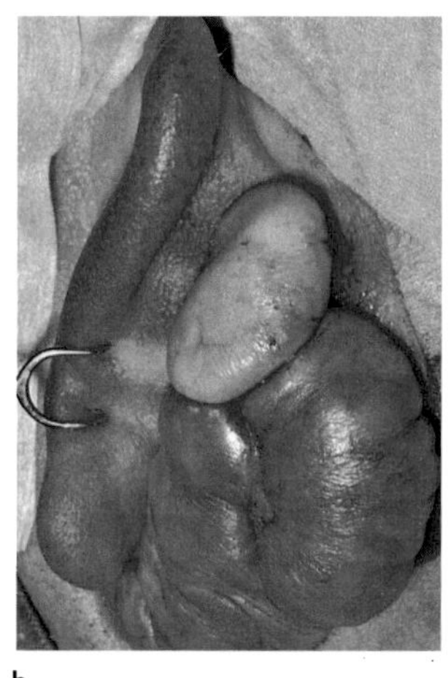
b

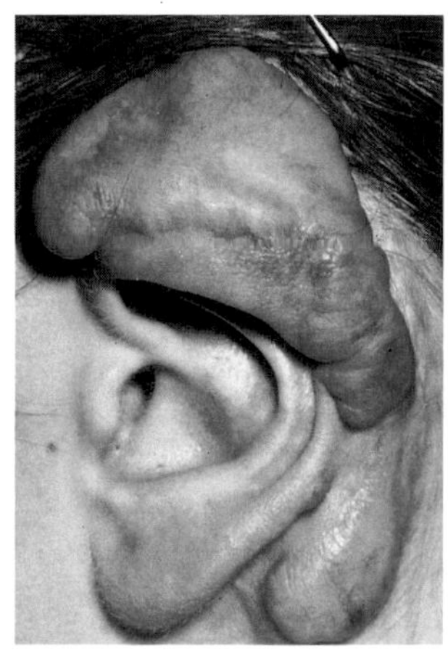
c

Fig. 2.**14** **Keloid.**
a "Spontaneous" keloid in the concha.
b, c Keloids following otoplasty (ear lobe see also p. 84).

Therapy

This is difficult. A keloid should only be excised using special surgical techniques because recurrence must be expected. Recently, photocoagulation by yellow-light laser (pulsed dye laser, copper vapor laser) has been used to sclerose pathological vessels. Intralesional administration of steroid crystal suspension or the local application of foils containing steroids can be attempted. Involution radiotherapy and the fitting of pressure dressings beneath a silicone patch are no longer considered useful.

We recommend excision of the keloid and a tension-free coverage with a skin graft, which is usually harvested from the groin (Fig. **5.58 b**, **d**). Superficial x-ray irradiation is administered on the day of surgery with a total of 20 Gy over 10 days (see also p. 146).

Prognosis

The rate of recurrence is high (see p. 146).

2.5 Neurofibroma (Fig. 2.15)

Synonyms: von Recklinghausen's disease, neurofibromatosis, generalized neurofibromatosis.

Definition

Generalized neurofibromatosis is an inherited autosomal dominant disorder with varying penetrance. In some cases of neurofibromas of the cranial nerve roots the vestibulocochlear and other cranial nerves are involved (with corresponding loss of function), whereas the auricle and external auditory canal can be affected by neurofibromas and café-au-lait spots without functional impairment. Neurofibromatosis type I mainly involves the skin; in type II, involvement of the nerve tissue is paramount (Fig. 2.**15**).

Histomorphology

Neurofibromas consist of myelinated and unmyelinated nerve fibers, Swann cells and fibroblasts.

Therapy

This consists of excision of troublesome neurofibromas, prophylactic tumor screening. In cases of very pronounced enlargement of the auricle, as in this child with von Recklinghausen's disease, we have undertaken surgical reduction and recanalization of the blocked auditory canal (Fig. 2.**15**).

Prognosis

Progression throughout life, rarely malignant degeneration.

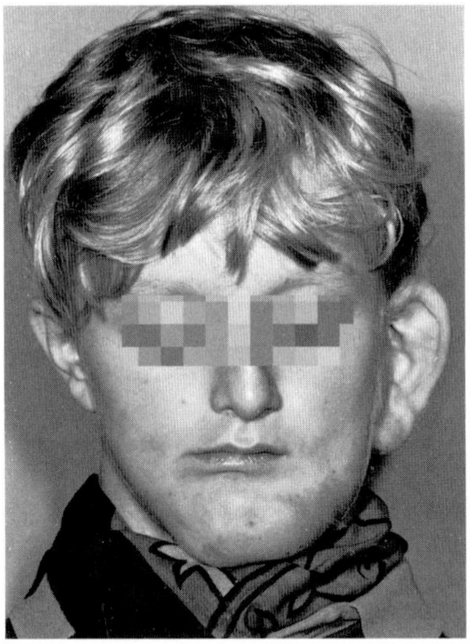

a

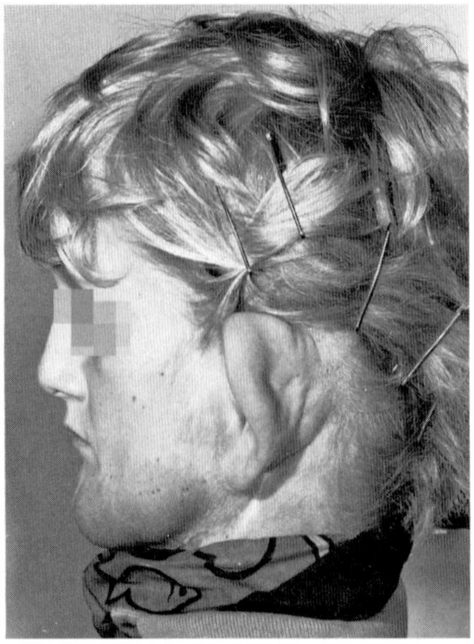

b

c

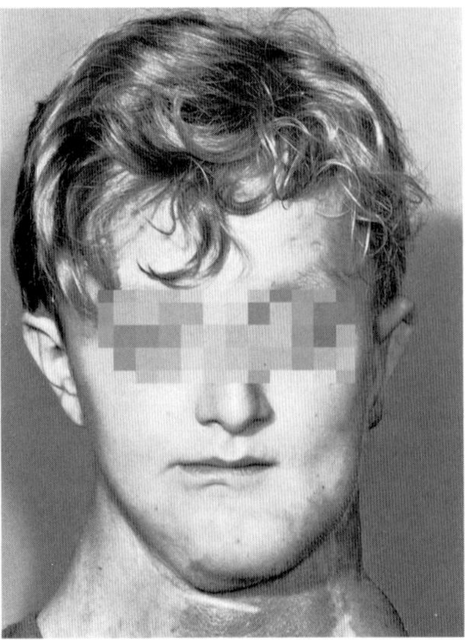

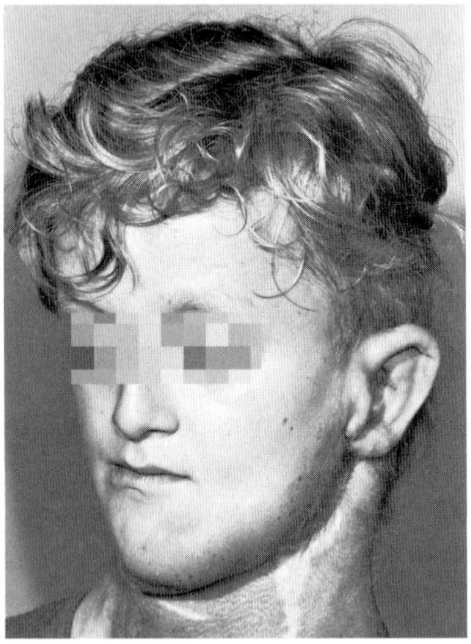

d

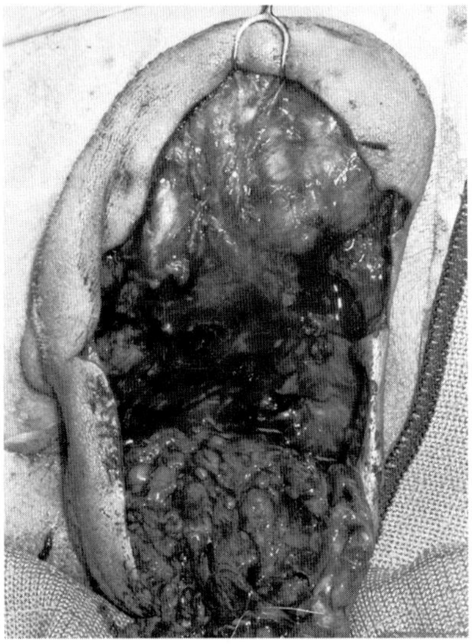

e

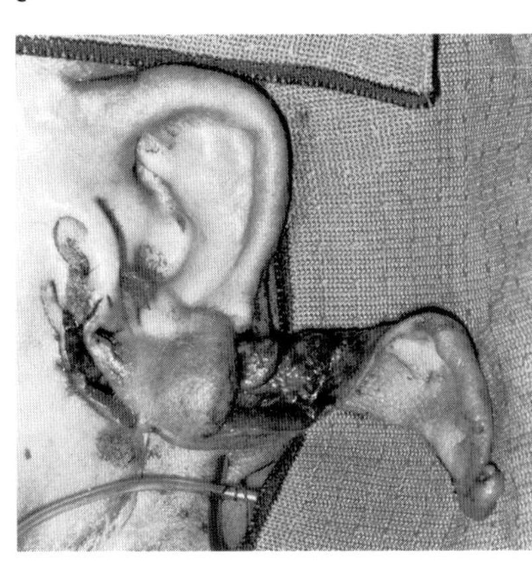

f

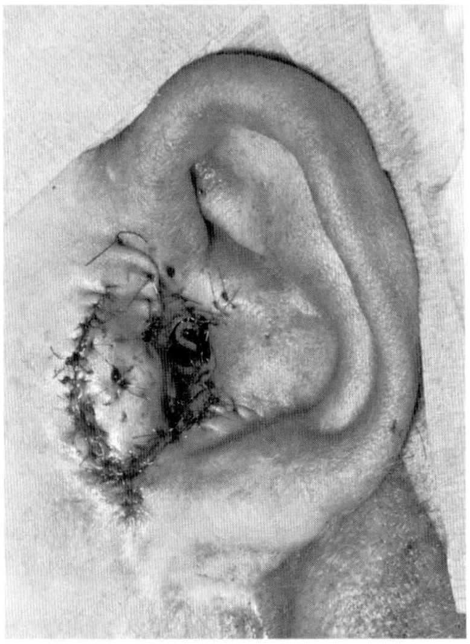

g

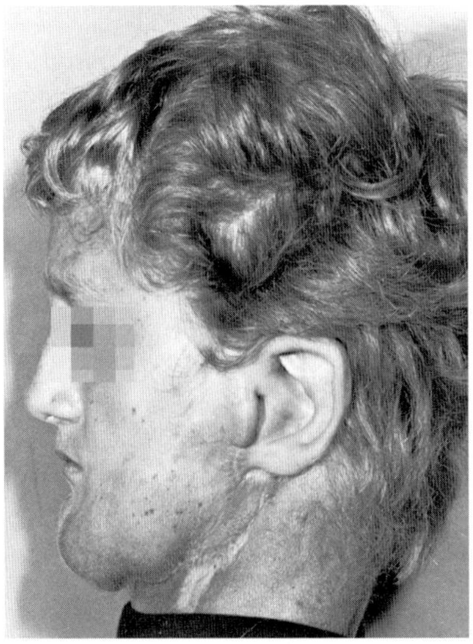

h

Fig. 2.**15** **v. Recklinghausen disease with gigantism of the external ear.**
a, b Preoperative finding.
c, d Postoperative finding.
e Resection of the neurofibromatous tissue.
f Reduction of the auricle, especially the earlobe, and trimming of the skin.
g Fine corrections to the tragus and widening of the stenotic auditory canal.
h Appearance after further forming of the earlobe and otoplasty (see also **d**).

2.6 Gout Tophi (Fig. 2.16)

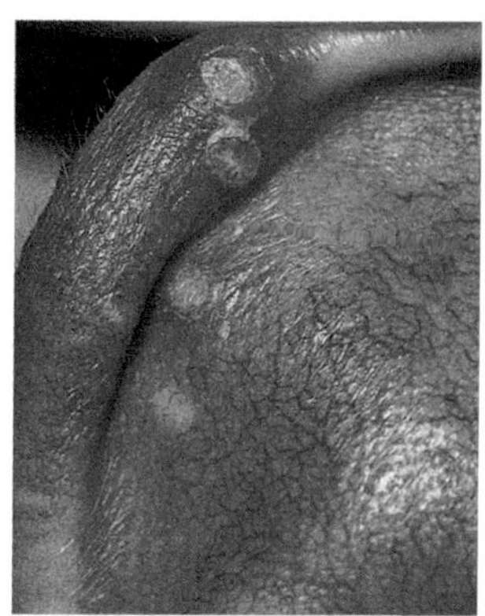

Fig. 2.16 **Gout tophus.**

Pathogenesis

Urate crystal deposits in the corium with concomitant inflammatory reaction in the course of hyperuricaemia.

Clinical Presentation

Painful, inflammatory, hard nodules in the region of the helix from which urate crystals can discharge (Fig. 2.16).

Histomorphology

Urate crystal deposits detectable in cryostat sections; amorphic, nodular, undyed masses in the corium, as seen in the formalin section, sometimes accompanied by an inflammatory reaction.

Therapy

Appropriate medical treatment of the underlying hyperuricaemia; local excision of the troublesome gout tophi.

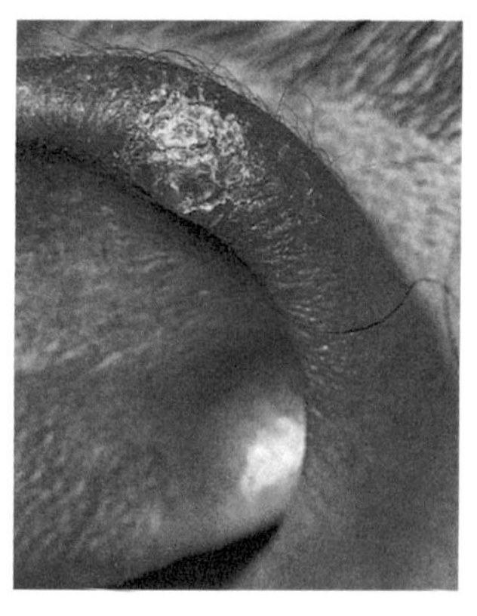

Fig. 2.17 **Chondrodermatitis nodularis chronica helicis.**

2.7 Chondrodermatitis Nodularis Chronica Helicis (Fig. 2.17)

Synonym: painful ear nodule.

Definition

Very painful, tender inflammatory nodule in the region of the helix.

Clinical Presentation

In the region of the corner of the helix, less frequently on the antithelix, there is a very painful, hard, skin-colored, slightly translucent nodule over the cartilage (Fig. 2.17).

Differential Diagnosis

Gout tophus, granuloma annulare, basal cell carcinoma, spinal cell carcinoma.

Histomorphology

Chronic, granulomatous inflammatory area with minimal necrosis and transepidermal perforation of elastic fibers in the region of the cartilage/cutis interface, extending into the cutis.

Therapy

Excision with adequate surgical margins prevents recurrence.

3 Trauma and Non-inflammatory Processes

H. Weerda

3.1 Acute Trauma of the Auricle

The exposed position of the auricle predisposes it to a large number of different injuries. Early treatment prevents defective healing and time-consuming secondary plastic reconstruction. Large parts of the external ear are endangered by infection after many types of trauma, because of the unusual construction of the auricle in the form of a three-layered composite graft with very thin skin and lack of subcutaneous fat on the anterior surface, its minimal total thickness (see Fig. 1.2), and the bradytrophic cartilage which lies embedded between the two layers of skin.

As a bradytrophic structure, the cartilage is dependent upon nutrition from its surrounding tissue.

3.1.1 Chemical Burns

Synonym: cauterization.

Acid burns result in superficial injuries to the auricle (coagulation necrosis), whereas alkali burns produce more penetrating injuries (liquefaction necrosis).

Therapy

Immediate irrigation with clear water helps to reduce damage. The application of sterile, moist, cool compresses prevents damage extending farther. Steroid ointments are used to stem local reactions.

Where the skin has been extensively destroyed and cartilage is exposed, the defect should be covered with skin from the local area. In cases where the auricle has suffered more extensive destruction, partial or total reconstruction will be necessary at a later stage, once the defects have healed (see Chapter 4; Braun-Falco et al. 1983; Steigleder 1986; Weerda 1991 a, 1994 c, 1996 a).

3.1.2 Thermal Injuries

Synonym: burns.

This group encompasses all tissue damage secondary to thermal effects. Frequent causes of thermal injury are scalds from hot liquids during childhood. Other possible causes include low-speed detonations, exposure to flames, gas explosions, steam, and burns from accidents.

The ears are involved in about 90% of all burns to the head and neck (Osguthorpe 1991).

First-degree Burns

Causes and Clinical Presentation

After very brief thermal exposure, only the superficial epidermal layer is affected. A painful erythema is apparent and sometimes swelling of the affected area is seen (Weerda 1994 g, 1996 a).

Therapy

Immediate cooling with water or ice should be commenced, although ice should not be applied directly to the skin. Steroid ointments reduce the chances of later damage. Analgesic therapy is also initiated.

Course

Complete recovery is usually observed within a few days, as the symptoms subside. As with operations on the ear, we use special fenestrated dressing gauze (see p. 223) or sponge dressings which leave the ear free (see Fig. 5.**39**, p. 131).

Radiation burns (Richter and Feyerabend 1996) are treated with powder (e. g., talcum), azulene, or baby oil. Moist dressings and ointments should be avoided.

Panthenol ointment should be used for erythema and dry desquamation. Antiseptics (2% gentian violet, hydrogen peroxide, etc.) should be daubed on areas of moist desquamation. Damaged tissue can be covered with steroid ointment, actihaemyl, or a collagen preparation. Skin infections will require antibiotic treatment and, if necessary, the skin should be cared for with antibiotic or antimycotic ointment (Richter and Feyerabend 1996).

Second-degree (Partial-thickness) Burns

Causes and Clinical Presentation

Second-degree burns can be **superficial (2 a)** or **deep (2 b)**.

- **Superficial dermal burns (2 a)** are frequently caused by scalds (hot liquids) and are associated with blistering and broken epidermis.

- **Deep dermal burns (2 b)** are associated with deeper dermal destruction (boiling liquids, brief exposure to flame), subepidermal blistering and destruction of two-thirds of the cutis, which may occur immediately or within hours.

Therapy

Therapy of **superficial second-degree** burns is the same as for first-degree burns. Healing usually occurs spontaneously within 14 days.

Therapy and complications of **deep second-degree** burns will be dealt with under third-degree burns.

Course

Here too, complete restoration can be expected within weeks; sometimes skin discoloration is observed.

Third-degree (Full-thickness) Burns

Causes and Clinical Presentation

Severe burns (open fire, electrical burns) produce full-thickness destruction and necrosis of the dermis and possibly even the cartilage. Depending on the depth of the destruction, a dry or moist eschar is later found and, after its removal, ulcers covered with granulation tissue are observed. There is a smooth transition from second-degree to third-degree burns.

Complications and Therapy

After third-degree burns the ear appears white to reddish-brown, leathery, or charred (Osguthorpe 1991).

As mentioned earlier, the cartilage is covered on its anterior surface only by thin skin. As a bradytrophic tissue, the cartilage is dependent upon a covering of nutrient tissue. After immediate cooling, further measures are therefore necessary to protect the cartilage. If the perichondrium is still intact, split skin can be harvested from the vicinity of the ear, e. g., from the hair-bearing scalp (see Fig. 5.**173**, p. 217), above the hair bulbs at a thickness of about 0.25–0.3 mm, not more.

Because burns are usually extensive and do not affect the ear alone, interdisciplinary cooperation with plastic surgeons in a burns unit or with other specialties is necessary. Resuscitation is indicated, and a careful covering of the ear with diluted povidone–iodine solution is essential in the acute phase.

It is also extremely important to cover exposed cartilage early enough (Grant et al. 1969). According to studies by Osguthorpe (1991), infections with ***Pseudomonas aeruginosa*** or ***Staphylococcus aureus*** occur in about 25 % of patients.

Closed wound treatment with sterile, possibly metal-coated or paraffin-containing dressing gauze is essential.

Broad-spectrum antibiotics are also administered to prevent infection with ***Pseudomonas aeruginosa***, staphylococci, ***Proteus***, or ***Klebsiella***, and also as a precaution against perichondritis.

Where parts of the ear are destroyed, these are debrided and the resultant tissue defects covered as early as possible with thick split skin or full-thickness skin harvested from the vicinity (see above). If perichondrium is missing, the cartilage is covered with a local flap (see Fig. 4.**16**). Where cartilage necrosis is more extensive, the remaining viable skin is secured to the scalp to prevent shrinkage. Once healing has set in, auricular reconstruction should be carried out as soon as possible (see Chapter 4).

It is occasionally necessary to cover the burned auricle with pedicled, parietotemporal fascia from the ipsilateral side or, if this has been destroyed, as a microvascular anastomosed free parietotemporal fascia graft from the contralateral side (see Figs. 4.**69**, 4.**108**, and 4.**109**). Thick split skin, harvested from the retro- and postauricular region of the contralateral side or from the ipsilateral scalp (0.2–0.3 mm thick), is then applied to the fascia as a form of epithelial coverage (Brent and Byrd 1983, see also p. 217). Reconstruction of the external ear after burn injuries can be extremely difficult, because the surrounding skin may also be severely damaged (Wellisz 1993; Weerda 1994 c, 1996 a; see also Fig. 4.**130**, p. 105).

Additional therapeutic measures. Pain control and tetanus prophylaxis are also essential, in addition to antibiotic therapy where secondary infection is present.

Partial reconstruction of the external ear, see pp. 43
Total reconstruction of the external ear, see pp. 90

Frostbite

As with burn injuries, frostbite is also divided into three degrees of severity.

Calcifications secondary to frostbite have been reported (Fig. 3.**1**; DiBartolomeo 1985; Blondell and Lelion 1991; Lautenschlager et al. 1994; Lehmuskallio et al. 1995).

3.1.3 Acute Otoseroma and Otohematoma

Hematoma of the ear, particularly its chronic form, was described in classical and medieval times. The treatment of auricular hematoma was even the subject of early surgical textbooks (Körner 1918; Passow 1923; Muck 1927).

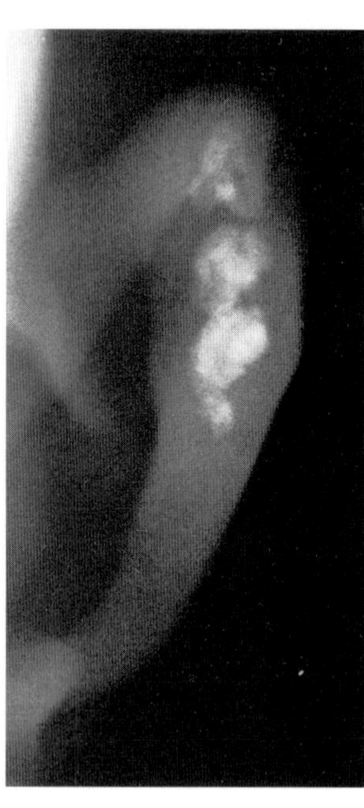

Fig. 3.1 **Calcifications after frostbite (radiograph).**

Cause

Otoseromas and otohematomas develop between the cartilage and the nutrient skin–perichondrium layer of the cartilage on the anterior surface of the external ear. About 80% are seen on the superior portion of the auricle, the rest in the middle region of the scapha and antihelix (Choi et al. 1984).

They are caused by tangential shearing movements during sports, such as boxing, wrestling, karate, and even water polo, when played without protective headgear (Weerda 1996 a).

Hematomas of the ear are found in the acute (Fig. 3.**2 a, b**; Fig. 3.3 **a–e**) or already fibrosed (chronic) state (cauliflower ear; Fig. 3.**4**).

Therapy

The treatment of acute otoseroma and otohematoma has been the subject of much discussion. Basic therapy encompasses:

- Removal of the seroma and hematoma
- Durable and secure adaptation of the skin–perichondrium flap onto the cartilage
- Prevention of renewed filling of the seroma cavity

Aspiration method. The simplest method is the aspiration of the seroma over its highest point (see Fig. 3.**2 a**).

Recommendation. Because our group has used the aspiration method with very little success, and we have frequently seen recurrences and infections, we are not inclined to recommend this method.

Surgical treatment. We prefer evacuation of the hematoma through an incision in the scapha over the anterior surface, or in the antihelical or conchal fold (see Fig. 3.**3 b**). The blood, which is commonly already clotted, is evacuated; damaged cartilage is removed; and if necessary granulation tissue is curetted (Kelleher et al. 1967; Weerda 1980, 1991 a, 1994 c). After cleansing, we adapt the skin with fibrin adhesive and carefully resect any excess skin. Skin closure is obtained using a 6–0 monofilament suture (see Fig. 3.**3 c**; Weerda 1980, Brusis 1982; Giffin 1985). Afterwards mild compression is applied for 1 week with mattress sutures (4–0, 5–0 monofilament) tied over a cotton bolster (see Fig. 3.**3 d**). When this technique is used recurrence is rare (Choi et al, 1984; Maurer et al. 1990) and only a barely visible scar remains (see Fig. 3.**3 e**).

We do not recommend the surgical approach from the **posterior surface of the ear** to remove anterior otoseroma and otohematoma (Herrmann 1968) because the otherwise

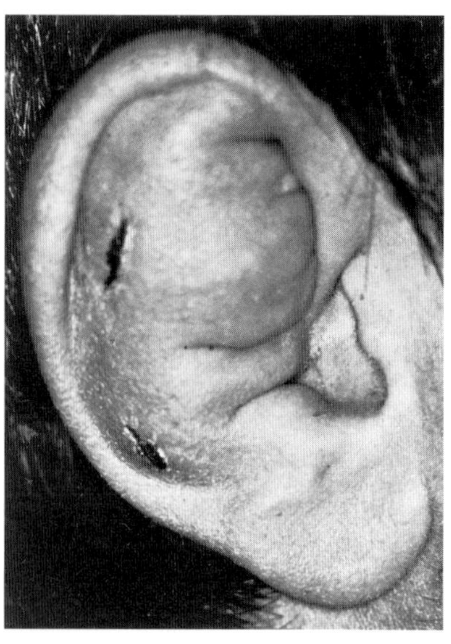

a

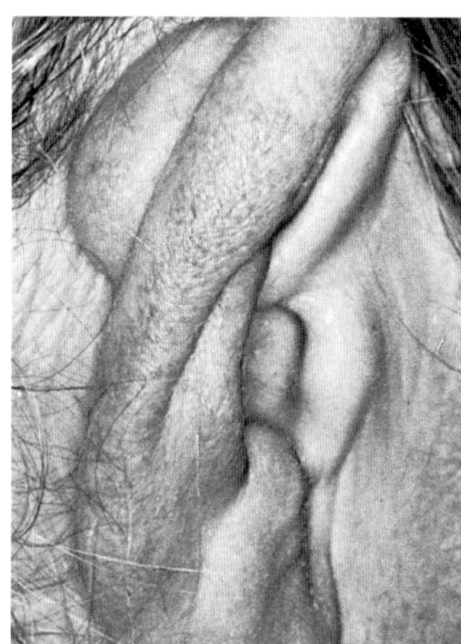

b

Fig. 3.**2** **Location of otohematomas.**
a Large otohematoma after unsuccessful aspiration and incision.
b Rare otoseroma of the posterior auricular surface.

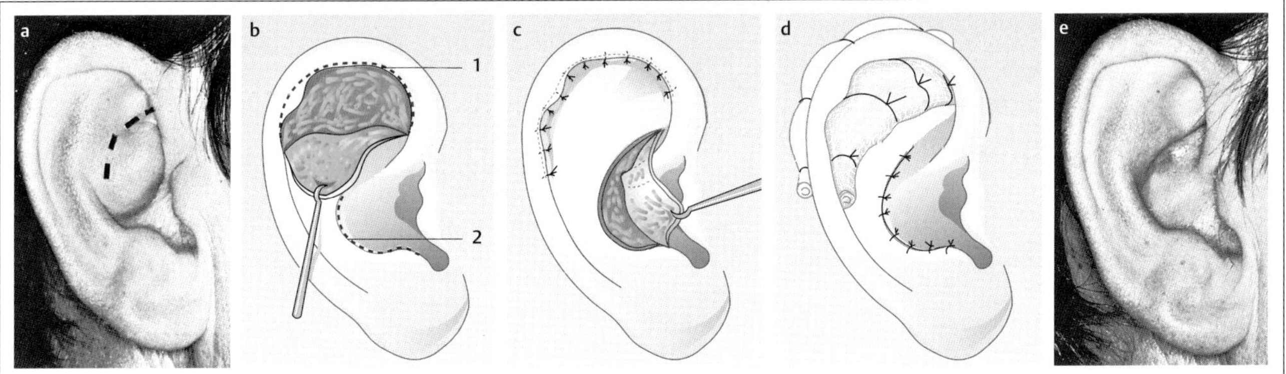

Fig. 3.3 **Approaches for surgical treatment of otohematoma (after Giffin 1985).**
a Conchahematoma.
b Incision in the scapha (1), beneath the antihelix for conchahematoma (2).
c Suture.
d Mattress sutures tied over cotton bolsters for mild compression after applying fibrin glue to the skin.
e Result of **a**.

partially intact cartilage needs to be extensively resected to gain access to the hematoma.

3.2 Chronic Otohematoma

Cause

If hematomas of the ear are not treated, organization and fibrosis occur initially. The auricular contours disappear (cauliflower ear; Fig. 3.**4 a**).

Later, calcifications of the fibrosed areas can develop (see Fig. 3.1, DiBartolomeo 1985; Blondell and Lelion 1991).

Therapy

This consists of incision of the severely thickened skin in the scapha or in the concha, thinning out of the callus-like thickenings, and remodeling of the cartilage with a scalpel or burr (Fig. 3.**4 b**). The skin is then readjusted with fibrin adhesive and any excess skin is removed with scissors. The area is secured with mattress sutures tied over a cotton bolster. The compression dressing is removed after 6–7 days at the earliest.

The aesthetic results are often not as good as those after treating acute otohematomas (Fig. 3.**4 c**).

3.3 Auricular Injuries

3.3.1 Bite Injuries

Causes

Human bites are very common in the region of the face (Fig. 3.**5**; Bardsley and Mercer 1983). Stucker et al. (1990) reported that 25 % of 32 bite injuries to the face were found in the region of the auricle. One such injury to the ear achieved fame after boxer Mike Tyson's attack on Evander Holyfield in June 1997 (Fig. 3.**6**).

The general recommendation is immediate wound care under antibiotic coverage (Lackmann et al. 1990; Agrawal et al. 1992; Weerda 1994 g, 1996 a; and see also pp. 30 and 34).

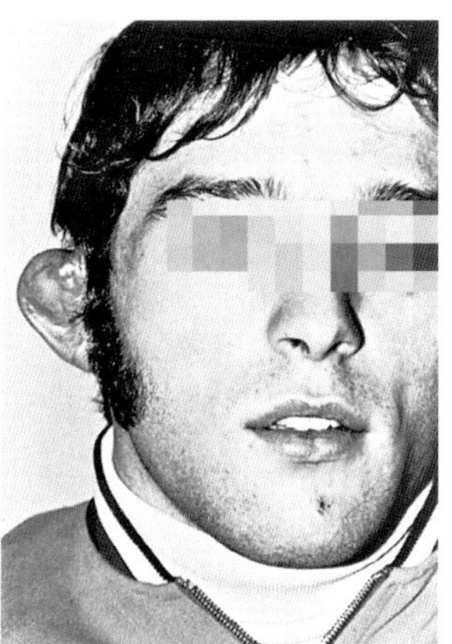
a

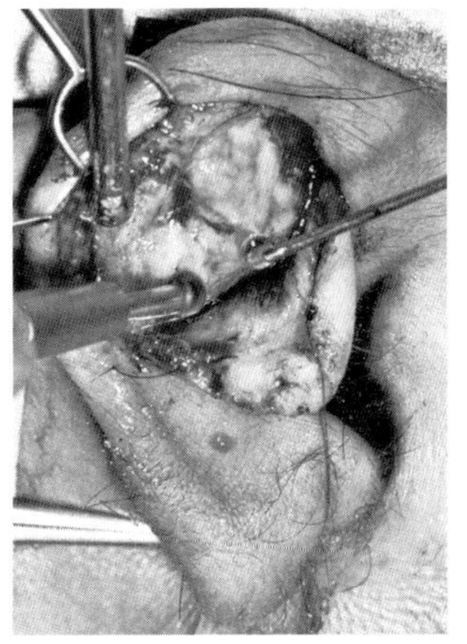
b

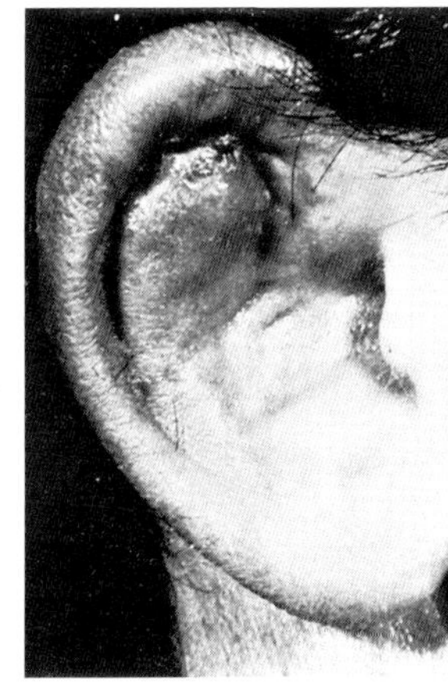
c

Fig. 3.**4** **Surgery of a chronic otohematoma.**
a Organized otohematoma, partially calcified.
b Incision in the scapha, remodeling of the cartilage (partly with the aid of a burr and a diamond drill).
c Result.

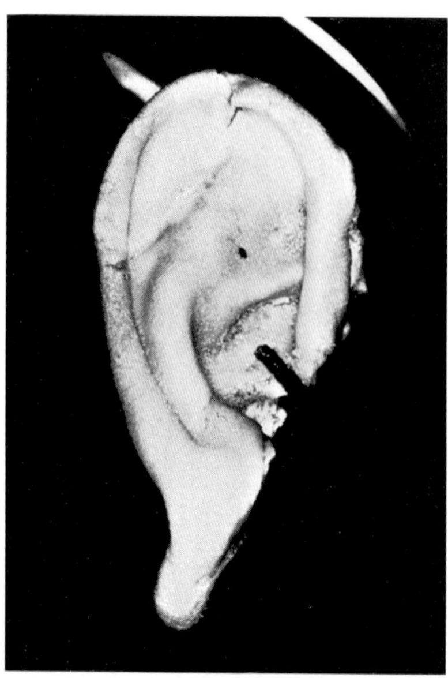

Fig. 3.5 **Ear bitten off in a psychiatric clinic; bite marks in the superior portion.**

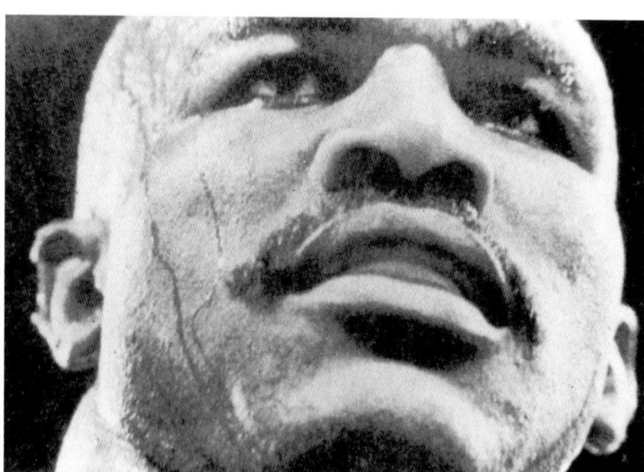

Fig. 3.6 **Bite wound inflicted on boxer Evander Holyfield by Mike Tyson.**

Table 3.1 Analysis of bacterial culture in bite wounds (Agrawal et al. 1992)

Time lapse (h)	No. of patients	Positive culture from avulsed tissue	Postoperative infection
0–24	24	2/13	1
24–48	9	3/6	2
48–72	2	1/2	–
> 72	1	1/1	–

In a study of bacterial cultures isolated in bite wounds, Agrawal and co-workers (1992) found that an infection only rarely occurs after early wound care (see Table 3.1). Earley and Bardsley (1994) found a tendency for anaerobes to be the cause of infections.

Therapy

This is our recommendation for the treatment of bite injuries:

- Wound swab culture
- Immediate cleansing and disinfection of the wound
- If necessary, scrubbing with diluted povidone–iodine solution or a similar antiseptic, especially with traumatic tattoos
- Immediate debridement, trimming of the wound edges, removal of devitalized tissue, and wound closure
- Coverage of any defects using plastic reconstructive techniques (see pp. 45)
- Antibiotic coverage for medicolegal reasons, compulsory in wounds more than 24 hours old

3.3.2 Piercing

Despite the overall high number of ear piercings (Fig. 3.7), some even in the region of the helix, and despite the subsequent frequent injury to the bradytrophic cartilage, inflammation associated with granulomatous chronic changes (Fig. 3.8) and loss of the auricle secondary to perichondritis (see Chapter 5, Fig. 5.65 b; p. 151) are in fact rare occurrences.

Therapy

Antibiotic treatment is indicated for infections. If possible, granulomas are removed, and any deformities will require reconstruction after healing.

Complete reconstruction will be necessary after auricular loss (see Chapter 4.2.7, p. 90).

3.3.3 Tears and Avulsions of the Auricle

Classification

We should like to modify the classification of Laskin and Donohue (1958) and suggest four degrees of severity:

- **First degree:** abrasions with mild cartilage involvement
- **Second degree:** tear with separation of a pedicled flap of tissue
- **Third degree:** avulsion without segmental loss (avulsed portion of the ear available):
  - Partial segment (see Figs. 3.15 and 3.16)
  - Total auricle loss (see Figs. 3.20 and 3.22)
- **Fourth degree:** avulsion with segmental loss (avulsed auricle is lost):

- Partial defect (see section on Surgery, p. 43)
- Total auricular loss (see section on Surgery, p. 90)

First-degree Auricular Injuries

Abrasions without significant cartilage involvement.

The wound is cleaned; an attempt is made to adapt the skin with subcutaneous and cutaneous sutures using fine 6-0 and 7-0 monofilament suture material. Smaller defects are closed with local flaps.

Short-term antibiotic coverage is advised, depending on the degree of contamination and cause of injury. A pressure-free dressing (see p. 131) should be used.

Sutures are removed after 7–8 days.

Second-degree Auricular Injuries

Tear with nutrient skin pedicle:

- Partial segment
- Entire auricle

Here too, re-adaptation should be attempted first (Fig. 3.**9 a, b**), with necrotic and poorly perfused skin areas requiring debridement. The auricular segment is reattached in its correct anatomical position. The posterior skin is adapted first, using a 6–0 monofilament suture, the cartilage is adapted with a 5–0 absorbable suture, and then the skin of the anterior aspect is closed with 6–0 monofilament suture material. Any residual defects are covered with skin from the vicinity (see Defect Surgery; p. 43).

Third-degree Auricular Injuries

Acute avulsion without segmental loss: replantation.

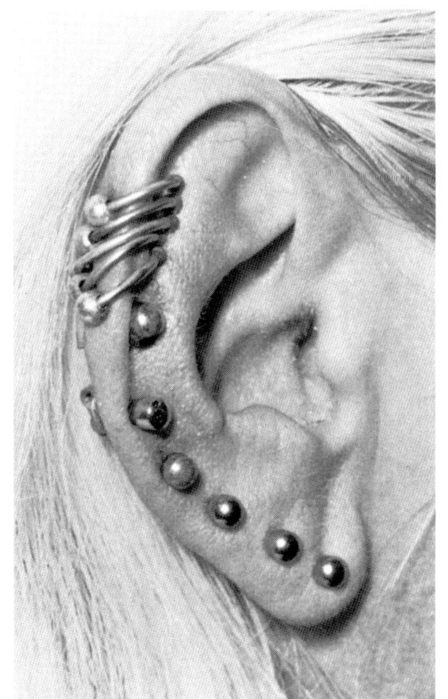

Fig. 3.**7** **Piercing in a young woman.**

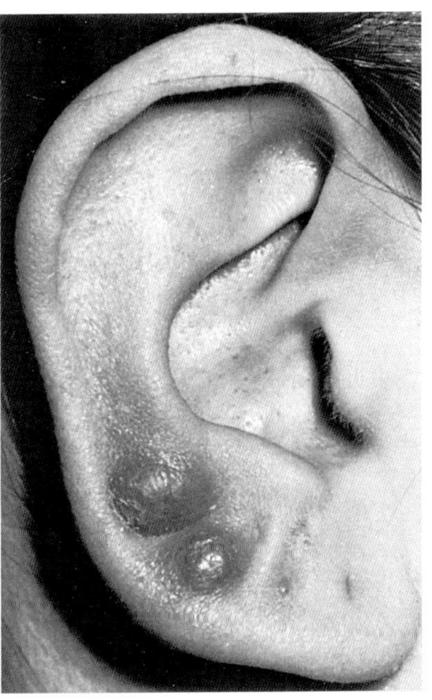

Fig. 3.**8** **Chronic inflammatory alterations after piercing, displaying in part scar hypertrophy, in part granulation tissue (Therapy, see pp. 28, 166).**

Historical Review

In early days, attempts were made to reattach avulsed parts of the ear.

St. Luke's Gospel (Luke 22:47) tells of Christ's miraculous reattachment of Malchus' ear after it had been severed by Simon Peter (Fig. 3.**10**).

In the seventeenth century the successful survival of a severed ear was reported, although Cocheril states in 1894: "No information is available about the fate of Burton's ear" (quoted from Kazanjian and Converse 1959). Replantations, i. e., the reattachment of severed parts such as noses and also ears, were attempted more and more often in the nineteenth century (by Barthelemy 1824, Magnin 1830, Manni 1834, Marini 1834, and Dornblüth 1836; Zeis 1838 b). The majority of these replantations were probably unsuccessful. Brown (1898) describes and documents a case of a successful replantation, and in the course of the twentieth century more and more individual cases of successful replantations were reported, e. g., by Brown (1898), Purcell (1898), Schmieden (1905), Lockwood (1929), von Zubriczky (1936) and increasingly also after World War II by Alexandrov (1964), Pierer (1967) and Brandt (1969). In the 1960s, 1970s, and 1980s

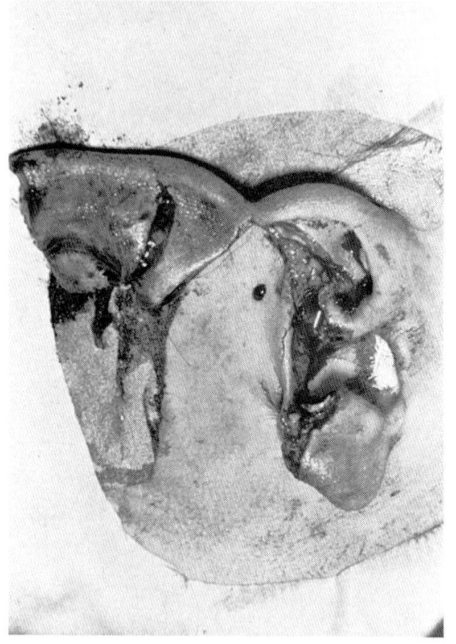

a

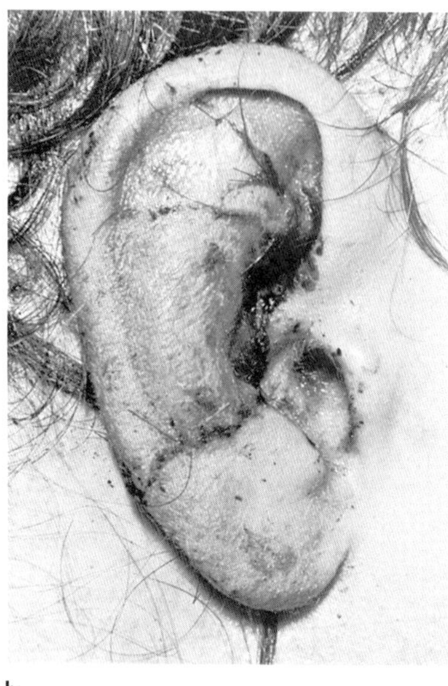

b

Fig. 3.9 **Second-degree auricular injury after Laskin and Donohue (1958).**
a Tear with nutrient skin pedicle.
b Appearance after suture and healing of the tear.

we then find more descriptions of replantations of various kinds, including individual successful cases of survival. As an excellent synopsis of the various procedures, I recommend the dissertation of one of my doctoral candidates, Ms. S. Schewior, Lübeck, 1995, entitled "Die Behandlung des Ohrmuschelabrisses: Ein geschichtlicher Überblick" (The treatment of the avulsed ear: a historical overview).

In 1902 König first specifically reported composite grafts for the purpose of nasal reconstruction. Haas and Meyer (1973 a) state that about 50% of these transplants were lost, but Walter (1966) puts the loss at 20%.

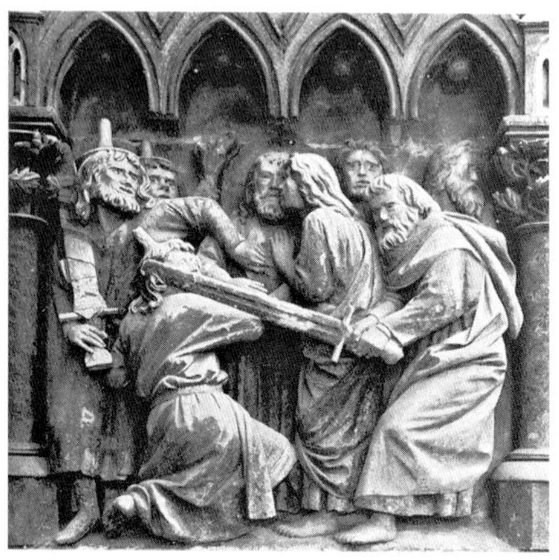

a

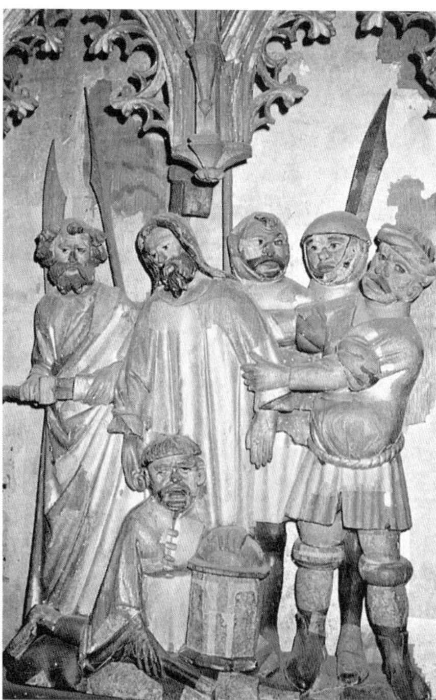

b

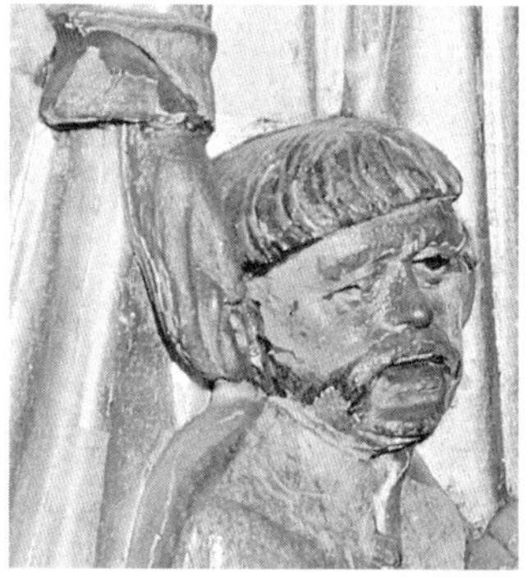

c

Fig. 3.10 **Biblical account of the severance of an ear (see text).**
a Simon Peter cuts off the ear of Malchus with a sword (Naumburg dome, Germany; 15th century).
b, c Christ reattaches the severed ear (Grönau altar, about AD 1430; St. Annen-Museum, Lübeck, Germany).

Epidemiology of Auricular Trauma

In a doctoral thesis, Steffen (2004) analysed all injuries to the external ear (with the exception of otseromas and othematomas) that were treated in Lübeck, Germany, between 1 January 1991 and 31 December 2001. In all, 141 sets of notes for a total of 197 treated patients were retrospectively assessed. Forty-three female and 98 male patients had been treated, a male-to-female ratio of 2:1; this compares with a ratio as high as 4:1 found in the literature. More than 60% of the injuries occurred to individuals between the ages of 10 and 40 years (Fig. 3.**11**, Table 3.**2**), with road traffic accidents being the cause in over 40% of the cases and domestic accidents in over 30% (Tables 3.**2**, 3.**3**). A similar trend was found on comparing an analysis of the available literature between 1885 and 2002 (Steffen 2004, Table 3.**3**), where the proportion of physical assaults (14%) was slightly higher than in our analysis.

The percentage of tears with preservation of a skin pedicle is slightly higher in our statistics than in the literature search (60% vs. 38% and 18%), but avulsion injuries were lower (40% vs. 82% and 62%) (Table 3.**4**). Partial and total avulsions are about equal (see Table 3.**7**).

One interesting observation is the large number of bite injuries, which amounted to approximately 30% of the total patient population (Table 3.**5**), with about half being human bite injuries.

Theoretical Principles

Usually partial or total auricular loss involves a three-layered avulsion, which may be repaired using various techniques.

When the entire external ear has been lost there is always the temptation to reattach the completely avulsed tissue segment, but, depending on the size of the replant, a high rate of loss must be expected due to trophic disturbances resulting from the very restricted nutrient base (Brown et al. 1946; Haas and Meyer 1973 a; Kotthaus et al. 1978; Schewior 1995).

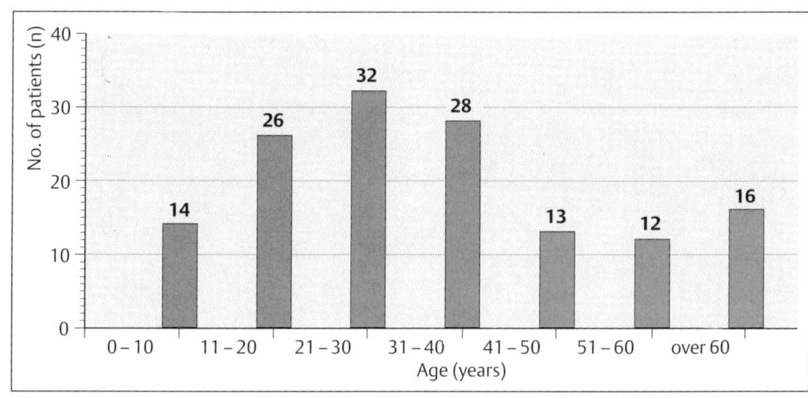

Fig. 3.**11** **Incidence of injury and age of the Lübeck patient population (1 January 1991 to 31 December 2001; n = 141).**

Table 3.**2** Absolute (n) and relative (%) values for cause of injury, incidence, and age of the Lübeck patient population (n = 141) (modified; from Steffen 2004)

Age (years)	0–10		11–20		21–30		31–40		41–50		51–60		Over 60		Total	
	n	%	n	%	n	%	n	%	n	%	n	%	n	%	n	%
Road traffic accidents	1	1.7	13	21.7	15	25	13	21.7	7	11.7	6	10	5	8.3	60	42.6
Domestic accidents	10	24.7	7	15.2	6	13	4	8.7	5	10.9	3	6.5	11	23.9	46	32.6
Physical assault	0	0	5	25	5	25	8	40	1	5	1	5	0	0	20	14.1
Miscellaneous	3	20	1	6.7	6	40	3	6.7	0	0	2	13.3	0	0	15	10.7
Total population	14	9.9	26	18.4	32	22.8	28	19.9	13	9.2	12	8.5	16	11.4	141	100
	0–40 years								> 40 years							
	100/141				70.9%				41/141				29.1%			

Table 3.3 Etiology of auricular trauma of the Lübeck patient population in comparison with the literature (Steffen 2004, modified)

	Lübeck population 01/01/1991–31/12/2002 141 patients		Literature analysis 1885–2002 135 patients		Bardsley and Mercer 1983 1975–1982 50 patients		Metanalysis 326 patients	
	n	%	n	%	n	%	n	%
Road traffic accidents	60	42.6	49	36.3	8	16	117	35.9
Domestic accidents	46	32.6	27	20.0	17	34	90	27.6
Physical assault	20	14.1	38	28.1	22	44	80	24.5
Industrial injuries	7	5.0	12	8.9	2	4	21	6.5
Leisure accidents	7	5.0	9	6.7	1	2	17	5.2
Miscellaneous	1	0.7	0	0	0	0	1	0.3
Total	141	100	135	100	50	100	326	100.0

Table 3.4 Tears and avulsion injuries of the Lübeck patient population in comparison with the literature (Steffen 2004, modified)

	Lübeck population 01/01/1991–31/12/2002 141 patients		Literature analysis 1885–2002 135 patients		Bardsley and Mercer 1983 1975–1982 50 patients		Metanalysis 1885–2002 326 patients	
	n	%	n	%	n	%	n	%
Tears	85	60.2	24	18	19	38	128	40
Avulsions	56	39.8	111	82	31	62	198	60
Partial avulsions	29	52	51	46				
Total avulsions	27	48	60	54				
Total	141	100	135	100	50	100	326	100

Table 3.5 Proportion of bite injuries in auricular trauma (Steffen 2004, modified)

Bite injuries	17/141 Lübeck population		54/135 Literature analysis 1895–2002		28/50 Bardsley and Mercer 1983 1977–1982		Total	
	n	%	n	%	n	%	n	%
Human	2	11.8	28	51.8	21	75	51	51.5
Dog	11	64.7	21	38.9	7	25	39	39.4
Horse	4	23.5	5	9.3	0	0	9	9.1
	17	100	54	100	28	100	99	100
	17/141	12.1	54/135	40	28/50	56	99/326	30.4

The one-centimetre rule. This states that, in cases of freely transplanted composite grafts, the distance from the nutrient transplant bed should be no more than 1 cm (Walter 1969).

Skin survival time. Webster (1944) and Matthews (1945) showed that freshly harvested full-thickness skin remained viable for up to 3 weeks when kept at 4 °C.

Cartilage survival time. When freshly harvested, elastic cartilage can retain its viability in Ringer's solution for 14 days at 3 °C (Krüger 1964).

Survival time of composite grafts. There are varying opinions regarding the period of time within which composite grafts (two-layered skin–cartilage grafts or three-layered skin–cartilage–skin grafts) should be transplanted and replanted. Walter (1966), for example, stated that the grafts should be replanted without undue delay. Boenninghaus (1979) regards 1 hour between harvesting and replantation as feasible, Spira (1974) considers a replantation within 2.5 hours as essential for the survival of the graft, and he also considers small segments of at most 15% of the auricle to be replantable. Clemons and Connelly (1973) regard a storage time of 5 hours to be possible.

Effect of drugs. In an animal study, Henrich et al. (1995) studied the survival of auricular segments, which were replanted using the classic procedure (see p. 35). They amputated and reimplanted the distal 2 cm of rabbit ears (Fig. 3.**12**) and studied the effects of various drugs, especially corticosteroids. After 3 weeks only 1.3% of the reimplanted tissue had survived in the untreated control group, while 23% of the composite grafts had survived in the group that had received corticosteroids ($p \leq 0.003$; Table 3.**6**, Fig. 3.**13**).

Hartman and Goode (1987), also using rabbit ears, found survival rates of 41% in reimplantations of round, three-layered composite grafts 2 cm in diameter (1 cm rule, see above) and a significantly improved survival rate of 75% after corticosteroid administration for 5 days after reimplantation. Mladick and Curraway (1973) found complete necrosis of the replants in a control group. Heparin produced no improvement in the survival rate.

Author's own animal studies. We were able to show in animal studies (see also p. 34) that replanted two-layered composite grafts survived completely after 24 hours of warm ischemia at 22 °C (Fig. 3.**14 b**), and survival was 75% after 30 hours (Fig. 3.**15**; Grüner 1985; Cannive 1985; Weerda 1986 c, 1994 g) using Baudet's technique (1972, cited in Weerda 1986 c; Figs. 3.**14**, 3.**15**). After this time there was a rapid decrease in the healing rate, resulting in almost complete necrosis after 36 hours. The same experimental regime also demonstrated that complete survival of the two-layered composite grafts, stored at 4 °C, could still be achieved within 1 week employing Baudet's technique. After an ischemic period of more than 1 week, partial or complete necrosis of the graft rapidly ensued (Fig. 3.**15**).

A significant conclusion of our trials was that, for the many failed replantations, it was not the warm or cold ischemia time of the auricle, i. e., the time between avulsion and replantation, that was the limiting factor—reimplantation was usually undertaken within 6–7 hours—but rather the difficult replantation technique and poor revascularization of the graft (1 cm rule, see p. 32).

Microvascular anastomosed replantations. In animal studies Kotthaus et al. (1978) were able to achieve a survival rate of 80% for ear replantations after storage for 2 hours at 20 °C, while only 50% of the replants survived after storage for 2 hours at 20 °C and a subsequent 2 hours at 4 °C. After more than 20 hours of ischemia, all the rabbit ear replants necrosed, even those that were kept cool. In contrast, however, survivals of cooled auricular replantations were reported by Katsaros et al. (1988) even after 7 hours and by Mutimer et al. (1987) after 8 hours.

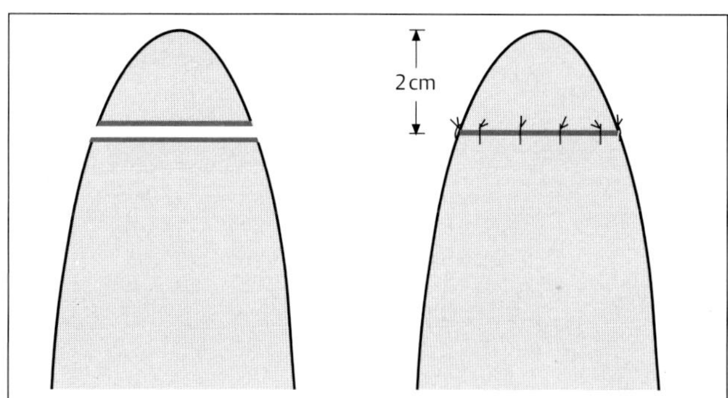

Fig. 3.**12** **Reimplantation of a three-layered composite graft comprising the distal 2 cm of the rabbit ear (after Henrich et al. 1995).**

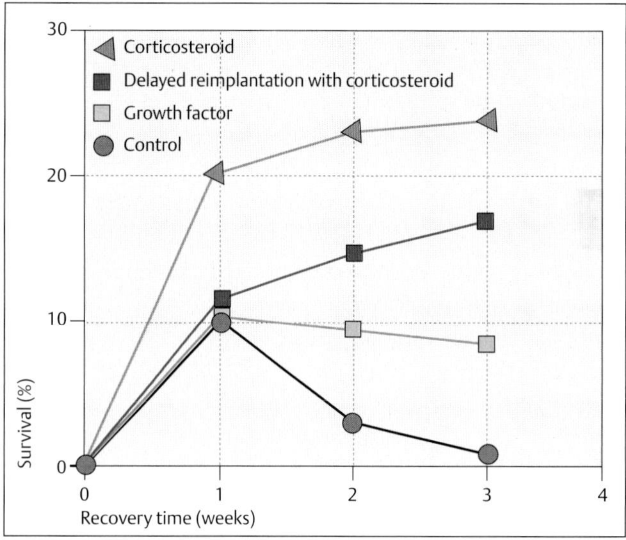

Fig. 3.**13** **Survival of composite grafts under different reimplantation conditions (from Henrich et al. 1995; delayed = stored in sterile saline solution for 90 minutes).**

Table 3.**6** Survival of composite grafts 1–3 weeks after reimplantation (Henrich et al. 1995)

Group	Survival (%) Week 1	Week 2	Week 3
Control	9.6	2.6	1.3
Corticosteroid	19.7	21.7	23.2
Growth factor	9.8	9.0	7.5
Delayed corticosteroid application	10.5	14.3	15.5

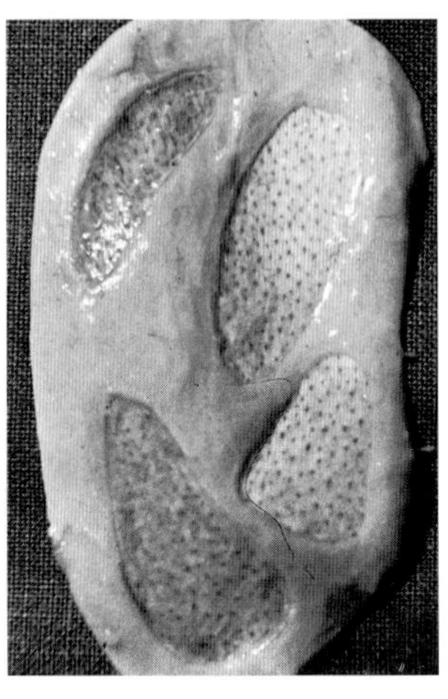
a

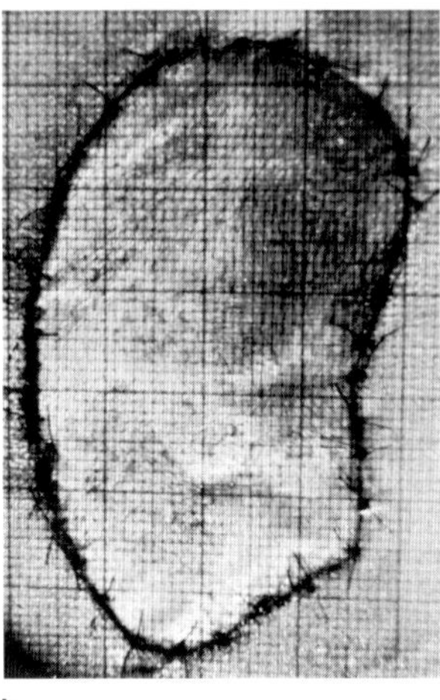
b

Fig. 3.**14** **Two-layered composite grafts replanted after Baudet (1972; 1780 mm²).**
a Replant in true auricular size; the cartilage is fenestrated.
b Replanted ear after 5 hours warm ischemia time at 22 °C (see Fig. 3.**15**): transplant survived completely.

Emergency Care of Auricular Avulsions

Emergency medicine has standardized guidelines for the treatment of amputations.

- If possible, the amputated ear should be transported in clean gauze inside a plastic replantation bag. By surrounding the inner bag with ice and water, the temperature is kept down to about 4 °C. Direct contact of the ice water with the tissue must be avoided because this would result in frostbite and necrosis (Sefrin 1991). If a transplantation bag is not available, a paper handkerchief soaked in clean tap water can also keep the amputated part clean, moist, and cool. The amputated part wrapped, in one or two paper handkerchiefs, is then placed in a plastic bag and handed to the patient for transport (Weerda 1994 c).
- The amputated part should be reattached as soon as possible, even though a warm ischemia time of 8–10 hours and a cold ischemia time of much longer than this can be tolerated by these composite grafts (Weerda et al. 1986, see p. 40; Fig. 3.**23**).

As already reported (Fig. 3.**15**), our studies showed that two-layered amputated tissues failed to survive only after a warm ischemia time of more than 48 hours or a cold ischemia time (storage at 4 °C) of more than 13 days after amputation. Fifty percent of the transplants survived with a warm ischemia time of up to 30 hours after graft removal and even with a cold ischemia of 10 days (see Fig. 3.**15**; Cannive 1985; Grüner 1985; Weerda et al. 1986; Mall 1989).

Given the generally unsatisfactory results of "classic replantation" (see p. 35; Table 3.7), many suggestions have been made on how to replant severed auricular segments or the entire auricle.

3.3.4 Replantation of the Auricle

Preoperative Care of the Amputated Part

The wound margins of the amputated part should, if necessary, be sparingly excised when tissue has been destroyed. Any contamination should be carefully brushed with povidone–iodine solution and removed. Careful hemostasis of the wound bed is required (Smith et al. 1972; Bernstein and Nelson 1982).

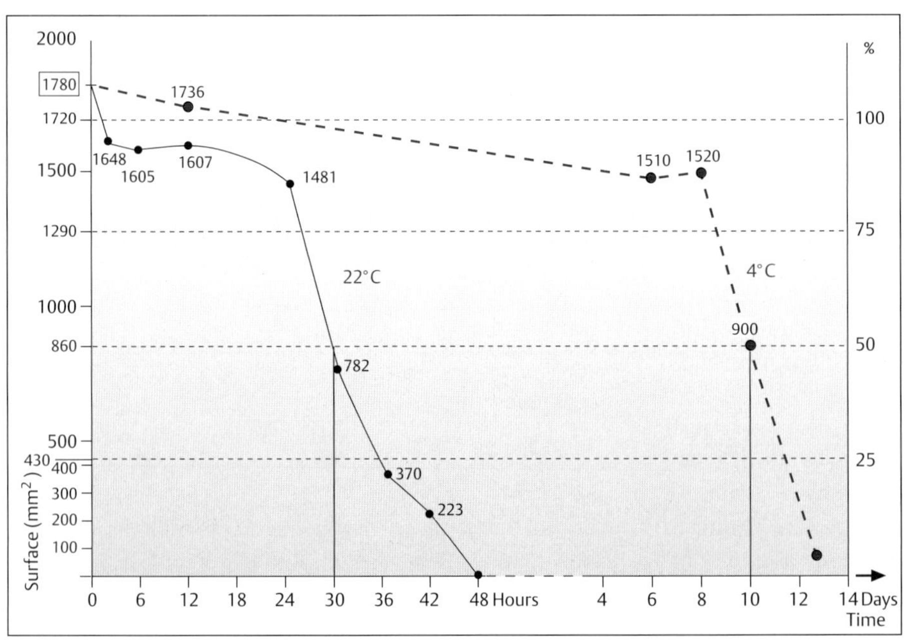

Fig. 3.**15** **Ischemia time before replantation (Weerda 1986 c; Weerda et al. 1986).**
Experimental studies on the replantation of fenestrated, two-layered composite grafts using the technique after Baudet using rabbit ears 64 ×34 mm in size (see Fig. 3.**14**).
x-axis: Storage time (ischemia time) until replantation.
y-axis: area of the survived composite grafts in mm² and %.
Continuous line: 80 (i. e., 8 × 10) transplants stored at room temperature (22 °C).
Interrupted line: 100 (i. e., 5 × 20) transplants refrigerated at 4 °C.

Table 3.7 Poor results of "classic replantation" in humans (Schewior 1995; see also Table 3.2)

	Case nos.	Complete survival	%	Incomplete survival[1]	%	Necrosis	%
Total avulsion	16	8	50	2	12	6	38
Partial avulsion	32	5	16	4	13	23	71
Total	48	13	27	6	13	29	60

[1]Replantation results with postoperative partial necrosis or shrinkage were classified as "incomplete survival."

Suture Technique

As few skin sutures as possible are inserted, beginning with the posterior surface and using monofilament suture material, e. g., 6–0, armed with an fine, atraumatic, needle. The cartilage is adapted with absorbable, braided or monofilament 5–0 suture material. The skin of the anterior auricular surface is closed last, using 6–0 or 7–0 monofilament sutures (Smith et al. 1972; Burgess et al. 1985). The dressing comprises povidone–iodine–petroleum jelly gauze swabs to cover the ear for 6–7 days without pressure, and a fenestrated sponge dressing. For immobilization we use an adhesive bandage for 1 week, covered by a head dressing (see p. 131).

Perioperative Measures

The overall poor survival rate of replanted auricular segments has prompted numerous attempts to improve the circulation and metabolism of the replanted ear with the aid of medications as well as the use of physical and anti-inflammatory means (Schewior 1995).

Cooling the replanted part was recommended by Alexandrov (1964), Pierer (1967), Gifford (1972), Clemons and Connelly (1973), Potsic and Naunton (1974), Lewis and Fowler (1979) and Fuleihan et al. (1987).

Rheological measures. Many authors have employed heparin (Clemons and Connelly 1973; Potsic and Naunton 1974). Other recommendations include spraying the replanted part with oxygen (Pierer 1967); the use of dextran (Pierer1967; Fuleihan et al. (1987); or stab incisions placed to avoid venous congestion (Clemons and Connelly; Fuleihan et al. 1987). An improvement in survival rate was reported with the use of corticosteroids (see Fig. 3.**13**). It is also essential to immobilize the transplanted part to guarantee revascularization. We therefore recommend an adhesive dressing, which should be left unchanged for at least 1 week (see p. 226; Fig. 5.**190**).

Replantation Techniques

Classic Replantation

By classic replantation, we mean the technique by which the three-layered amputated part is reattached in three layers to the remnant of the auricle as a composite graft. Although there must certainly have been a multitude of avulsions and replantations worldwide—just in our clinic we have attempted replantations on over 50 patients (Tab. 3.**4**, p. 32) the literature is not very forthcoming on this topic. We found (Weerda 1994 a; Schewior 1995) that of 48 replantations of this type reported in the literature, 13 (27 %) survived fully, 13 % survived incompletely, and 60 % became completely necrotic (Table 3.**3**). Of the 56 replantations documented in our clinic, only 1 replanted ear with a length of 2.6 cm and a width of 0.8 cm finally survived, with a central necrosis (Fig. 3.**16 a–c**; Weerda 1987, 1994 a). Other partial transplantations or complete replantations failed (Fig. 3.**17**).

The "classic" replantation of all three tissue layers is the oldest replantation technique (Brown 1898; Purcell 1898; Schmieden 1908, among others). The preconditions for survival are unfavorable because of the narrow nutrient base. Observing the 1 cm rule provides some improvement. Good immobilization for more than a week, i. e., a good form of dressing, also plays a decisive role. The ischemia time, which usually amounts to less than 6–7 hours, does not play any significant role in survival (Clodius 1968; Weerda 1986 c; Weerda et al. 1986, see Fig. 3.**15**).

Pocket Techniques

Given the poor survival rates with classic replantation, attempts have been made over the last 50 years to develop improved techniques to save the replanted parts by allowing them to heal in a cutaneous pocket. The following pocket techniques have been employed:

- **Distant banking:** abdominal pocket (Fig. 3.**18**; Conway et al. 1948; Musgrave and Garrett 1967), supraclavicular pocket (Gerow 1973; Spira 1974), cervical pocket (Conroy 1972)
- **Banking beneath retroauricular mastoid skin:** Sexton 1955; Converse 1958; Spira and Hardy 1963; Mladick et al. 1971; Tarabey 1981 (see p. 59, Fig. 4.**40 a**)
- **Flap coverage:** local flaps (Elsahy 1986 a), platysma flaps (Ariyan and Chicarilli 1986), temporoparietal fascial flaps (Fox and Edgerton 1976; Brent and Byrd 1983)

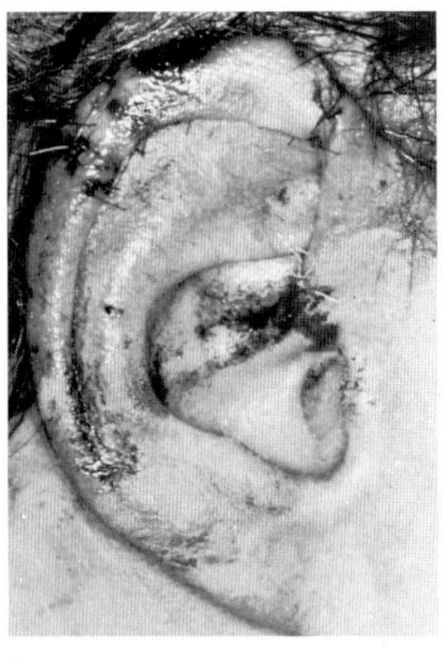
a

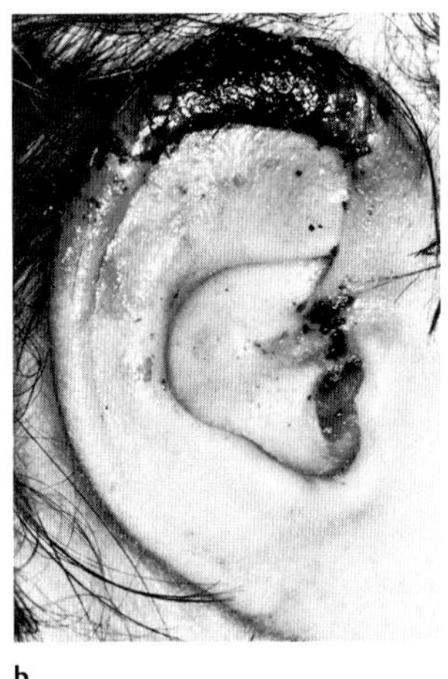
b

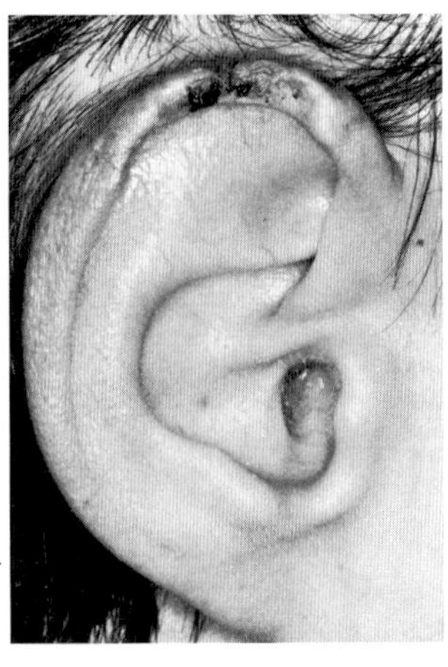
c

Fig. 3.**16** **Helical replantation.**
a 24 hours after replantation.
b Partial necrosis after 3 weeks.
c Defect healing after 3 months.

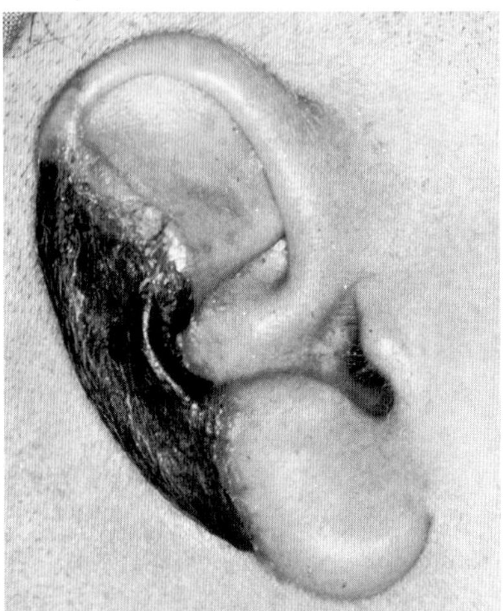

Fig. 3.**17** **Classic replantation. Necrosis of a medium sized replant (see p. 70, Fig. 4.64).**

Distant Banking

All techniques of distant cartilage banking have usually resulted in the cartilage framework, void of skin, becoming distorted and eventually unsuitable for auricular reconstruction (Fig. 3.**17**).

Banking Beneath Retroauricular Mastoid Skin

Sexton's Technique

As with the usual technique of reconstructing the avulsed auricle (see Chapter 4, p. 65), Sexton (1955) removed the skin of the anterior and posterior surface and buried the cartilage framework in a retroauricular pocket beneath mastoid skin. An additional flap was used for coverage if there was not enough skin.

The skin of the pocket also formed the anterior surface of the new auricle. In one case described, the framework survived and, after exteriorization, the posterior auricular surface was covered with split skin harvested from the thigh. The earlobe required additional reconstruction; the entire reconstruction was documented with photographs. Converse (1958) describes a similar technique.

Mladick's Technique

The term "pocket technique" was first used by Mladick et al. (1971). Unlike the previous authors, Mladick did not remove the skin, but dermabraded the amputated part on both surfaces and then inserted the reattached part in its correct anatomical position.

First operative stage (Fig. 3.**19**). The severed part is cleaned; the edges of both severed part and auricular stump are debrided. Both skin surfaces of the severed part are then dermabraded. The epidermis is removed and the dermis remains intact (Fig. 3.**19 a**). A subcutaneous postauricular pocket is then developed, the amputated ear is inserted in its correct anatomical position, its cartilage is attached to the stump cartilage, and the skin of the pocket is sutured to the anterior skin of the stump (Fig. 3.**19 b–d**). A light pressure dressing is applied for 10–14 days and prophylactic antibiotics given.

Second operative stage (Fig. 3.**20**). After about 4 weeks, the reattached ear is freed from the subcutaneous pocket by opening the pocket at the stump and exposing the buried auricle. After exteriorizing the ear, the skin is returned to its old retroauricular bed (Fig. 3.**20**).

The dermabraded auricular parts of the anterior and posterior surfaces, which are initially nourished by the enveloping pocket and the mastoid bed, begin to reepithelialize. If there is no sign of any spontaneous epithelialization, the raw area is covered with a split-thickness skin graft.

Following animal studies conducted by Mladick et al. (1971), Mladick and Curraway (1973) subsequently modified and improved the pocket technique.

Modification of Mladick's Technique

A traction mattress suture flattens out the skin onto the replanted auricular framework. Apart from improved nutrition for the reattached ear, Mladick expected reduced tendency for shrinkage. The pockets of three of the replanted ears were already opened after 14 days, and the three reported cases (Mladick and Curraway 1973; Lehmann and Cervino 1975) showed good results. Only once was a poorly epithelialized region observed.

Summary. Between 1956 and 1980, 14 different techniques of "pocket replantation" were reported (Table 3.8). It is not possible to make a reliable assessment of these techniques because of the small numbers reported. One advantage is certain: even if the reattached auricle is lost, the skin of the postauricular pocket—albeit slightly scarred—remains intact for reconstruction with a costal cartilage graft (Fig. 4.40, p. 59).

Complications. These include lack of spontaneous re-epithelialization, hypertrophic scarring in the region of the auricle and mastoid with deformation, and lack of contour-

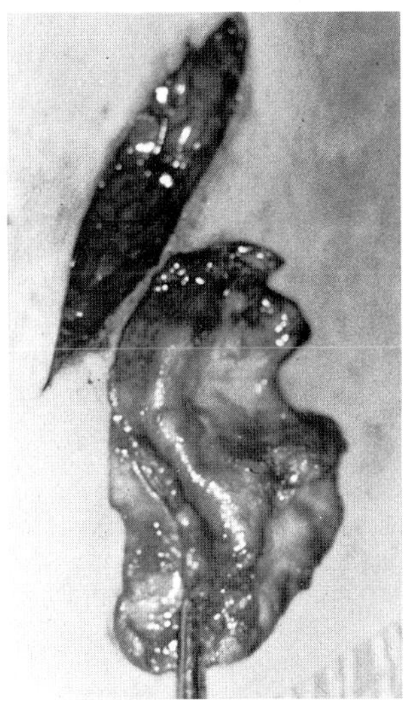

Fig. 3.18 **Shrinkage and partial resorption after banking of the cartilage framework in an abdominal pocket (posterior aspect).**

Table 3.8 Survival after the various "pocket techniques" (Schewior 1995): examples from the literature

	Case nos.	Complete survival	%	Incomplete survival[1]	%	Necrosis	%
Total avulsion	8	6	75	2	25	–	–
Partial avulsion	6	3	50	3	50	–	–
Total	14	9	64	5	36	–	–

[1]Replantation results with postoperative partial necrosis or shrinkage were classified as "incomplete survival."

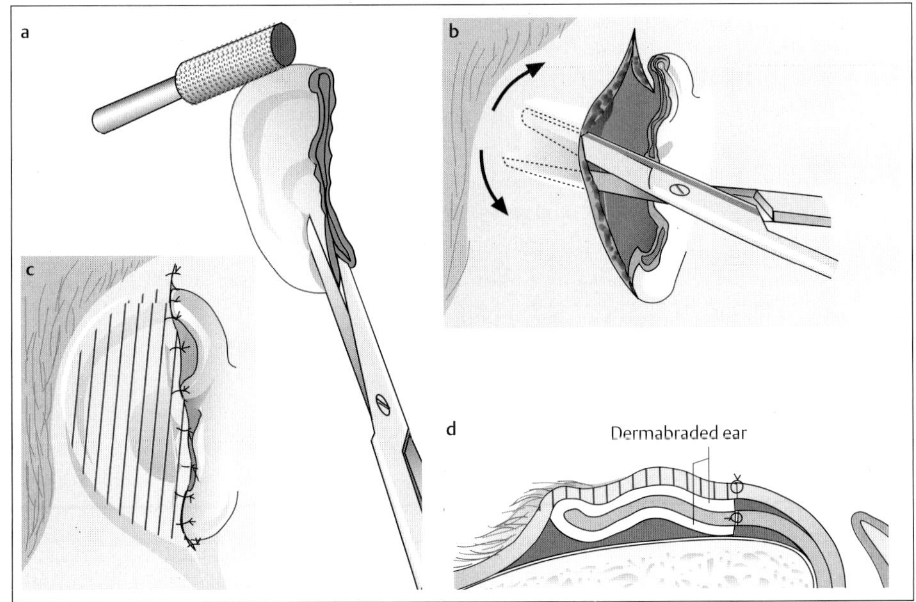

Fig. 3.19 **Replantation beneath retroauricular mastoid skin using the "pocket technique" for reattaching the severed ear. First stage (after Mladick et al. 1971):**
a Debridement and dermabrasion.
b Development of a subcutaneous pocket over the mastoid.
c Replantation of the ear, which has been dermabraded on both sides, into the pocket (hatched area): suture of the cartilage onto the cartilage stump (5–0 braided suture), suture of the skin onto the skin of the stump (6–0 monofilament suture).
d Cross-section.

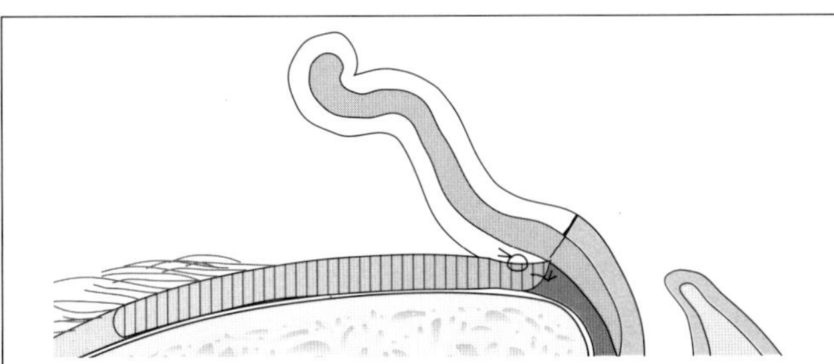

Fig. 3.20 **Replantation beneath retroauricular mastoid skin using the "pocket technique" for reattaching the severed ear (after Mladick et al. 1971).**
Second stage: Exteriorization of the replanted ear from the pocket in cross-section (see text).

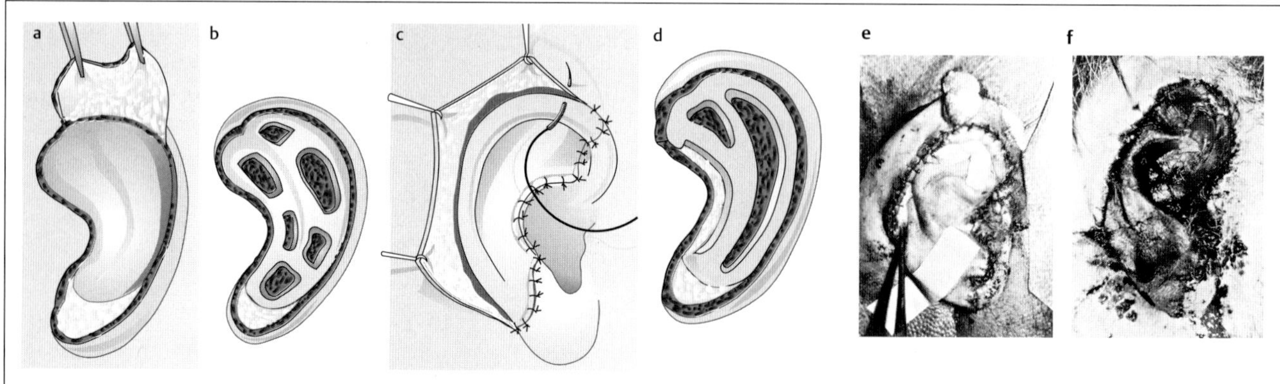

Fig. 3.21 **Replantation using the technique of Baudet et al. (from Converse and Brent 1977).**
a Removal of the posteromedial skin from the amputated part.
b Fenestration of the cartilage with preservation of the anterior perichondrium.
c Dissection of the auriculomastoid recipient bed and reattachment of the amputated part with sutures and fibrin adhesive. Sponge tie-over dressing for 1 week (see p. 216, plaster dressing, see p. 222).
d Fenestration of the cartilage using Brent's technique (1977).
e Replantation using the technique of Baudet et al (1972).
f Replant necrosis after which the patient was referred to us (see p. 94, Fig. 4.**109**).

ing of the scapha, concha, and the soft elastic cartilage. Shrinkage of the entire auricle, as well as partial and total resorption, have also been reported.

Flap Coverage

Coverage of the reattached cartilage with **local skin flaps** is described later in the book when dealing with auricular reconstruction after loss of individual parts, because the coverage and the flaps used there are employed in a similar way, regardless of any loss of the supportive framework (see Chapter 4, pp. 43).

Dufourmentel (1958 b), Fox and Edgerton (1976), Tegtmeier and Gooding (1977), Erol et al. (1981), Brent and Byrd (1983) and others have reported on **temporoparietal fascial flaps** (synonym: fan flap, see Figs. 4.**108**, 4.**109**; pp. 92 and 93) for various indications of auricular reconstruction. The technique is described in more detail in Chapter 5 (p. 214, Fig. 5.**171**).

Other Techniques of Replanting Auricular Parts

After loss of parts of the auricle, e. g., the superior auricle, the cartilage is sutured to the cartilage stump with monofilament or braided 4–0 or 5–0 sutures, after removal of the skin. Care should be taken when removing the skin that it remains intact throughout, i. e., the anterior and posterior surfaces remain joined together, because, if it is kept largely intact, this full-thickness skin graft may be used to cover the fascia.

For the replantation of the **entire auricle** using the fan flap see pp. 74, 93, and 94.

Baudet's Replantation of the Auricle

(Fig. 3.**20**)

Together with many others, Baudet and co-workers were also dissatisfied with the "classic" reimplantation of the ear as a three-layered graft and its exceptionally poor survival rates. They described their technique as the reimplantation of a "two-layered composite graft with fenestrated cartilage" (Baudet 1972, Baudet et al. 1972 a, b). They hoped to have developed a safe and reliable technique.

First operative stage (Fig. 3.**21**). The severed part is denuded of its skin on the posterior surface, but the perichondrium is left. The incision of the postauricular skin courses behind the helix, this skin being subsequently discarded (Fig. 3.**21 a**). Those parts of the cartilage not needed to support the ear are excised from a posterior approach, leaving the perichondrium on the anterior surface (Fig. 3.**21 b**). The cartilage is sutured to the stump cartilage using a 5–0 braided suture, the anterior skin of the severed part to the skin of the stump using a 6–0 suture, and the mastoid skin to the skin on the posterior surface of the helix (Fig. 3.**21 c**). In addition, we recommend gluing the entire reattached part to the mastoid wound bed with fibrin adhesive to condition the vessels into revascularizing into the anterior skin through the fenestrations (Weerda 1980, 1986 a, b). We further recommend a sponge tie-over dressing to achieve light compression and prevent the reimplanted ear from lifting off its bed. The sterile sponge is then secured to the skin with strips of adhesive plaster and left for at least 1 week (see Fig. 5.**185 c**, **d**, p. 223). Brent (1977) recommends fenestrating the cartilage in the triangular fossa and in the whole of the scapha (Fig. 3.**21 d**; Converse and Brent 1977).

This Baudet procedure has been used by many authors, sometimes with modifications (Arfai 1974, cited in Weerda

Table 3.9 Survival after replantation using the techniques of Baudet et al. and Arfai (Schewior 1995): examples from the literature

	Case nos.	Complete survival	%	Incomplete survival	%	Necrosis	%
Total avulsion	7	2	29	3	43	2	29
Partial avulsion	6	3	50	2	33	1	17
Total	13	5	38	5	38	3	23

1986c; Larsen and Pless 1976; Salyapongse et al. 1979; Gemperli et al. 1991). Destro and Speranzini (1996) replanted the base component according to Baudet's technique; they also removed the anterior skin of the lateral part near the helix and inserted the cartilage beneath the non-hair-bearing skin of the mastoid.

Second operative stage. After about 4–6 weeks, the posterior auricular surface is exteriorized and the defects covered with free skin grafts (see Chapter 4, p. 72; Fig. 4.**66 d–f**). The earlobe often requires additional reconstruction (see Fig. 3.**23 c**, **e**).

The literature reports 5 complete survivals from 13 replants (38 %). Five (38 %) survived incompletely, and 3 (23 %) were lost entirely (Fig. 3.**21 e**, **f**; see Table 3.**9**; Salyapongse et al. 1979; Bardsley and Mercer 1983; Cannive 1985; Grüner 1985; Mall 1989; Gemperli et al. 1991; Schuffenecker 1991).

Animal studies by Weerda et al. Our animal studies involving Baudet's technique have already been explained in detail (see pp. 33 and 34). We were able to show that it is not the time between amputation of the ear and its reimplantation (which is reported in the literature as being 2–8 hours on average) that is the cause for replant loss, but the exceptionally poor revascularization into the nutrient tissue (see also p. 38) and inadequate or missing immobilization of the replant for 1 week.

Arfai's Modification of the Baudet Technique (Figs. 3.**22**, 3.**23**)

In 1974 Spira reported on a technique with which Arfai is supposed to have tried to retain the postauricular skin. The operative procedure is shown in Figs. 3.**22** and 3.**23 a–e** (Arfai 1974, Weerda 1979 a).

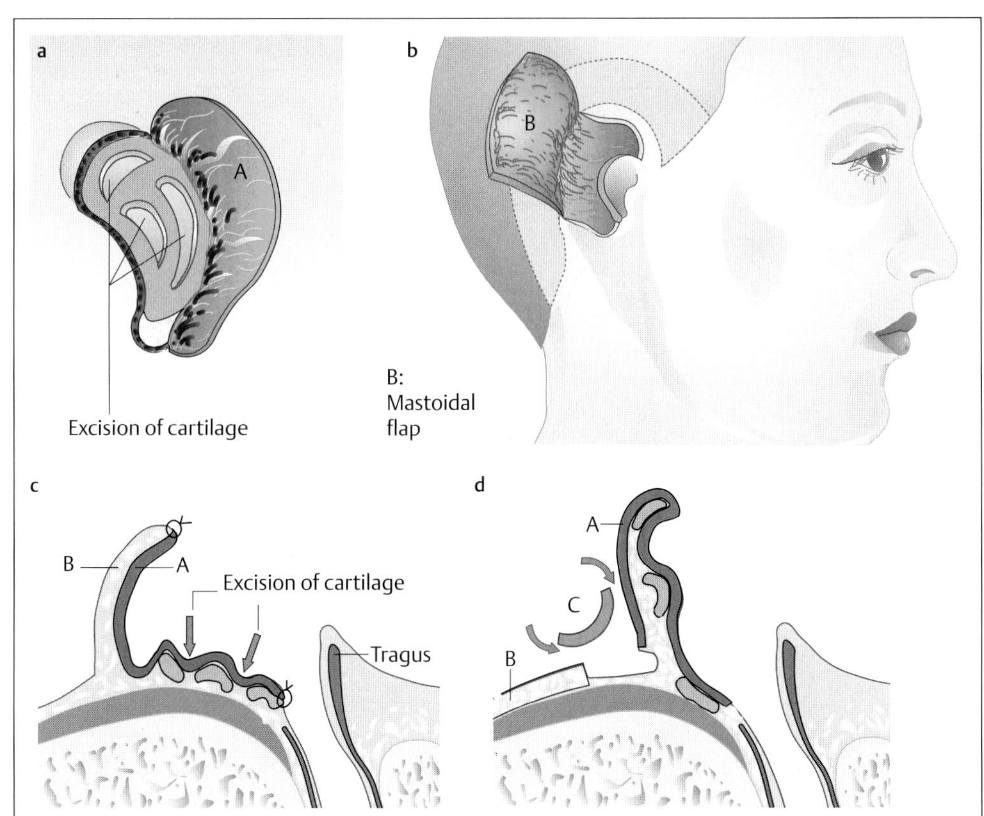

Fig. 3.**22** **Replantation of an avulsed auricle using the technique of Baudet as modified by Arfai (after Weerda 1979 a, 1999 a, 2001; see Fig. 3.23).**
a Dissection of the avulsed posteromedial surface: Dissection of the skin and perichondrium back to the helical rim as a full-thickness flap (A). Fenestration of the auricular framework by removing parts of the cartilage down to the perichondrium of the anterolateral auricular surface.
b Dissection of the recipient bed out of the auriculomastoid skin: flap (B) raised towards the scalp, enlarging the wound surface.
c **First stage:** Reattachment of the cartilage to the recipient bed with sutures and tissue glue, the flap raised from the posterolateral auricular surface (A) is glued with fibrin adhesive and sutured onto the dissected mastoid flap (B).
d **Second stage:** After 3 weeks the two flaps (A and B) are separated before the posterolateral auricular surface is exteriorized. The posterolateral auricular flap (A) and the mastoid flap (B) are returned to their original positions. Residual defects are covered with split skin (C).

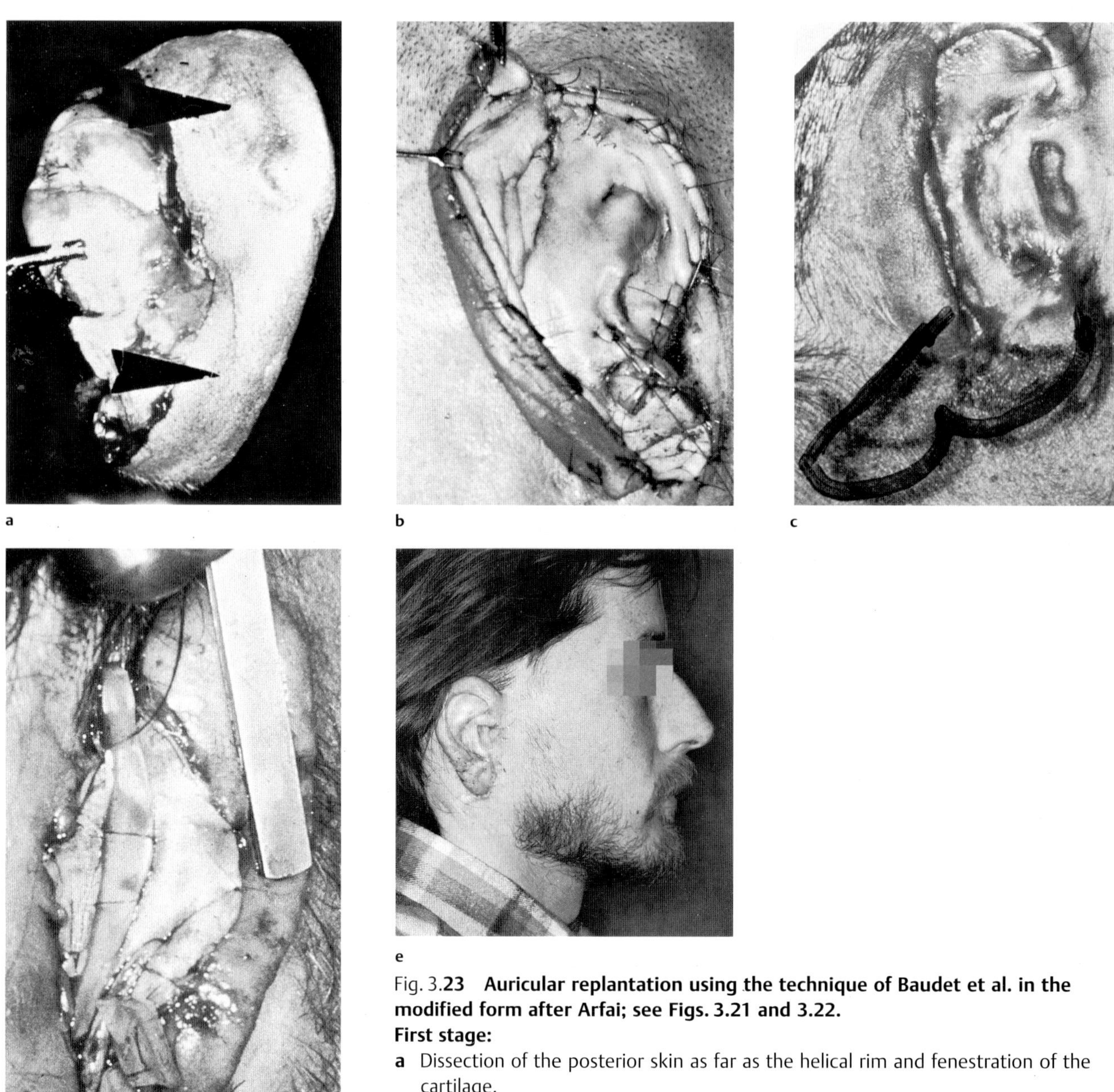

Fig. 3.23 **Auricular replantation using the technique of Baudet et al. in the modified form after Arfai; see Figs. 3.21 and 3.22.**
First stage:
a Dissection of the posterior skin as far as the helical rim and fenestration of the cartilage.
b Reattachment of the cartilage with sutures and fibrin adhesive
Second stage:
c After about 6 weeks the auricle is exteriorized and the earlobe reconstructed with a Gavello double flap (see also pp. 75 and 76).
d Coverage of the posterior surface with a thick split-skin graft.
e Result 1 year after the operation.

Summary. Between 1972 and 1993, 13 cases employing Baudet's technique and its modifications were reported in the literature (Table 3.9). This includes the technique after Larsen and Pless (1976). The longest ischemic time was 8 hours, although this reimplanted ear was in fact cooled preoperatively (Schuffenecker 1991).

Microvascular Ear Replantation

Although the first microsurgical vascular anastomoses were performed at the beginning of the twentieth century (Carell and Guthrie 1912, cited in Dongen 1987), Buncke and Schulz first reported on replantation trials with microvascular anastomoses of rabbit ears in 1966. Further animal studies are known to have been undertaken by Tsai (1975) and

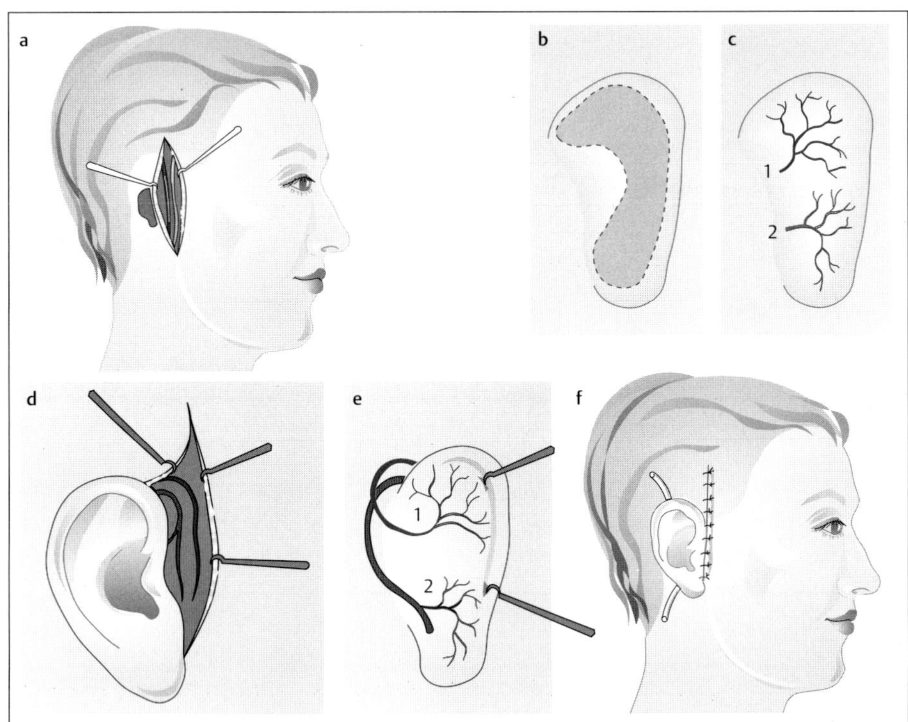

Fig. 3.**24** **Microvascular replantation: operation diagram after Juri et al. (1987).**
a Preauricular incision to dissect the superficial temporal vessels.
b Deepithelialization of the posterior auricular aspect.
c Dissection of the vessels: arteries (1), veins (2).
d Transposition of the superficial temporal vessels to the posterior aspect of the auricle.
e End-to-end anastomosis of the arteries (1) and end-to-end anastomosis of the veins (2).
f Final suture and placement of two drains.

Hausamen et al. (1977). Pennington et al. reported on the first successful human replantations in 1980.

A well-trained team is essential for this type of surgery. We ourselves have only conducted this type of microvascular repair using vein grafts once, in a case of an incomplete avulsion where the circulation of the replanted part was tenuous. We do not intend to discuss here the techniques of microvascular anastomosis and its complications, given that there is enough literature on the subject (including Weerda 1999 a; 2001). The various animal studies on this technique show that the survival times of the replanted part depends on the suture technique and the study conditions. Thus the work by Buncke and Schulz (1966) demonstrate a high rate of tissue loss, whereas in later animal studies the improved techniques employed by Tsai (1975), Hausamen et al. (1977), and above all Kotthaus et al. (1978) and von Giesen et al. (1983) show better results. Here the survival rate of the transplants was increased to 100% by storing them at 4 °C for 24 hours (von Giesen et al. 1983; Strauch et al. 1983; Mutimer et al. 1987; Schoenich and Biemer 1987; van Beek 1988; Katsaros et al. 1988; Anthony et al. 1989; Sadove 1990; Rapaport et al. 1993; Safak et al. 1993).

It is important to observe the following procedure when undertaking microvascular replantation of the external ear:

- The vascular sutures should be inserted using 9–0 or 10–0 suture material. Vein grafts are usually necessary (Pennington et al. 1980), harvested from the dorsum of the foot, the hand, the lower arm region (Turpin 1987; Turpin et al. 1988), or the neck region. The anastomoses are done using a retroauricular end-to-end technique, or as an end-to-side anastomosis if otherwise impossible (Juri et al. 1987; Tanaka and Tajima 1989; Remmert et al. 1999, 2001; Fig. 3.**24** **a–f**).
- The replants should be stored moist and cool. They should also be carefully and gently cleaned with peroxide or (diluted) povidone–iodine before doing the anastomosis.
- The general rules of microvascular surgery must be observed (Remmert et al. 1999, 2001).

Summary. With an almost 60% complete survival rate, auricular replantation using microvascular anastomosed vessels gives the best results (Table 3.**10**; p. 42). After avulsion of the ear, the small vessels are difficult to identify, given their small caliber and the often traumatized auricle. In addition, the majority of clinics do not have a replantation team at their disposal. However, an attempt at this technique of reattachment should always be made.

Concluding Summary and Assessment of Replantation Techniques

Complete survival was achieved in 40% of cases and incomplete survival in 24% of all replantations (51 partial and 50 total avulsions), but there was a complete loss in 37% of cases (Table 3.**11**).

It is well worth considering replantation as a suitable technique for auricular reconstruction in cases of clean-cut avulsions with small stump surfaces. With a success rate of

Table 3.**10** Survival after auricular replantation with microvascular anastomosis (Schewior 1995): examples from the literature

	Case nos.	Complete survival	%	Incomplete survival[1]	%	Necrosis	%
Total avulsion	16	10	63	1	6	5	31
Partial avulsion	3	1	33	2	66	–	–
Total	19	11	58	3	16	5	26

[1]Replantation results with postoperative partial necrosis or shrinkage were classified as "incomplete survival."

Table 3.**11** Survival rates for auricular replantations using all techniques found in the literature up to 1995 (Schewior 1995)

Replantation technique	Avulsion	Case nos.	Complete survival	%	Incomplete survival	%	Loss	%
Classic replantation	Total	16	8	50	2	13	6	38
	Partial	32	5	16	4	13	23	72
Pocket techniques	Total	8	6	75	2	25	–	–
	Partial	6	3	50	3	50	–	–
Flap coverage	Total	4	1	25	3	75	–	–
	Partial	3	1	33	2	67	–	–
Techniques after Baudet/Arfai	Total	7	2	29	3	43	2	29
	Partial	6	3	50	2	33	1	17
Microvascular reanastomosis	Total	16	10	63	1	6	5	31
	Partial	3	1	33	2	67	–	–
Total no. of cases	Total	51	27	53	11	22	13	25
	Partial	50	13	26	13	26	24	48
Total of total and partial avulsions		101	40	39.6	24	23.7	37	36.7

almost 60% for microvascular anastomosed replantation and a 16% partial survival, it is without doubt the technique of choice.

The Arfai technique also demonstrates good replantation results, although it does produce scarring of the mastoid skin, resulting in difficulties for the reconstruction of the ear using costal cartilage and adjacent skin should the transplant fail. The same applies to the pocketing techniques.

The technical demands of the "classic" replantation may be low, but the expected failure rate is high (see Table 3.**11**). **For this reason, selection of the method of treatment should be directed towards avoiding additional injury to the skin in the form of adhesions. This would allow secondary reconstruction using local skin and autologous costal cartilage should replantation fail** (Steffen 2004; see p. 66, Fig. 4.**54**; p. 70, Fig. 4.**64**; p. 94, Fig. 4.**109**).

4 Classification and Surgery of Auricular Defects

H. Weerda

4.1 History

The mutilation of parts of the face as a consequence of war or for reasons of punishment has been known throughout human history. In the Roman Empire it was customary to mutilate the ears of slaves as a form of identification (Mündnich 1962 a). The earlobes were pierced and the perforations enlarged with heavy chains and rings. Thus Celsus (25 BC–AD 30) describes the reconstruction of partial auricular defects, as cited in Zeis (1863):

> Mutilations to the lips, the nose and the ears can be treated if they are small, even if there are two small injuries of this kind; if they are large, either they are not susceptible of treatment, or else may be so deformed by it that the site from which material is harvested may quite easily become even more deformed than the region to be treated. But where the earlobes, in a man for instance, have been pierced and have become offensive, it is enough to pass a red-hot needle quickly through the hole in order to blister its margins superficially.

Sushruta (around AD 1000) writes:

> A surgeon can reconstruct the earlobe in a person devoid of them by slicing off a patch of living flesh from that person's cheek in a manner so as to have one of its ends attached to the cheek. Then the part where the artificial earlobe is to be made should be slightly scarified and the living flesh should be made to adhere to it (Zeis 1863).

Antonius Branca, like his father, reconstructed noses and ears from skin of the arm (Joseph 1931). The oldest known illustrations date back to Tagliacozzi (1546–1599; Fig. 4.1 **a, b**) who later became professor of anatomy and medicine in Venice and in 1597 described the techniques in his work ***De curtorum chirurgia per insitionem***.

In later centuries, the French surgeons Paré (1509–1590) and Roux in 1894 tended to prefer treating ears with prostheses (Fig. 4.2). Even the surgeon Dieffenbach (1845 a) described only the reconstruction of the upper and lower auricle, and advised against reconstruction of the entire ear because of the less than satisfactory results (Fig. 4.3 **a, b**). In his book (1845 a) he writes: "I consider the replacement of the whole ear to be an entirely inappropriate experiment because it will be impossible to lend the ear its necessary form. Regardless of all efforts at reconstruction, the ear will remain an unshapely, disfigured lump."

In 1870 Szymanowsky reported a reconstruction of the upper and lower ear. He is also credited with the reconstruction of the entire auricle (Fig. 4.4 **a, b**). However, it is most unlikely that he ever employed this technique with any degree of success.

With Szymanowsky also began the era of reconstruction for the complete loss of the ear. Körte (1905) was the first to use a composite graft of the contralateral ear. Schmieden in

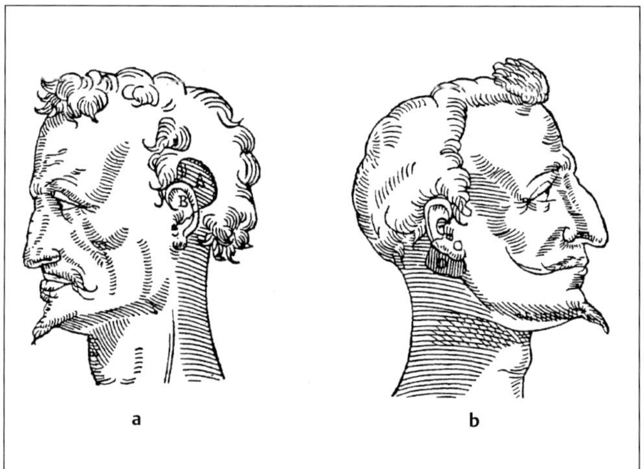

Fig. 4.1 **Partial auricular reconstruction as described by Tagliacozzi (1597; in Joseph 1931).**
a Reconstruction of the upper auricle.
b Reconstruction of the lower auricle.

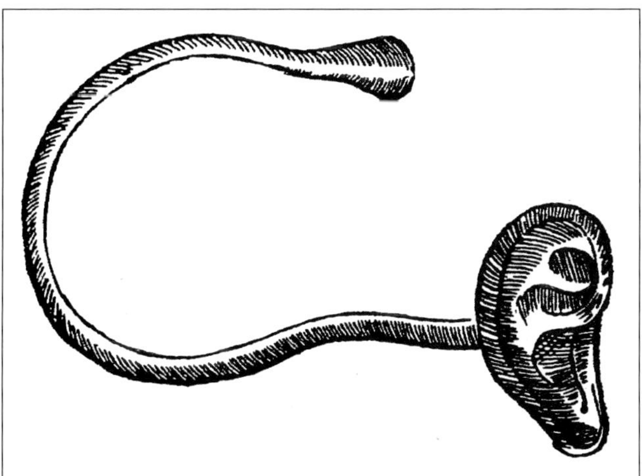

Fig. 4.2 **Auricular prosthesis as designed by Ambroise de Paré, c.1579 (in Roberts 1971).**

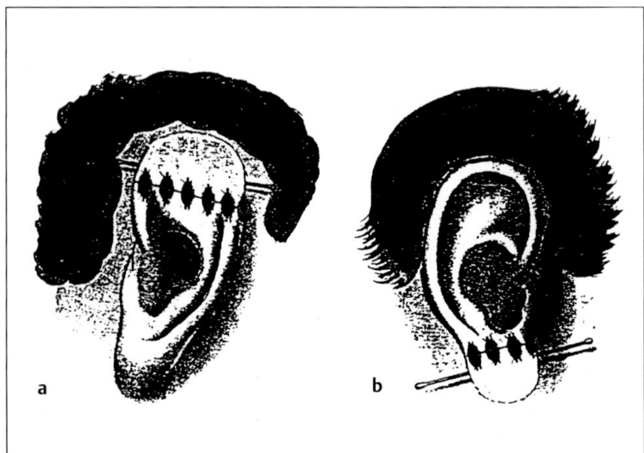

Fig. 4.3 **Reconstruction of partial auricular defects by Dieffenbach (1845; in Fritze and Reich 1845).**
a Reconstruction of the upper segment.
b Reconstruction of the earlobe.

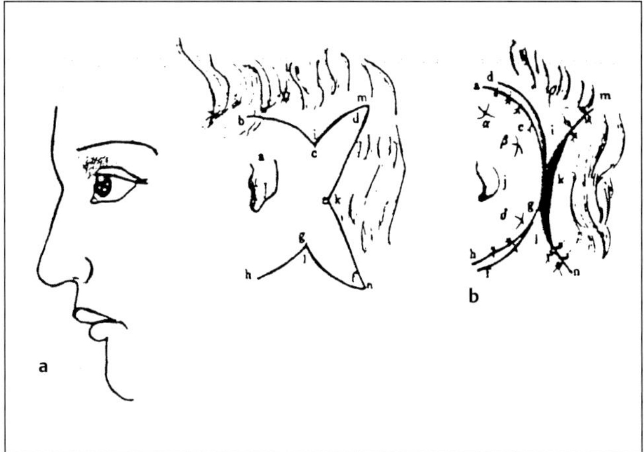

Fig. 4.4 **Total auricular reconstruction as described by Szymanowsky (1870).**
a Plan of reconstruction; the skin for the posterior auricular surface is situated in the hair-bearing region.
b Result after folding in the skin. Note that the earlobe was reconstructed with a bilobed flap which was later attributed to Gavello (as cited in Nelaton and Ombredanne 1907).

1908 describes for the first time the use of a cartilaginous framework (p. 198).

In his dissertation "Die Totalrekonstruktion der Ohrmuschel" (The total reconstruction of the ear), Toplak (1986) described in detail the reconstruction of the entire auricle using many forms of framework. Even though quite good results for total reconstruction of the auricle are to be found occasionally during the first half of the twentieth century, it is not until after World War II that the various stages of reconstruction are described in detail in the comprehensive works by Tanzer (1959, 1963 a, b and c, 1965, 1977), Converse (1950, 1958, 1977), Brent (1974, 1977, 1983, 1999 b), and Nagata (1993, 1994 a, b and c). The work of these authors will be referred to in more detail later when total auricular reconstruction is dealt with.

4.2 Classification (Table 4.1)

Although there will inevitably be overlaps when attempting to classify auricular defects, we still regard it as worthwhile to classify the defects for didactic reasons, in order to offer a system of surgical reconstruction (Weerda 1980, 1984 b, 1987, 1989 c, 1994 d, 1999 a, 2001; Mellette 1991) (Table 4.1).

Table 4.1 Classification of auricular defects (Weerda 1980, 1987)

1 Central defects
- Concha
- Antihelix–scapha
- Combined central defects

2 Peripheral defects (helix and helical crus)
- Reconstruction with auricular reduction
- Reconstruction without auricular reduction

3 Partial reconstructions
- Upper third of the auricle:
  - Reconstruction with auricular reduction
  - Reconstruction without auricular reduction
- Middle third of the auricle:
  - Reconstruction with auricular reduction
  - Reconstruction without auricular reduction
- Lower third of the auricle

4 Earlobe
- Traumatic earlobe cleft
- Reduction of the earlobe (hyperplasia)
- Defects of the earlobe
- Loss of the earlobe (hypoplasia and aplasia)
- Hypertrophic scar formation
- Keloids

5 Posterior defects
- Postauricular defects (posterior surface of the ear)
- Retroauricular defects (mastoid region)
- Combined post- and retroauricular defects

6 Subtotal defects

7 Reconstruction after total auricular loss

8 Preauricular defects

9 Defects of the auricular region

10 Burns

4.2.1 Central Defects: Recommended Defect Coverage (Fig. 4.5)

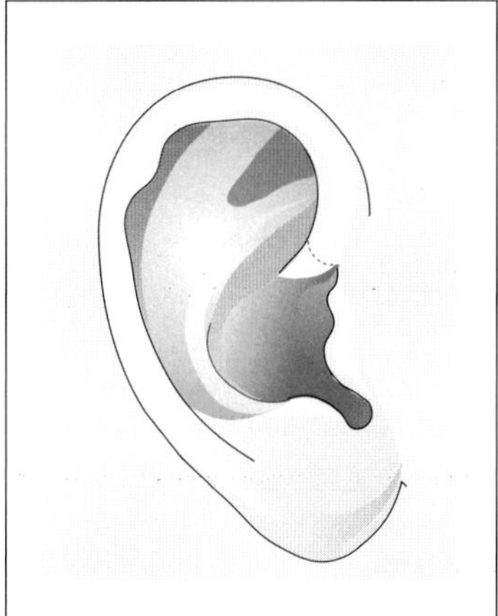

Fig. 4.5 **Central defects: concha–antihelix–combined defects.**

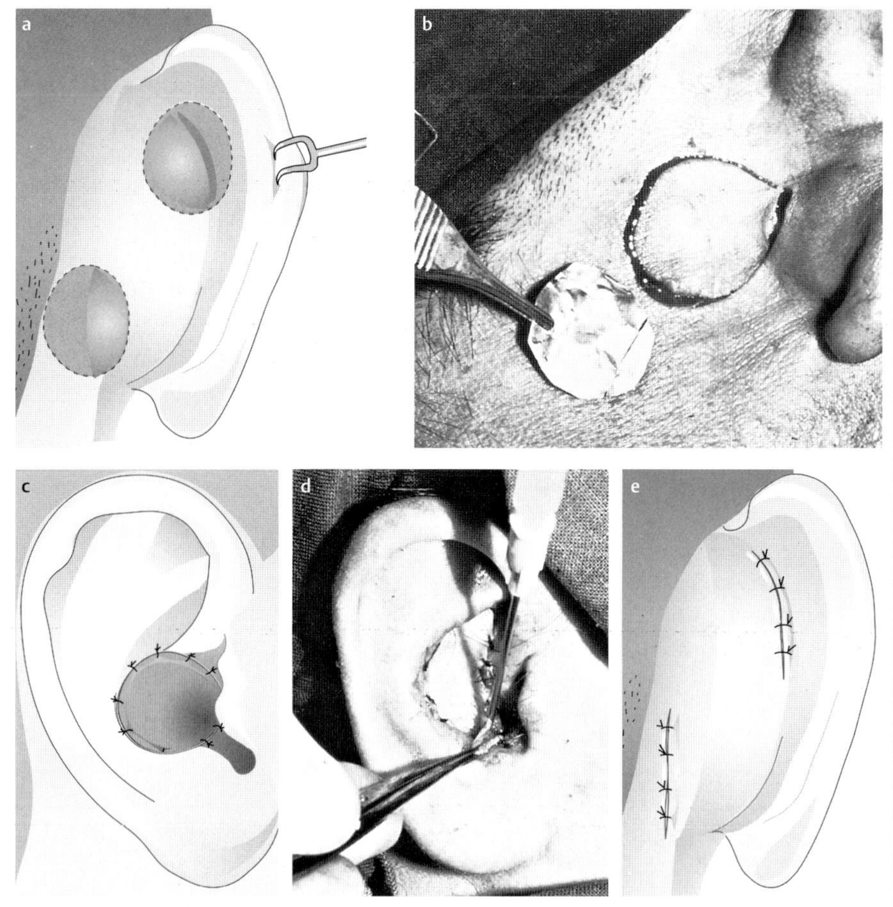

Fig. 4.6 **Coverage of a central defect with full-thickness skin.**

a, b Full-thickness skin graft harvested from the sulcus or mastoid region and fashioned by means of a template.

c, d Inset using a few approximation sutures (6–0 monofilament) and fibrin adhesive.

e Primary closure of the wound.

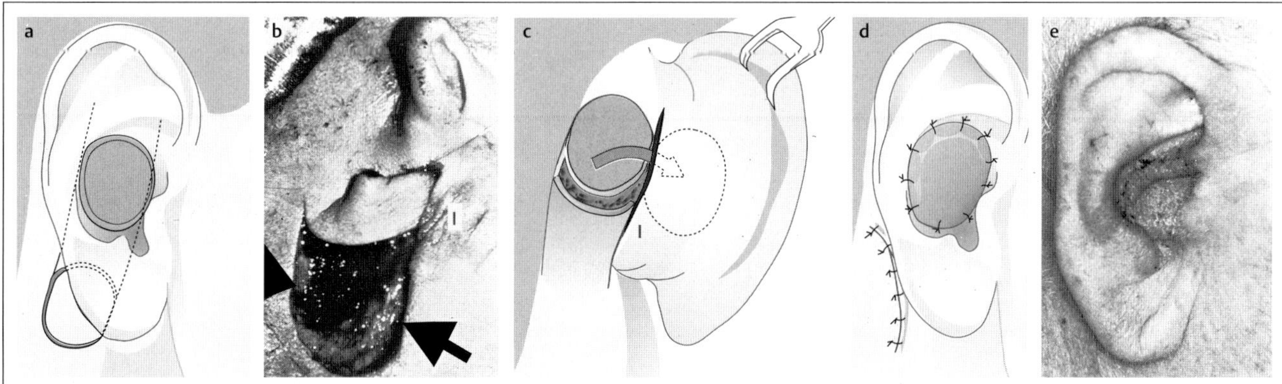

Fig. 4.7 **Two-layer defect of the concha: coverage using a superiorly or inferiorly based transposition flap.**

a, b Retroauricular, superiorly based transposition flap with de-epithelialized area located beneath the tunnel (I).

c Inferiorly based transposition flap (alternative technique to **a**).

d Closure of all defects. In a second session after about 3 weeks, the pedicle usually requires separation and incorporation (see Fig. 4.**16**; Weerda 1999 a, 2001).

e Result.

Conchal Defects

Reconstruction with a Full-thickness Skin Graft
(Fig. 4.6)

Since large parts of the concha adjoin the mastoid region, full-thickness skin is an option for reconstructing the concha. Reconstruction with a full-thickness skin graft is shown in Fig. 4.6 a–e.

Transposition Flap and U-shaped Advancement
(Fig. 4.7)

When the defects are situated somewhat higher or extend into the antihelix, it is possible to use superiorly or inferiorly based transposition flaps, de-epithelialized at the site that comes to lie beneath the tunnel when passed anteriorly (**pull-through technique**) (Fig. 4.7 a–e).

Reconstruction with Island Flaps
(Figs. 4.8–4.10)

"True" island flaps are flaps which are supplied by an artery but disconnected from the surrounding tissue (Kazanjian 1958; Weerda 1999 b, 2001). The following techniques are used:

- Reconstruction of a two-layer defect using a **myocutaneous island flap** based posteriorly on the posterior auricular artery (Krespi et al. 1983; Weerda 1999 a, 2001; Fig. 4.8 a–f)
- Chen and Chen (1990) also use an island flap based posteriorly on the posterior auricular artery
- Large **island flap based on a dermal pedicle** (as described by Masson 1972; Renard 1981; Koopman and Coulthard 1982; Jackson 1985 b; Fig. **4.9 a–g**).
- Island flap as described by Park et al. (1988; Fig. 4.**10 a, b**).

Park and Chung (1989) have pointed out that the direction of blood flow is reversed after the flap is inset. The donor site is covered with a split- or full-thickness skin graft.

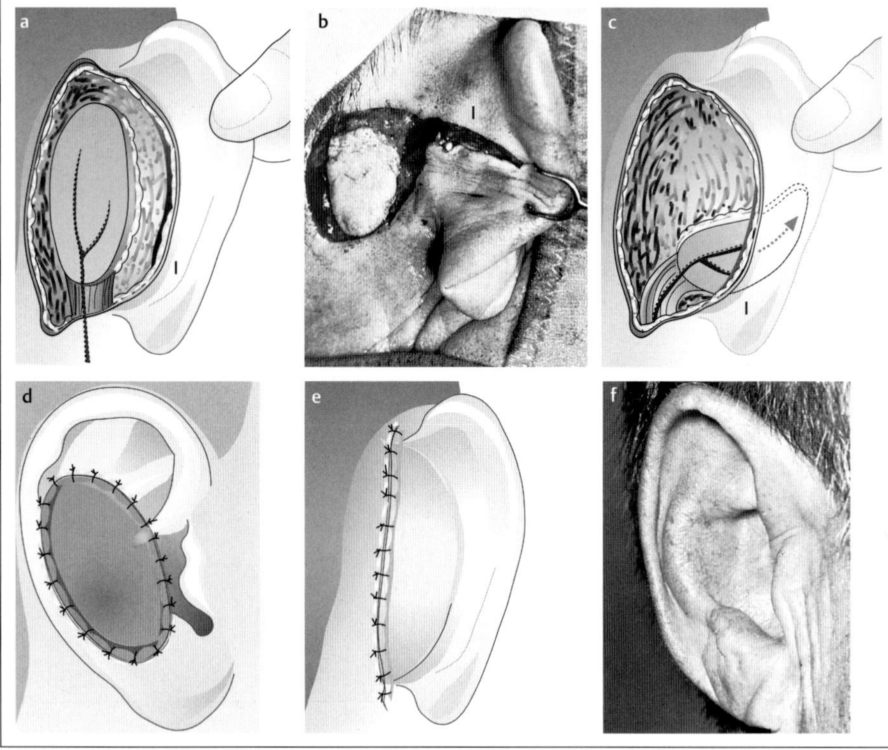

Fig. 4.8 **Two-layer central defect: coverage using a myocutaneous island flap based on the posterior auricular artery (in Krespi et al. 1983).**

a, b The flap is incised according to a template of the defect, while protecting both the vessels arising from beneath as well as the muscular pedicle.

c The postauricular skin is undermined as far as the anterior defect.
(I = tunnel)

d, e The flap is inset into the anterior defect and the posterior wound is closed (red: island flap).

f Result after healing onto the concha.

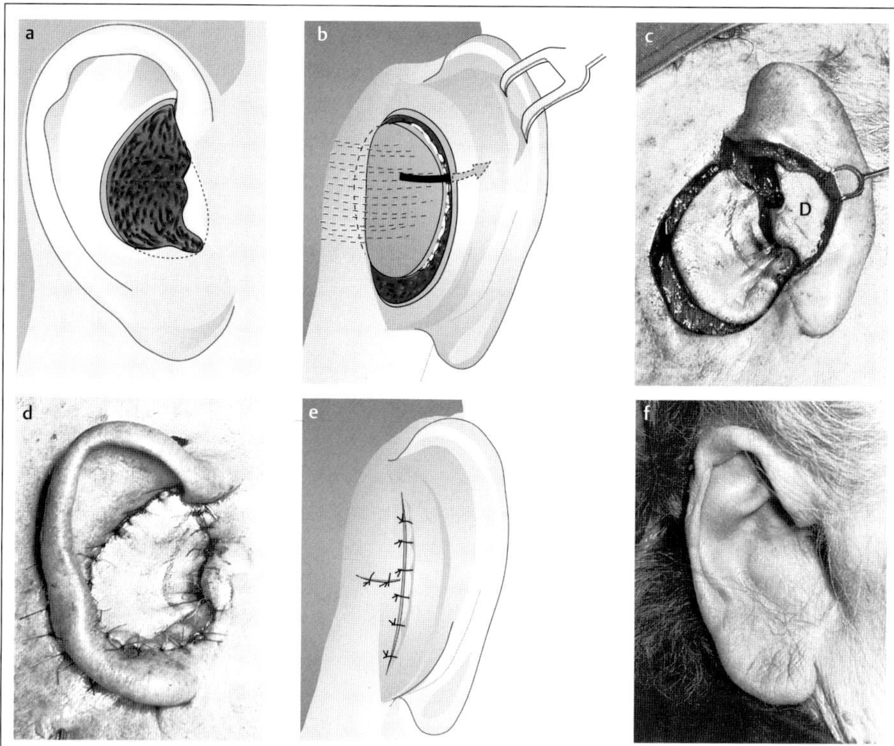

Fig. 4.**9** **Coverage of a full-thickness conchal defect using a two-layer island flap based on a dermal pedicle.**
a Defect in the concha, antihelix.
b, c Retro- and postauricular island flap, based on a dermal pedicle (D = defect in concha and antihelix).
d The island flap is brought out anteriorly onto the defect and sutured (anterior surface).
e Suture of the secondary defect (posterior surface).
f Result (considerable reduction of the sulcus, see **c** and **e**: the postauricular surface is sutured onto the defect on the mastoid surface) (see Fig. 4.**97**, p. 86).

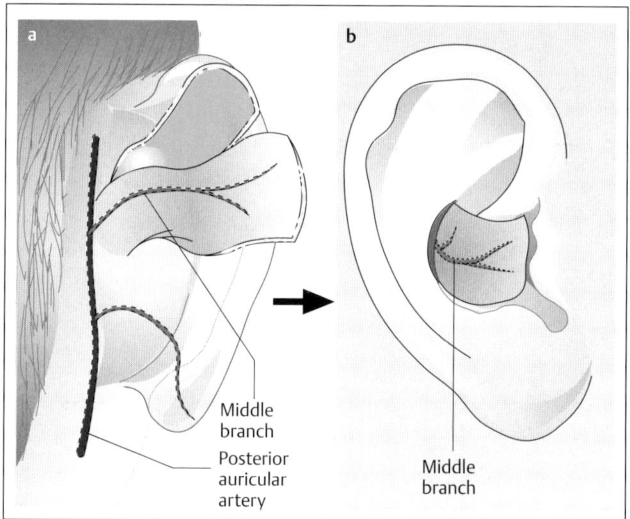

Fig. 4.**10** **a, b Reconstruction of an anterior defect using a postauricular island flap as described by Park et al. (1988).** The vessels are identified using Doppler ultrasound and the flap is elevated. The flap is brought out anteriorly and sutured onto the defect.

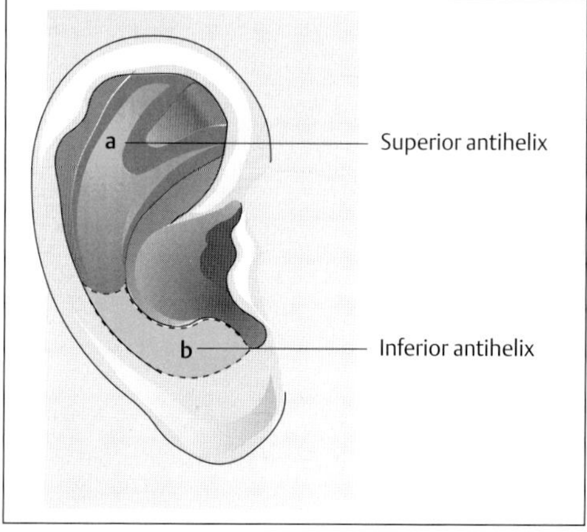

Fig. 4.**11** **Antihelical defects.**
(Transposition flap: see Figs. 4.**7** and 4.**14**; island flap: see Fig. 4.**8**; U-shaped advancement flap: see Fig. 4.**15**).
a Superior antihelix.
b Inferior antihelix.

Defects of the Antihelix and Combined Central Defects

(see also pp. 69 ff)

In particular, posterior transposition flaps and island flaps based posteriorly on a dermal pedicle or on the posterior auricular artery can be used (see Figs. 4.7–4.**9**) for the reconstruction of defects in the antihelical region (Fig. 4.**11 a, b**) or for more extensive central defects (combined central defects; Fig. 4.**12**), as previously described (see pp. 45 and 46).

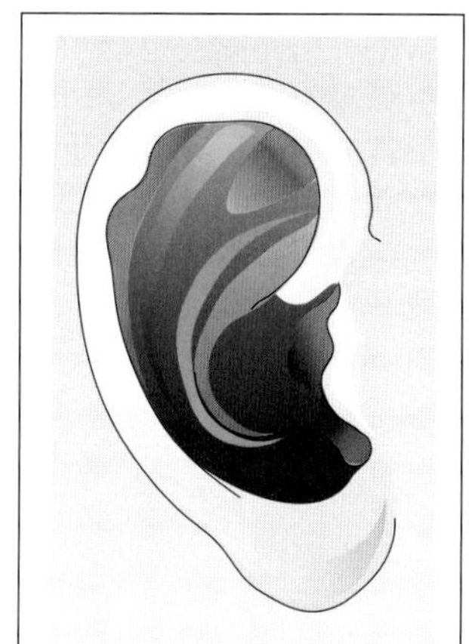

Fig. 4.**12** **Combined central defects.**
Flaps as used for conchal and antihelical defects (see Figs. 4.**9** and 4.**17**).

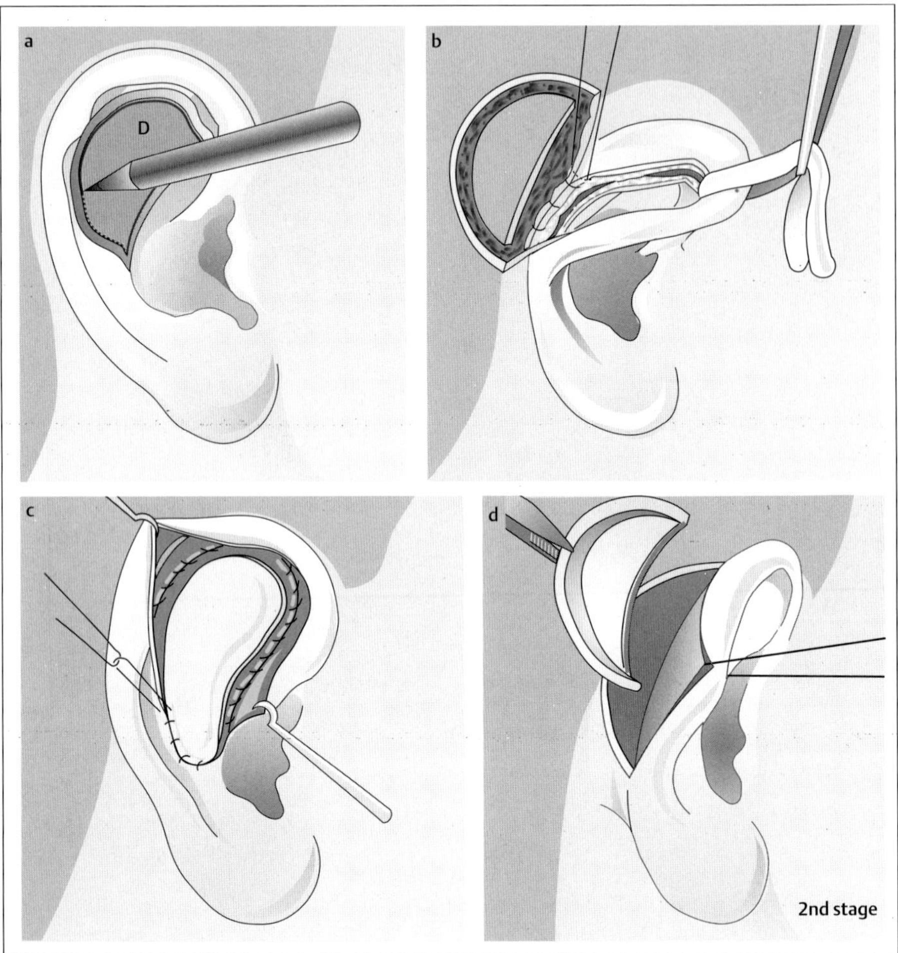

Fig. 4.**13** **Reconstruction with a large island flap (in Converse and Brent 1977).**
First stage:
The defect (D) is outlined on the mastoid skin (**a**). Incision around the flap, minimal mobilization of the margins of the flap and the mastoid skin (the flap remains pedicled to the mastoid). The mastoid skin is sutured to the skin of the posterior auricular defect (**b**). The island flap is sutured to the margins of the anterior defect (**c**).
Second stage:
Elevation after 3 weeks and insertion of a framework.
(**d**: Conchal cartilage from the ipsi- or contralateral side or from costal cartilage).
Third stage:
After a further 3–4 weeks the framework, together with its fibrous coating, is elevated and the defect is covered with a split- or full-thickness skin graft (see Fig. 4.**66 d–f,** p. 72).

Converse and Brent's Three-stage Reconstruction of Full-thickness Defects of the Antihelix
(Fig. 4.**13**; Converse and Brent 1977)
The flap can be extended onto the postauricular skin to cover large defects of the concha and antihelix (Jackson 1985 b; see Fig. 4.**9**, p. 47).

Superiorly or Inferiorly Based Transposition Flap
(Fig. 4.**14**; see also Fig. 4.**7**)

First-stage operation. A large, superiorly based, retroauricular transposition flap is raised which, depending on the size of the defect, can be extended to the neck (Fig. 4.**14 a**). The flap is de-epithelialized at the site where it is brought through, and then inset (Fig. 4.**14 b**). Behind the ear, the flap may also be used to cover the postauricular defect (Weerda 1994 b; see Fig. 4.**7**).

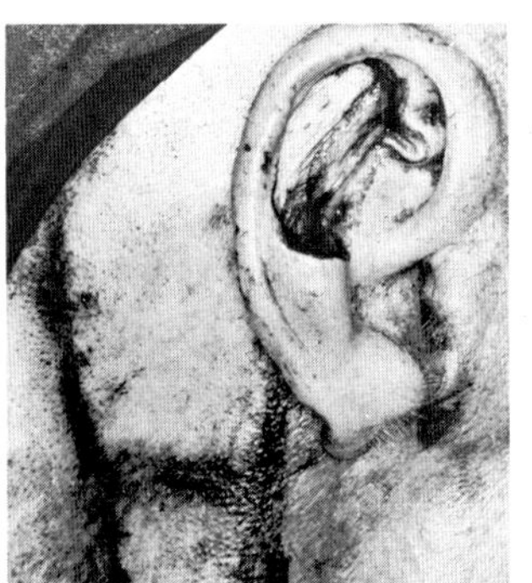
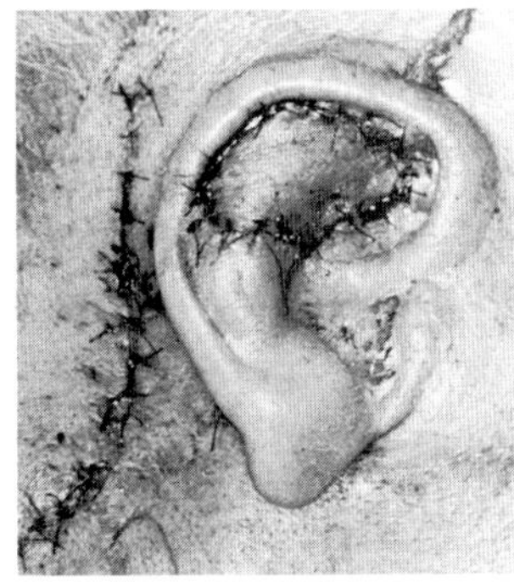

a b

Fig. 4.**14** **Single-stage coverage of a large central defect using a superiorly based transposition flap.**
a The superiorly based transposition flap is outlined and de-epithelialized at the site which will come to lie beneath the tunnel when passed anteriorly.
b The flap has been set into the defect (see Fig. 4.**7**).

Second-stage operation. The flap pedicle can be divided after 3 weeks. The remnants of the pedicle are thinned out and incorporated into the mastoid surface, and the wound is closed in two layers. Full-thickness defects which are not too large can be covered on their postauricular surface with a split- or full-thickness skin graft. Double-rotation (see also Fig. 4.**98**) or transposition-rotation flaps (see also Fig. 4.**104**) can be used for the single-stage resurfacing of particularly large central defects (see also pp. 87 to 89).

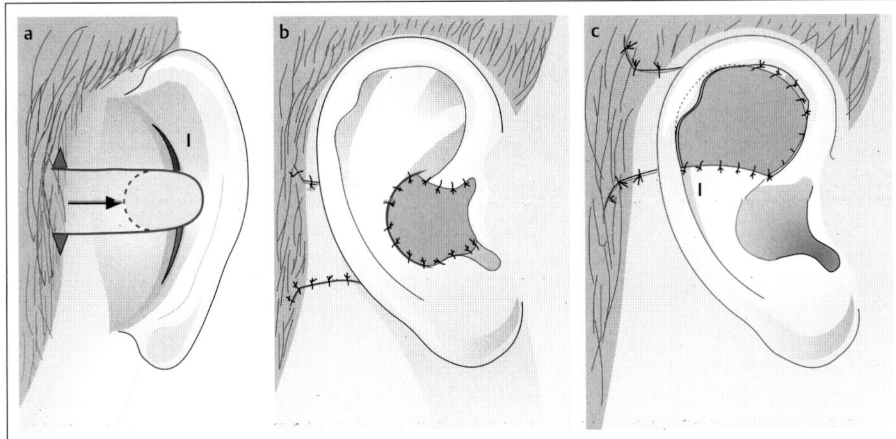

Fig. 4.**15** **U-shaped advancement flap as described by Gingrass and Pickrell (1968; see also Fig. 4.64, p. 70).**
a Defect in the concha, U-shaped advancement flap to be drawn anteriorly to close the defect and Burow's triangles (l = tunnel).
b Coverage of the conchal defect.
c Reconstruction of the fossa region.

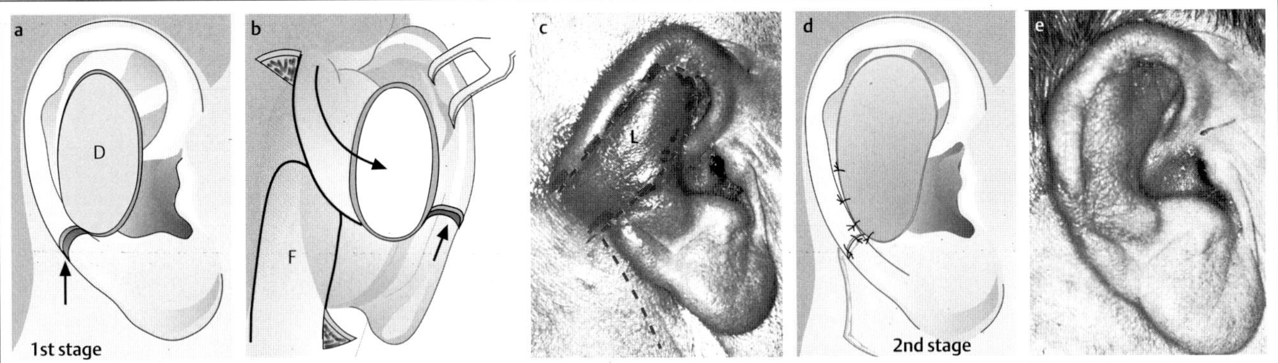

Fig. 4.**16** **Temporary repositioning of the helix for a large two-layer or full-thickness auricular defect (in Weerda 1984 b, 1999).**
a Defect and helix divided inferiorly above the earlobe (arrow).
b Inferiorly based transposition flap (F) to cover the anterior surface, rotation flap to cover the posterior surface (a thick split-thickness skin graft may also be used here).
c The flaps have been inset.
d Separation of the transposition flap and replacement of the helix after about 3 weeks.
e Appearance after healing.

Gingrass and Pickrell's U-shaped Advancement Flap
(Fig. 4.**15**; Gingrall and Pickrell 1968)
After about 3 weeks the pedicle is divided and the post-auricular wound closed. This flap is also suitable for defects in the region of the posterior auditory canal and the antitragus.

Weerda's Reconstruction with a Transposition Flap and Temporary Repositioning of the Helix
(Fig. 4.**16**; Weerda 1984 b).

Weerda's Bilobed Flap as a Transposition–Rotation Flap
(Fig. 4.**17**; Weerda 1981; see also pp. 87, 89)
As will later be described in detail, a bilobed flap (Fig. 4.**17 b**, **c**) can also be used for larger, full-thickness antihelix–conchal defects (Fig. 4.**17 a**). The flap is de-epithelialized below the helix and supported with cartilage (Fig. 4.**17 d**).

Weerda's Scaphal Reconstruction with a U-shaped Advancement Flap
(Fig. 4.**18**)

Preauricular Flaps
Many authors use preauricular flaps for smaller central defects.

Tebbetts's Superiorly Based, Preauricular Flap for the Triangular Fossa
(Fig. 4.**19**; Tebbetts 1982)

Mellette's Preauricular Flap Based Superiorly on the Helical Crus
(Fig. 4.**20**; Mellette 1991)
This technique is also suitable for the reconstruction of the helical crus. The flap is pedicled on the ascending limb of the helical crus and can be used to cover defects in the region of the concha and the entrance to the auditory canal. Sometimes improvements can be made to the helical crus in a second stage (Weerda 1999 a, 2001).

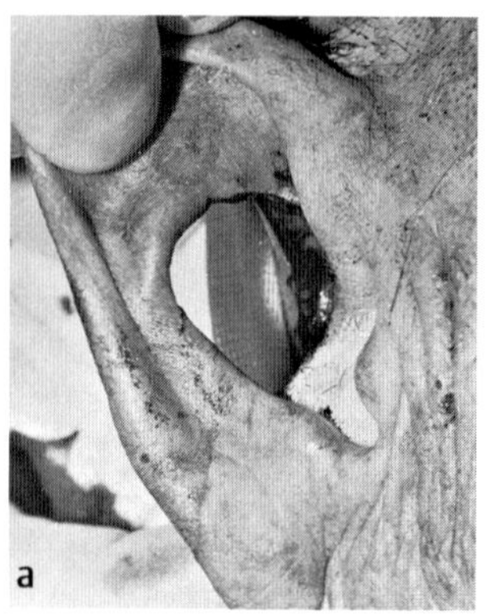

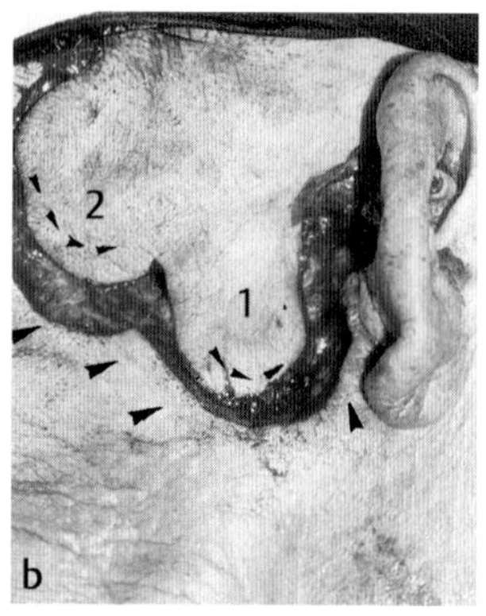

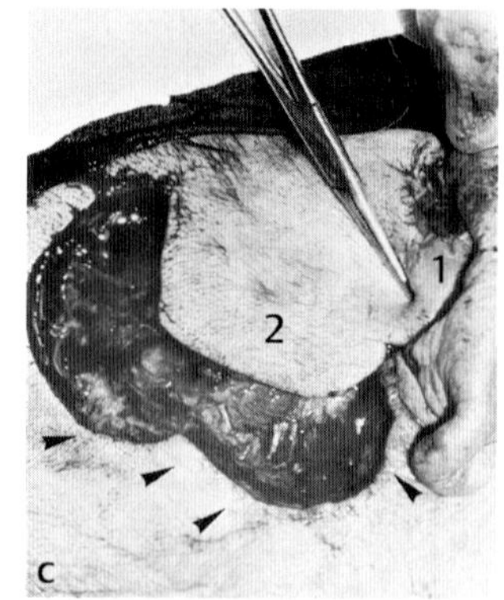

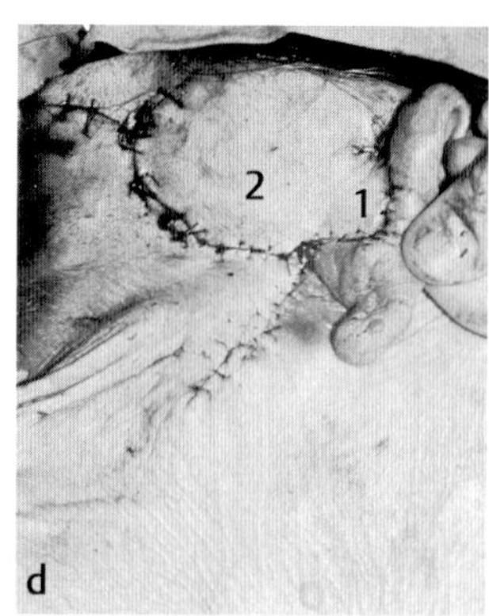

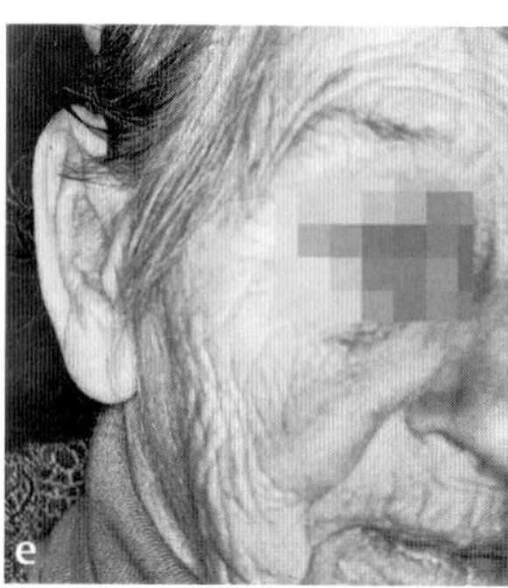

Fig. 4.**17** **Reconstruction of large, full-thickness defects with a bilobed flap (transposition–rotation flap; in Weerda and Münker 1981 and Weerda 2001).**

a Defect.

b Incision of the non-hair-bearing transposition flap (reconstruction flap 1) and hair-bearing rotation flap (transport flap 2).

c, d The flaps are inset after de-epithelialization beneath the helix, the cartilaginous strut is inserted, and the primary and secondary defects are closed.

e Result.

1: Transposition (reconstruction) flap.

2: Rotation (transport) flap.

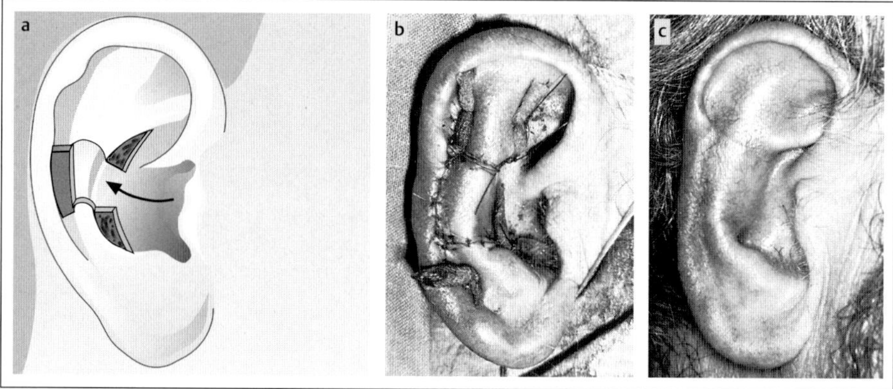

Fig. 4.**18** **Weerda's technique of scaphal reconstruction using a U-shaped advancement flap from the concha.**

a Defect in the scapha, skin incision over the antihelix, Burow's triangles in the concha, cartilage strut from the concha.

b The defect is closed by U-shaped advancement, the flap is adapted with mattress sutures (5–0 monofilament, P3 or PS 3 needle) tied over small cotton bolsters.

c Result.

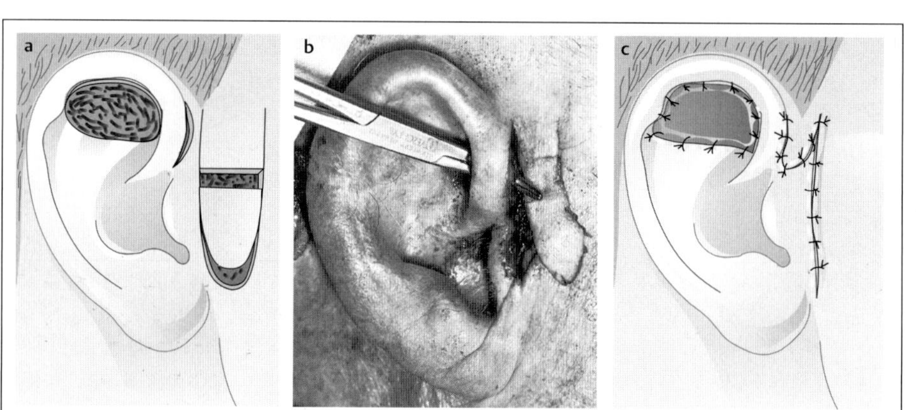

Fig. 4.**19** **Technique by Tebbets for coverage of the triangular fossa using a superiorly based preauricular flap (1982).**

a, b Elevation of the flap and de-epithelialization at the site that will come to lie beneath the tunnel.

c The flap has been inset.

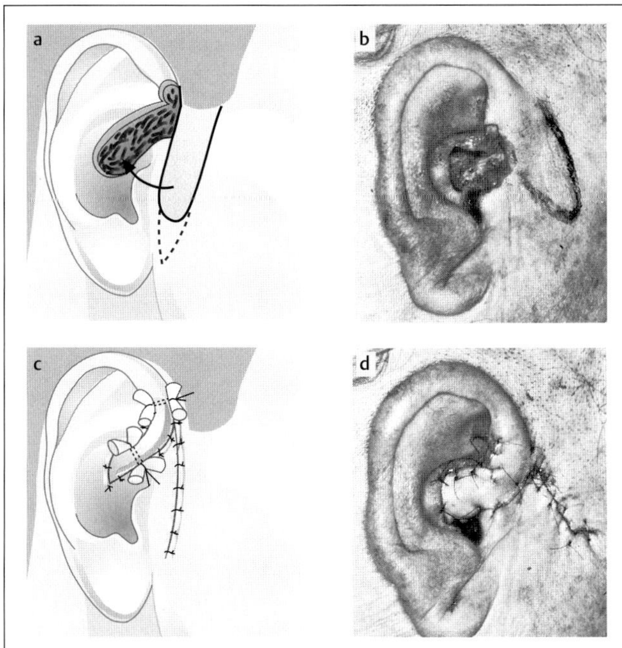

Fig. 4.**20** **Reconstruction of the helical crus (Weerda 1999 a, 2001).**
a, b Elevation of the flap adjacent to the helical stump.
c, d Closure of the defects.

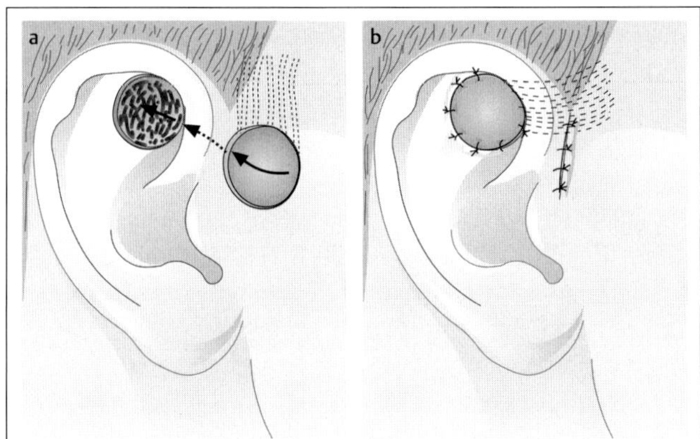

Fig. 4.**21** **Subcutaneous pedicled island flap as described by Barron and Emmet (1965).**
a Elevation of the flap and development of a tunnel.
b Inset and closure of the secondary defect.

Critique. Here too, techniques which preserve the size of the auricle should usually take preference.

The techniques of reconstruction described here for conchal defects and defects of the antihelix can also be used for larger **combined defects of the concha and antihelix** (see also pp. 72).

Barron and Emmet's Subcutaneous Pedicled Flap
(Fig. 4.**21**; Barron and Emmet 1965)

Inferiorly Based Preauricular Flap
(Fig. 4.**22**)
An inferiorly based preauricular flap can be used for covering the intertragic notch, the inferior concha, for the posterior surface of the tragus and the lateral auditory canal.

Tenta and Keyes's Excision of the Triangular Fossa with Reduction of the Auricle
(Fig. 4.**23**; Tenta and Keyes 1981)
After full-thickness excision (Fig. 4.**23 a**), the helix is used to cover the defect (Fig. 4.**23 c**; see also Fig. 4.**29**), as with Gersuny's technique (1903; Fig. 4.**23 b**; see also Figs. 4.**27**, 4.**32**, and 5.**74**, p. 155).

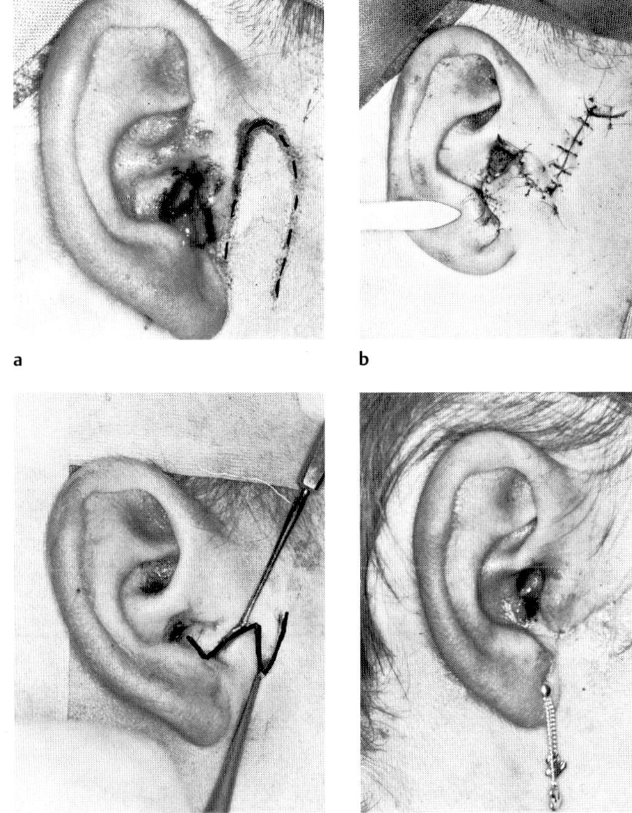

Fig. 4.**22** **Reconstruction of the intertragic notch.**
First stage:
a, b Reconstruction of the intertragic notch, lower concha, lateral auditory canal using an inferiorly based transposition flap.
Second stage:
c, d After the notch has been widened in this way, it is subsequently reduced with the use of a Z-plasty.

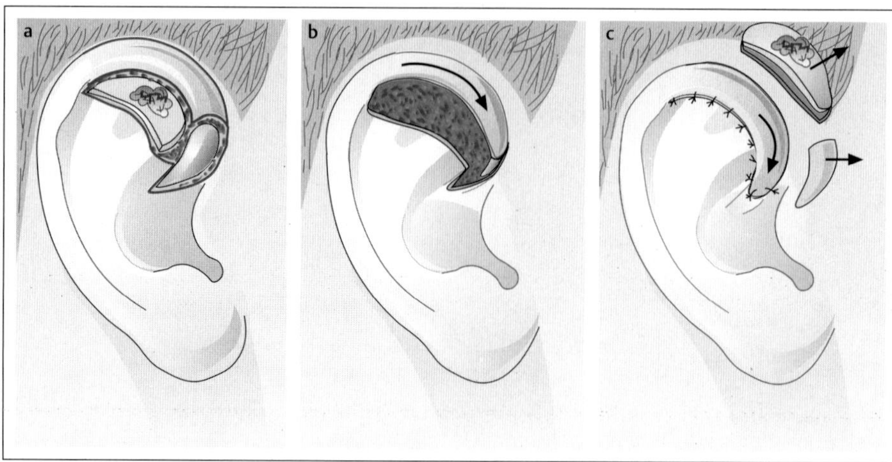

Fig. 4.**23** **Tumor excision in the triangular fossa with reduction of the auricle as described by Tenta and Keyes (1981; see Figs. 4.29, 4.33, 5.74).**

a Excision of a tumor in the triangular fossa.
b Excision of the skin behind the tumor, including part of the helical crus.
c Closure of all defects.

4.2.2 Peripheral Defects

Peripheral defects refer in particular to defects located on the helix (Fig. 4.**24**).

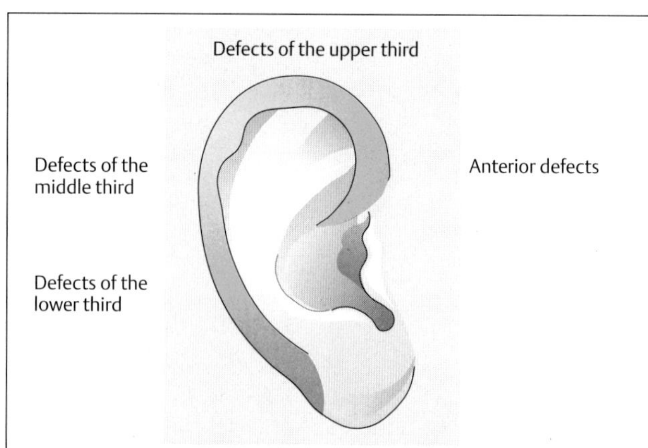

Fig. 4.**24** **Peripheral defects: helical defects.**

Helix Reconstruction with Auricular Reduction

The techniques described for the reduction of the auricle during correction of macrotia are very well suited for treating defects of the helix secondary to tumor excision or trauma (see for example Di Martino 1856, as cited in Joseph 1931; Trendelenburg 1886, as cited in Joseph 1931; Cocheril 1894, as cited in Tanzer 1977; Joseph 1896, 1931; see also operations for the correction of macrotia, p. 153). If the age and general condition of the patient allow it, some of these operations can be performed under local anesthesia on an outpatient basis.

Recommended Defect Reconstruction

Wedge excisions and reconstruction with advancement of the helix can be recommended.

Simple Wedge Excisions

(Fig. 4.**25**)

For small helical lesions or small defects, a simple extension of the wound in the form of a wedge excision is enough to achieve an adequately pleasing aesthetic result.

Wedge Excision and Burow's Triangles

(Fig. 4.**26**)

Because irregularities in form and contour can result from simple wedge excision, Trendelenburg (1886; as cited in Joseph 1931) recommended the removal of Burow's triangles. This procedure has since been modified in many ways (see for example Trendelenburg 1886; Joseph 1896; Goldstein 1908; Lexer 1933; see also Fig. 5.**69**). Whenever possible, we place the Burow's triangles in the scapha (Fig. 4.**26 e**) or along the border between the concha and its transition to the antihelix (Fig. 4.**26 a**; Converse and Brent 1977).

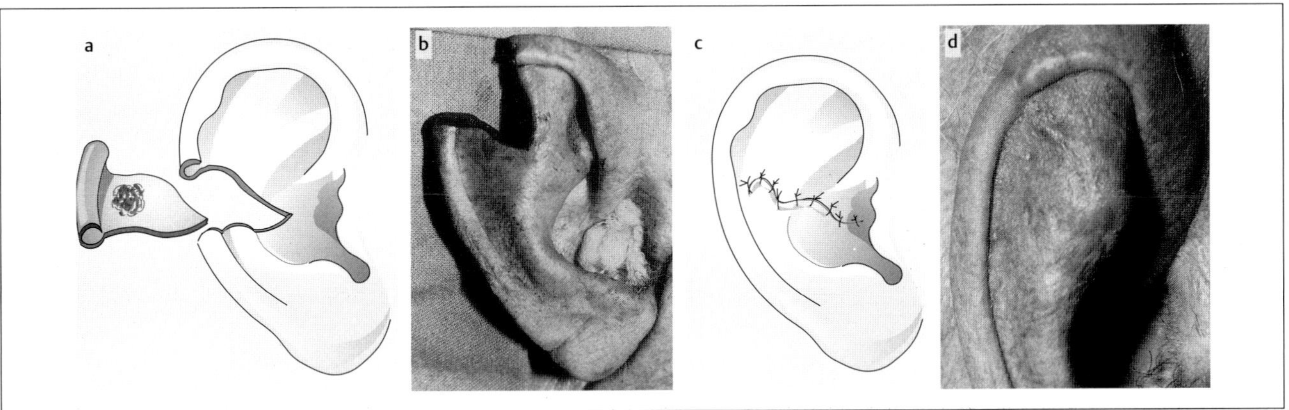

Fig. 4.25 **Wedge-shaped excision without Burow's triangles (for defect sizes up to about 1 cm).**

a, b Wedge-shaped excision.
c Closure.
d Result.

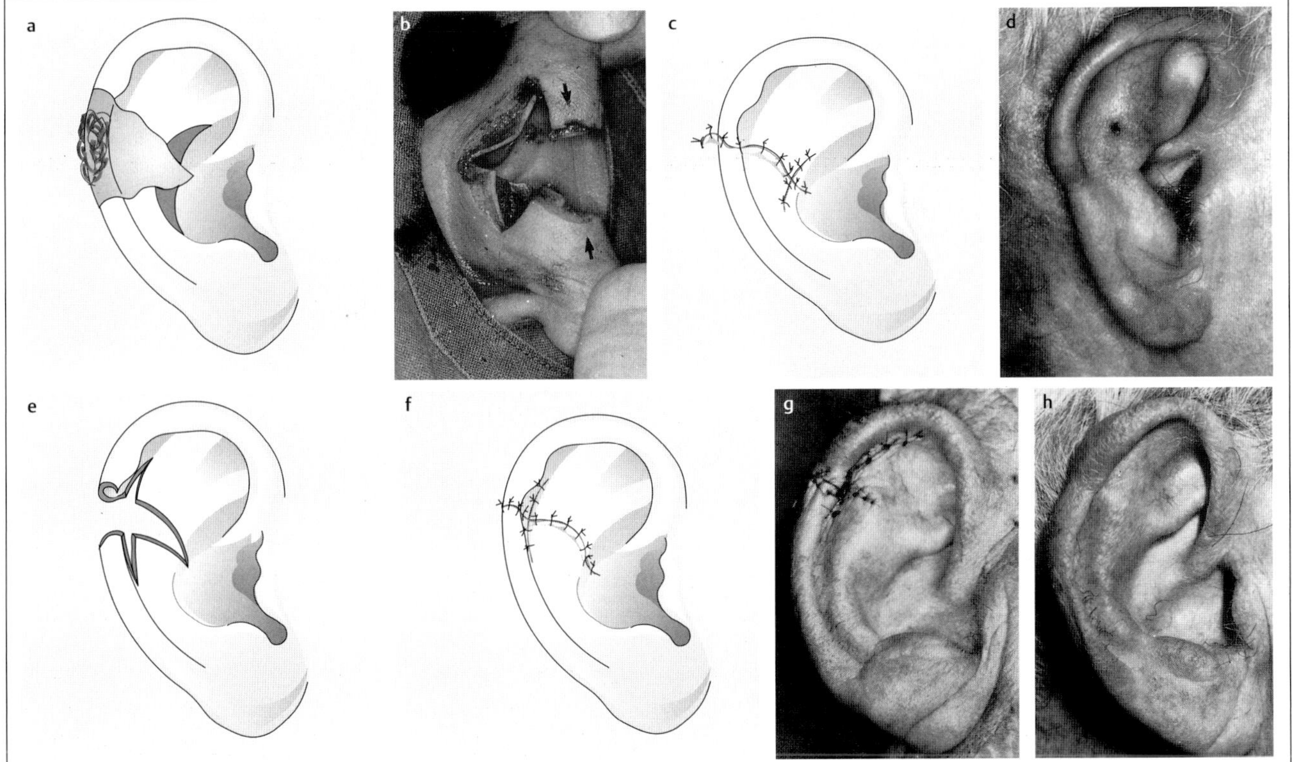

Fig. 4.26 **Wedge-shaped tumor excisions with Burow's triangles (for defect sizes up to about 2 cm).**

a–d Excision with Burow's triangles in the concha (Joseph 1896).
e–g Burow's triangles in the scapha.
h Result.

Gersuny's Technique of Defect Closure by Transposition of the Helix

(Fig. 4.**27**; Gersuny 1903)

Gersuny performed a full-thickness crescent-shaped excision in the scapha of a female patient who had sustained a helical lesion, and transposed the helix into the resultant defect (Fig. 4.**27 a, b**). This elegant method has been modified in a number of different ways.

Modification of the Gersuny Technique by Weerda and Zöllner

(Fig. 4.**28**; Weerda and Zöllner 1986)

Similar to Antia and Buch (1967, 1974) and in contrast to Gersuny (1903; see Fig. 4.**27**), we made only a two-layer, crescent-shaped excision in the scapha after excision of the tumor and dissected the skin on the posterior auricular surface (Fig. 4.**28 b, d, e**).

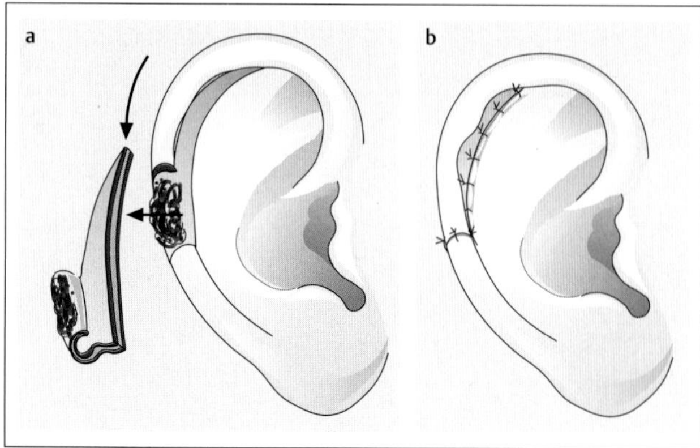

Fig. 4.**27** **Gersuny's technique for full-thickness tumor excision (Gersuny 1903).**
a Tumor excision and full-thickness, crescent-shaped upper scaphal excision.
b Closure of the defect by rotating the helix downwards.

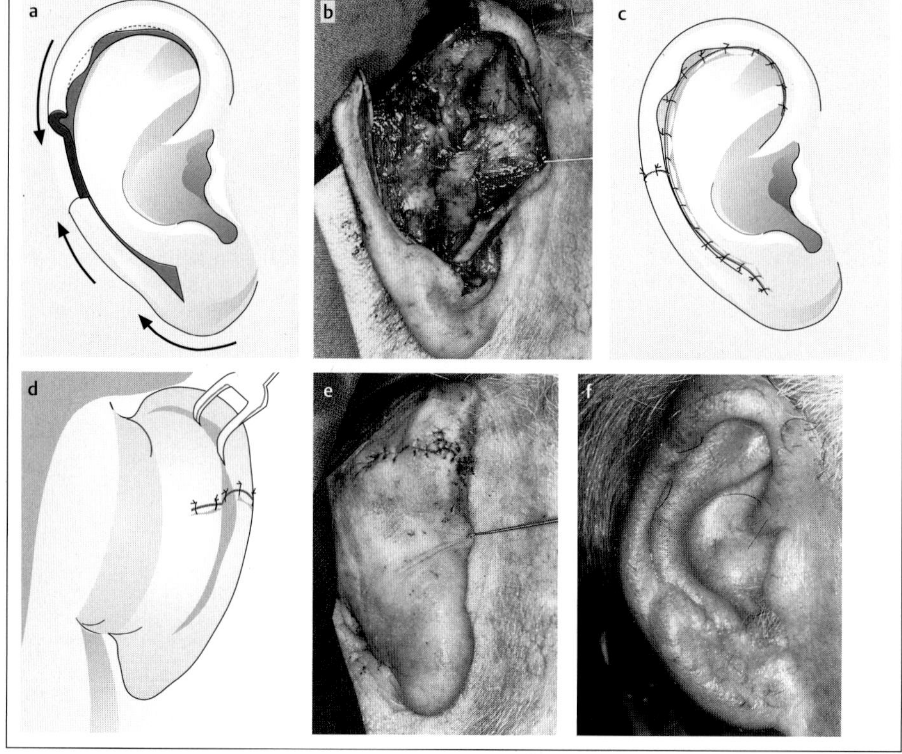

Fig. 4.**28** **Excision of small defects in the helical region and closure using Gersuny's technique (Gersuny 1903), modified after Antia and Buch (1967, 1974) and Weerda and Zöllner (1986).**
a Tumor excision and two-layer, crescent-shaped excision in the scapha with a Burow's triangle in the earlobe.
b, c Mobilization of the entire helix on the postauricular skin and closure of the wounds.
d, e Excision of a dog-ear on the postauricular surface and suture.
f Result.

Antia and Buch's Modification with Mobilization of the Helical Crus

(Fig. 4.**29**; Antia and Buch 1967, Antia 1974)

In a modification for larger defects, the helical crus was additionally incised (it remains pedicled posteriorly and superiorly).

Lexer's Modification

(Fig. 4.**30**; Lexer 1933)

Full-thickness crescent-shaped excision from the scaphal and antihelical margin after excision of the tumor. The postauricular skin is excised slightly higher and then elevated. The defects are slid into each other and the auricle is reduced by closing cartilage and skin (Fig. 4.**30 b**; Ginestet et al. 1967).

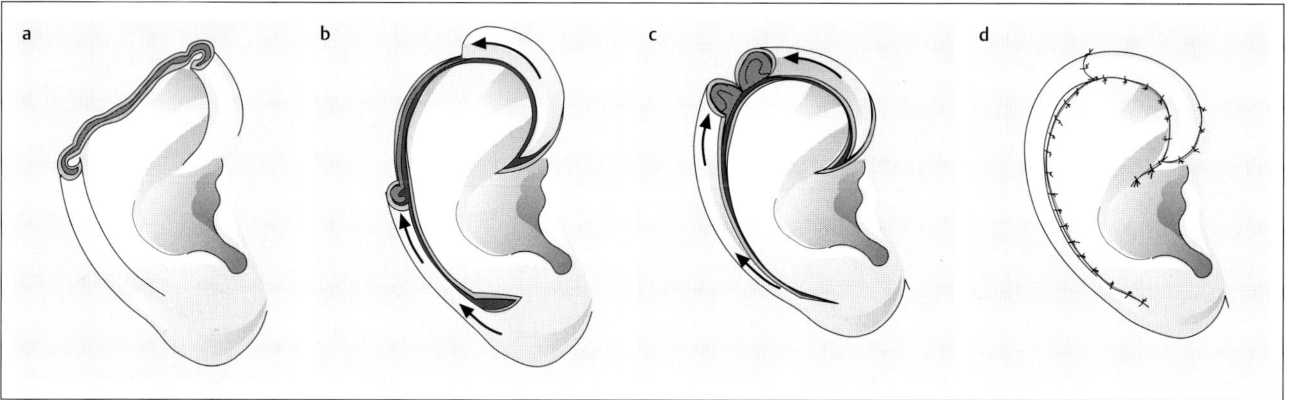

Fig. 4.29 **Helix reconstruction of a small defect; in Antia and Buch (1967).**
a Debridement of the wound margins.
b Incisions around the helical crus and dissection of the postauricular skin pedicled on the entire helix extending from the scapha, incision within the scapha down to the earlobe where a small Burow's triangle is excised.
c, d Closure of all defects with transposition of the helical crus with reduction of the auricle (see Fig. 4.**28**).

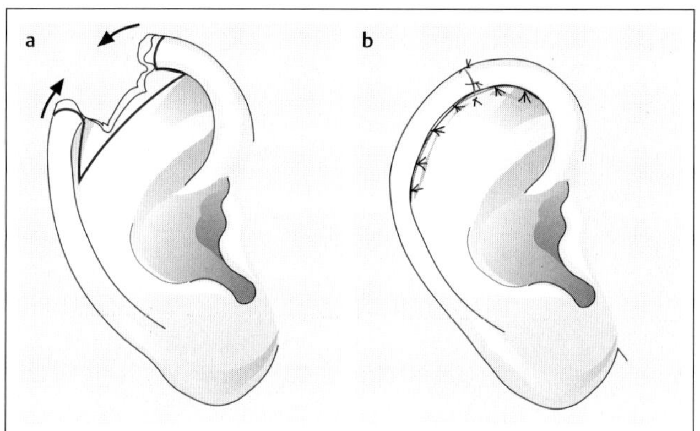

Fig. 4.**30** **a, b Lexer's method for reconstruction of a helical defect with scaphal excisions (Lexer 1933; Ginestet et al. 1967).**

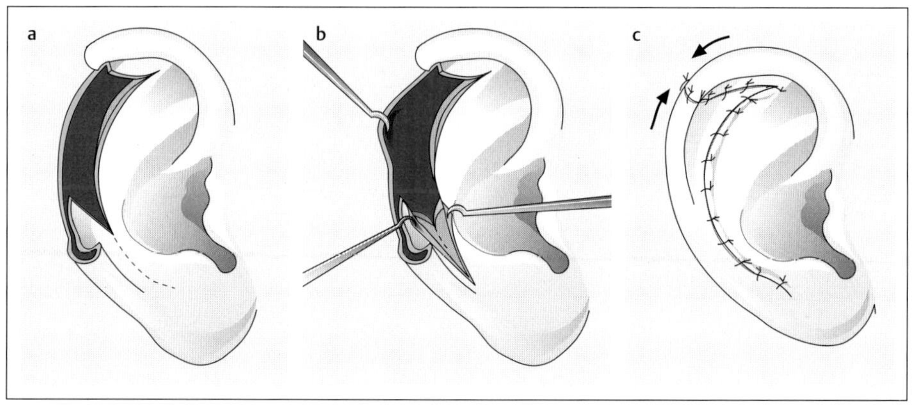

Fig. 4.**31** **Ear reduction (defect reconstruction) using the technique of Argamaso and Lewin (1968).**
a Tumor excision, crescent-shaped, two-layer excision from the scapha (antihelix).
b Elevation of the postauricular skin and excision of the cartilage towards the earlobe.
c Closure of all defects, excision of a dog-ear from the earlobe and the postauricular skin.

Argamaso and Lewin's Technique of Ear Reduction and Defect Reconstruction

(Fig. 4.**31**; Argamaso and Lewin 1968)
For smaller defects, a Z-plasty is performed by transposing the inferior portion into the superior segment (Fig. 4.**31 c**) in the form of a chondrocutaneous flap (Fig. 4.**31 a, b**).

Meyer and Sieber's Modification of the Technique

(Fig. 4.**32**; Meyer and Sieber 1973)
The concha or the preauricular defect can be treated together with tumors of the ascending helix (Fig. 4.**32 a–d**; Argamaso 1989).

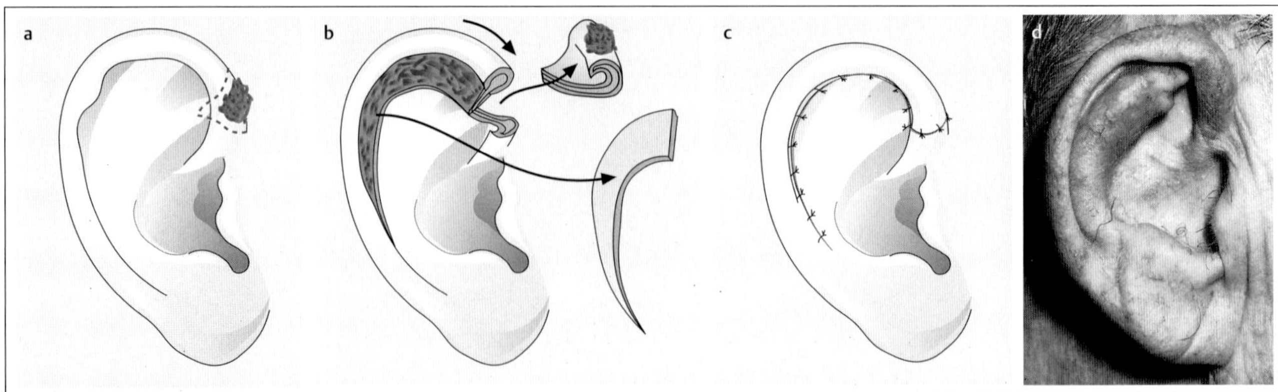

Fig. 4.**32** **Wedge excision of an anterior tumor of the helix and closure with auricular reduction as described by Meyer and Sieber (1973).**

a Tumor excision.
b Crescent-shaped, two-layer excision from the scapha.
c Closure.
d Result (see Fig. 4.**27**, 4.**28**).

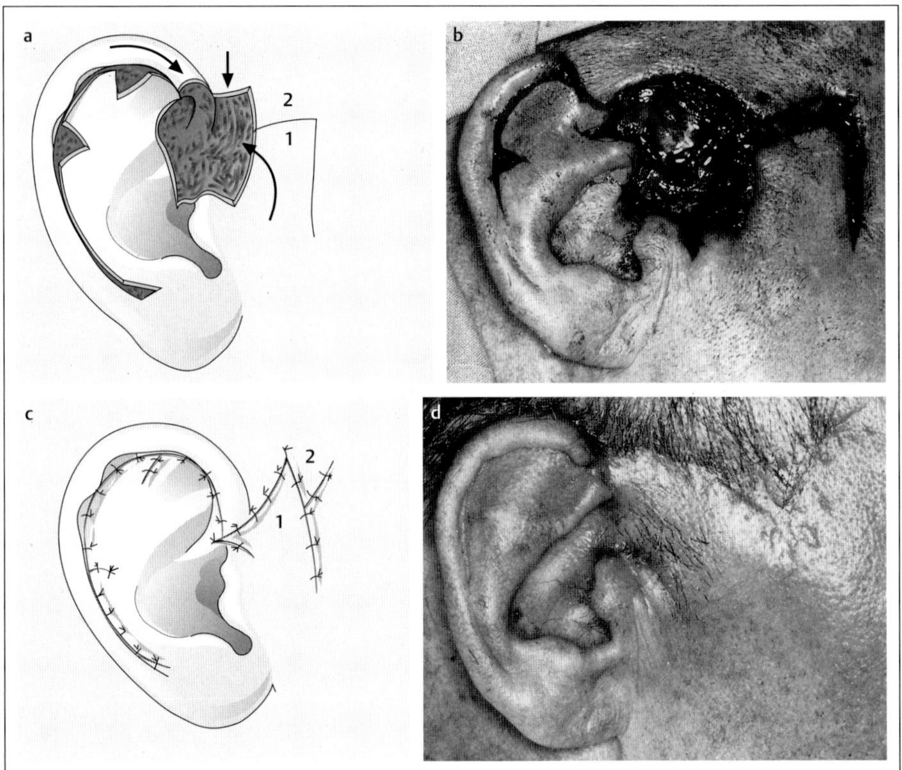

Fig. 4.**33** **Defect of the preauricular region and in the region of the helical crus and anterior helix.**

a, b Elevation of a preauricular Dufourmentel flap (see Fig. 4.**48**, p. 63) and anterior transposition of the helix as a Gersuny plasty (see Fig. 4.**27**).
c Closure of all defects.
d Result (see also Fig. 4.**32**).

Weerda and Zöllner's Technique for Defects of the Helical Crus and Preauricular Region

(Fig. 4.**33**; Weerda and Zöllner 1986; Weerda 1988 d; see also Fig. 4.**49**)

The entire helix can be rotated anteriorly to treat tumors in the region of the anterior ascending helix, the helical crus, and the preauricular region, with the preauricular defect subsequently being covered by a Dufourmentel rhomboid flap (see also p. 63).

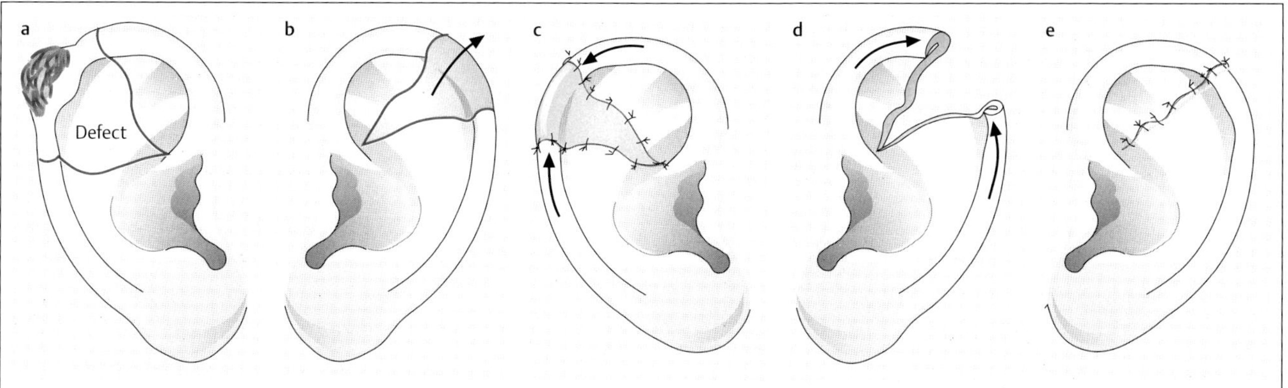

Fig. 4.**34** **Wedge-shaped composite graft from the contralateral ear as described by Pegram and Peterson (1956); red: graft.**
a Tumor excision (defect).
b Full-thickness cartilage wedge (half the size of the tumor wedge) from the contralateral ear.
c Transplantation of the composite graft and suture (5–0 braided cartilage suture and 6–0 monofilament skin suture).
d Donor defect in the contralateral ear.
e Closure (ears are of equal size).

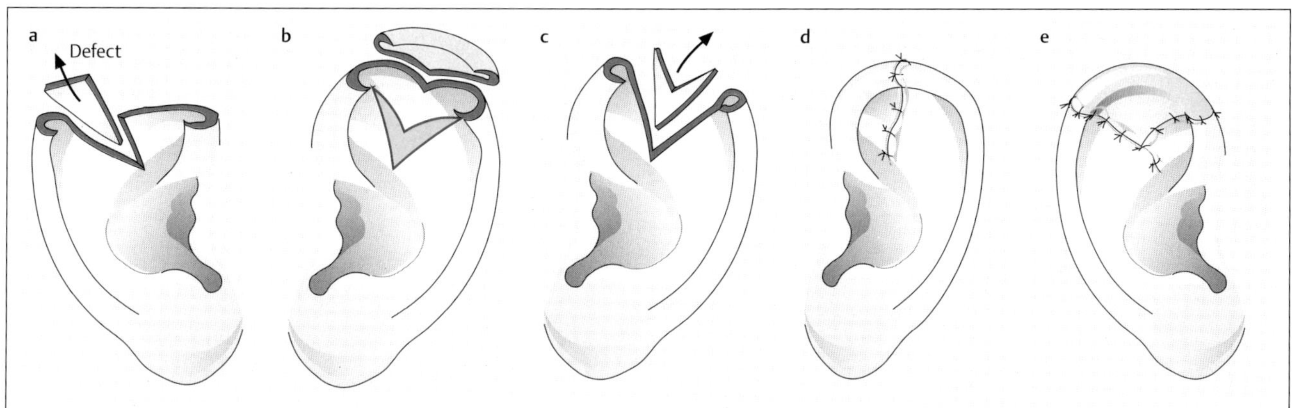

Fig. 4.**35** **Nagel's modification (Nagel 1972); red: graft.**
a Defect, excision of a Burow's triangle for reduction of the defect.
b A composite graft half the size of the defect is harvested from the contralateral ear.
c, d Removal of a Burow's triangle and closure of the contralateral side.
e Closure of the defect with the composite graft of the contralateral side (ears are of equal size).

Nonrecommended Methods of Defect Reconstruction

Pegram and Peterson's Reconstruction with a Free Full-Thickness Composite Graft from the Contralateral Ear

(Fig. 4.**34**; Pegram and Peterson 1956; see also section "Middle third of the auricle," p. 69, and Fig. 4.**63**, p. 70).
Even Körte (1905) and Lexer (1910) had previously used composite grafts for reconstruction of the ear. Similar techniques to reconstruct partial defects are described by Day (1921), Melchior-Breslau (1928 as cited in Joseph 1931), Wachsberger (1947), Pegram and Peterson (1956), Nagel (1972), Brent (1975), and Converse and Brent (1977). The margins of the defect are freshened or the tumor excised (Fig. 4.**34 a**), a wedge-shaped, full-thickness composite graft of half the defect size is removed from the contralateral ear (Fig. 4.**34 b**), inset into the defect, the cartilage is adapted with a 5–0 braided suture and the skin closed with a 6–0 or 7–0 monofilament suture (Fig. 4.**34 c**). The wedge defect of the contralateral side is closed in a similar fashion (Fig. 4.**34 d, e**).

Nagel's Modification

(Fig. 4.**35**; Nagel 1972)
By this technique of taking a wedge from the contralateral side of only half the size of the defect, both ears again become of equal size and the donor side is reduced by only half of the defect size (Fig. 4.**35 a–d**).

Critique. These techniques may be suitable, if at all, for smaller defects (see Fig. 3.**16**, p. 36) because adequate nutrition of larger, freely transplanted composite grafts cannot be guaranteed. We see a high rate of graft loss, especially when

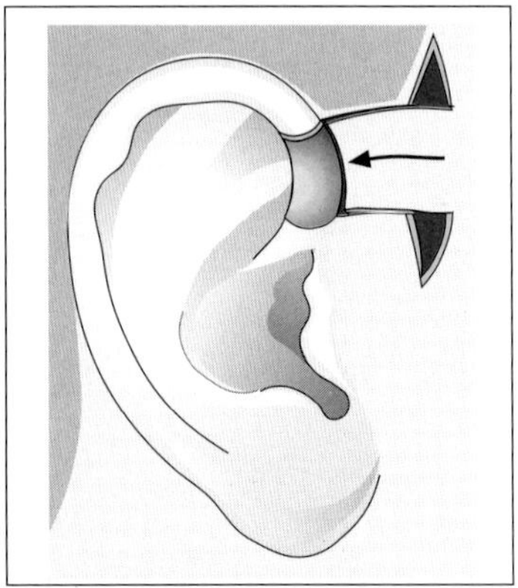

Fig. 4.**36** **U-formed advancement flap to cover a defect of the ascending helix.**

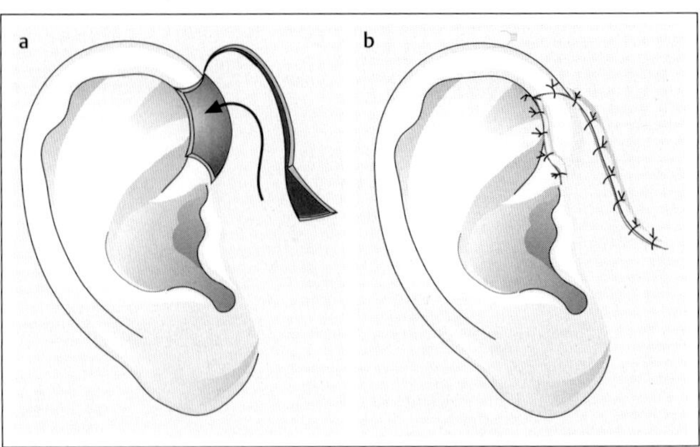

Fig. 4.**37 a, b** **Coverage of the ascending helix with an inferiorly based rotation flap (helical crus, see Fig. 4.60).**

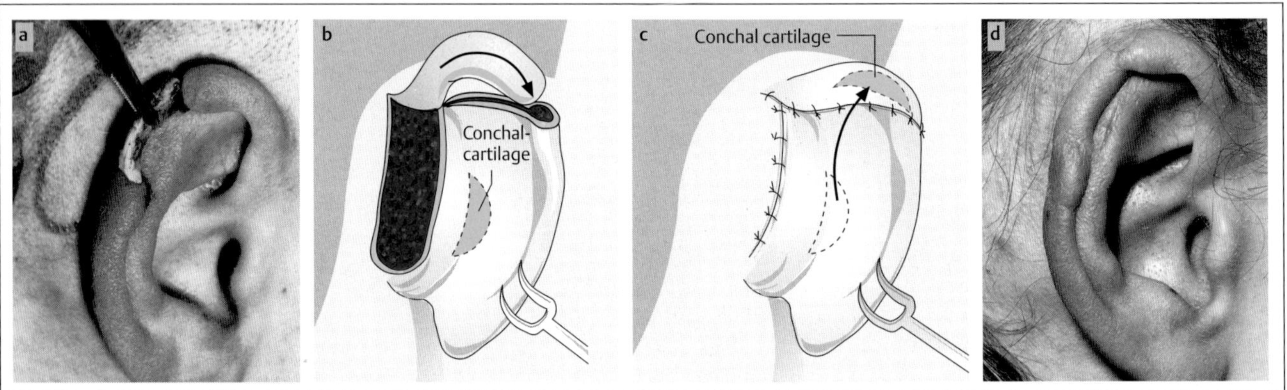

Fig. 4.**38** **Reconstruction of the superior helix with a posterosuperiorly based transposition flap.**
First stage:
a The superiorly based transposition flap is marked, the helix supported by a conchal cartilage strut.
b, c The flap is brought into position.
Second stage:
After at least 3 weeks the base of the flap is inset in a fish-mouth manner (see Figs. 4.**44** and 4.**45**).
d Result.

this technique is performed by less experienced surgeons. For example, a child was referred to our clinic on whom this technique had been attempted for correction of grade II microtia and where subsequently the full-thickness composite graft did not survive. In addition, the healthy ear was also deformed (see p. 192, Fig. 5.**140**).

Helix Reconstruction without Auricular Reduction

Since the defects (see Fig. 4.**24**; p. 52) frequently involve more than one region, reference will be made in the text and in the figure legends to similar reconstructions in other chapters.

Anterior Defects: Helical Crus And Ascending Helix (Figs. 4.36, 4.37)

The ascending helix as well as the helical crus can be reconstructed with a small U-shaped advancement flap (Fig. 4.**36**), a rotation flap (Fig. 4.**37 a**, **b**), or a preauricular, superiorly or inferiorly based transposition flap (see Fig. 4.**20**; p. 51).

Superior and Middle Thirds of the Helix

Superiorly Based Postauricular Transposition Flap
(Fig. 4.**38 a–d**; Weerda 1999 a, 2001)
A superiorly based posterior flap is raised in the sulcus patterned from a template made from aluminum foil (Pennisi et al. 1965; Tebbetts 1982; Mellette 1991; Weerda 1999 a, 2001).

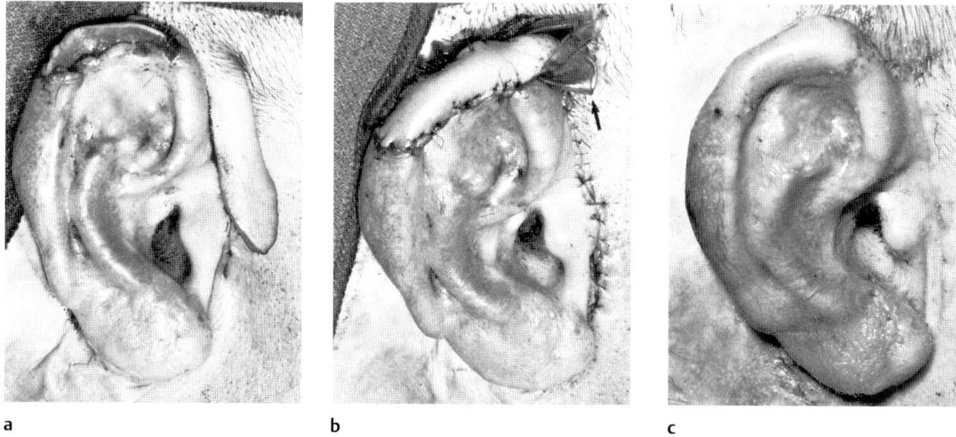

Fig. 4.39 **Reconstruction of the superior helix with a preauricular flap secondary to necrosis of this region after total auricular reconstruction following an avulsion injury.**

a Total reconstruction, necrosis of the superior helix: the superior helix has been reconstructed with cartilage from the contralateral concha and the preauricular tubed flap has been incised (it must be of adequate length; see Figs. 4.**43**–4.**45**).

b The flap is brought into position and attached in a fish-mouth fashion; the non-epithelialized end of the flap is protected with a small silicone plate (arrow).

c Result after the flap pedicle is inset, about 3 weeks later.

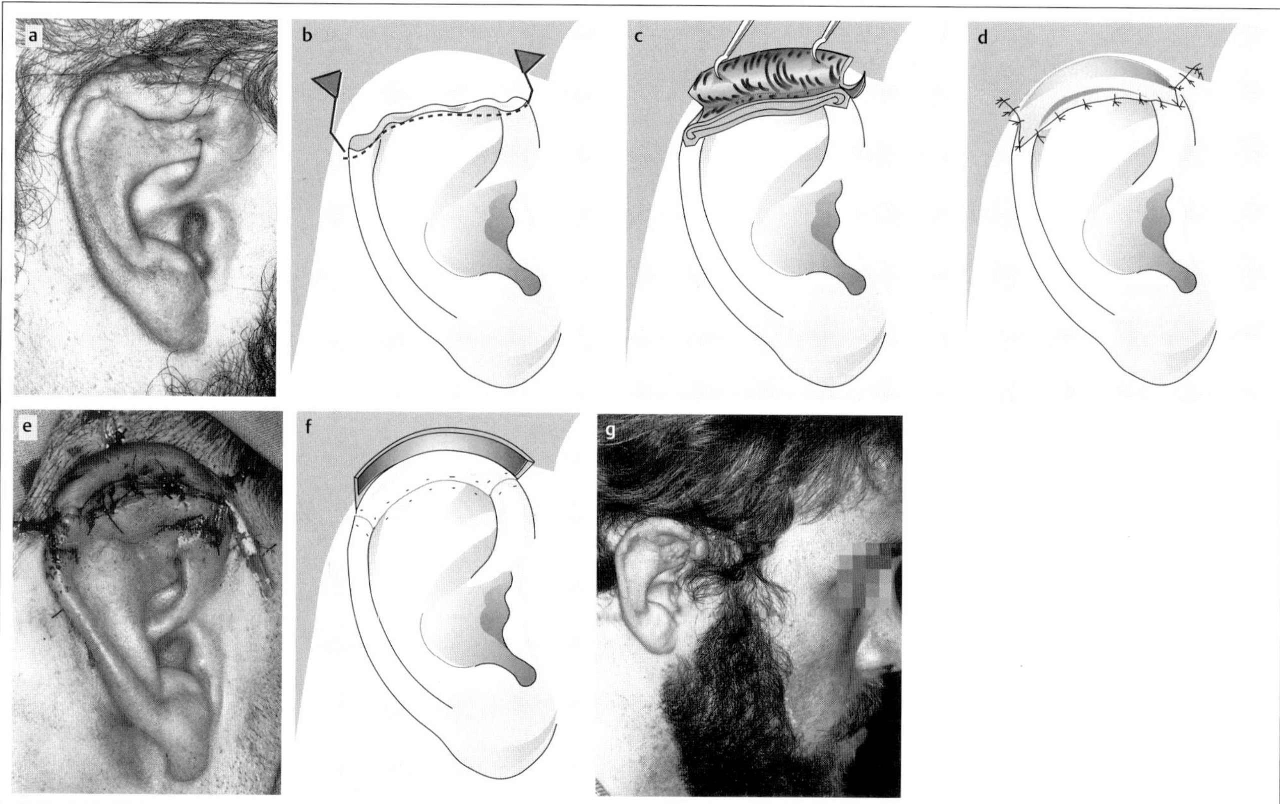

Fig. 4.**40** **Coverage of the superior, middle, and inferior helix with a broad-based superiorly pedicled retroauricular flap as described by Smith (1917).**

a Resorption of the cartilage after insertion of the denuded cartilage placed into a cutaneous pocket (see Fig. 4.**52**) secondary to an avulsion injury.

First stage:

b The flap is outlined.

c Incision and dissection.

d, e Inset with cartilage strut (pink) in a fishmouth manner onto the helix (see Fig. 4.**44 d**).

Second stage:

f After about 3 weeks, separation from the mastoid skin and posterior inset, coverage of the mastoid defect with thick split skin (Nagata 1994 a–d; see Fig. 5.**172 a–d**, pp. 215, 216).

g Result after second stage.

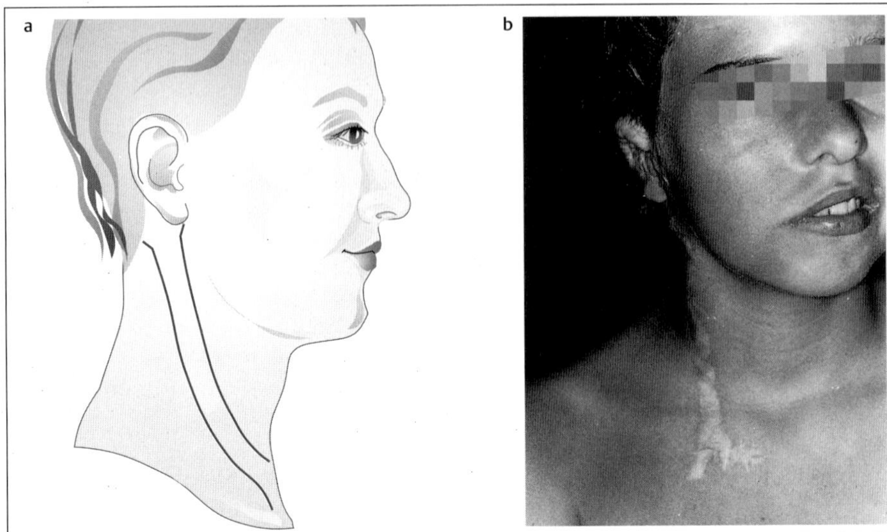

Fig. 4.**41** **Tube-pedicled flap from the neck as described by McNichol (1950): a technique no longer used.**

a Reconstruction of the helix with a tube-pedicled flap from the neck.

b Unsightly scar on the neck after a reconstruction by the author in the early 1970s (see also Fig. 5.**151**, p. 199).

Preauricular Transposition Flap

(Fig. 4.**39**)

As with the posterior flap, a patterned preauricular flap is used to reconstruct the superior helix (Fig. 4.**39 a–c**).

Smith's Retroauricular Flap

(Fig. 4.**40**; Smith 1917)

The upper (middle) third of the auricular helix is reconstructed with a broad-based, superiorly pedicled retroauricular flap (see Fig. 4.**64**, p. 70 and Fig. 4.**66**, p. 72).

Tube-pedicled Flap

(Fig. 4.**41**)

Pre-, post-, and retroauricular tube-pedicled flaps can be employed for all regions of the helix. Tube-pedicled flaps of the neck (Fig. 4.**41 a**; Pierce 1925; Hamblen-Thomas 1938; McNichol 1950; Converse 1958; Cosman and Crikelair 1966; Pitanguy and Flemming 1976; Davis 1987), can usually no longer be recommended, given that they produce conspicuous hypertrophic scars in the neck region (Fig. 4.**41 b**). "Migrating" flaps of the supraclavicular region are better (see pp. 198, 199, Figs. 5.**149**, 5.**151**).

Defects of the upper, middle, or lower third of the helix can be reconstructed with a tunneled (bipedicled) or tube-pedicled flap which is raised in the sulcus and initially based superiorly and inferiorly (see Fig. 4.**43**; Streit 1914; Troha et al. 1990; Dujon and Bowditch 1995).

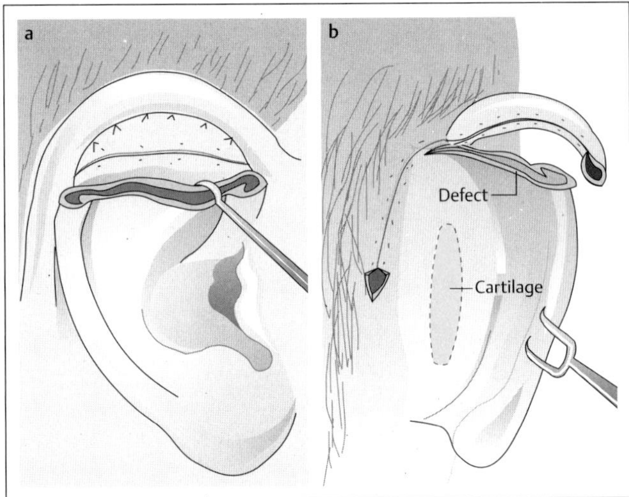

Fig. 4.**42** **Reconstruction of the superior helix with a tube-bipedicled, tunneled flap.**

First stage:

a Incision of the tunneled flap, pedicled both anteriorly and posteriorly to the ear along the hairline, closure of the wound beneath the flap (see Fig. 4.**44 c**).

Second stage:

b Incision around the posterior flap base after 3 weeks and inset into the defect (alternatively: inset during the first stage and separation of the flap in the second stage; see Figs. 4.**43**, 4.**44**).

Third stage:

After a further 3 weeks, the second end of the flap is inset. If necessary, cartilage is also inserted as a strut (see Fig. 4.**39**).

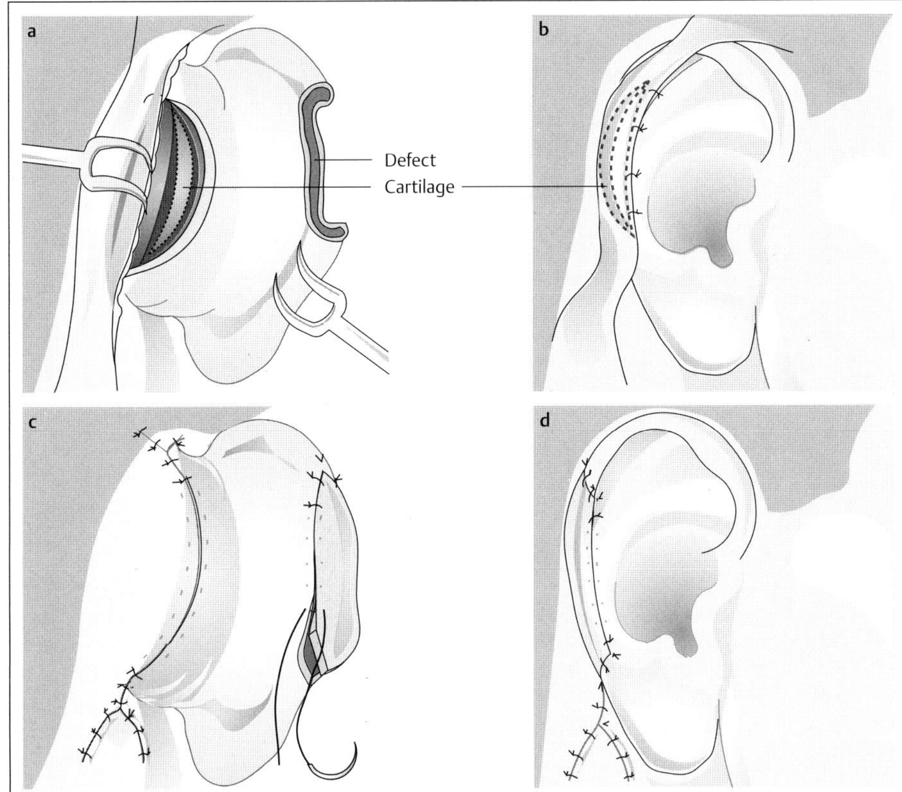

Fig. 4.**43** **Reconstruction of a longer helical defect with a tube-bipedicled, tunneled flap in two stages (see text; Weerda 1999 a, 2001).**

First stage:

a Cartilage harvested from the concha, access via the donor defect of the tunneled flap in the sulcus.

b After suturing in the cartilage strut, the wound margins are freshened before the tunneled flap is inset onto the defect.

Second stage:

c Three weeks after reconstruction, the flaps are separated and inset onto the helical defect at an acute angle. The remains of the tunneled flap are incorporated into the mastoid surface (see Figs. 4.**44**, 4.**45**).

d Result at the end of the second stage.

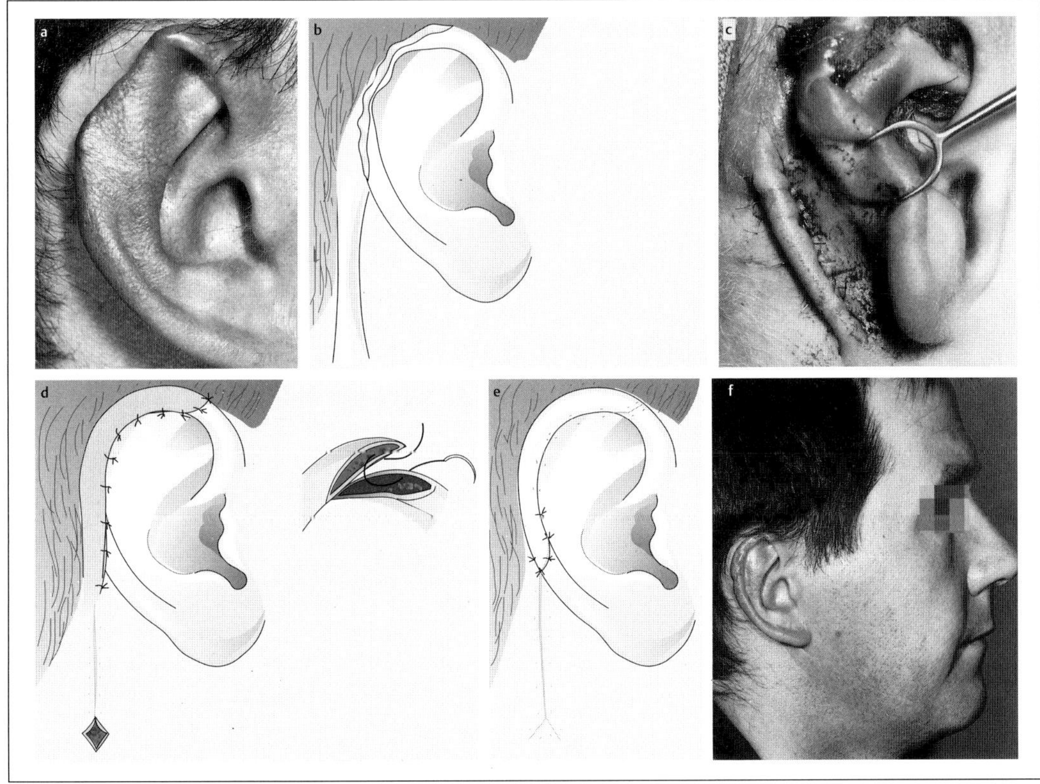

Fig. 4.**44** **Reconstruction of the helix with a tube-bipedicled flap in three stages as described by Steffanoff (1948).**

a Defect.

First stage:

b, c The flap is incised and rolled up; if insufficient skin is available, the flap is enclosed in a silicone foil (0.2 mm thick).

Second stage:

d After 3 weeks, separation of the flap base inferiorly and incorporation into the defect in a fish-mouth manner. If necessary, a cartilage strut may be incorporated.

Third stage:

e After about 3 further weeks, incorporation of the remaining flap.

f Result (operating surgeon: R. Siegert).

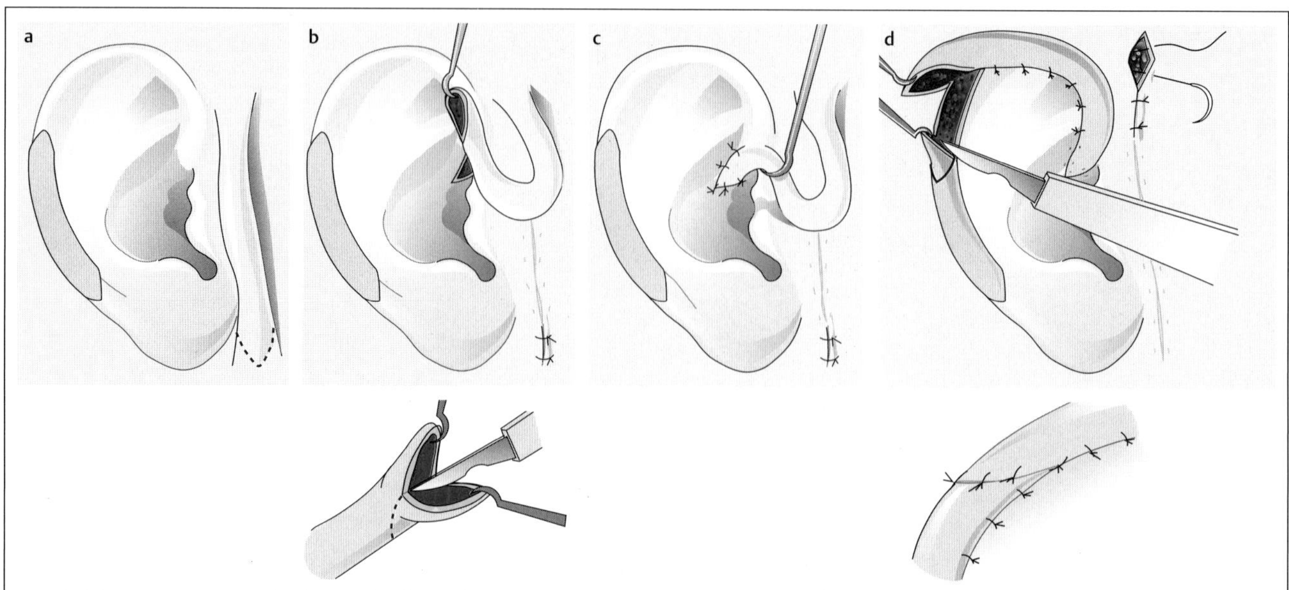

Fig. 4.**45** **Reconstruction of the entire helix with a tube-bipedicled flap, modified from the technique of Converse and Brent (1977).**

First stage:

a The posterior helix is reconstructed (see Fig. 4.**43**), a preauricular tube-bipedicled flap can be raised concurrently.

Second stage:

b, c Incorporation of the flap as a helical crus.

Third stage:

d After 3 weeks at the earliest, incorporation of the flap (see Fig. 4.**44 d**) into the helix (for a similar technique of flap elevation in two stages, see Fig. 4.**39 a, b**).

Recommended Techniques for Defect Reconstruction

Tube-pedicled Flap for the Superior Helix

(Fig. 4.**42**; see also p. 59, Fig. 4.**39**)

The tube-pedicled flap for the superior helix can also be used as a tube-bipedicled (tunneled) flap (see also p. 61, Fig. 4.**43**).

Tube-bipedicled flap for Defects of the Superior and Middle Thirds

(Fig. 4.**43**)

Three-stage Reconstruction of a Defect of the Middle Third with a Tube-Pedicled Flap

(Fig. 4.**44**; Steffanoff 1948; Converse and Brent 1977; Weerda 1999 a, 2001)

Unlike reconstruction with a tunneled flap (see Fig. 4.**42 a**), the tube-pedicled flap is first raised and rolled into a tube (Fig. 4.**44 b, c**). If there is not sufficient skin for closure, we use split skin for coverage or wrap the exposed tube-pedicled flap with silicone foil (see also Fig. 4.**39 b**).

Converse and Brent's Reconstruction with a Preauricular Tube-pedicled Flap

(Fig. 4.**45**; Converse and Brent 1977)

Similar to the flap previously described, a preauricular tube-pedicled flap can be raised for defects of the anterior and superior helix as well as for the helical crus (Berson 1948; Converse 1958; Converse and Brent 1977).

Reconstruction with a Superiorly Based Posterior Flap

(see Fig. 4.**38 b**)

Inferior Helix

These reconstructions are similar to those of the superior and middle thirds of the helix; further reconstructions are discussed under "Lower partial reconstructions" (see pp. 74 ff).

4.2.3 Partial Reconstruction of the Auricle

Although a number of reconstructions are similar or identical for the upper and middle thirds of the auricle, and in part also for the lower auricle, as well as for subtotal and total defects, a distinction will be made between upper, middle, and lower auricle, to make it easier for the surgeon to select options for reconstructions in particularly problematic cases. When necessary, reference is made to reconstructive procedures found in other chapters of this book.

Upper Third Auricular Defects (Fig. 4.46)

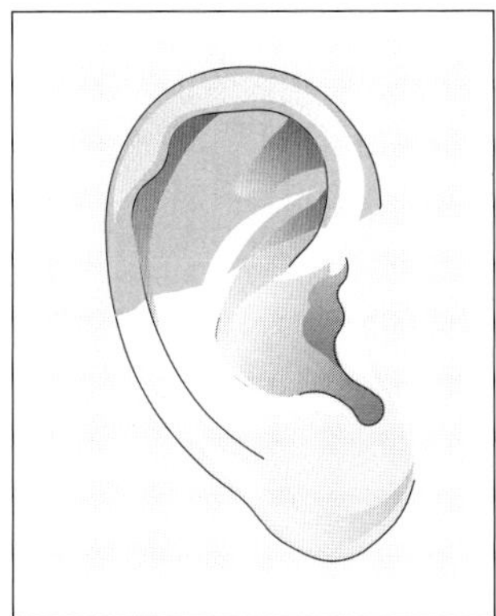

Fig. 4.46 **Superior third of the auricle.**

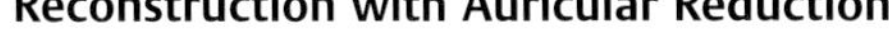

Reconstruction with Auricular Reduction

Reconstructions of the auricle with reduction of the ear are appropriate only in rare cases, e. g., for auricular lesions in elderly patients, or for very large ears.

Wedge Excisions

(Fig. 4.**47**; see reconstruction of peripheral defects with auricular reduction; Figs. 4.**25**, 4.**26**).

Wedge Resections with or without Burow's Triangles

(see p. 154; Fig. 5.**70**; and for example Joseph 1931; Berson 1948).

Antia and Buch's Helical Sliding Flap

(Figs. 4.**48**, Fig. 4.**49 a**, **b**; Antia and Buch 1967)

This technique lends itself for reconstructions with auricular reduction (see Fig. 4.**29**) as a modification of Gersuny's technique (1903; see Figs. 4.**27** and 4.**28**).

Full-thickness Composite Grafts of the Contralateral Ear as Described by Pegram and Peterson

(see Fig. 4.**34**; Pegram and Peterson 1956)
Replacement of wedge-shaped defects with a full-thickness composite graft taken from the contralateral ear.

Critique. There is a danger of losing the composite graft and deforming the other ear (see pp. 57, 70, 192).

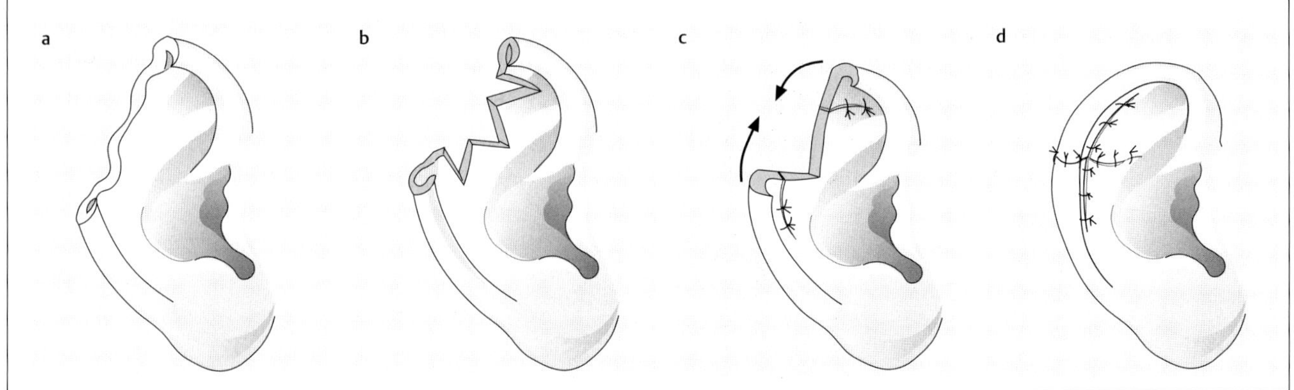

Fig. 4.**47** **Reconstruction by auricular reduction with wedge resection and Burow's triangles (see also Fig. 4.26).**

a Defect.
b Burow's triangles in the scapha.
c, d Closure of the defects.

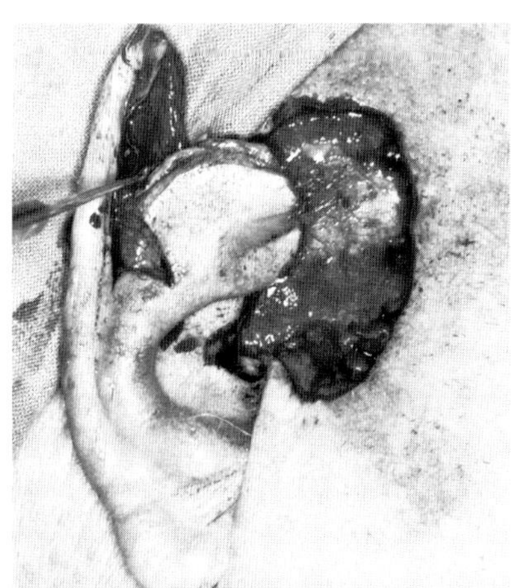

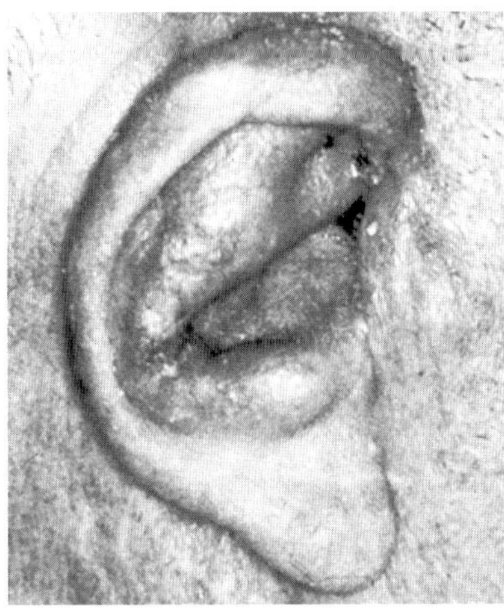

a b

Fig. 4.**48** **Helical sliding flap and Dufourmentel rhomboid flap (see also Fig. 4.33, p. 56).**

a Preauricular defect and defect of the superoanterior auricle.
b Coverage with a helical sliding flap and a rhomboid flap with considerable reduction of the auricle.

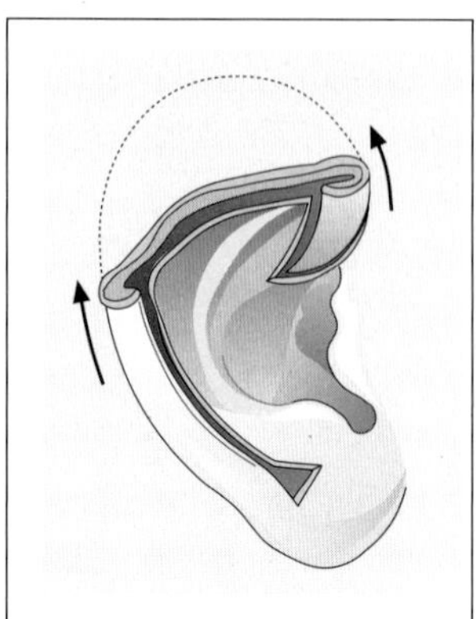

Fig. 4.**49** **Coverage of a superior defect with a posterior and anterior helical sliding flap (Gersuny technique) modified from the technique of Antia and Buch (1967).** Two-layer incision in the scapha, continued around the helical crus with a Burow's triangle in the earlobe, postauricular skin mobilization (explained in more detail in Fig. 4.**29**; p. 55).

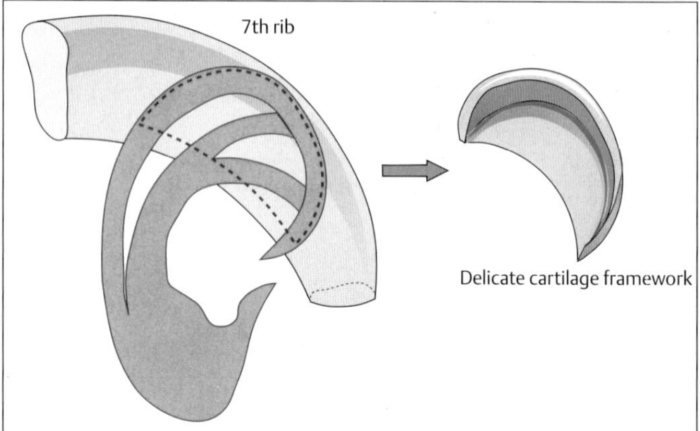

Fig. 4.**51** **Carving of a delicate cartilage framework patterned from a template (6th, 7th, or 8th rib).** The template is reversed (see Fig. 4.**50**). The framework is 2–3 mm smaller (dotted) than the auricular segment to be reconstructed.

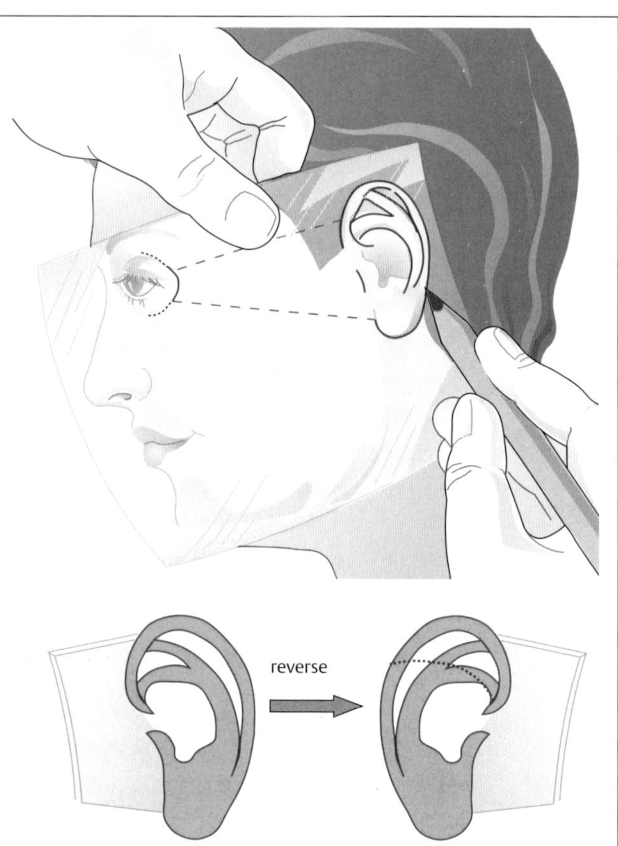

Fig. 4.**50** **A template based on the healthy ear, made from transparent material (e. g. x-ray film).** Place the film on the orbital margin, outline the auricle and excise the scapha, the triangular fossa, and the concha (a template of the auricle alone will suffice for partial defects). The size of the defect is marked out on the template (dotted line).

Reconstruction without Auricular Reduction

Historical review. Although there are reports of attempts at auricular reconstruction dating back to ancient and medieval times (Goedecke 1995), it was not until Tagliacozzi in 1597 (see Fig. 4.1), Dieffenbach in 1845 (see Fig. 4.3), and Szymanowsky in 1870 (see Fig. 4.4) that reconstructive techniques were first described; however, these almost certainly resulted in very contracted reconstructions (see Section 5.4.3, p. 197).

Schmieden (1908) was the first to use autologous cartilage; he reconstructed part of the ear by suturing a square-shaped, pedicled flap from the ipsilateral arm to the margin of the defect (see Fig. 5.**149**). However, the results of such distant flaps are still poor in terms of color and texture match (Mündnich 1962 a; Toplak 1986; Goedecke 1995).

It was Gillies (1920) who first used a carved autologous costal cartilage framework for reconstruction.

Recommended Reconstruction

Reconstruction with a Costal Cartilage Framework and Skin Pocket

Informed consent. Detailed and extensive informed consent should be obtained before the reconstruction.

Positioning. Supine. The contralateral ear should also always be prepped; any possible harvesting of full-thickness skin and/or conchal cartilage should also have been included in the informed consent.

Fabrication of a template. Before the operation, a template of the healthy ear (Fig. 4.**50**) should be fashioned from transparent film material (unexposed x-ray film or thick transparent foil). The contours are outlined with a marker pen and then cut out and reversed. The reversed template is placed over the injured ear and the margins of the defect are outlined. Usually the position of the auricle can be determined exactly from the position of the residual ear, which is why the fabrication of a template the size of the healthy auricle with the defect outlined should suffice (see also p. 90, Fig. 4.**106**).

Harvesting of costal cartilage. We have the harvesting performed by a second team (see p. 204; Fig. 5.**157**). The cartilage framework is carved about 2–3 mm smaller than the part of the ear to be reconstructed (see also p. 202, Fig. 5.**154** and p. 203, Fig. 5.**156**).

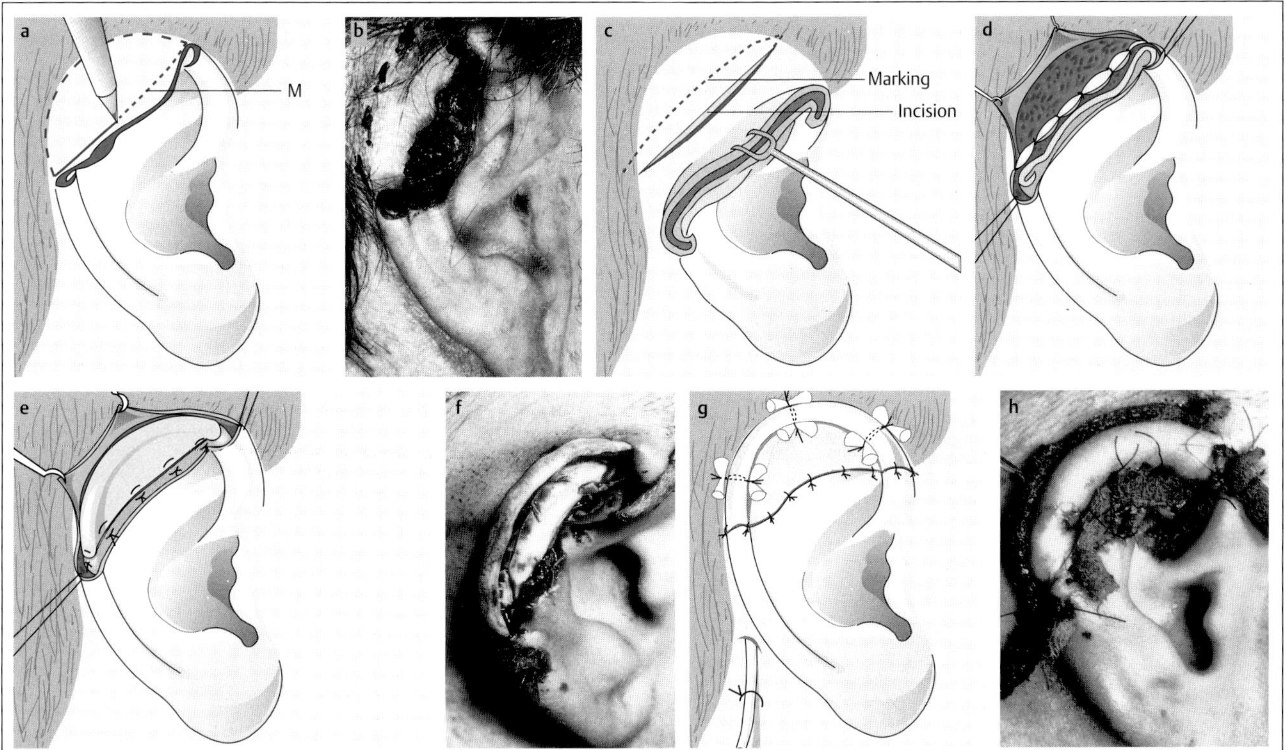

Fig. 4.52 **Reconstruction of the upper auricle with a subcutaneous pocket over the mastoid (as described by Converse and Brent 1977; see Fig. 2.12, p. 19).**
First stage:
a, b The height of the stump (M) is marked on the skin of the mastoid surface and the superior auricular rim is outlined according to the template (see Figs. 4.**50** and 4.**51**).
c The skin is incised about 3–4 mm lower than the marked height of the stump.
d A subcutaneous pocket is developed, about 1 cm larger than the height of the superior helical margin, and the postauricular stump skin is sutured to the lower margin of the incision.
e, f The framework (amputated ear denuded of skin or carved cartilage framework, 2–3 mm smaller in size) is attached using a 5–0 braided suture and inserted into the pocket.
g, h Closure of the skin wound, vacuum drainage, mattress sutures without pressure (see text; second stage: Fig. 4.**53**).

Fabrication of an auricular framework. A second template, about 2 mm smaller, is cut to fabricate the framework. The framework, which should be as delicate as possible (see p. 64) and made entirely of costal cartilage (Fig. 4.**51**), is carved with the aid of appropriate instruments and kept moist until the pocket over the mastoid surface has been developed and is ready to receive it.

Implantation of the cartilage framework. The first-stage operation is shown in Fig. 4.**52 a–h** (see also Fig. 4.**64**).

Possible errors. It is essential to reconstruct the auricular profile, i. e., the cartilage framework must be attached to the stump in such a way as to ensure that it does not become folded during insertion into the pocket. The pocket must therefore be made sufficiently large, and the auricular stump may need to be set back and attached to the mastoid surface.

Second-stage operation: Elevation of the auricle (Fig. 4.**53 a–d**). The auricle is elevated after 6–8 weeks (some surgeons do it even later). For this purpose, according to the suggestions made by Nagata (1994; see p. 72, Fig. **4.66 d** and pp. 215, 216, Fig. 5.**172**), a thick split-thickness skin flap about 8–10 mm in width is elevated above the helix and above the hair follicles in the direction of the helix, leaving some fibrous tissue on the helical cartilage (Fig. 4.**53 a**). Next, the entire postauricular surface is exposed in such a way that a good layer of fibrous and granulation tissue remains on the framework. The postauricular surface and the mastoid surface are covered with a thick split- or full-thickness skin graft taken from the thorax donor site, the groin area, or the buttocks (Fig. 4.**53 b–d**, Fig. 4.**54**; Ombredanne 1931; Cronin 1952; Converse 1958; Musgrave and Garret 1967; Converse and Brent 1977; Weerda 1984 a, 1999 a, 2001).

Reconstruction by Insertion of an Expander (see pp. 231 ff) —— Where there is insufficient skin or after burn injuries, a 35-ml expander is implanted (Fig. 4.**55 a, b**) and inflated continually twice a week over a period of about 8 weeks. The expanded skin is then used for reconstruction (Fig. 4.**55 c**).

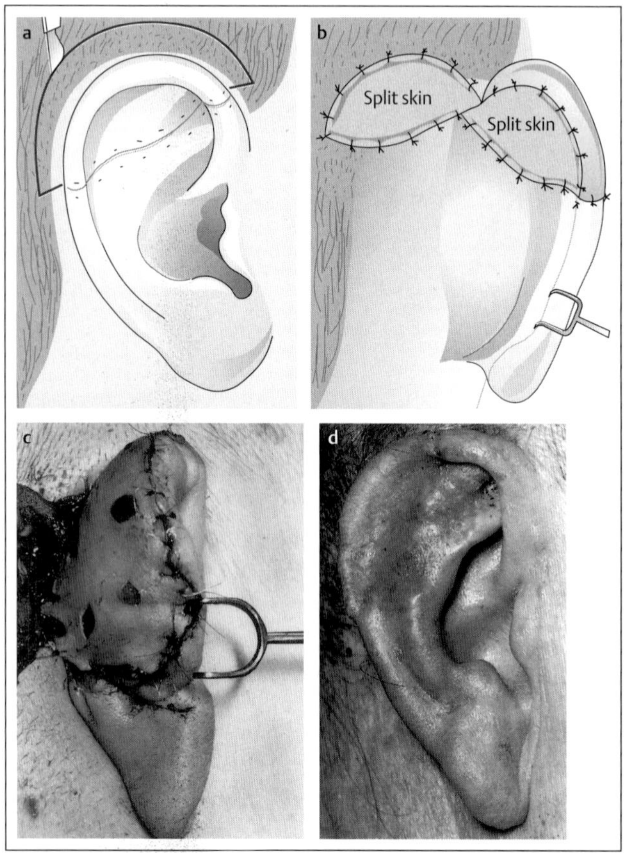

Fig. 4.**53** **Second stage of the reconstruction of the upper auricle: elevation of the auricle as described by Nagata (1994b).**

a Incision of a full-thickness skin flap pedicled on the helix (see Fig. 5.**172a**, pp. 215, 216), above the level of the hair follicles. Fibrous tissue is left behind on the periosteum (see Fig. 5.**172f**) and on the posterior surface of the auricle.

b, c Coverage of the remaining defects with thick split skin which is secured with sutures and fibrin glue. Dressing (see p. 223).

d Result.

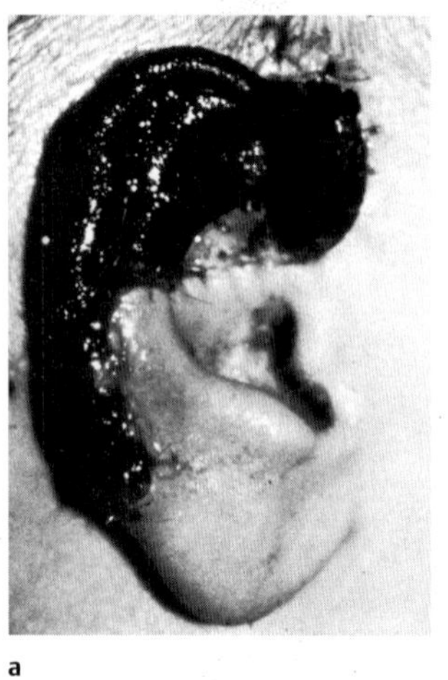

a

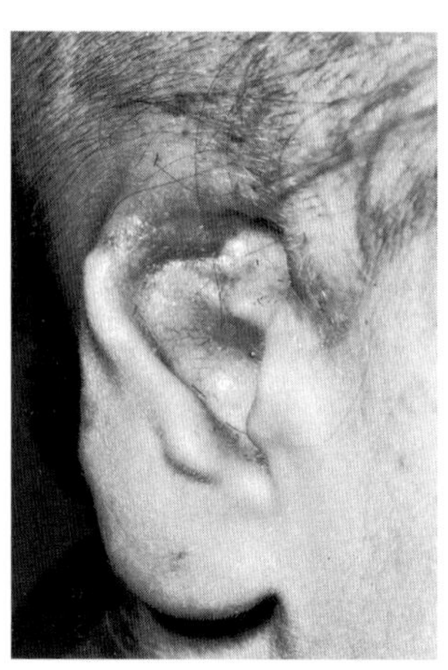

b

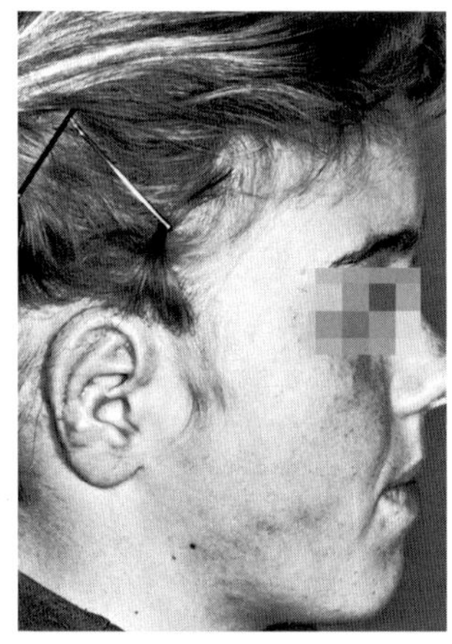

c

Fig. 4.**54** **Reconstruction of the superior auricle after failed classic replantation (see Figs. 4.52, 4.53).**

a Necrosis after replantation.

b Defect.

c Result after two-stage reconstruction (surgeon: R. Siegert).

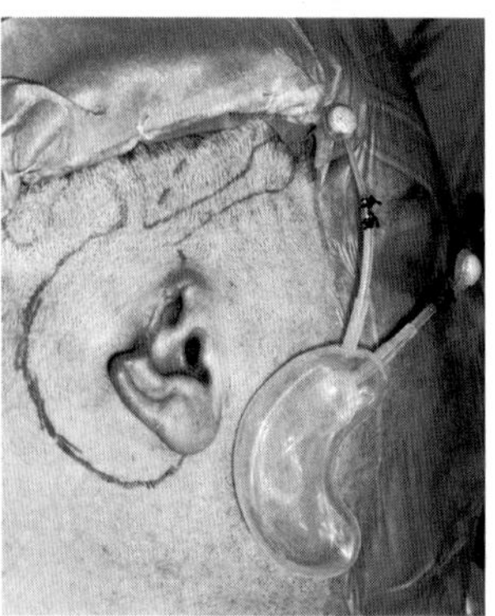

a

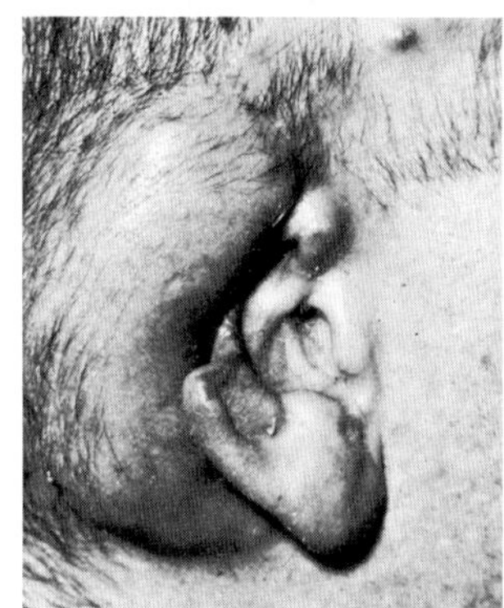

b

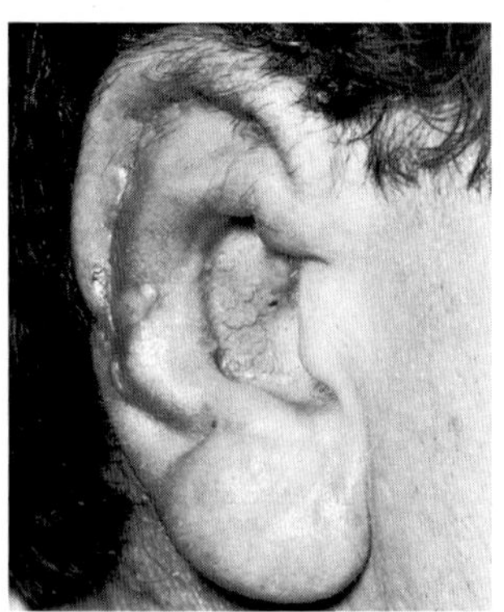

c

Fig. 4.**55** **Additional skin expansion before reconstruction.**

a Outline of the 35 ml expander.

b Appearance after implantation (via an incision through hair-bearing skin) and expansion.

c Reconstructed ear; epilation is intended (surgeon: R. Siegert).

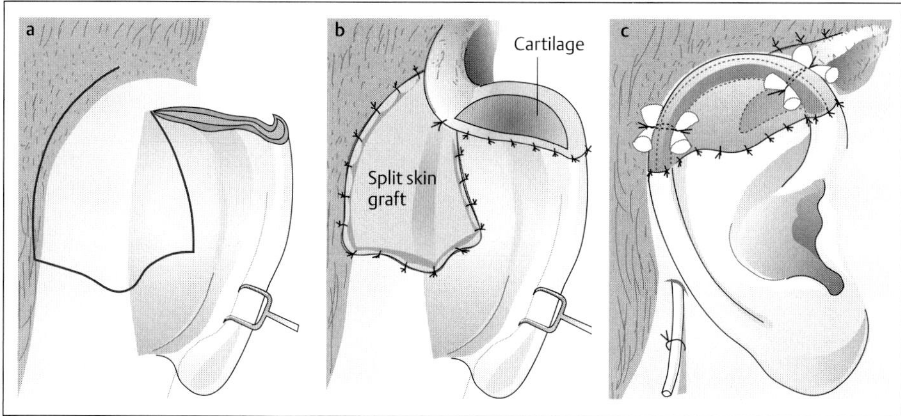

Fig. 4.**56** **Anterosuperiorly based retroauricular and postauricular transposition flap as described by Crikelair (1956).**
a Elevation of the flap.
b Incorporation of the patterned framework, coverage of the secondary defect with a thick split-thickness skin graft.
c Mattress sutures are used to form the contours and a drain is inserted.

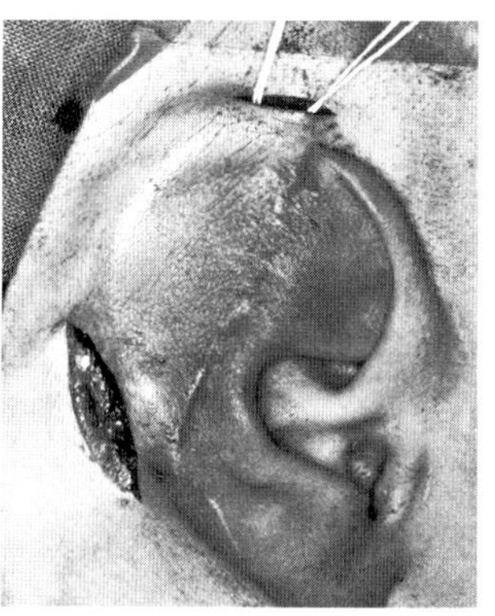
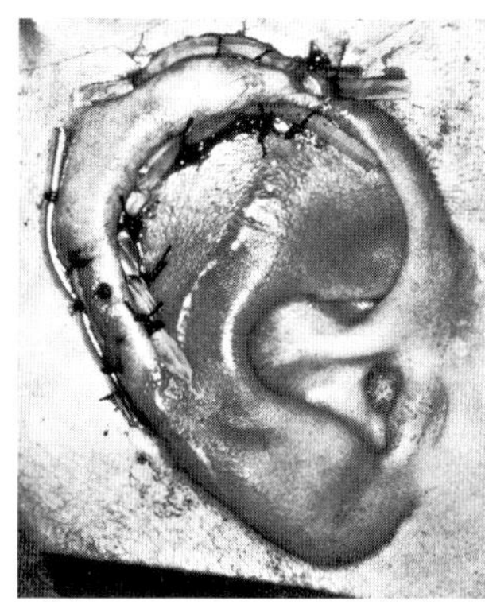

a b

Fig. 4.**57** **Secondary reconstruction with a pocket after earlier debridement and closure of the wounds (reconstruction from the early 1970s after primary wound closure in another institution; see Fig. 4.67).**
a Development of the pocket via a lateral incision and insertion of the costal cartilage framework (here cartilage was stored in merthiolate).
b Skin closure and molding with mattress sutures (see Fig. 4.**67**).

Crikelair's Reconstruction using an Anterosuperiorly Based Posterior Flap

(Fig. 4.**56**; Crikelair 1956)

The anterior and posterior auricular surfaces can be reconstructed with the flap described by Crikelair which is superiorly based and includes the skin of the mastoid and postauricular regions (Fig. 4.**56 a–c**). In cases with larger defects and insufficient skin, only the anterior surface of the ear need be reconstructed in a first stage, with the posterior surface then being raised in a second stage after 6–8 weeks and covered with a free thick split-thickness skin graft (see Fig. 4.**66 d–f**).

Methods of Reconstruction Described in the Literature

Primary management involved suturing the skin of the stump to the mastoid skin (see Fig. 4.**52**; see also reconstruction of the middle third of the auricle).

Secondary Reconstruction Using a Pocket

(Fig. 4.**57**)

Critique. Here the cartilage framework is not attached accurately to the stump, and the cosmetic results are not so good. It is better to revise the scar and insert the cartilage framework, as with the pocket method.

Ombredanne's Second-stage Reconstruction Using a Flap Pedicled Superiorly on the Defect

(Fig. 4.**58**; Ombredanne 1931)

Ombredanne dissected the mastoid skin in a second stage and folded it back, pedicled on the helix, to cover the posterior surface (Fig. 4.**58**).

Critique. Usually there is not enough skin to fold it back, even in cases of defects of the middle third. The method recommended by Nagata (see Fig. 4.**66 d**) is also possible, even when the new helix is situated in the region of the hairline, and provides good cosmetic results.

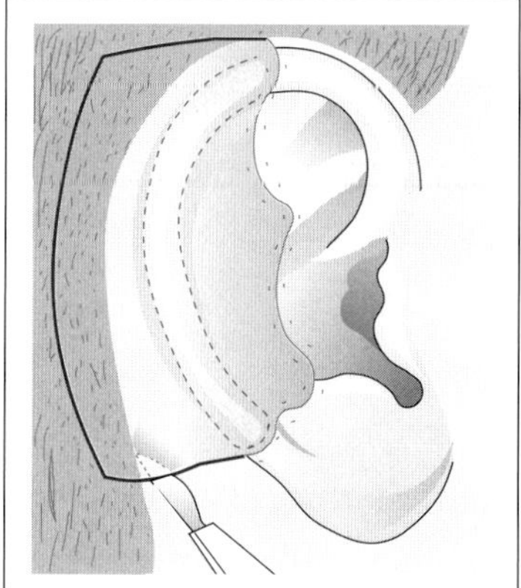

Fig. 4.**58** **Second stage: Reconstruction using Ombredanne's technique (Ombredanne 1931) with a flap pedicled on the helix.** After the flap has healed (see also Fig. 4.**64**), it is divided and folded over to cover the posterior surface. The Nagata method is better (see Fig. 4.**66**).

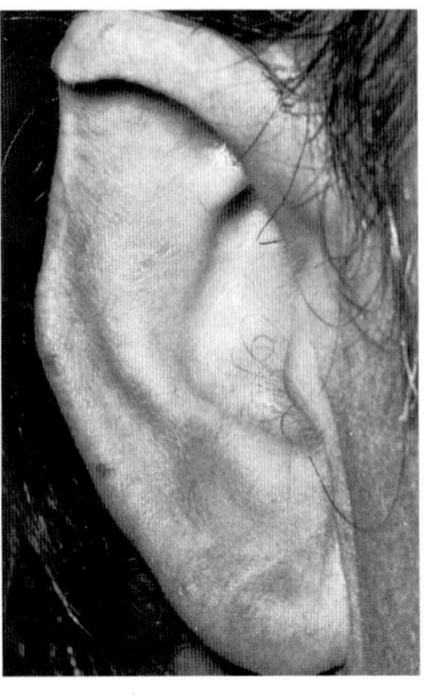
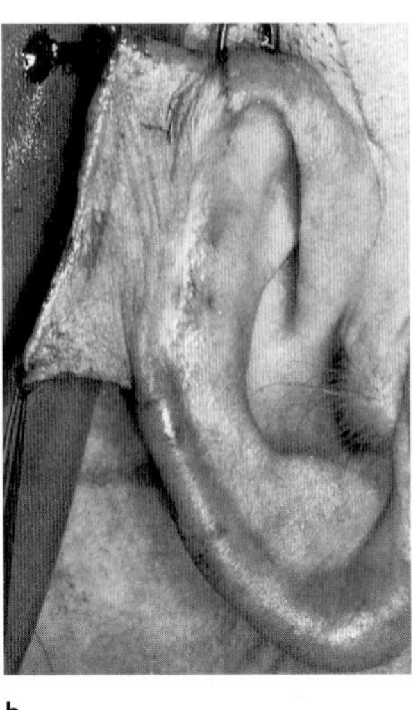
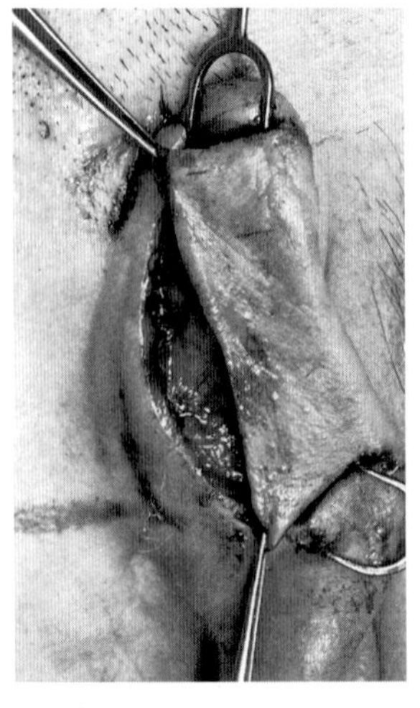
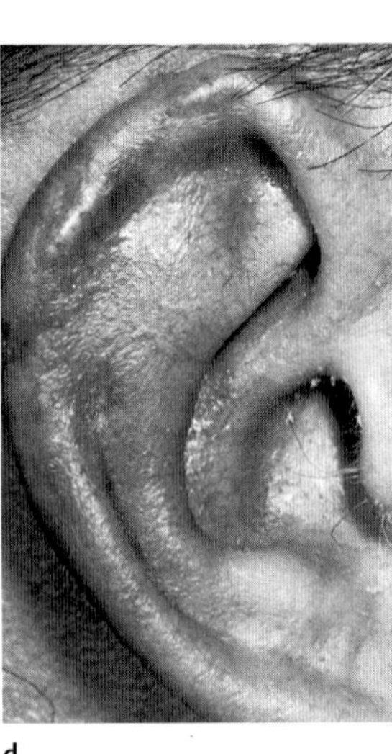

Fig. 4.59 **Secondary reconstruction with a postauricular flap pedicled on the helix.**
a Defect.
b Posteriorly raised flap, pedicled on the scar. Placement of a strut fabricated from costal or conchal cartilage.
c The flap is sutured to cover the cartilage. Closure of the residual defect with a U-shaped advancement flap (see Fig. 4.**64 b**) or thick split-thickness skin graft (see Fig. 4.**64 f**).
d Outcome (surgeon: R. Katzbach).

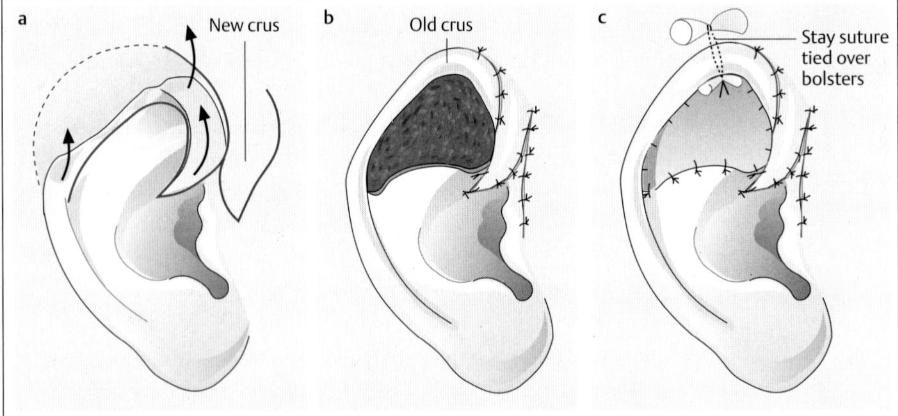

Fig. 4.**60** **Lueder's reconstruction of the superior auricle with a chondrocutaneous flap (1966; particularly suited for burn injuries).**
a Two-layer incision in the scapha around the helical crus and dissection on the mastoid (the presence of resilient skin is a prerequisite). Incision of the "new helical crus."
b Based on a template of the contralateral ear, the contracted helix is transposed superiorly together with the "old crus," and the "new crus" is sutured into the defect. Closure of the defects.
c A full-thickness skin graft, patterned from a template of the defect (**b**) on the mastoid surface, is harvested from the sulcus of the contralateral side and sutured and glued in with fibrin adhesive.

Secondary Reconstruction Using a Postauricular Flap Pedicled on the Helix

(Fig. 4.**59**)

Reconstruction of the Ear Secondary to Burn Defects Using Lueders' Chondrocutaneous Flap

(Fig. 4.**60**; Lueders 1966)

Partial Reconstruction with a Temporoparietal Fascial Flap (Fan Flap)

(see Fig. 4.**69**)

The use of a fascial flap for the reconstruction of the superior auricle is described in detail later (see pp. 93, 94). This flap is particularly suitable when the skin is exhausted, after burns or after previous futile operations (Park and Roh 2001).

Middle Third Auricular Defects (Fig. 4.61)

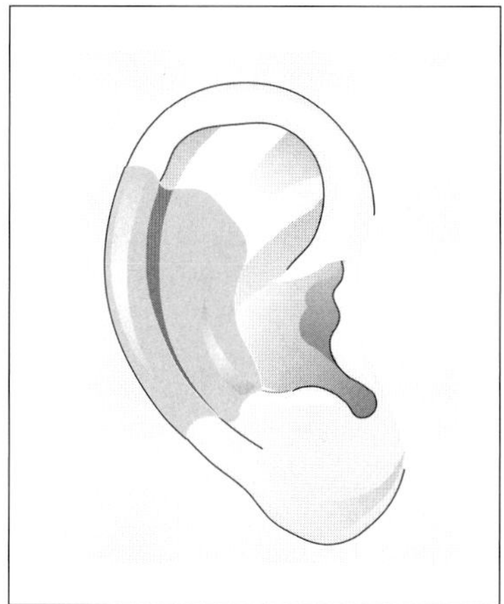

Fig. 4.61 **Middle third of the auricle.**

Reconstruction with Auricular Reduction

The methods described under partial reconstruction of the upper auricle (see pp. 52 ff) can also be employed in the region of the middle third of the ear (see also pp. 63 ff). Mention should be made of:

- reconstruction of wedge-shaped defects with Burow's triangles (see Fig. 4.47)
- techniques as described by Antia and Buch (1967) (see Fig. 4.29)
- techniques as described by Day (1921) and Pegram and Peterson (1956) among others (see Fig. 4.34).

Reconstruction of the Middle and Lower Thirds as Described by Templer et al.
(Fig. 4.62; Templer et al. 1981)
The authors freshen the wound margins. The contour of the ear is restored by rotating the lower part into the defect (Fig. 4.62 a–d).

Brent's Technique
(Fig. 4.63; Brent 1975)
Brent reconstructs using a full-thickness composite graft of half the defect size, taken from the contralateral ear. Consequently, both ears are slightly reduced in size (see p. 57; Figs. 4.34 and 4.35).

Critique. Composite grafts have a non-survival rate of about 20%, tend to contract, and the contralateral ear has to be operated upon (see p. 35, Tab. 3.7): **not to be recommended.**

Reconstruction without Auricular Reduction: Recommended Methods of Reconstruction

Advancement and transposition flaps of the retroauricular region are the most frequently used, extending on occasion beyond the sulcus to include the postauricular region.

Retroauricular U-shaped Burow Advancement Flap
(Fig. 4.64)
First-stage operation (Fig. 4.64 b–e). A wide, posteriorly based, retroauricular flap can be used for defects of the middle third of the helix. The hair should be generously shaved before the operation (Fig 4.64 b).

After suturing in the cartilage (C) (Fig. 4.64 b, c), the height of which should be 2–2.5 mm lower than that of the defect and which is sutured onto the cartilage stump with a 4–0 or 5–0 braided suture, the flap can be advanced into the defect and sutured to the anterior and posterior skin of the defect with 6–0 monofilament. The form of the helix can then be molded with two deep mattress sutures (Fig. 4.64 d, e).

Second-stage operation (Fig. 4.64 f, g). After about 3 weeks the flap is divided from the posterior skin of the defect and its superior part incorporated. The residual defect is covered with a split-thickness skin graft after freshening its margins and returning the U-shaped flap into its original position (Fig. 4.64 f, g; Nelaton and Ombredanne 1907, 1931; Berson

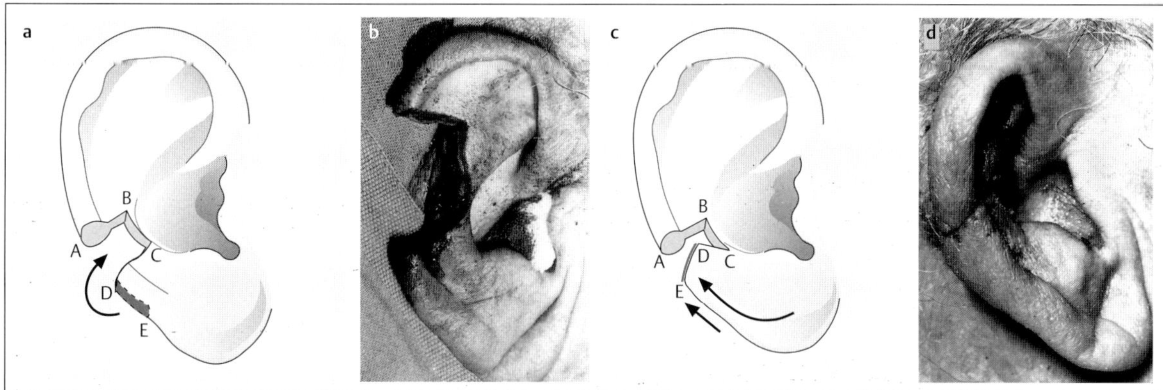

Fig. 4.62 **Reconstruction of the middle third of the auricle as described by Templer et al. (1981).**

a, b The margins of the defect and the lower helical region are freshened, D–E.
c The inferior auricle is rotated into the defect.
d Result.

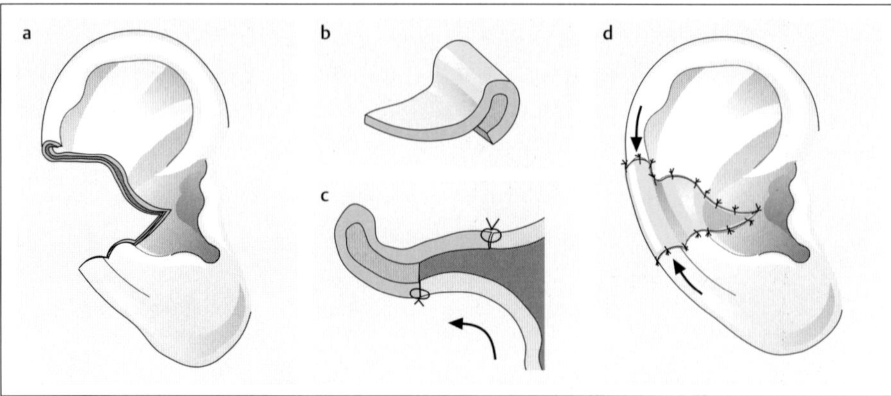

Fig. 4.**63** **Modification of Brent's technique of reconstruction using a full-thickness composite graft from the contralateral ear (Brent 1975; in Converse and Brent 1977).**

a The margins of the defect are freshened.

b Removal of the posterior skin from a full-thickness wedge taken from the contralateral auricle and measuring one half the size of the defect.

c Insertion of the full-thickness composite graft. The posterior auricular skin is advanced towards the helical margin, only the helical region remains full-thickness.

d The composite graft is inset (not to be recommended; see Fig. 4.**64 a**).

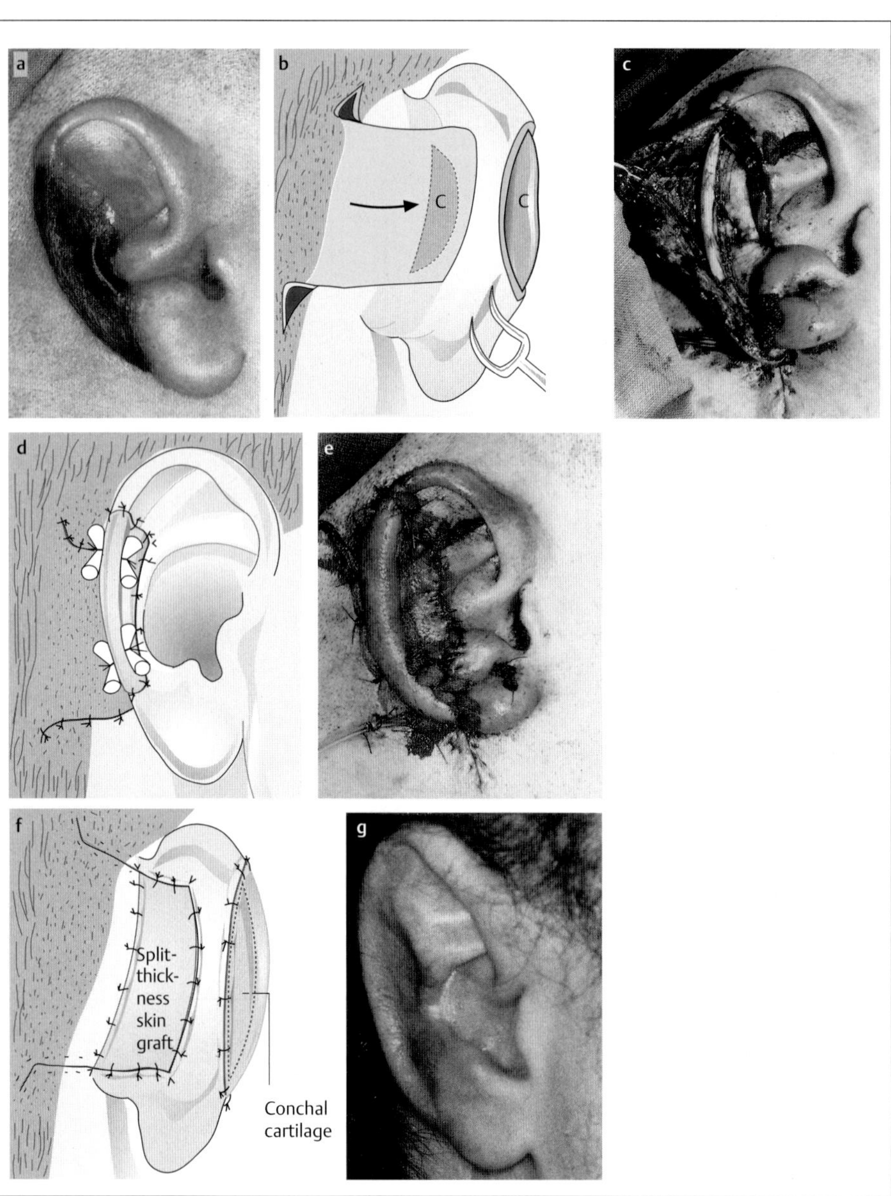

Fig. 4.**64** **Smaller and larger defects of the middle third of the auricle; coverage with a U-shaped advancement flap (see Fig. 4.66 b).**

a Loss of the middle third of the ear after "classic replantation" (see Fig. 3.**16**).

First stage:

b, c The wound margins are freshened and a cartilage framework (C) is inserted. A postauricular U-shaped flap is incised posterior and anterior to the sulcus and remains pedicled in the region of the scalp.

d, e This flap is sutured to the anterior skin of the stump and the contours molded with mattress sutures.

Second stage:

f The flap is divided after 3 weeks and incorporated into the postauricular region; if necessary, split-thickness graft is used to cover the residual defect (Fig. 4.**66 d**).

g Result (see also p. 152, Fig. 5.**67**; p. 189, Fig. 5.**136**).

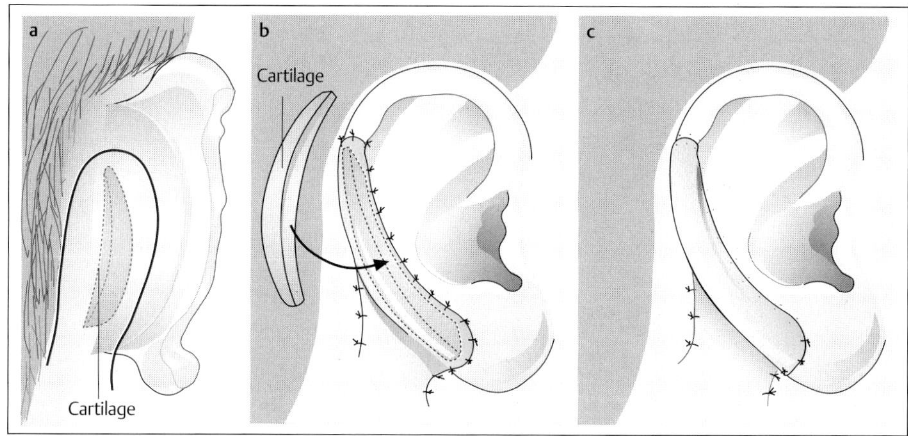

Fig. 4.**65** **Retro-postauricular inferiorly based transposition flap as described by Scott and Klaasen (1992).**
a Elevation of the patterned flap, harvesting of a patterned strut fabricated from concha and anterior antihelix (see Figs. 4.**16 b**, **c**, 4.**56**, 4.**71**).
b The strut is placed in position and sutured with 4–0 or 5–0 braided suture material, and the transposition flap is sutured to the trimmed wound margins.
c Separation and incorporation of the flap pedicle after 3 weeks.

1948; Musgrave et al. 1967; Converse and Brent 1977; Weerda 1981, 1999 a, 2001; Jackson 1985).

Avulsed auricular cartilage can also be denuded of skin and used as a strut, as can cartilage from the concha of the contralateral ear (see Figs. 4.**38**, 4.**39**; Musgrave et al. 1967).

Scott and Klaasen's Inferiorly and Superiorly Based Transposition Flap

(Fig. 4.**65**; see also Figs. 4.**56**, 4.**71**; Scott and Klaasen 1992)

A superiorly based transposition flap was described by Joseph (1931). It should have sufficient length when raised (see Fig. 4.**71 c**).

Reconstruction with a Rotation Flap

(see Figs. 4.**68**, 4.**98**; see also p. 190)

Likewise, a superiorly based rotation flap can be used if the hairline here does not allow reconstruction with a U-shaped advancement flap. **It is important to use a template to determine the form of the flap precisely, in advance of the reconstruction.**

Reconstruction with a Subcutaneous Pocket or a U-shaped Advancement Plasty

(Fig. 4.**66**; see also Figs. 4.**52**, 4.**53**)

This procedure is used for larger defects of the upper and middle thirds of the auricle.

First-stage operation. As previously described for smaller defects, here the retro- and postauricular skin is incised and dissected towards the hairline. An auricular template is patterned from the healthy ear, the defect is outlined (see p. 64) and, based on this template, a costal cartilage framework is carved to achieve a contour about 2–3 mm smaller than that of the expected reconstruction. A vacuum drain is secured with a suture for 6 days (Fig. 4.**66 b**, **c**).

Second-stage operation. Following suggestions made by Nagata, after 3–4 weeks a thick split-thickness skin flap is raised about 1 cm above and parallel to the posterior margin of the frame, but not quite reaching it (see also Fig. 4.**66 d–f**).

The scapha can be formed in a further stage. Some later refinements can be made to improve overall form and contour (Fig. 4.**66 h–j**).

Reconstruction with a Pocket as a Tunneled Flap

(Fig. 4.**67**; see also Fig. 4.**57**; Millard 1966; Converse and Brent 1977; Weerda 1980, 1991 a)

Second-stage operation. (see Fig. 4.**66 d–f**). After about 5–6 weeks the reconstructed part can be divided, the posterior surface dissected using Nagata's technique, and the secondary defect reduced. The residual defects are then resurfaced with a thick split-thickness skin graft.

Caution: Thin scar tissue and poor vascularity can result in necrosis (see also Fig. 4.**57**).

Critique. Excise the scar if it is hypertrophic, and proceed as shown in Fig. 4.**66 b**. The transitions from stump cartilage to framework cartilage are not always satisfactory.

Weerda's Rotation–Transposition Flap

(Fig. 4.**68**; see also Figs. 4.**98** and 4.**104**; Weerda 1980, 1984 c, 1991 a, 1999 a, 2001)

A second stage is not usually required, but if necessary some fine tailoring can be undertaken 3–4 weeks after the operation (see Fig. 4.**68 f**).

Critique. This procedure involves more extensive skin mobilization and increased scar formation. We have therefore used it only on rare occasions in recent years.

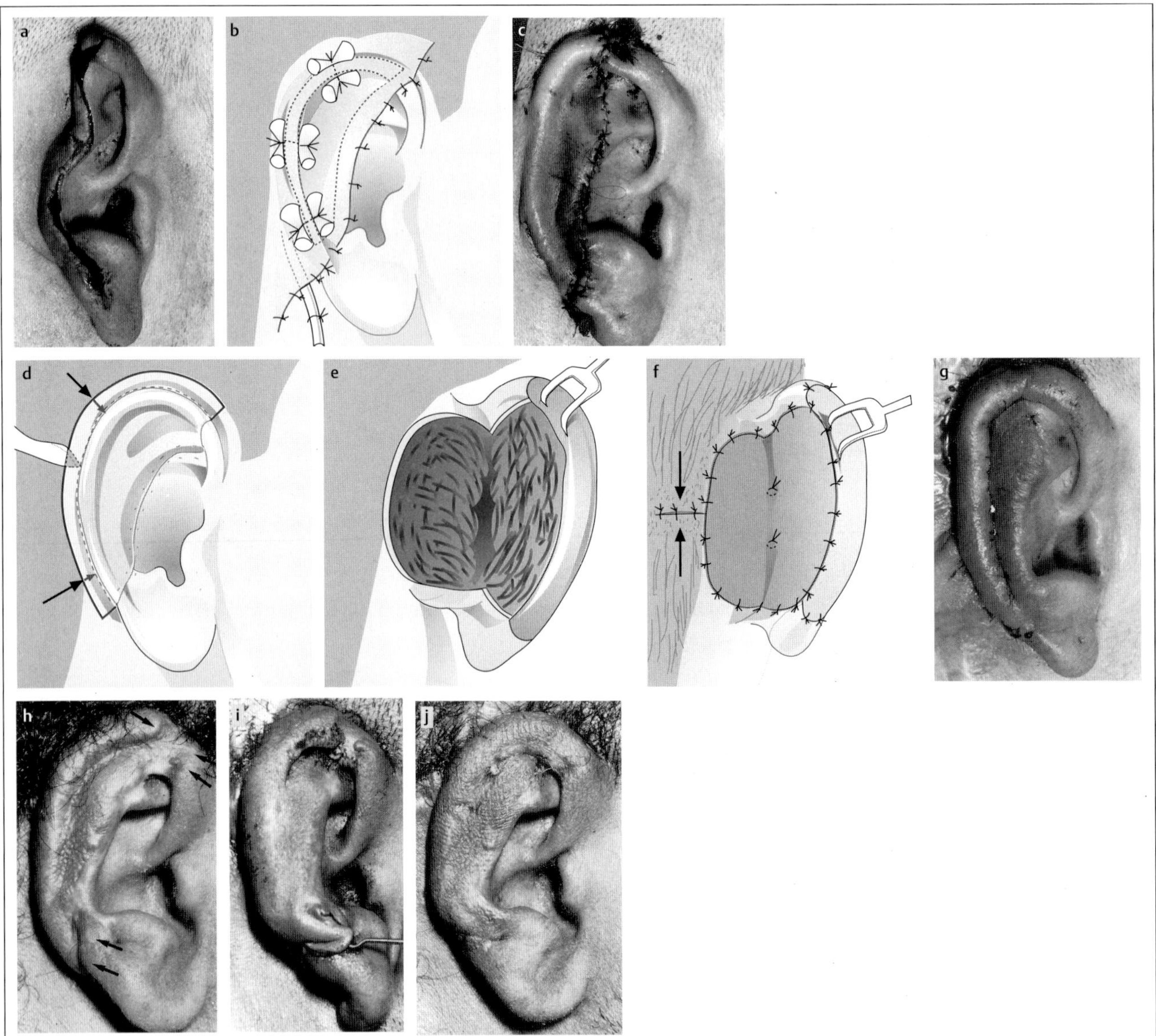

Fig. 4.66 **Reconstruction of a large defect of the upper and middle thirds of the auricle with a subcutaneous pocket (or a U-shaped advancement flap).**

First stage:

a The wound margins of the defect are freshened. The delicate cartilaginous framework is put into place (see Figs. 4.**50,** 4.**51**, 4.**52**, 4.**52 e, f**).

b, c The skin surrounding the defect is mobilized and sutured to the anterior skin of the auricular stump, a vacuum drain is inserted, and the auricle molded into shape (if necessary, large U-shaped advancement flap, see Fig. 4.**64 b, d**).

Second stage:

d Incision placed 1–1.5 cm behind the cartilage margin and a thick split-thickness skin flap extending near to the helical margin is dissected with a size 15 blade (as described by Nagata 1994 a–d, see pp. 211, 212).

e Careful dissection of the new postauricular surface, leaving behind a layer of fibrous tissue on the cartilaginous framework. The dissected split-thickness flap is draped over the raw surface of the posterior helix.

f Reduction of the defect over the mastoid (arrows) and coverage of the residual defect with a split-thickness skin graft (taken from the scalp, groin, buttocks, or the old thoracic wound) which is glued with fibrin adhesive and sutured with 6-0 monofilament, while 5-0 sutures with a P3 needle are used for molding the sulcus (Weerda 1999 a, 2001).

g Result after molding the scapha in the third stage (see p. 210).

Final refinements, if necessary:

h Small defects of contour are seen superiorly and at the transition to the earlobe in another reconstructed auricle (arrows).

i The defect is filled out with cartilage (above) and Z-plasty performed (below).

j Result.

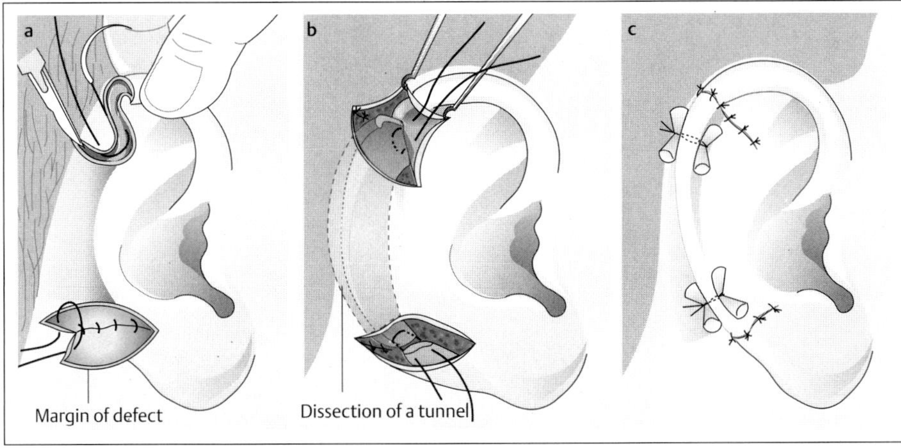

Fig. 4.67 **Secondary reconstruction after earlier simple debridement and closure (after Converse and Brent 1977; see also Fig. 4.57).**

a Incision slightly above and below the margins of the auricular defect. Dissection of a tunnel extending just beyond the hairline.

b A delicate framework (see Fig. 4.**57**) carved from costal cartilage (conchal cartilage) is drawn into the tunnel and attached to the stump with 4–0 (5–0) braided suture material.

c Closure of all wounds with 6–0 monofilament sutures and molding of the helix with mattress sutures.

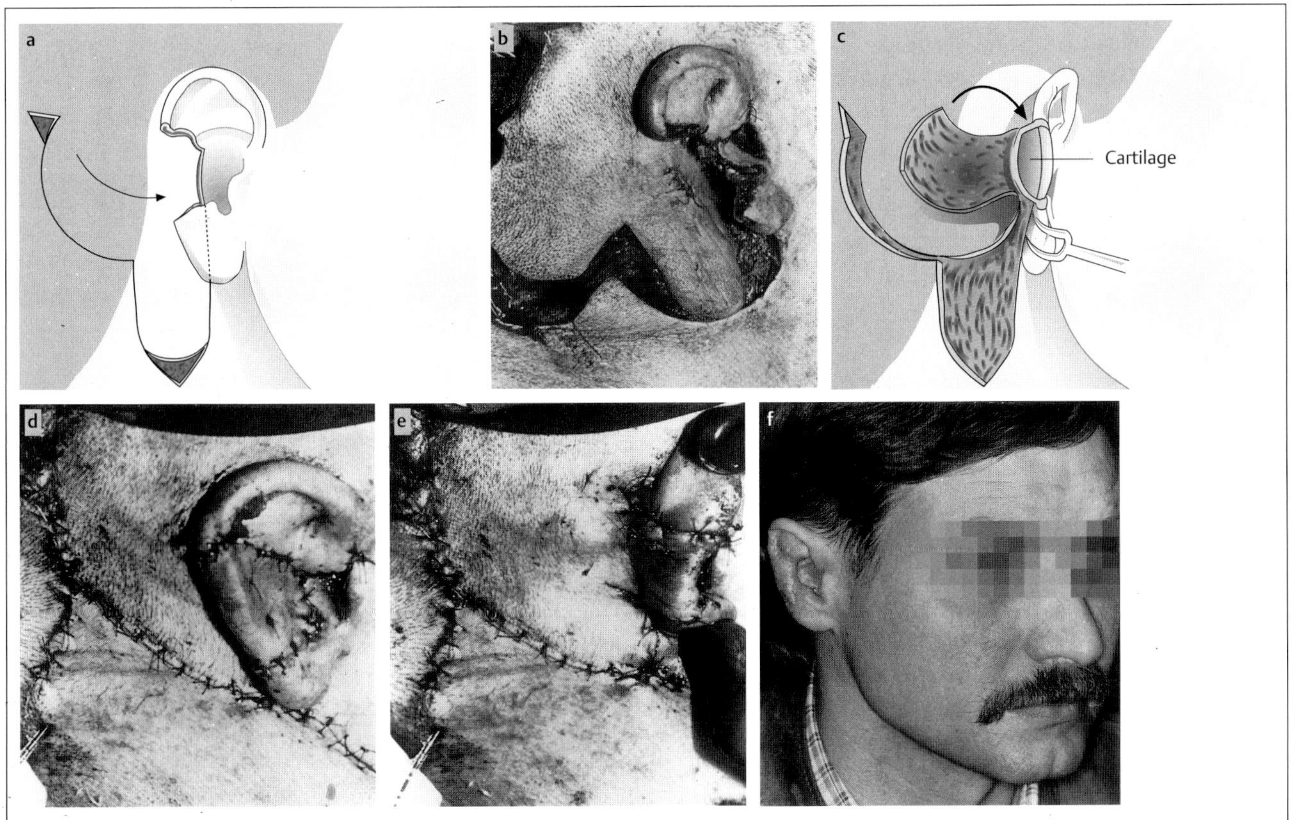

Fig. 4.**68** **Reconstruction of a larger defect of the middle third of the auricle with a Weerda rotation–transposition flap (1978, 1981).**

a, b The rotation–transposition flap is outlined. The hairless retroauricular transposition flap (**reconstruction flap**) is transported into the correct retroauricular position by the hair-bearing rotation flap (**transport flap**).

c The transposition flap now lies behind the defect. The cartilaginous strut spans the defect and is 3 mm less in height. Mobilization of the area surrounding the secondary defect.

d, e Appearance after reconstruction of the anterior and posterior surfaces in one stage (the suture line runs along the hairline).

f Result (later contouring of the helix was recommended).

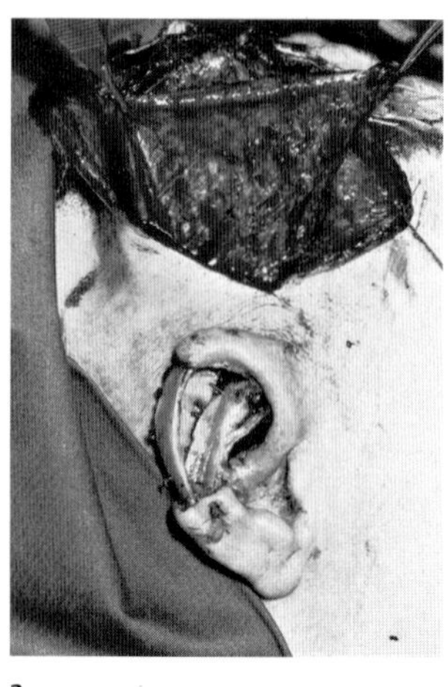
a

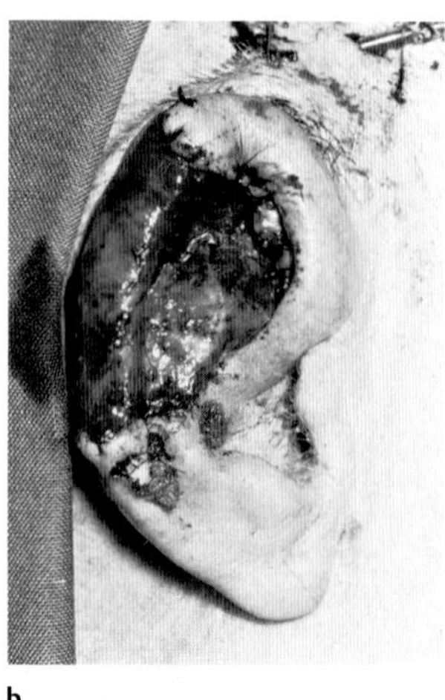
b

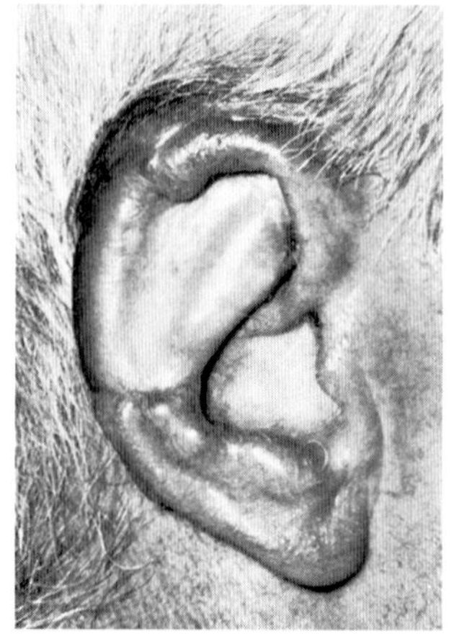
c

Fig. 4.69 **Reconstruction of the middle third of the auricle with a temporoparietal fascial flap (fan flap).**
a Elevation of the vascular-pedicled fascia.
b The flap is inset and covered with a full-thickness skin graft harvested from the posterior region of the contralateral ear (coverage of the secondary defect with split-thickness skin graft).
c Appearance after healing (surgeon: R. Siegert; see also Figs. 4.**108**, 4.**109**; pp. 93, 94).

Other Types of Flaps Described in the Literature

Posterior Auricular Flap Based on Scar Tissue

(see also Figs. 4.**58**, 5.**59**; Navabi 1964; Millard 1966; Davis 1987)

This is used for defects of the middle third of the auricle which have scar adhesions to the postauricular skin. A postauricular flap, pedicled on the scar and extending into the sulcus, is raised according to the size of the defect, with dissection continued in a superior direction. The secondary defects are closed by mobilizing the surrounding skin.

Reconstruction with a Fan Flap (Temporoparietal Fascial Flap) – (Fig. 4.**69**)

These flaps and their usage are described in detail on p. 93.

Reconstruction with Tubed Flaps

These flaps are described in detail under reconstruction of the upper third of the auricle (see pp. 60 ff).

Lower Third Auricular Defects (Fig. 4.70)

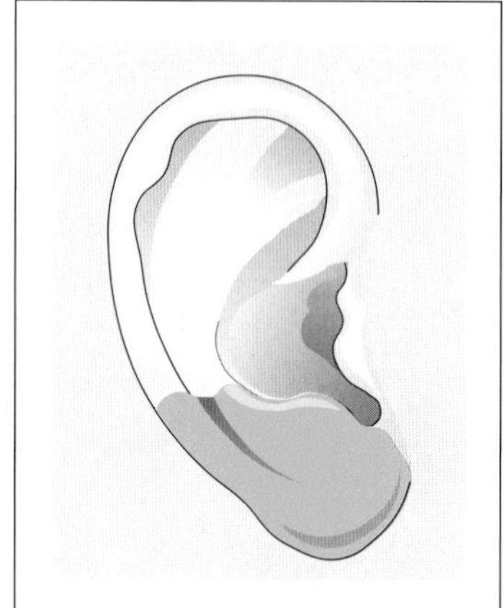

Fig. 4.**70** **Lower third of the auricle.**

Recommended Methods

Superiorly and Inferiorly Based Transposition Flap

(Fig. 4.**71**)

First-stage operation. As with the reconstruction of central defects (see Fig. 4.**14**) or of the upper auricle (see Fig. 4.**56**), coverage can also be achieved in the region of the lower third in two stages using a superiorly or inferiorly based transposition flap. Cartilage from the concha or from a rib is also used in the lower auricular region to prevent any significant contracture of the flap (Fig. 4.**71 a–e**).

Second-stage operation. The flap is inset after 3 weeks at the earliest (Fig. 4.**71 f, g**).

Reconstruction of the Entire Lower Auricle Using a Modified Gavello Flap

(Fig. 4.**72**; Gavello 1907, as cited in Nelaton and Ombredanne 1907).

A flap for the reconstruction of the earlobe was originally devised by Gavello and previously mentioned by Szymanowsky in 1870 (see Fig. 4.**4**; p. 44). Brent (1976) has described a similar flap for the reconstruction of larger defects of the lower auricle. We have modified this flap slightly. In order to prevent contracture of the lower reconstructed auricle, a framework carved from costal cartilage is inserted into the lower auricle and earlobe. The costal cartilage is attached to the cartilage stump of the auricle with a 4–0 braided suture after its wound margins have been freshened. The patterned flap is raised and sutured to the anterior and posterior skin of the auricular stump. The suture is placed slightly behind the earlobe to achieve a good

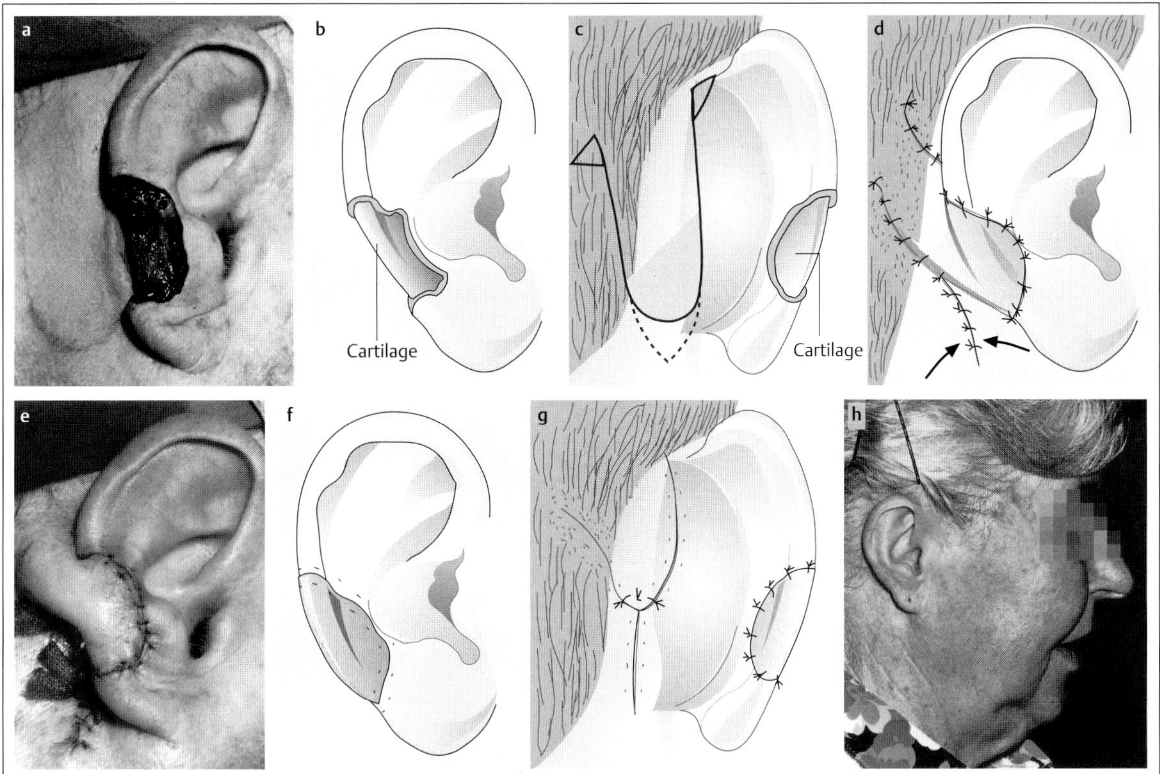

Fig. 4.**71** **Reconstruction of the lower third of the auricle with an (inferiorly or) superiorly based transposition flap (see also Figs.** 4.**16**, 4.**38**, 4.**65**).

First stage:

a Defect; flap outlined.

b Defect with incorporated cartilaginous strut from the ipsi- or contralateral ear, harvested following a template.

c Transposition flap.

d, e Flap inset over the cartilaginous framework.

Second stage:

f, g After about 3 weeks, division of the flap and incorporation into the postauricular surface and incorporation of the flap base.

h Result.

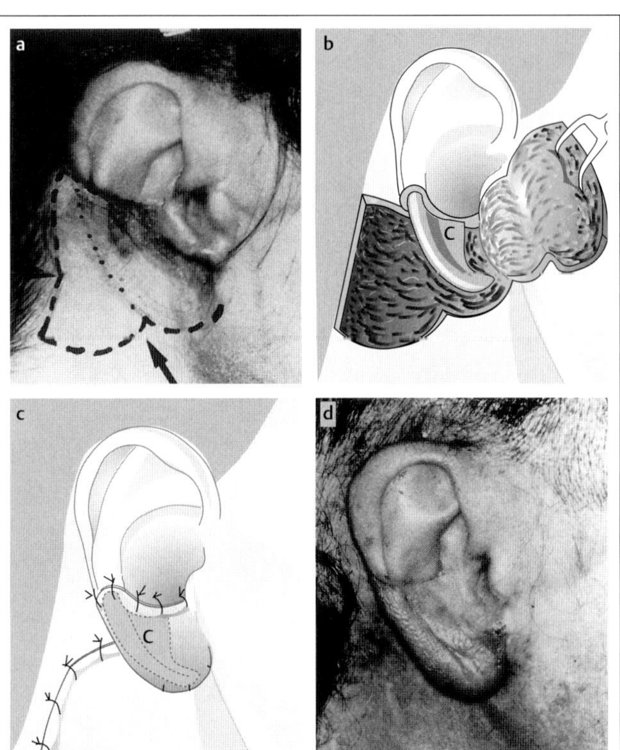

Fig. 4.**72** **Gavello and Brent's reconstruction of the lower auricular third (modified by Weerda, 1989 d).**

a The bilobed flap is planned and outlined.

b A large, anteriorly based, bilobed Gavello flap is elevated and, after preparation of the flap, the costal cartilage framework (C) is sutured into place.

c The framework (C) is enveloped by the flap and all defects are closed (see text).

d Result after a single-stage reconstruction (see p. 193).

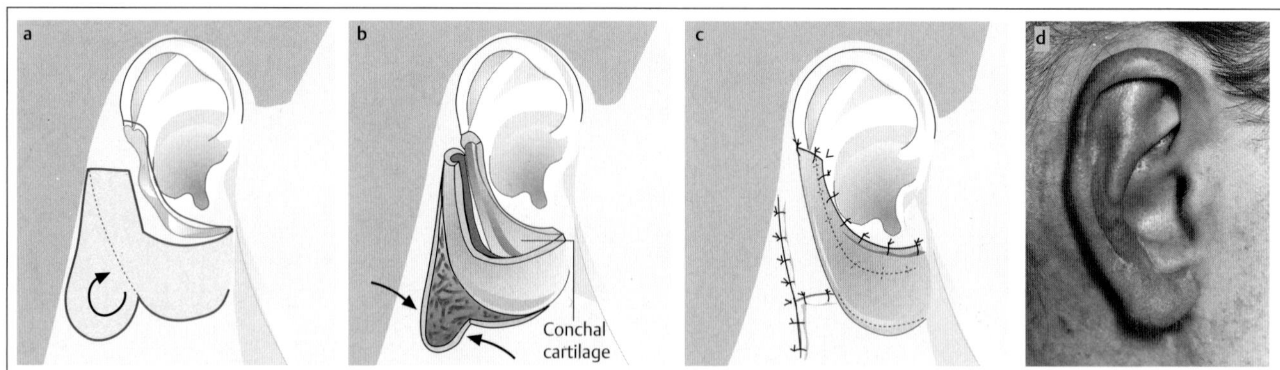

Fig. 4.73 **Modification of the Szymanowsky–Gavello flap for a single-stage reconstruction of the helix and lower auricle after failure of primary reconstruction.**

a Defect. The flap is outlined, designed from the previously prepared template (see Fig. 4.**84**: low insertion of the double flap due to the split-skin graft which had previously been placed behind and below the auricle in another instituion).

b The wound margins have been freshened, the flap is raised, the patterned cartilage harvested from the contralateral concha (or carefully carved from the costal cartilage) is sutured to the cartilage stump with a 4–0 (5–0) braided suture.

c Closure of all defects.

d Result.

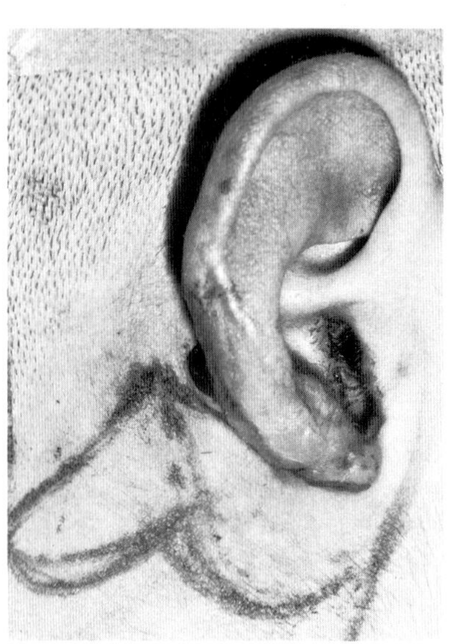
a

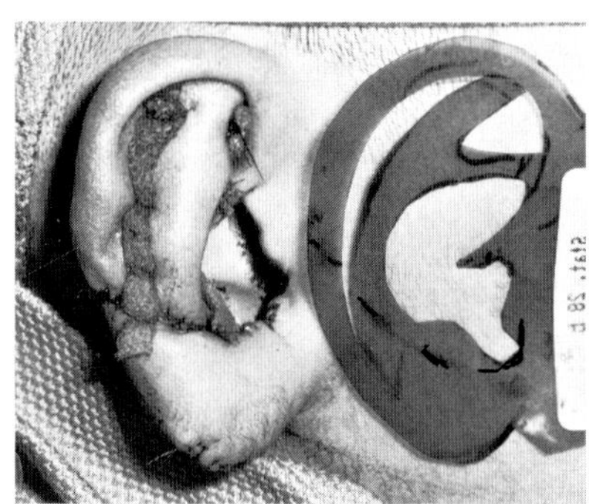
b

Fig. 4.**74** **Reconstruction of the lower auricular third with a Gavello flap (see also Fig.** 4.**73**).

a Defect; the flap is outlined. Conchal cartilage as a strut, harvested according to template 2. Mobilization of the flap.

b The reconstruction is checked with the previously prepared template 1 fashioned from the healthy ear. See also Figs. 4.**50**, 4.**51** (p. 64), 5.**141** (p. 193), and 5.**154**–5.**157** (pp. 202–204).

round curvature in the anterior region. A good round curvature of the earlobe is achieved if the earlobe curvature incised for coverage in the lower region is slightly larger than the earlobe curvature of the second flap.

Modified Gavello Flap

(Fig. 4.73; Fig. 4.74 **a**, **b**; Weerda 1999 a, 2001)

If, in addition to the earlobe, parts of the helix are also missing, the latter can be reconstructed with a modified Gavello flap (Fig. 4.73 **a–d**). After carving a costal cartilage framework or harvesting conchal cartilage from the contralateral auricle patterned from a template, it is attached to the cartilage stump with 4–0 braided sutures after freshening the wound margins. The raised Gavello flap is then draped around the frame and sutured to the anterior and posterior wound surfaces, thus reconstructing the earlobe and helix. With the additional aid of a slightly larger anterior flap, the curvature of the earlobe can be given a somewhat better form (see also Fig. 4.**84**). All the defects can be closed primarily by mobilizing the surrounding skin. This type of reconstruction was used for a female patient in whom the postauricular region had previously been resurfaced elsewhere with a split-skin graft (Fig. 4.73 **d**; a similar reconstruction is shown in Fig. 4.74 **a**, **b**).

Reconstruction with a Tunneled Gavello Flap

(Fig. 4.75)

The posterior surface can also be covered with a thick split-thickness skin graft.

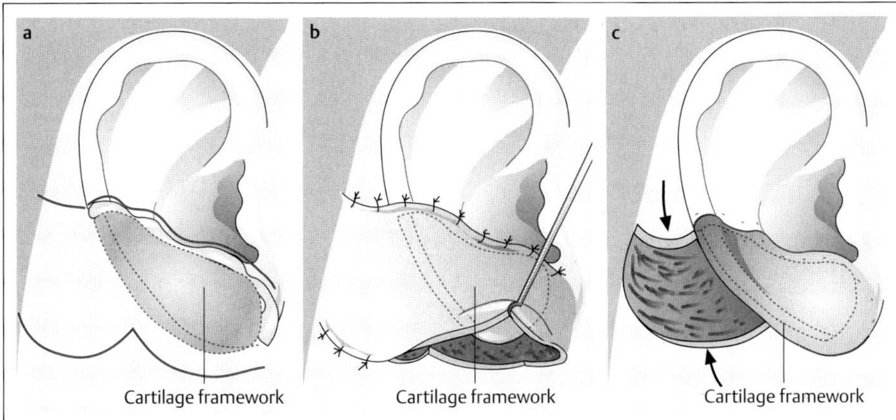

Fig. 4.**75** **Modified Gavello bilobed, bipedicled flap.**
First stage:
a The anteriorly and posteriorly based tunneled flap is raised, the margins of the stump are freshened and the framework, carved from a template, is sutured on with 4–0 braided suture.
b The skin flap is sutured to the skin of the anterior surface of the stump and replaced to its original position.
Second stage:
c After about 3 weeks, division of the posterior flap and reconstruction of the posterior surface, suture to close the secondary wound (see also Fig. 4.**72**).

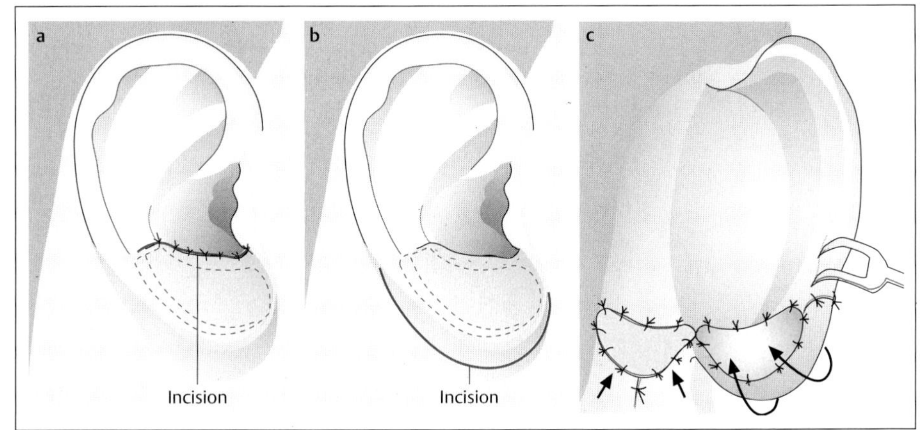

Fig. 4.**76** **Brent's reconstruction (1987 a).**
First stage:
a Incision in the concha–antitragus region and development of the earlobe pocket. Excision of a conchal cartilage from the ipsi- or contralateral site patterned from a template, insertion into the pocket, and suture.
Second stage:
b After about 3–4 weeks incision around the earlobe, about 3 mm below the cartilage, elevation of the earlobe.
c The cartilaginous margin is enveloped with skin (arrows) and the defect covered with a thick split-thickness skin graft. Reduction of the mastoid defect and closure of the residual defect with split-thickness skin.

Reconstruction with a Subcutaneous Pocket
(Fig. 4.76; Brent 1987)
As with partial or total reconstructions, the anterior surface is reconstructed during the first stage (Fig. 4.76 a) and the posterior surface during the second stage (Fig. 4.76 b, c; see also under "Partial reconstruction," p. 65, Fig. 4.52).

4.2.4 Reconstruction of the Earlobe (Fig. 4.77)

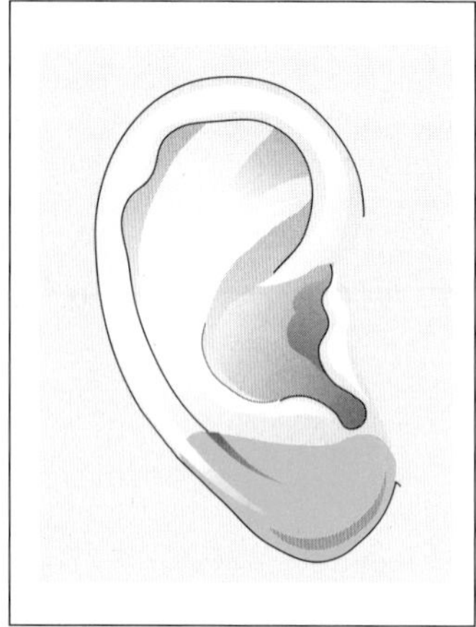

Fig. 4.77 **Earlobe.**

Since the earlobe, unlike the lower third of the auricle, contains no cartilage, procedures can differ from those to reconstruct the lower auricle (see p. 74). Operations to repair tears as well as procedures for reconstruction will be presented. See also the descriptions of surgical correction of **hypoplasia** (see p. 80) and hyperplasia in the chapter on malformations (pp. 166 ff).

Traumatic Earlobe Cleft

Example: Earring avulsions.

Historical note. In many cultures it is customary to wear earrings, and sometimes extremely heavy or large pieces of jewellery are inserted into the earlobe (Fig. 4.78).

Thus Celsus (25 BC–AD 30, in Zeis 1863) writes:

> If the hole in the earlobe is large, as it tends to be in those who wear heavy ornaments in their ears, then the remaining bridge should be divided and the margins of the hole additionally freshened with a knife. The wound margins are then sutured and a medication to promote adhesion is applied (Goedecke 1995).

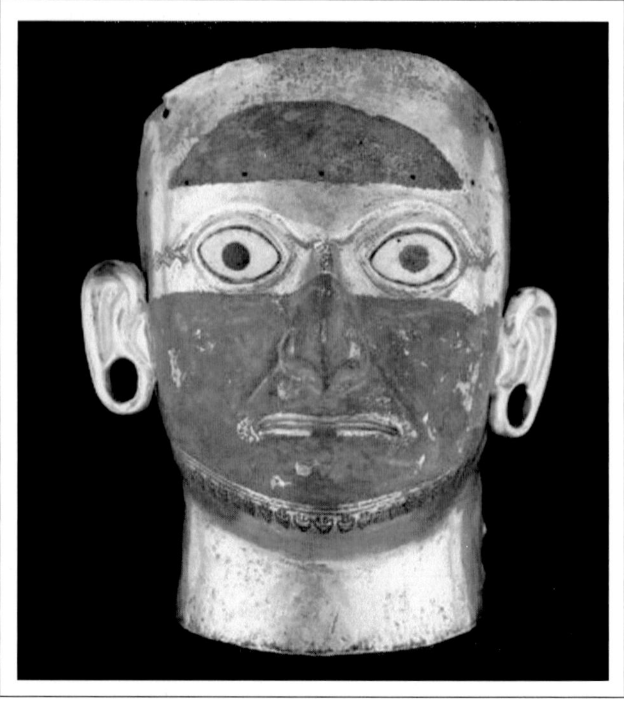

Fig. 4.78 **Earlobe defects in a mask of a king of the Moche culture, Northern Peru, 300–400 AD (Linden Museum, Stuttgart, Germany; photograph by A. Dreyer).**

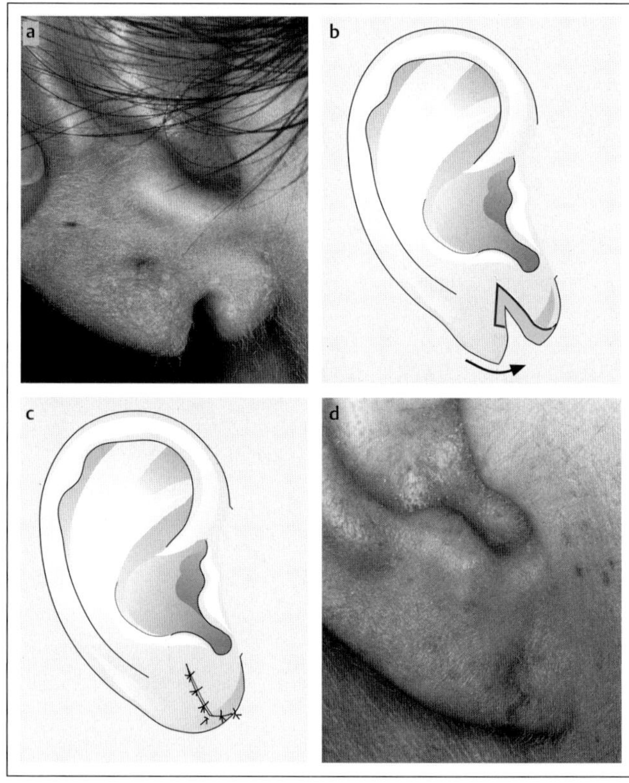

Fig. 4.79 **Passow's reconstruction of a cleft earlobe (in Mündnich 1962 a).**
a Defect after avulsion injury.
b L-shaped freshening of the margins.
c Suture without reconstruction of the earring perforation.
d Delicate, L-shaped scar.

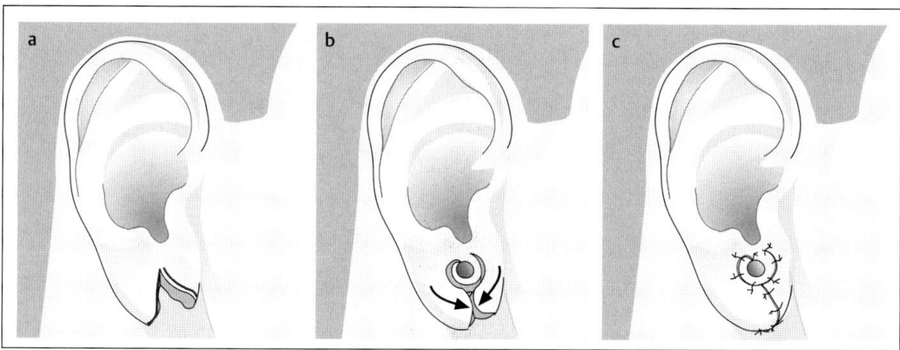

Fig. 4.**80** **Reconstruction of a torn earlobe with preservation of the perforation for an earring, as described by Pardue (1973).**

a An epithelialized flap is prepared and the wound margins are freshened.

b, c The flap is rolled in upon itself and the wounds are closed with 6–0 (7–0) monofilament sutures.

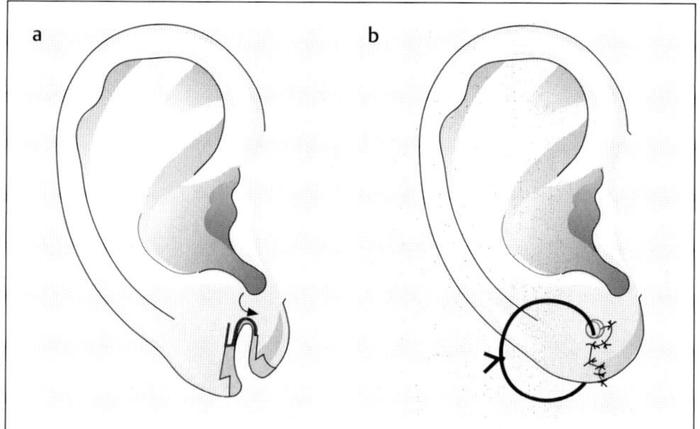

Fig. 4.**81** **L-plasty reconstruction with preservation of the earring hole as described by Fatah (1985).**

a An epithelialized flap is incised and the wound margins are freshened to form an L-shape.

b Closure in layers with placement of a small silicone rubber spacer.

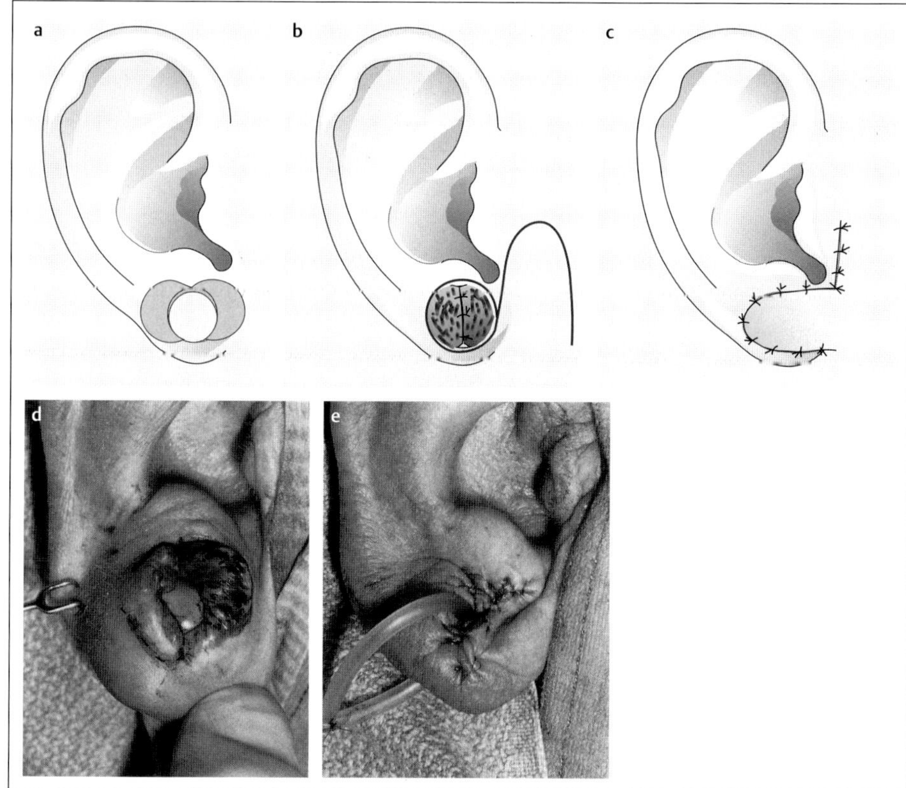

Fig. 4.**82** **Reconstruction of a central earlobe defect using the technique of Mohan et al. (1978).**

a Hinge flaps to resurface the posterior surface.

b Elevation of a small, inferiorly based preauricular transposition flap patterned from a template.

c Closure of the defect.

d Hinge flaps for the reconstruction of the posterior surface, small transposition flap to reduce the hole.

e Appearance after reconstruction with preservation of the hole for an earring.

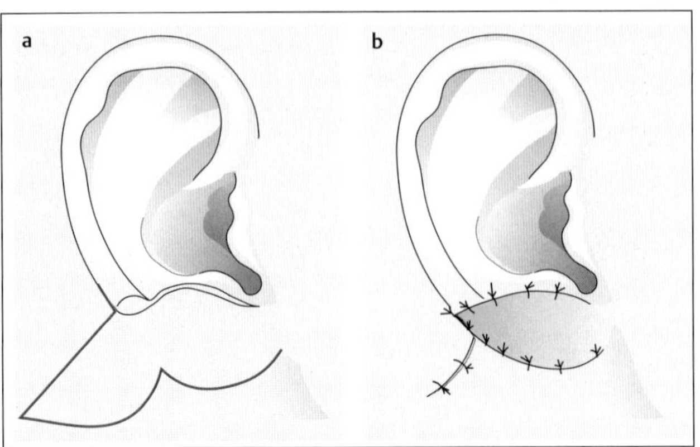

Fig. 4.83 a, b **Reconstruction of the lower auricle with a bilobed flap (corresponding to the Gavello flap, see pp. 75, 76; in Szymanowsky 1870).**

Reconstruction without Preservation of the Earring Perforation

Like Celsus about 2000 years ago, McLaren (1954) also freshens up the margins of the defect within the split earlobe and then closes the margins in layers.

Passow's Procedure

(Fig. 4.**79**; as cited in Mündnich 1962 a)
After avulsion injury, the wound margins are excised in a stepwise fashion (Fig. 4.**79 b**) and the earlobe subsequently reconstructed (Fig. 4.**79 c**, **d**).

Reconstruction with Preservation of the Earring Perforation

The perforation also requires reconstruction in order to allow further wearing of earrings.

Pardue's Method of Reconstruction

(Fig. 4.**80**; Pardue 1973)
A superiorly based epithelial flap is incised within the perforation (Fig. 4.**80 a**), the opposite side is de-epithelialized and the flap is folded in on itself (Fig. 4.**80 b**). The defects are then closed (Fig. 4.**80 c**).

Fatah's Stepwise Reconstruction with Resection of the Epithelial Layer

(Fig. 4.**81**; Fatah 1985)
Various other modifications have been described. The techniques suggested here can also be used without preservation of the perforation.

Reduction of the earlobe will be discussed under malformations of the earlobe (see pp. 165 ff).

Defects of the Earlobe

These can be resurfaced with local flaps.

Mohan et al.'s Reconstruction of a Central Defect

(Fig. 4.**82**; Mohan et al. 1978)
After closure of the posterior defect with two hinge flaps, a preauricular transposition flap is raised adjacent to the defect, which is subsequently covered (see also section on partial reconstructions of the lower auricle, p. 75, and of the earlobe, p. 76).

Loss of the Earlobe

Example: hypoplasia or aplasia.

Historical note. Sushruta (1000 AD, as cited in Zeis 1883; Meyer and Sieber 1973; Davis 1987) reports on the reconstruction of the earlobe which had most likely been performed in this manner for hundreds of years:

> A surgeon can reconstruct the earlobe in a person devoid of them by slicing off a patch of living flesh from that person's cheek in a manner so as to have one of its ends attached to the cheek. Then the part where the artificial earlobe is to be made should be slightly scarified, and the living flesh should be made to adhere to it.

The first description of a pedicled flap from the vicinity of the defect has from that time on been referred to as the "Indian method" (Goedecke 1995). In 1597 Tagliacozzi also described the reconstruction of the lower auricle (see Fig. 4.**1**, p. 43; Mündnich 1962 a).

The reconstruction of the earlobe is described in a similar way by Dieffenbach (1845 b, see Fig. 4.**3**). After freshening the margins of the defect, the infra-auricular skin is incised, elevated, and sutured into position. After 3 weeks this flap is divided inferiorly and folded over to cover the posterior surface.

For his "total auricular reconstruction," Szymanowsky (1870) incised around the earlobe in a manner similar to a Gavello flap (Fig. 4.**83**; see also Fig. 4.**84**).

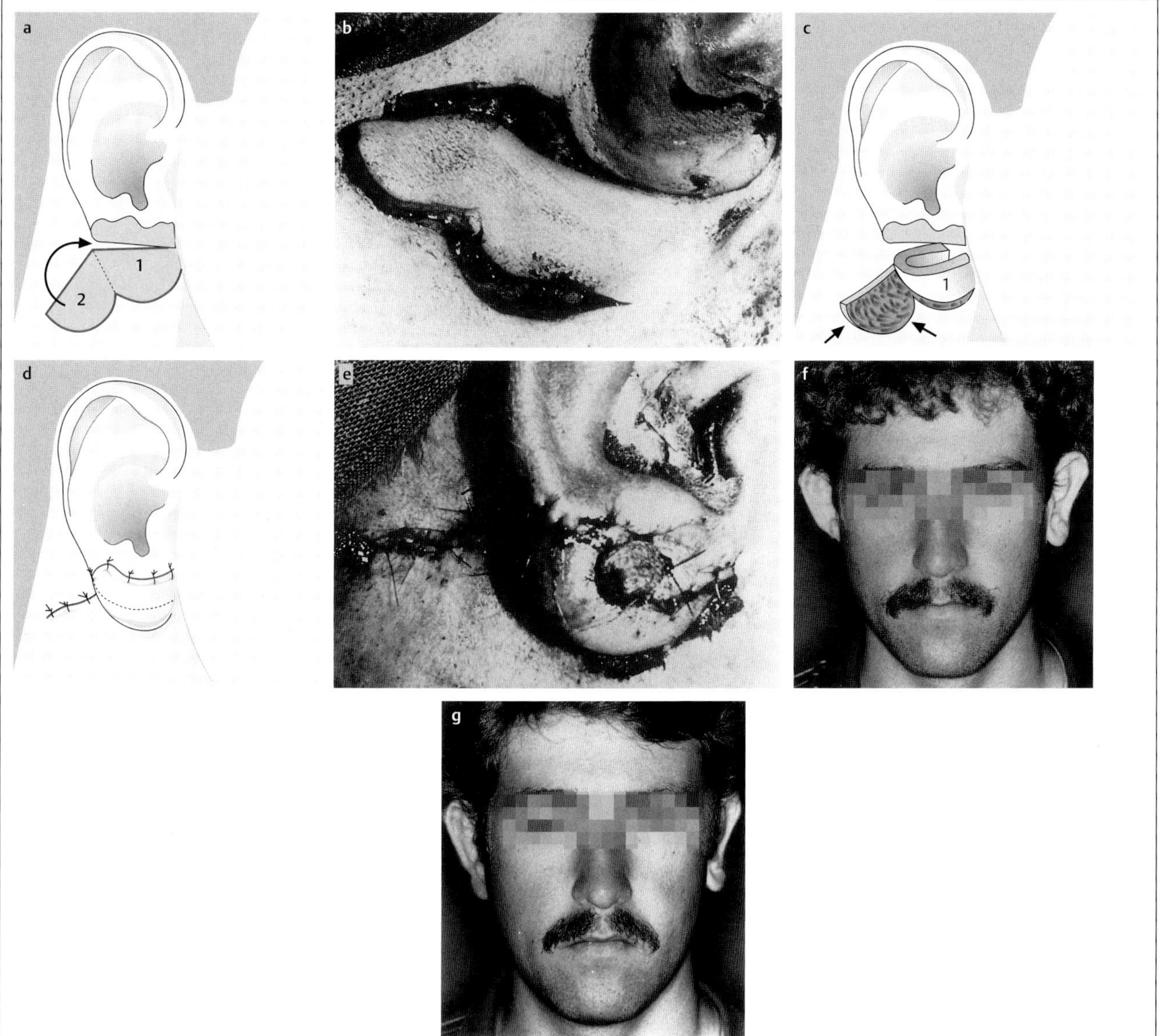

Fig. 4.**84** **Earlobe reconstruction using a Gavello flap (1907; in Szymanowsky 1870; see Fig. 4.83).**

a, b Anteriorly based, bilobed flap (1, 2) is raised below the auricular defect after fashioning a template as descıbed earller.

c The second flap (2) is folded over behind the first (1).

d, e Closure of the wounds (by mobilizing the inferior skin, the scar of the donor region comes to lie behind the auricle).

f, g One of my first Gavello flaps, from the early 1970 s: before the operation (**f**), result (**g**) (see also Fig. 4.**73**, and p. 193).

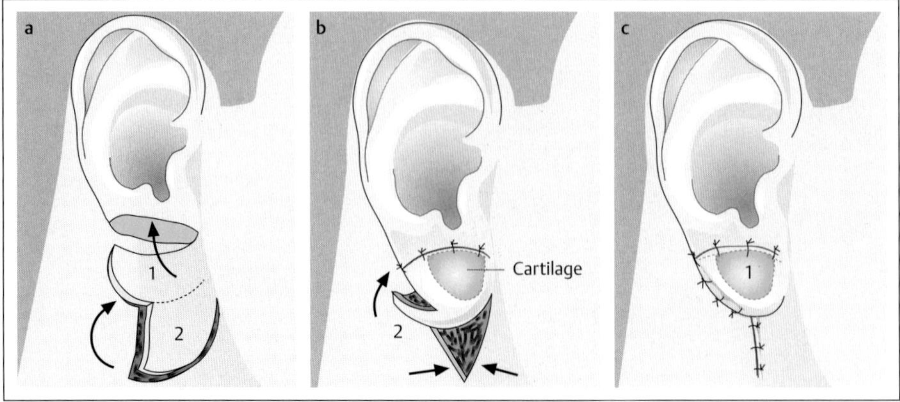

Fig. 4.**85** **Earlobe reconstruction as described by Alanis (1970), modified.**

a The margins of the defect are freshened and the anterior surface (1) is incised, the posterior surface is incised inferiorly(2). The anterior flap (1) is slightly larger than the second flap.

b Flap 1 is sutured into place and flap 2 is folded over a piece of cartilage harvested from the concha or a rib to cover the posterior surface.

c Closure of all defects (slight disadvantage: the scar beneath the earlobe is visible). This technique is similar to that reported earlier by Sanvenero-Roselli (1932).

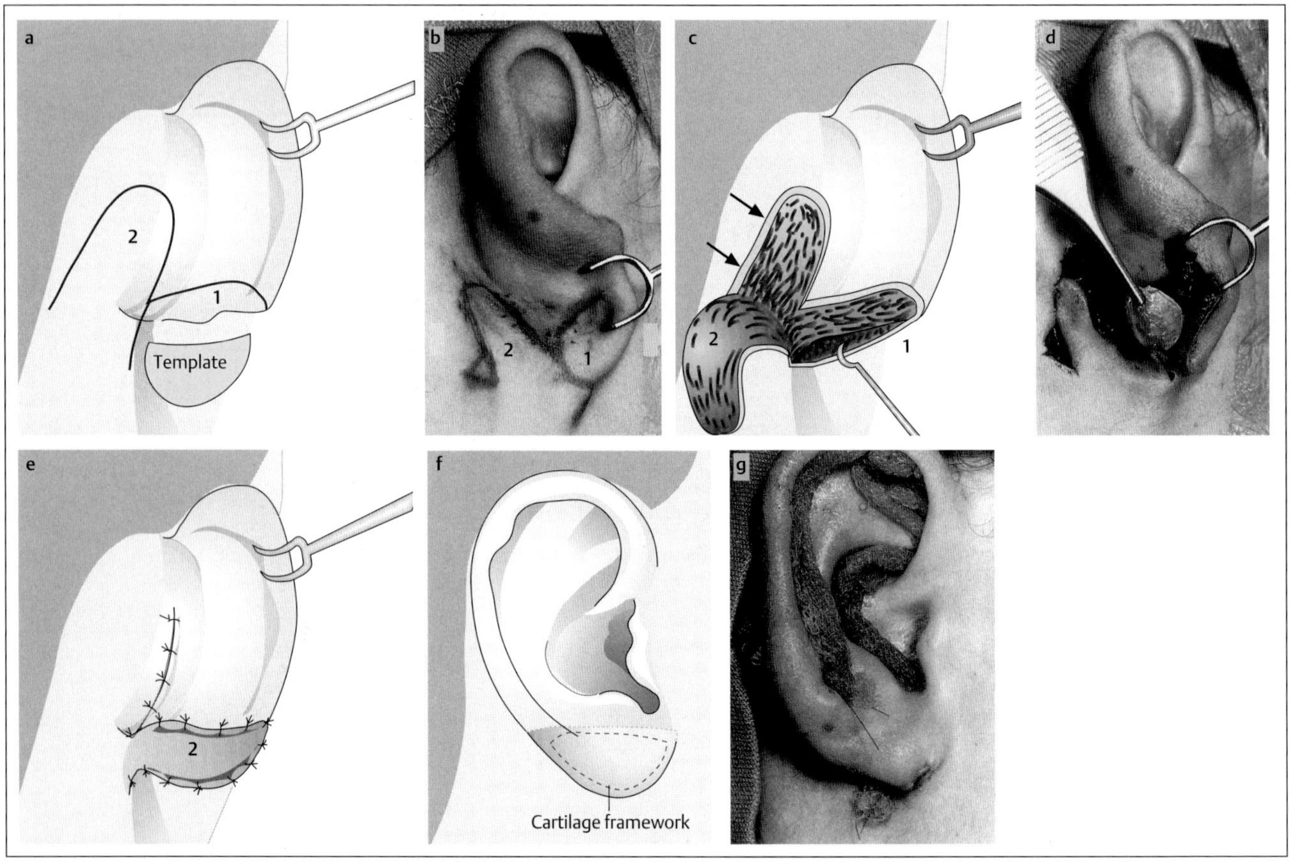

Fig. 4.**86** **Reconstruction of the earlobe with a turnover flap (1) designed from a template and an inferiorly based transposition flap (2) as described by Converse and Brent (1977).**

a, b Turn-over flap (1) designed from a template and an inferiorly based transposition flap (2).

c–e The flaps are dissected and inset and in addition a small conchal cartilage is inserted as a strut.

f, g Reconstructed earlobe at the end of the operation and otoplasty (surgeon: R. Katzbach).

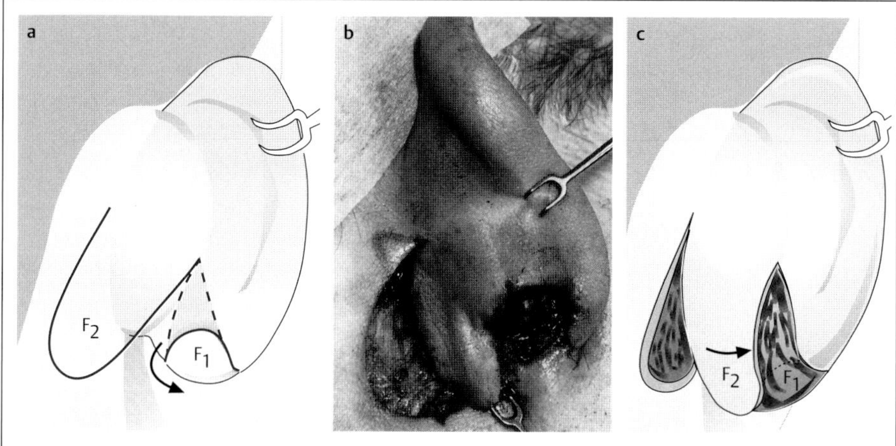

Fig. 4.**87** a–c **Reconstruction of the earlobe using a turnover flap (F_1) and a superiorly based transposition flap (F_2), modified after Bethmann and Zoltan (1968).**

Recommended Operations

Gavello's Method of Earlobe Reconstruction

(Fig. 4.**84**; as cited in Nelaton and Ombredanne 1907)

As previously described for the reconstruction of the lower auricle, we often use the double-flap method reported by Gavello for reconstruction of the earlobe (see also Figs. 4.**72**–4.**75**), previously described by Szymanowsky (1870; see Fig. 4.**83**). After freshening the margins of the defect, the flap is raised, patterned from a template made of aluminum foil or similar material, and folded over. For this purpose the anterior flap (Fig. 4.**84** **a**, **b**; 1) is chosen slightly larger than the second flap, bringing the lower suture line to lie on the posterior surface of the new earlobe.

The secondary defect is then closed by mobilizing the surrounding skin. Larger defects will require a cartilaginous framework, harvested from the ipsi- or contralateral concha, which is sutured into the flap (see Figs. 4.**71**, 4.**72**, pp. 75, 76).

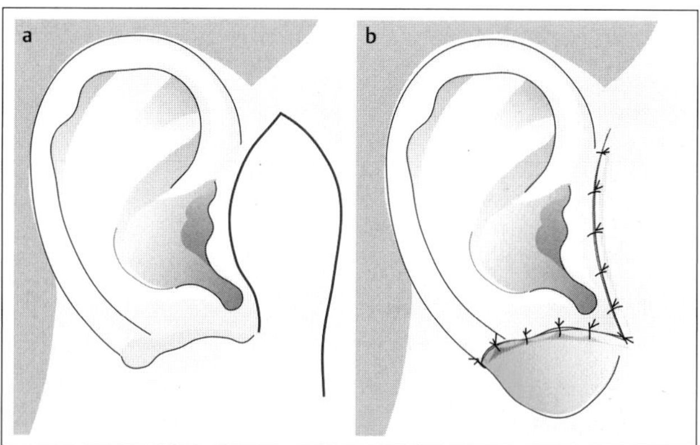

Fig. 4.**88** **Preauricular flap as described by Pitanguy and Flemming (1976).**
a Incision of a flap designed from a template.
b The flap is raised, rotated, and sutured in place before all defects are closed.

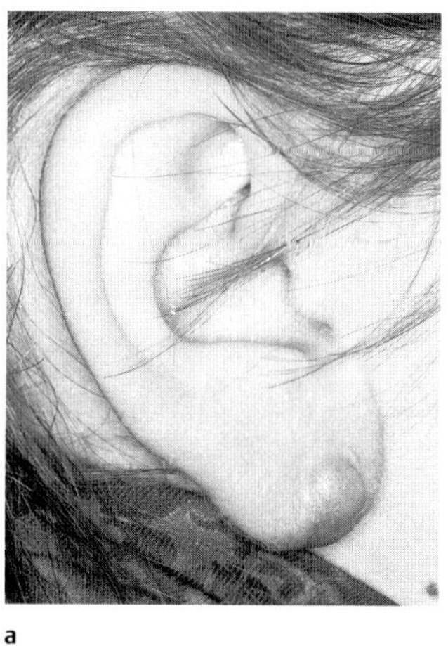
a

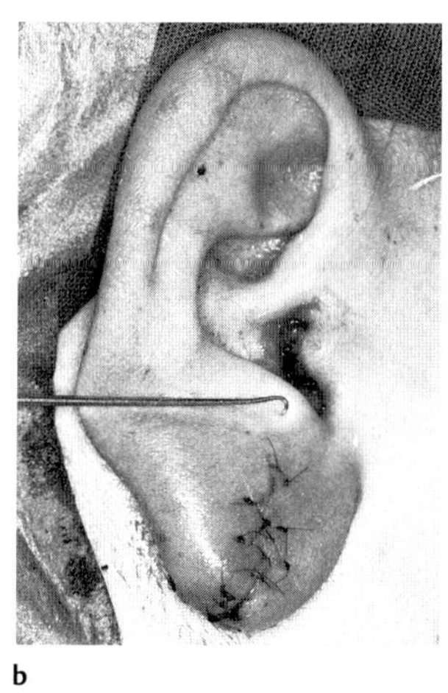
b

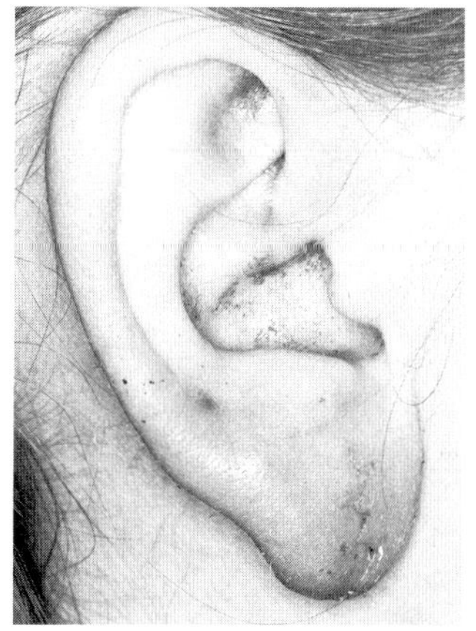
c

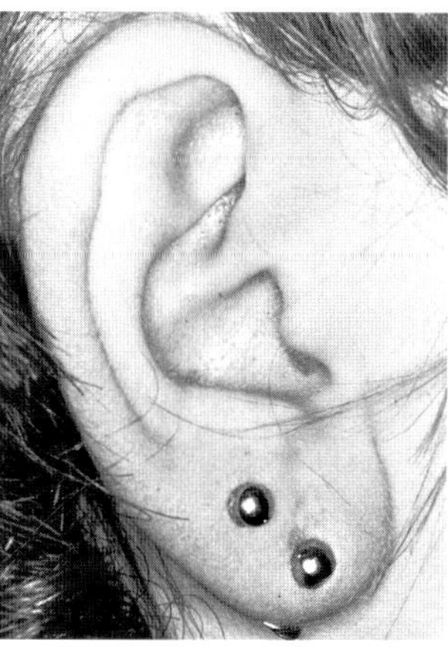
d

Fig. 4.**89** **Scar revision and staggering with a W-plasty or the broken line technique (see Weerda 1999 a).**
a Hypertrophic scarring of the earlobe.
b Excision and staggering of the scar with a W-plasty.
c Result after 14 days (steroid solution was infiltrated).
d Result after 1 year, with ear studs.

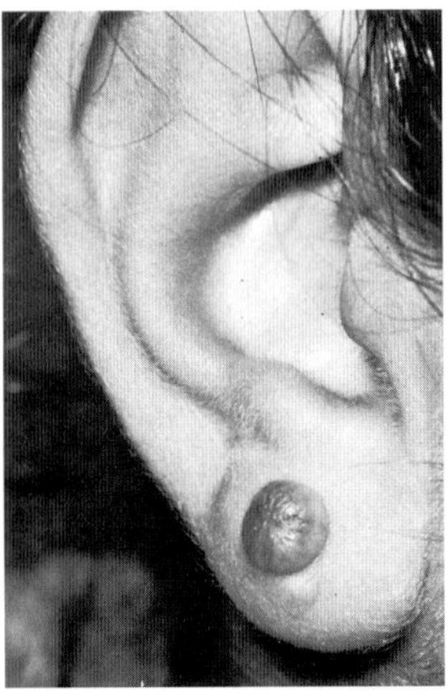
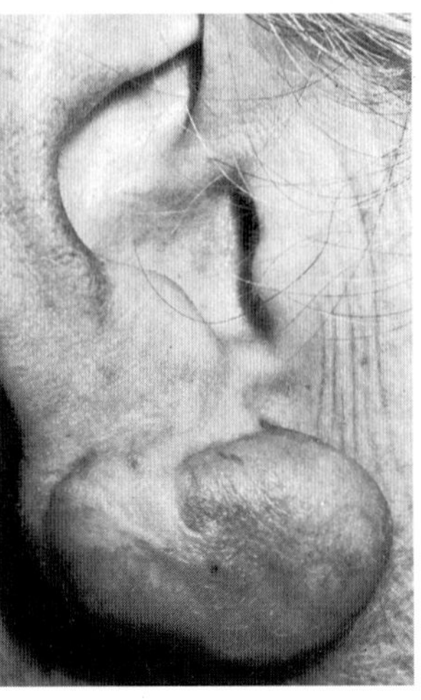

a b

Fig. 4.90 a, b **Keloids of various sizes secondary to piercing.**

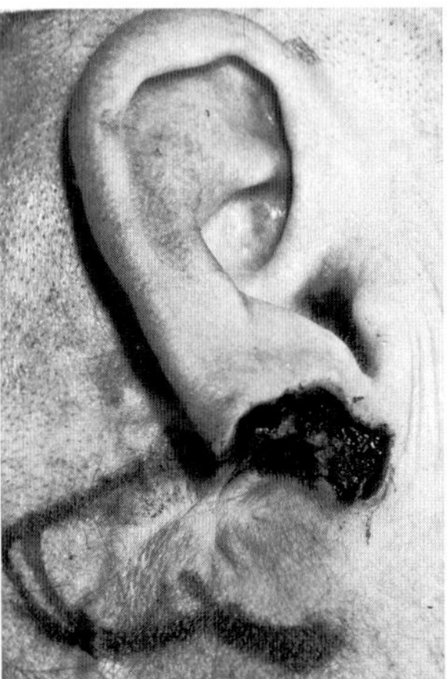
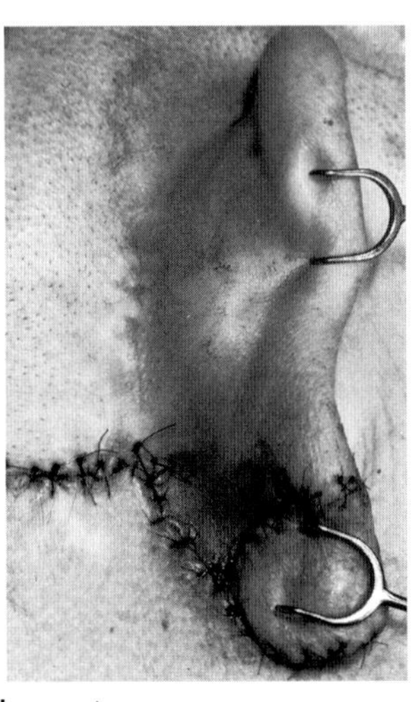

a b

Fig. 4.91 **Excision of the earlobe secondary to a large keloid (see Fig. 4.90 b) with reconstruction using a Gavello flap.**
a The keloid is excised and the Gavello flap outlined.
b Closure of all defects (see also Fig. 4.84 and p. 81).

Alanis's Reconstruction of the Earlobe
(Fig. 4.85; Alanis 1970)

Critique. The disadvantage of this method is that the scar comes to lie in front of the earlobe rather than behind it.

Converse and Brent's Reconstruction with a Hinge Flap and an Inferiorly Based Transposition Flap
(Fig. 4.86; Converse and Brent 1977)

Critique. A superiorly based transposition flap is more favorable (see Fig. 4.87).

Reconstructions Described in the Literature

Bethmann and Zoltan's Superiorly Based Transposition Flap — In 1968 Bethmann and Zoltan reported a similar method employing a superiorly based transposition flap (Fig. 4.87 a–c).

Pitanguy and Flemming's Preauricular flap
(Fig. 4.88 a, b; Pitanguy and Flemming 1976)
This flap must be raised relatively large, so it can occasionally prove to be inadequate to reconstruct a larger earlobe. It should only be used for small defects.

The methods described here will usually suffice to close all such defects. The many other methods described in the literature (Nelaton and Ombredanne 1907; Joseph 1931; Sanvenero-Rosseli 1932; Converse 1958, among others) are more time-consuming and effortful and do not provide such aesthetically good results.

Hypertrophic Scar Formation on the Earlobe

If possible, hypertrophic scars, which tend to settle down with time, but still remain unsightly, are excised and the wound closed with a W-plasty or the broken line technique. The results after 1 year are good (Fig. 4.89 c, d).

With lesions of the posterior surface, the skin of the anterior surface can usually be left untouched and the auricle is then closed with a transposition flap from the retroauricular region or from the sulcus (see p. 82).

For larger lesions with loss of the entire earlobe, reconstruction is accomplished—if possible—using Gavello's technique (see Figs. 4.84, 4.91).

Earlobe Keloids

Keloids can result from ear piercing (Fig. 4.90 a, b). Keloids are removed, and reconstruction depends upon the defects (see p. 146). Here too we like to use the Gavello flap (Fig. 4.91 a, b; see also p. 80 and Fig. 4.84).

4.2.5 Posterior Defects

The simplest method is to use thick split-thickness or full-thickness skin grafts if the perichondrium or periosteum is intact (see Fig. 4.103).

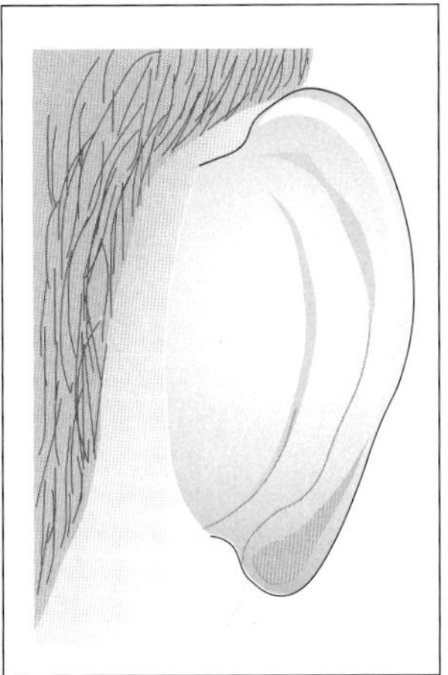

Fig. 4.92 **Postauricular defects.**

Postauricular Defects (Fig. 4.92)

Recommended Methods

Small Flaps

(Figs. 4.93, 4.94)

Smaller, two-layer defects can be closed with an inferiorly or superiorly based **rotation flap** (Fig. 4.93) or with a transposition flap. An additional island flap can be used for small, full-thickness defects (Fig. 4.94).

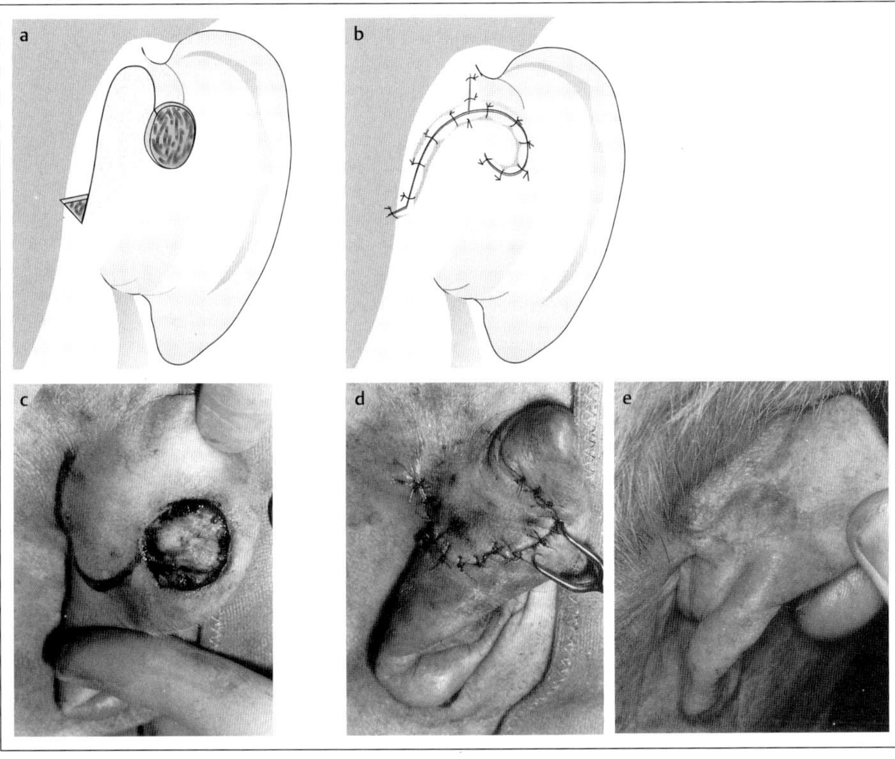

Fig. 4.93 **Closure of a two-layer defect with a small inferiorly (a, b) or superiorly (c–e) based rotation flap.**

a, b Incision of the inferiorly based rotation flap and coverage of the defect.

c Incision of the superiorly based rotation flap.

d Closure.

e Result.

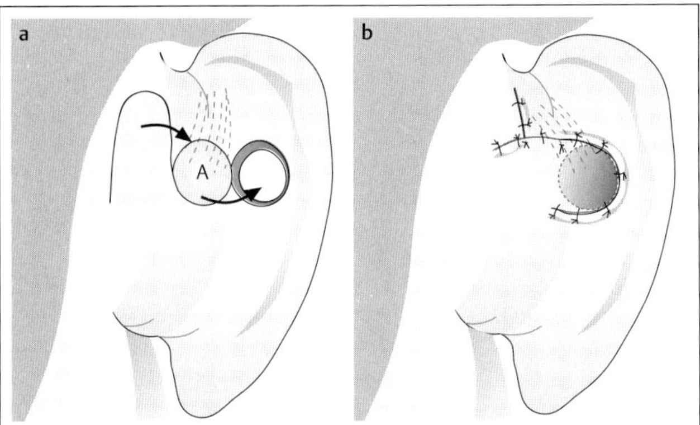

Fig. 4.94 **Closure of a full-thickness defect with an island flap and a transposition flap.**

a Elevation of an island flap (A) (see p. 47), which needs to be rotated, and the transposition flap.

b Closure of the defects (see also Fig. 4.93 **a, b**).

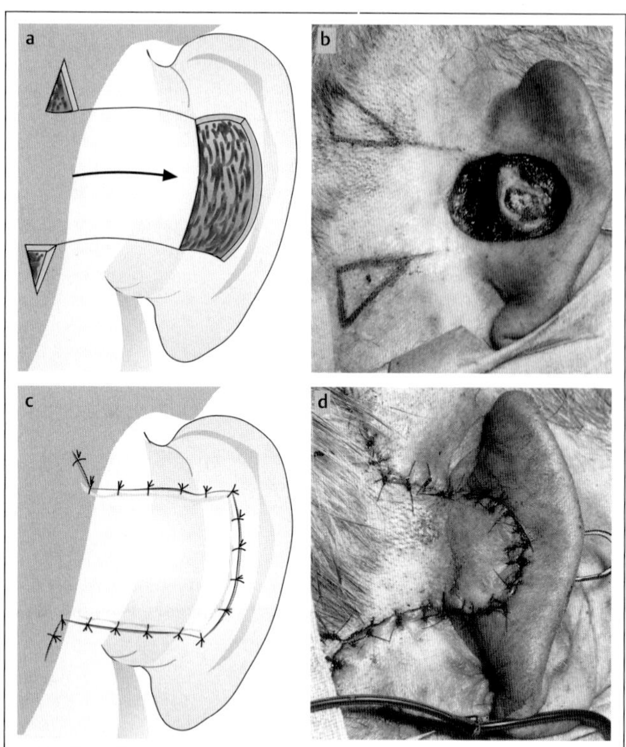

Fig. 4.**95** **Closure of a two-layer defect with a U-shaped Burow advancement flap (1853, as cited in Weerda 1991 a).**
a, b Elevation of the flap with Burow's triangles in the hair.
c, d Closure of the defects.

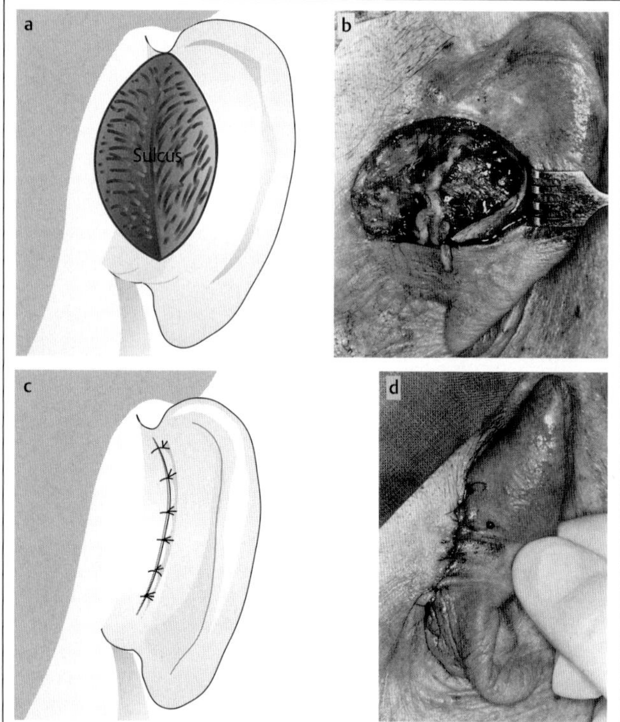

Fig. 4.**97** **Tumor excision or skin harvest, and primary closure by coverage with the auricle.**
a, b Defect after tumor excision.
c, d Closure using the entire auricular defect (and consequently reduction of the sulcus). The posterior helix should remain free.

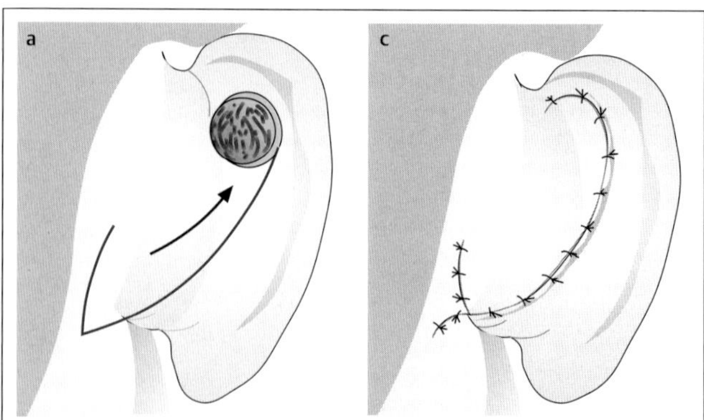

Fig. 4.**96 a, b** **VY-advancement (Petres and Rompel 1996) for a two-layer defect.**

U-formed Advancement Flap
(Fig. 4.**95**)
Advancement flaps are also suitable for covering a large number of two-layer defects (Fig. 4.**95 a–d**), as we have already previously encountered with the reconstruction of partial auricular defects (see Fig. 4.**64**).

VY-advancement
(Fig. 4.**96 a, b**)

Closure of Defects Caused by Skin Harvesting
(Fig. 4.**97**)
Wounds caused by tumor excision, skin harvesting (Fig. 4.**97 a, b**), island flap elevation (see p. 46), or similar procedures can be closed primarily, particularly in the sulcus. After excision of the entire post- and retroauricular skin, especially in the sulcus, the defect can be resurfaced with split-thickness skin (see Fig. 4.**103**), or the auricle can be sutured to the mastoid surface (Fig. 4.**97 c, d**). At least the helix should remain free (see Fig. 4.**105**).

Weerda's Bilobed Flaps
The hair-bearing transport flap transports the reconstruction flap which is raised behind the defect (see Fig. 4.**105**).

Weerda's Rotation–Transposition Flap
(Weerda and Münker, 1981, 1983 a, 1999 a; see p. 73, Fig. 4.**68**)

If sufficient skin is not available for a transposition or rotation flap, then a transposition flap based on a hair-bearing rotation flap can be used as a bilobed flap.

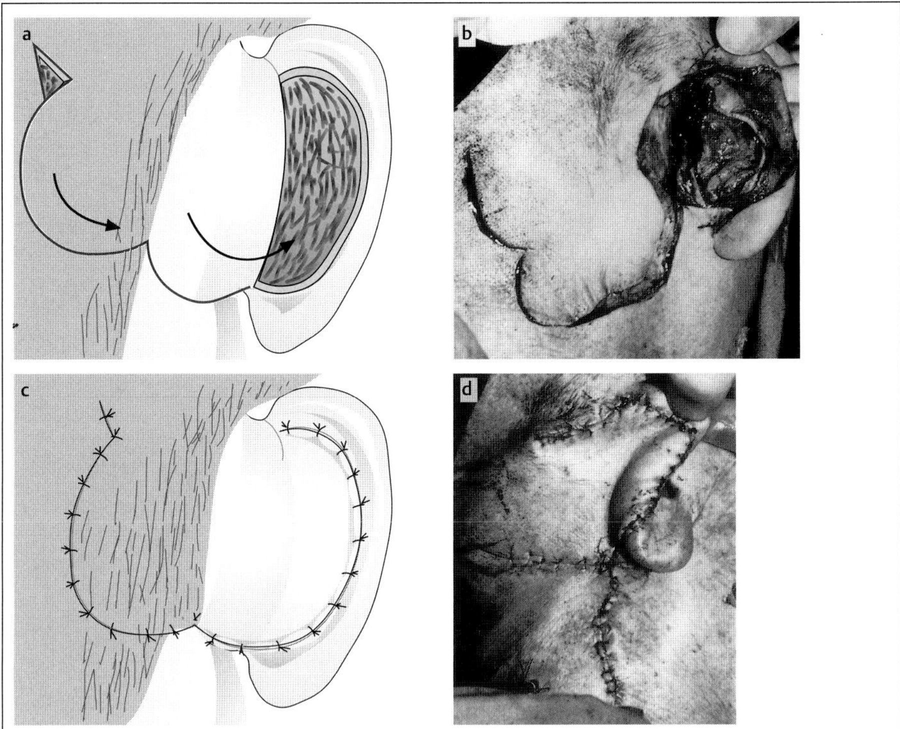

Fig. 4.**98** **Single-stage reconstruction of a posterior auricular defect using Weerda's double rotation flap (1983 a).**
a, b Defect; the hairless reconstruction flap and the hair-bearing transport flap are outlined.
c, d Mobilization and closure of the defects.

Weerda's Double Rotation Flap
(Fig. 4.**98**; Weerda 1983 a)
As with the flap described above, a double-rotation flap can be employed for large posterior defects (Fig. 4.**98 a–d**).

Retroauricular Defects (Fig. 4.99)

If primary closure is not possible for defects of the mastoid region, a split- or full-thickness skin graft can be used in the "ear's shadow" (see Fig. 4.**103**).

Elliptical or W-shaped Excisions and Primary Closure
(Fig. 4.**100**)

Preauricular Transposition Flap
(Fig. 4.**101**)

Coverage with Skin of the Postauricular Surface and Rotation of the Cavum
(see Fig. 4.**97**)

Free Skin Grafts
(see Fig. 4.**103**)
For larger defects, or for harvesting skin to cover defects of the face, we use split-thickness or full-thickness skin grafts from the thorax, abdominal, groin, or thigh regions for coverage (see Fig. 4.**103**).

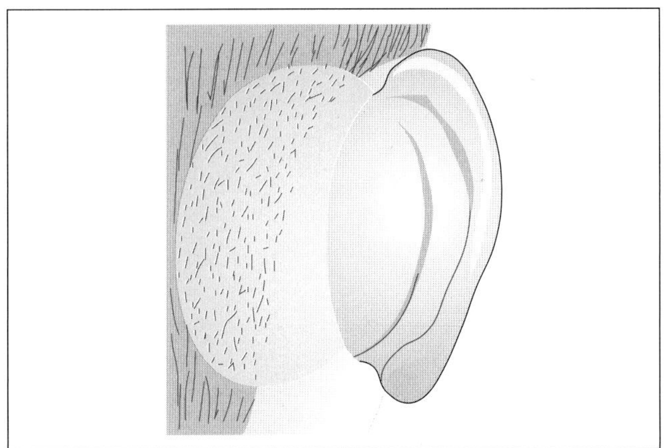

Fig. 4.**99** **Retroauricular (mastoid) defects.**

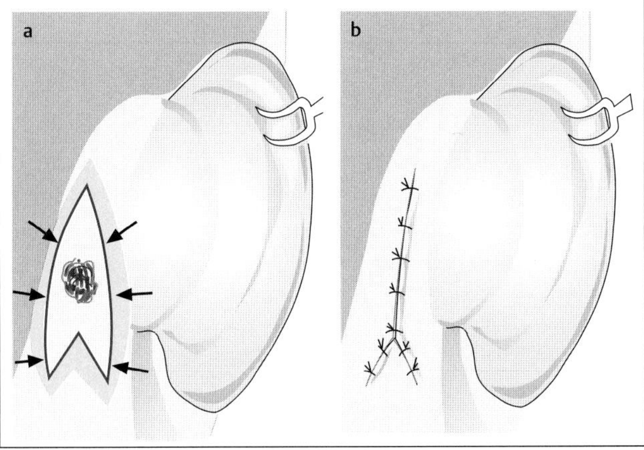

Fig. 4.**100 a, b** **Elliptical or W-shaped excision and primary closure (Petres and Rompel 1996).**

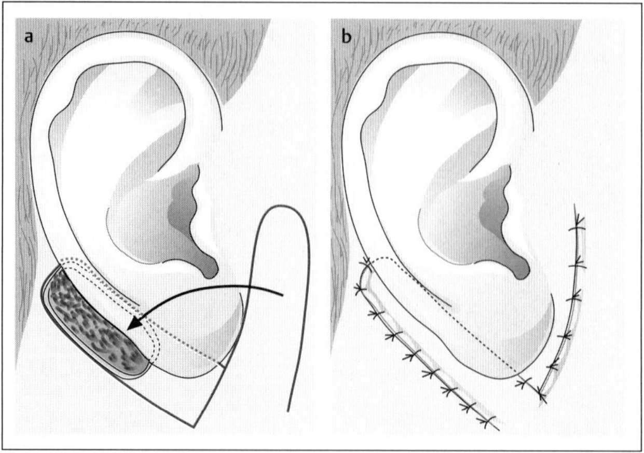

Fig. 4.**101** **Preauricular flap.**
a Preauricular, inferiorly based transposition flap.
b Appearance after closure (Pennisi et al. 1965).

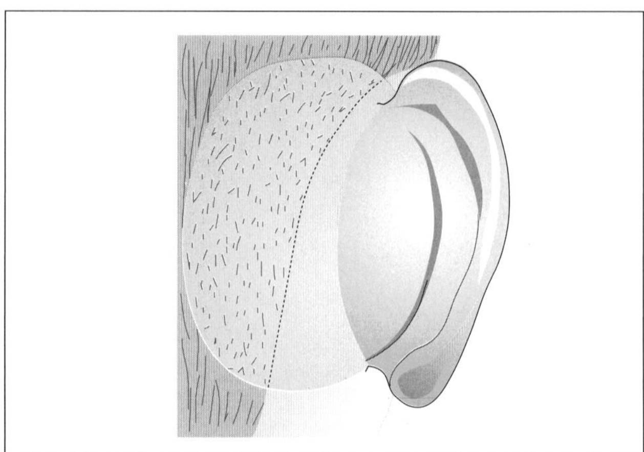

Fig. 4.**102** **Combined post- and retroauricular defects.**

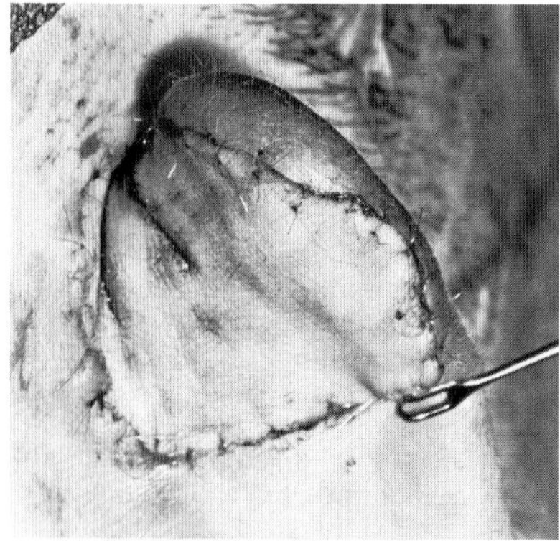

Fig. 4.**103** **Coverage of a post- and retroauricular defect with a free full-thickness skin graft, sutured and glued with fibrin adhesive.**

Combined Post- and Retroauricular Defects (Fig. 4.102)

Here we use free split-thickness or full-thickness skin grafts (Fig. 4.**103**) and the same flaps as described on pp. 85–88 for coverage.

More extensive defects are dealt with in the section on "Subtotal defects."

4.2.6 Subtotal Defects

Depending on their site, subtotal auricular defects can be managed in the same way as reconstructions of the upper segment (see p. 63), the middle auricular third (see p. 69), or the lower auricle (see p. 74).

Special Reconstructive Techniques

These special techniques may be useful for cases where the helix and earlobe have been preserved.

Single-stage Reconstruction with Weerda's Bilobed Flap as a Transposition–Rotation Flap

(Fig. 4.**104**; see Fig. 4.**68**; Weerda and Münker 1982, 1999 a, 2001)

After a full-thickness, subtotal defect with loss of the mastoid skin and preservation of the helix and earlobe (Fig. 4.**104 a–e**), a framework is first fashioned in the usual manner (see pp. 202–204). Next, using a rotation–transposition flap, the part of the **reconstruction flap** beneath the helix is de-epithelialized, and this flap is then transported into the defect via the rotation flap (**transport flap**). It is thus possible to close all the defects in a single stage.

Two hairless transposition flaps (Fig. 4.**104 a–c**; 1 and 2) are raised as reconstruction flaps to close the secondary defect. These flaps are transported into the defects by the hair-bearing rotation flap (Fig. 4.**104 a, d, e**).

Single-stage Reconstruction of the Anterior Surface with a Bilobed Flap

(Fig. 4.**105**)

A carcinoma invading the auricular soft tissue, the petrous bone, and the surrounding skin was removed. The patient, was left with only the auricular frame comprising helix, earlobe, and tragus. This huge defect was covered with a double rotation flap over which the auricular frame was placed (Fig. 4.**105 a, b**). The outcome was a good aesthetic result (Fig. 4.**105 c**).

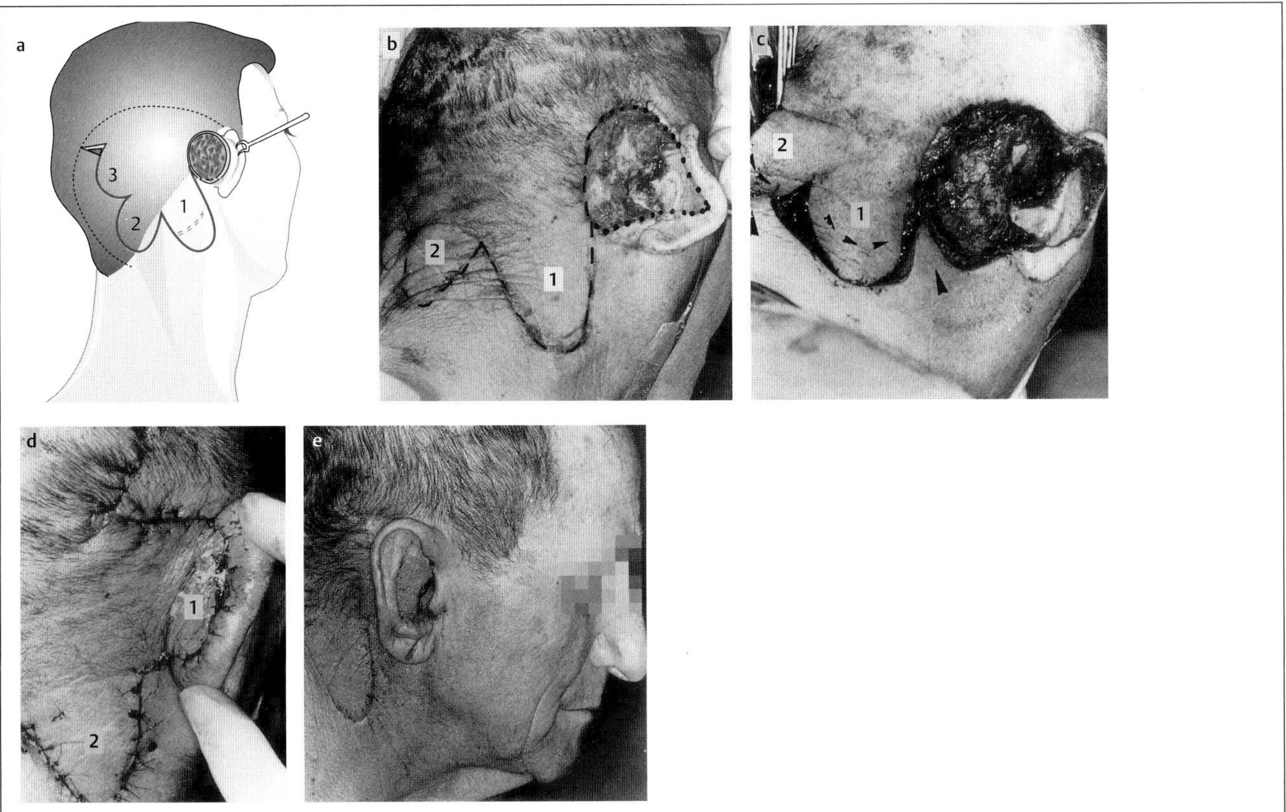

Fig. 4.**104** **Single-stage reconstruction of a subtotal auricular defect and a defect of the mastoid surface with a Weerda bilobed or trilobed flap (1982).**

a–c The two hairless transposition flaps (1, 2 = reconstruction flaps) are used for reconstruction of the auricle (1) over a cartilage framework and for coverage of the secondary defect (2). The rotation flap (3 = transport flap) transports the flaps into the correct position. Flap 1 is deepithelialized at the site which comes to lie beneath the tunnel when passed anteriorly (broken lines).

d Closure of the defect: posterior region.

e Reconstructed ear and resurfaced adjacent region.

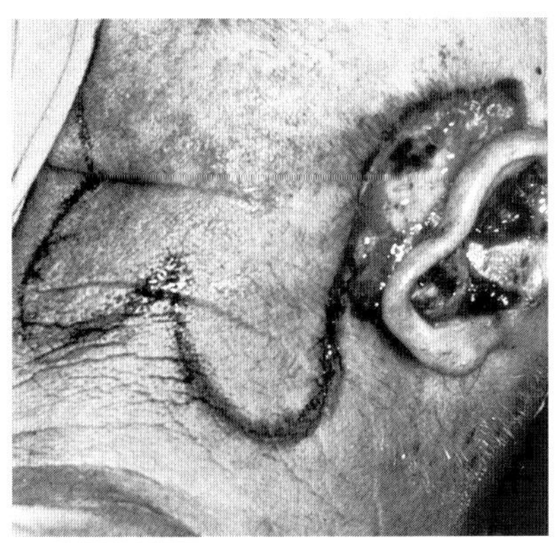

a

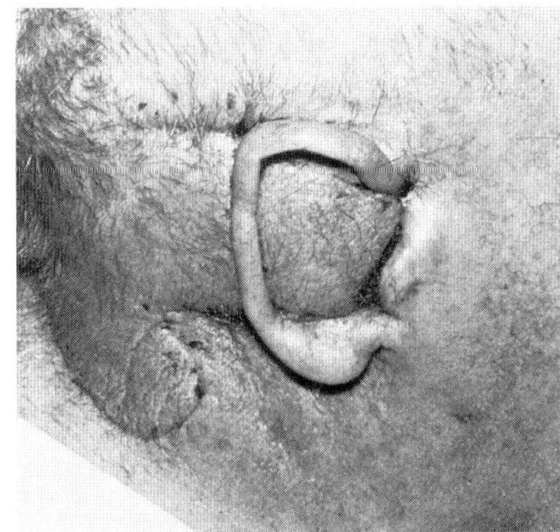

b

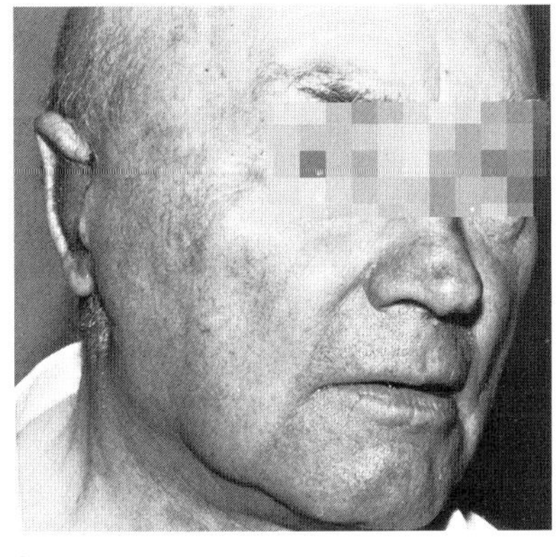

c

Fig. 4.**105** **Single-stage reconstruction of the anterior auricular surface with a bilobed flap in a case with preservation of the auricular frame and a large defect of the periauricular region.**

a Defects of the mastoid region and the central auricle after tumor excision. Helix, tragus, and earlobe still intact. Elevation of a bilobed flap.

b Healed appearance after placing the “frame” over the flap, which has been de-epithelialized along the corresponding margin.

c Good cosmetic result in half-profile in a patient over 80 years of age.

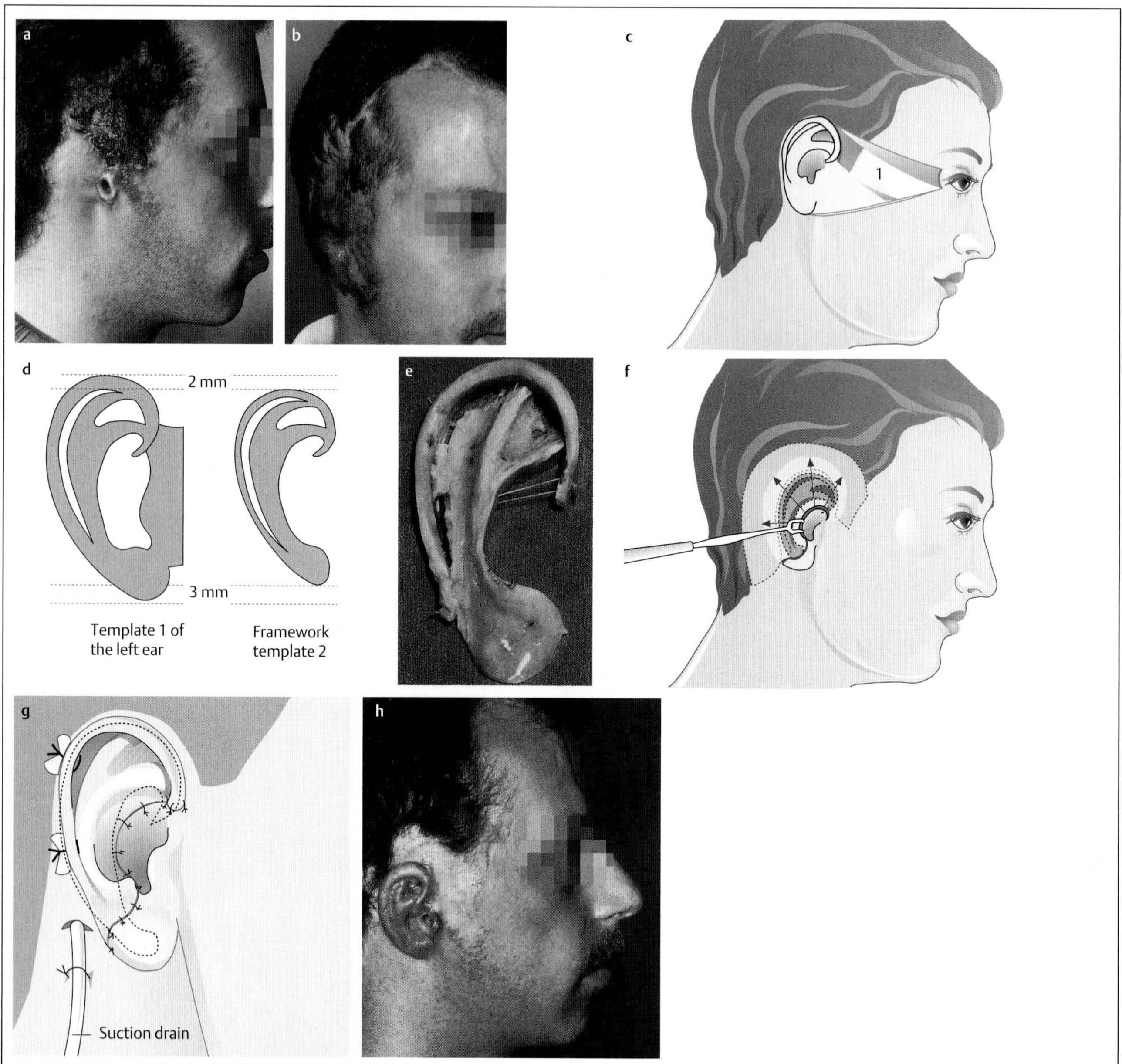

Fig. 4.**106** **Total auricular reconstruction (avulsion injury sustained in a road traffic accident).**
First stage:
a Total auricular loss with severe abrasions and scar formation.
b Prolonged expansion required because of the presence of severe scar tissue (see p. 231).
c The template designed from the contralateral side (see p. 64, pp. 202–204) is placed over the stump remnants, and the future position of the ear is outlined, which is usually well defined by the stump remnants.
d–f A slightly smaller framework is carved using template 2 (see also p. 64) and placed in its anatomically correct position (for template see also Fig. 5.**156**).
g Vacuum drain and closure.
h Result after three stages (see reconstruction for grade III dysplasia, pp. 209, 210, 213 ff).

4.2.7 Reconstruction After Total Auricular Loss

(see also pp. 197 ff, grade III microtia)

Definition. After total auricular loss, at most only the remnants of the earlobe, helical crus, ascending helix, and tragus are preserved.

Reconstruction with Local Skin

(Figs. 4.**106**, 4.**107**)

Depending on the condition of the skin in the region where the ear has been lost, it may be possible to reconstruct the auricle using local skin (otherwise with a temporoparietal fascial flap, see Figs. 4.**69**, 4.**108** and 4.**109**).

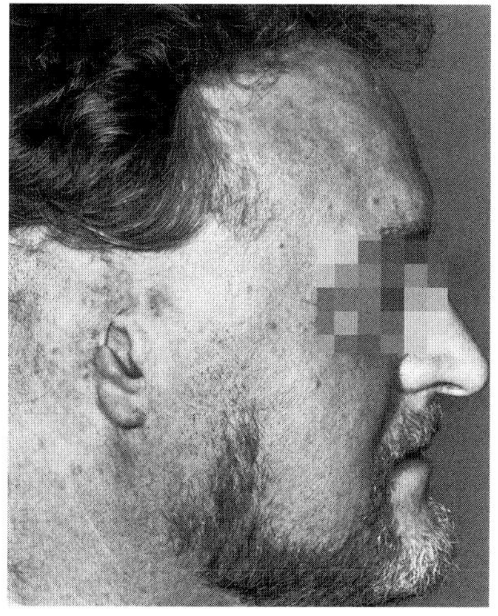
a

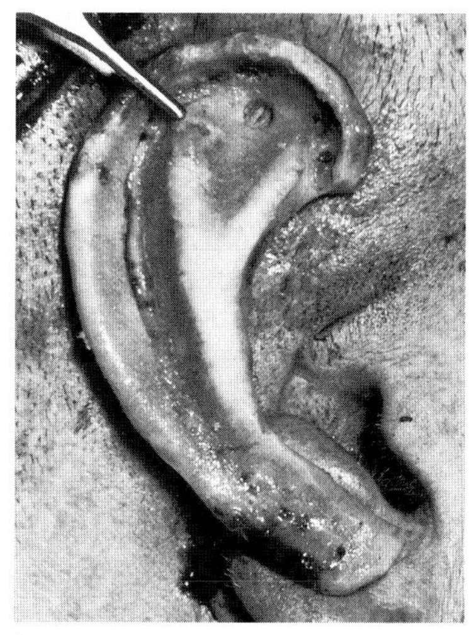
b

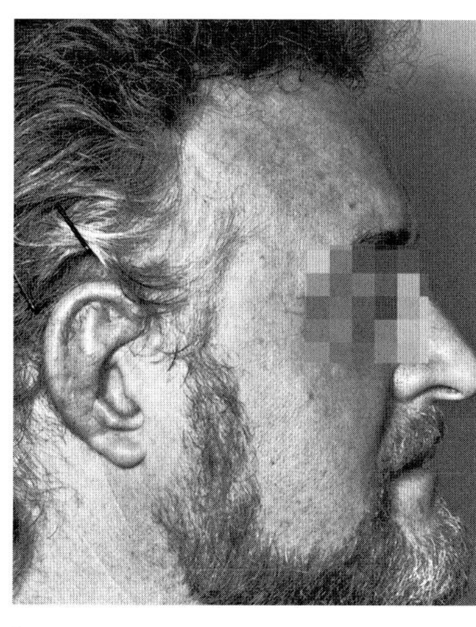
c

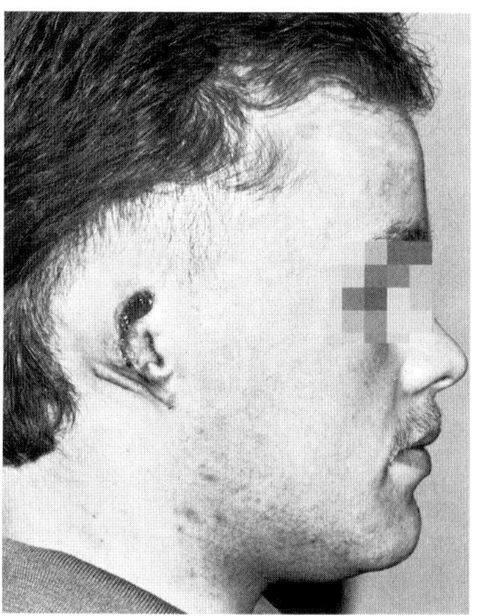
d

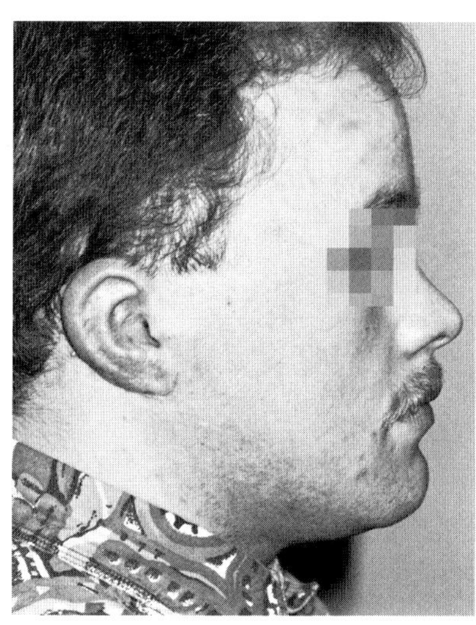
e

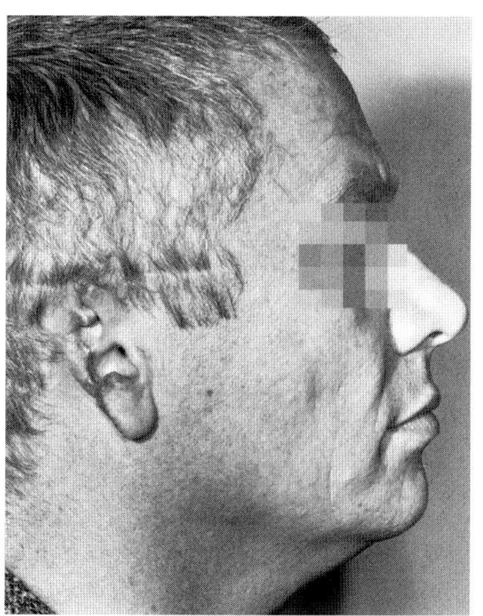
f

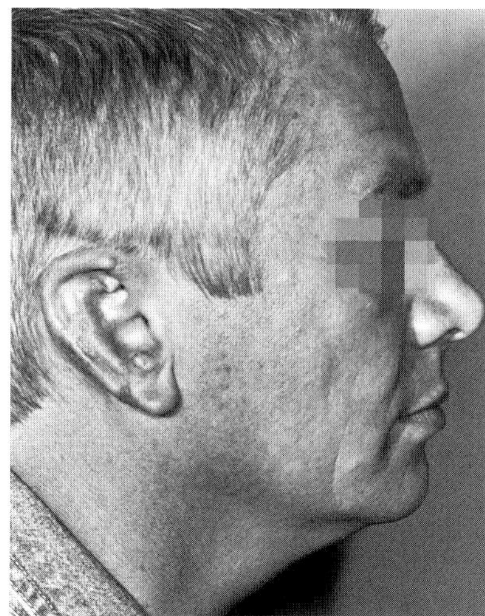
g

Fig. 4.**107** **Total reconstruction after avulsion.**
a Defect with residual earlobe and tragus.
b Frame and position of the frame.
c Appearance after two reconstruction stages.
d–i Examples of reconstruction. (see also Figs. 4.**39**, 4.**106**, 4.**109**).

Fig. 4.**107** **h, i** ▷

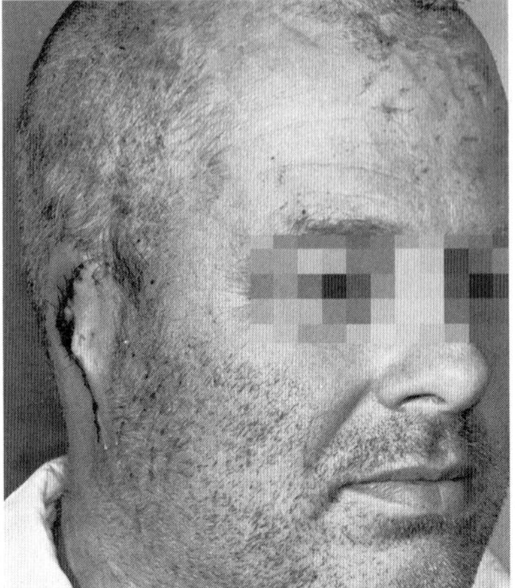
h

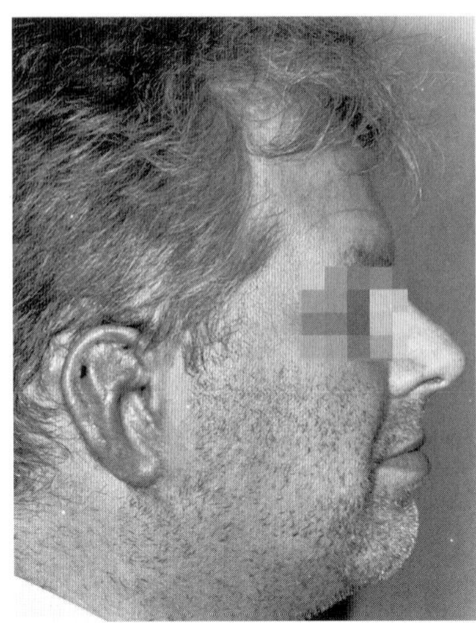
i

Fig. 4.**107 h, i**

Fabrication of templates. In a manner similar to that used for partial defects (see Fig. 4.**50**), a template is first fashioned from the healthy side (Fig. 4.**106 c**, **d**, template 1; see also pp. 64, 202–204). The position of the intact part of the auricle is then traced onto the region of the missing ear, with the position of the auditory canal, the tragus, the helical crus, and the remnants of the earlobe providing orientation in establishing the correct position of the new auricle (see also section on grade III dysplasia, pp. 209, 210, 216). We usually use the first template, which is based on the original size of the healthy ear, to fashion a second template which is about 2 mm smaller in every dimension (Fig. 4.**106 d**; 2). The templates are sterilized and taken into the operating room.

Preparations on the day before the operation. The patient's scalp is shaved to a width of 5–7 cm around the ear, the hair is washed the day before, and the region of the ear is prepped and draped. The contralateral site is shaved to a width of 1–1.5 cm, prepped and draped.

Informed consent. Both ears are prepped and draped because cartilage or skin is occasionally required from the healthy ear. The informed consent must take this into consideration.

Positioning. The patient is usually intubated and positioned supine.

Harvesting costal cartilage. The thorax is also prepped and draped (on the side where the surgeon is situated, with the anesthetist on the other side) in order to harvest the costal cartilage (6th, 7th, 8th, occasionally 9th rib).

First-stage operation. A second team harvests the cartilage while the ear is being dissected (see pp. 204, 205).

After the costal cartilage is obtained, it is used to make a lightweight cartilage framework patterned on the second (smaller) template, following the suggestions made by Tanzer (1974 a) and Brent (1987 b, 1998) (Fig. 4.**106 e**).

Preparation of the ear. In cases of severe burn injuries and significant scar formation an expander can be implanted initially to condition the skin and increase the amount available (see Fig. 4.**55**, p. 66, and Chapter 5.4.5, p. 231).

In the region of the auditory canal, the old scar is incised from the helical crus around the auditory canal, and if necessary excised. From here a pocket is carefully developed with dissection scissors according to the outline of the ear based on the first previously fashioned template. The dissection extends about 1 cm beyond the normal contour. From this incision, which extends from the auditory canal, the auricular framework (Fig. 4.**106 e**) is inserted into the pocket in the correct anatomical position (Fig. 4.**106 f**, **g**; see also Fig. 4.**107 b**). If necessary, the margins of the earlobe are freshened and the mastoid skin incised at the appropriate site (Fig. 4.**106 g**). The lower wound margin of the incision (see Fig. 4.**106 g**) is sutured to the posterior part of the earlobe, a pocket is dissected inside the earlobe, the inferior portion of the auricular framework is inserted into this pocket, and the anterior margin of the earlobe is sutured to the upper margin of the incision with a 6–0 monofilament suture. After placing a size 6 or 8 vacuum drain, the remaining wound is closed with a 6–0 monofilament suture. Two or three cotton bolsters secured by mattress sutures can be used to mold the skin to the contour of the helix (Fig. 4.**106 g**).

Second-stage operation. See second stage of auricular reconstruction for grade III dysplasia, pp. 207, 215 ff.

At the earliest 6–8 weeks after the first stage, as with procedures for correction of auricular malformations, an inci-

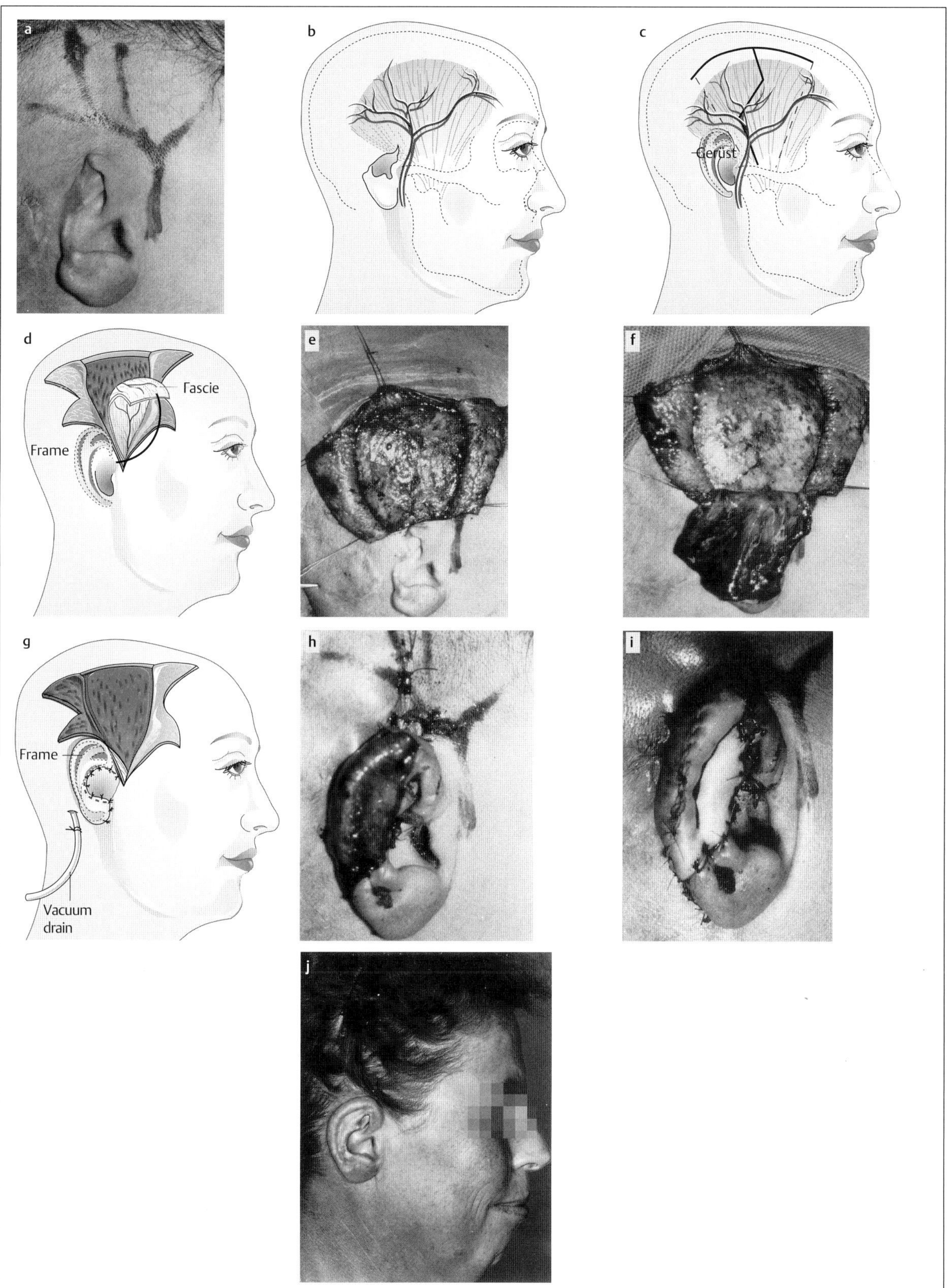

Fig. 4.**108** **Reconstruction with a temporoparietal fascial flap (fan flap) pedicled on the superficial temporal artery and vein above the thicker temporal fascia (as described by Weerda 2001 a).**

a, b Ear loss (see Fig. 4.**69**, p. 74). The superficial temporal artery and vein are identified using Doppler ultrasound.

c The temporoparietal fascia and vessels are exposed through a zigzag incision.

d–f The fascia is raised together with its vascular pedicle.

g, h The cartilage frame is covered with vascularized fascia.

i Then coverage with a thick split-thickness or full-thickness skin graft harvested from the retro- and postauricular region of the contralateral side, or from a similar site (see text, Abul-Hassan et al. 1986) and closure of all wounds (see Fig. 4.**97**, p. 86 and Fig. 4.**103**, p. 88).

j Result (surgeon: R. Siegert).

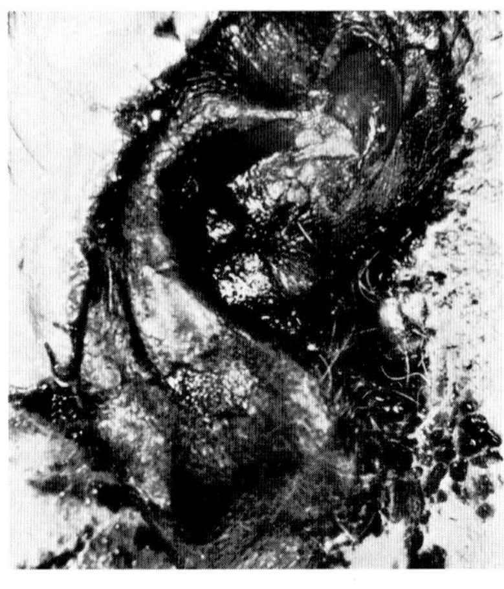

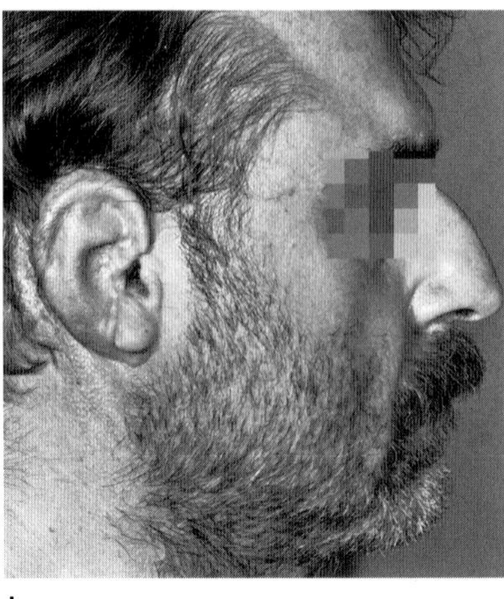

a b

Fig. 4.**109** **Reconstruction with a fan flap (see Fig. 3.21 e, f, p. 38).**
a Loss of an ear following avulsion and replantation performed in another institution using Baudet's technique (1972).
b Appearance after reconstruction with a fan flap.

sion is made around the auricle which is then elevated as in Nagata's operation for dysplasia (see pp. 215, 216). Using a size 15 blade, a full-thickness skin flap about 1 cm wide is incised above the hair follicles (see Fig. 5.**172 b**, pp. 215, 216) towards the framework, in order to achieve a good texture and color match of the helix after elevating the ear.

A piece of cartilage prepared during the first stage and stored at the donor site in a subcutaneous thoracic pocket (see Figs. 5.**164**, 5.**165**, p. 210) is inserted as a spacer and covered with a fascial flap (see Fig. 5.**172 d–i**). Then the primary defect over the mastoid is reduced after mobilizing the surrounding skin, a vacuum drain is inserted, and the residual defects are covered with thick split-thickness skin (see Fig. 5.**172 j–l**, pp. 215, 216). Further fine corrections may be made, if necessary, to improve the aesthetic result (see pp. 218 ff). Figures 4.**106 h** and 4.**107** show the results of this type of reconstruction following complete avulsion and loss of the auricle.

Reconstruction Using an Approach via an Incision in the Hair-bearing Scalp

(see Fig. 5.**182**, p. 221)
Sometimes a superior approach is chosen. We select this approach if we do not wish to revise the scars around the auditory canal, as well as for low hairlines, with the purpose of simultaneously removing the hair follicles.

Reconstruction with a Fan Flap

(Figs. 4.**108**, 4.**109**)

Reconstruction for total auricular loss using a temporoparietal fascial flap (fan flap; see Fig. 4.**69**, p. 74; Fox and Edgerton 1976; Brent and Byrd 1983).

A posteriorly and broadly based temporoparietal fascial flap will suffice for smaller defects in the upper auricular region, when there is not need to worry about blood supply. For total auricular avulsion and insufficient local skin, after multiple attempts at reconstruction with exhaustive use of the skin, or secondary to burn injuries, the fan flap requires dissection of the nutrient superficial temporal artery and vein (see Fig. 4.**108 a–c**). The fascia should be pedicled on these vessels and draped over the anterior and posterior surfaces of the cartilage framework (see Fig. 4.**108 g**).

Preparation. The appropriate half of the scalp is shaved around and above the ear in the region of the temporalis muscle, and the temporal vessels are plotted using Doppler ultrasound. The course of the vessels is mapped using the Doppler probe and marked (Fig. 4.**108 a, b**). The shaved side of the head is washed with povidone–iodine solution on the day before the operation and covered with a sterile dressing. The vascular markings should not be removed.

Positioning. The patient is positioned supine. On the evening before the operation a 1 cm margin is shaved around the contralateral ear as for a total reconstruction; the ear is prepped and also draped for the operation ready to harvest full-thickness skin from the retro- and postauricular region.

Approach to the fascia and dissection. The zigzag incision extends superior to and down anterior to the ear, with a transverse incision above the temporalis muscle. The incisions should just enter the adipose tissue layer, not deeper (Fig. 4.**108 c, e**). The temporoparietal fascia is dissected just deep to the hair follicles using a size 15 blade or dissecting scissors (see Fig. 5.**171**, p. 214), taking care not to damage the vessels (Brent and Byrd 1983; Abul-Hassan et al. 1986; Park et al. 1999; Fig. 4.**108 d, f**).

An incision is made in the region of the auditory canal or the concha (Fig. 4.**108 g**). The residual auricle, residual cartilage secondary to burns injuries, residual earlobe, etc. are freshened. The size of the fascia is generously outlined using the auricular template, ensuring that enough fascia is harvested to completely envelope the framework (Fig. 4.**108 f, g**). A transverse incision of the fascia is made above the temporal fascia and, corresponding to the template, anterior and posterior incisions in the direction of the vessels (Fig. 4.**108 d**). After inserting the supportive framework (Fig. 4.**108 e–g**) in its correct anatomical position, both the posterior and anterior surfaces of the auricle are draped with fascia. A vacuum drain allows the fascia to be fitted closely to the framework. The vessels should not be twisted or kinked (Fig. 4.**108 g, h**).

The anterior surface of the auricle is covered by a full-thickness skin graft taken from the post- and/or retroauricular region of the contralateral side to achieve as similar a color and texture match as possible. The free grafts are affixed securely with fibrin adhesive (Fig. 4.**97**, p. 86 and Fig. 4.**103**, p. 88).

The posterior surface may be resurfaced with a split-thickness skin graft (see Fig. 4.**103**, p. 88) harvested from the groin, abdominal, or gluteal region (Fig. 4.**108 i, j**; Fig. 4.**109 a, b**; Erol et al. 1981; Abul-Hassan et al. 1986).

Dressing. The auricle remains covered under mild compression for 1 week (see Fig. 5.**185 c, d**; p. 223).

The defects of the postauricular region and the contralateral side are reduced and the residual defects resurfaced with thick split-thickness skin grafts (see Fig. 5.**172 j–l**, pp. 215, 216).

These methods were first published by Fox and Edgerton (1976). The variable courses of the superficial temporal artery were studied by Park et al. (1999) on 123 fan flaps.

Complications. The following complications are possible:

- **Vascular injury.** The commonest complication is injury to the nutrient vessels, which is why dissection should always be performed just deep to the hair follicles. Park et al. (1999) report 21 vascular injuries (22.6%) in 93 flap dissections, involving the artery in 5 cases, the vein in 14, and both the artery and the vein in 2. Attempts were initially made to repair the injury by direct suture; veins were interposed in a number of cases, or the injured part of the vessel was excised and an end-to-end anastomosis performed.
- **Other injuries.** Hair loss can result from injury to the hair follicles. Infections have also been reported, and Park et al. (1999) report injury to the frontal branch of the facial nerve.
- **Flap necrosis.** Of the 12 fascial flap reconstructions with vascular dissection that we have performed, there was one partial necrosis and on one occasion flap necrosis resulted when, after initially good perfusion of the flap, the vascular pedicle was injured while elevating the auricle during the second-stage operation. Park et al. (1999) report 5 partial necroses and 2 total necroses, in all about 6% of 122 flap dissections.

Contralateral Temporoparietal Fascia as a Free Microvascular Graft

If the fascia has been totally lost, or after loss of the fascia due to burns, it is also possible to raise the fascia of the contralateral side as a free flap and perform microvascular anastomosis to the stump of the superficial temporal artery and vein of the injured side (Erol et al. 1981; Brent and Byrd 1983; Nakai et al. 1984; Brent et al. 1985; Turpin et al. 1988; Quatela and Cheney 1995; Giraldo-Ansio et al. 1998).

4.2.8 Upper (and Lower) Preauricular Defects (Fig. 4.110)

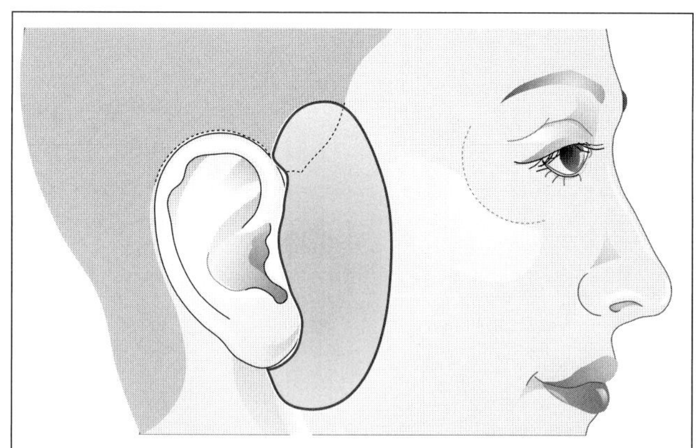

Fig. 4.**110** **Superior and inferior preauricular region.**

Small Defects

Scars are staggered along the **relaxed skin tension lines** (RSTLs) using a W-plasty or the broken-line technique (see Weerda 2001).

Attempts should be made to manage small defects with local sliding, rhomboid, advancement, transposition, or rotation flaps (see also Fig. 4.**33**, p. 56)

Larger rhomboid flaps are used for larger defects with partial loss of the auricle, while narrower defects in the preauricular region can be closed by cheek advancement (see Fig. 4.**115**). Dissection in the superior region should proceed along the fatty layer of the cheek to protect the frontal branch of the facial nerve. Subcutaneous wound closure is accomplished with 5–0 or 6–0 braided sutures and the skin is closed with 6–0 or 7–0 monofilament suture material (see Appendix 2; see Fig. 4.**115**).

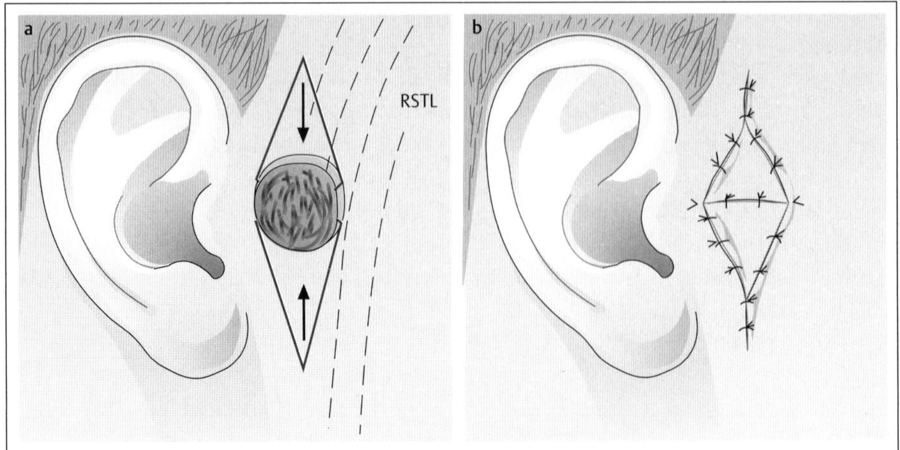

Fig. 4.**111 a, b** **Sliding flap using VY-advancement (island flap; as described by Lejour 1975) for a preauricular defect; RSTL: relaxed skin tension lines.**

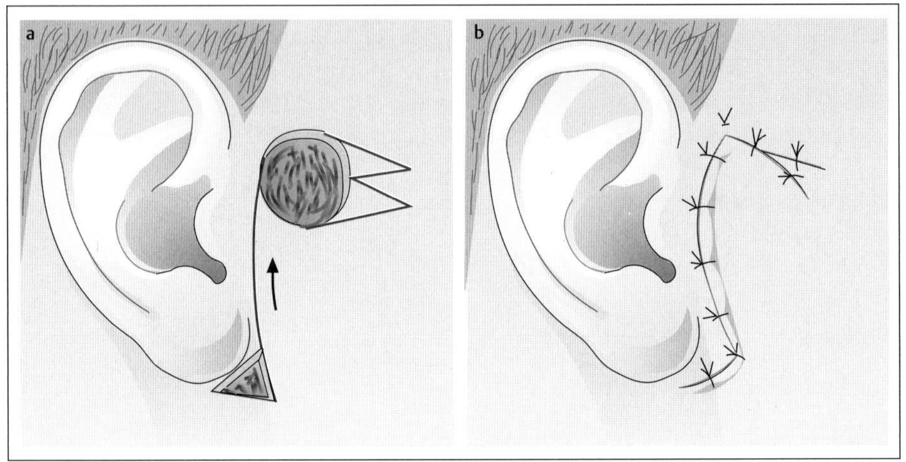

Fig. 4.**112 a, b** **Burow's L-advancement (Leemans et al. 2000).**

Lejour's Sliding Flap ("Island Flap") with VY-Advancement
(Fig. 4.**111**; Lejour 1975)

Simple L-shaped Burow Advancement Flap Plasty
(Fig. 4.**112**)
Round or wedge-shaped defects can be covered by simple Burow advancement (Fig. 4.**112 a, b**). Posteriorly or anteriorly based rotation flaps can be used for rounded defects (Leemans et al. 2000).

Limberg's or Dufourmentel's Rhomboid Flap
(Fig. 4.**113**; see Limberg 1967; Dufourmentel 1950; Weerda and Zöllner 1986)

Small defects can be covered with these flaps in such a way that the scars come to lie more or less in the RSTLs (Fig. 4.**113 a–d**).

Rhomboid Flap in Association with Gersuny Technique for Reconstruction of the Upper and Lower Auricle
(see pp. 54 and 55; Weerda and Zöllner 1986)
To achieve reconstruction, the auricle is considerably reduced before the preauricular defect is closed.

Reconstruction of the Tragus (Figs. 4.114, 4.115)

Defects of the tragal region are covered with an inferiorly (or superiorly) based transposition flap (Fig. 4.**114 a, b**). A Burow advancement flap is also an option for resurfacing the defect (Fig. 4.**115 a, b**). Reconstruction of the tragus using cartilage is described on pages 97 and 219.

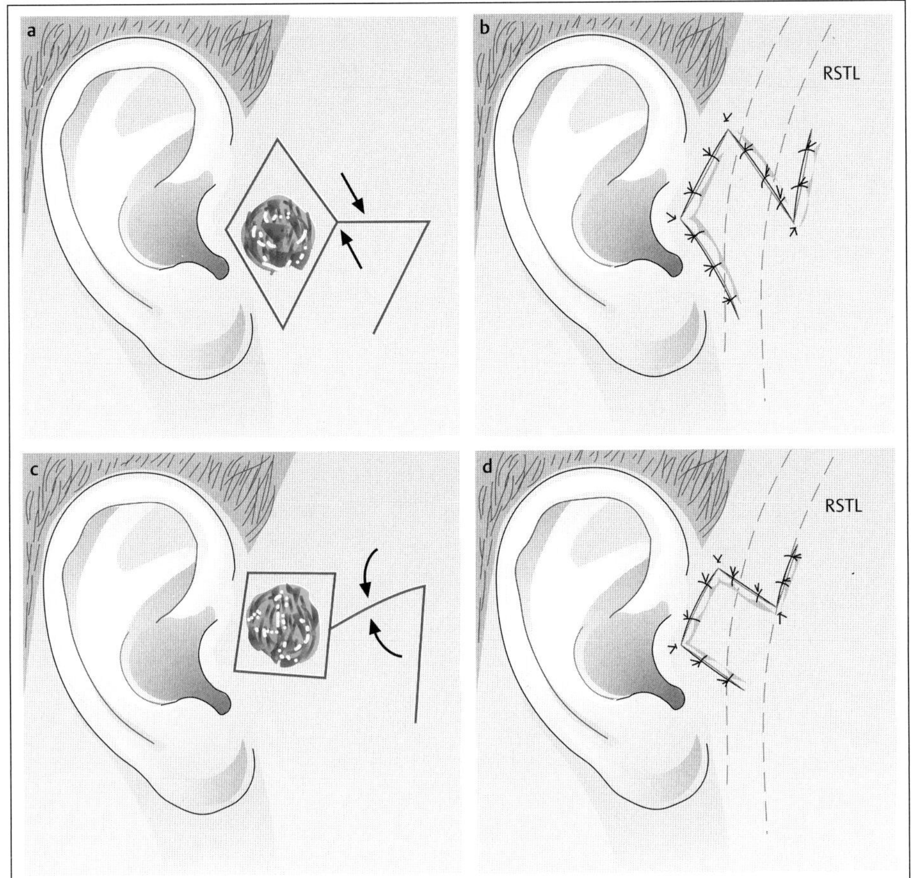

Fig. 4.**113** **Rhomboid flaps.**
a, b Limberg rhomboid flap (1967).
c, d Dufourmentel rhomboid flap (1950), modified; RSTL: relaxed skin tension lines (broken lines, see Weerda 1999 a).

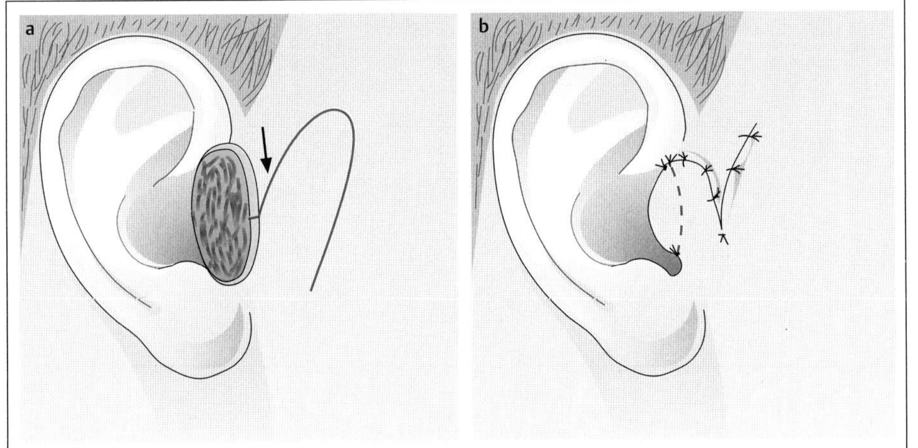

Fig. 4.**114** **a, b Tragus reconstruction with an inferiorly (superiorly) based transposition flap (see also p. 219).**

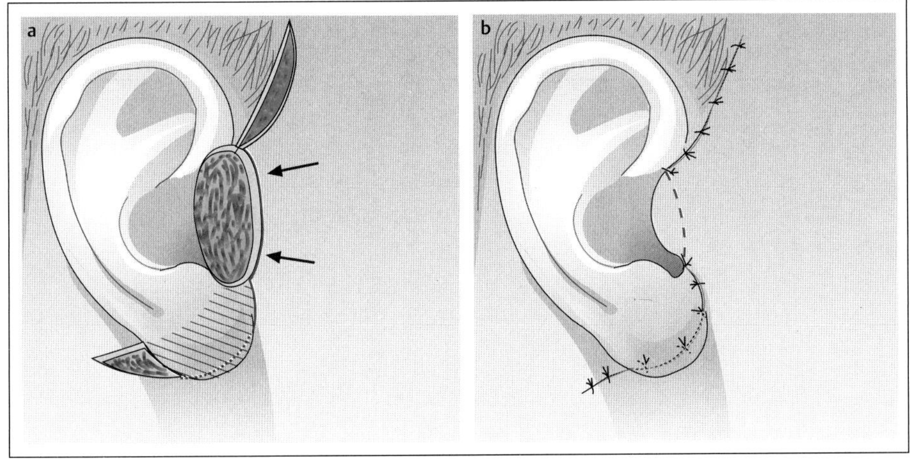

Fig. 4.**115** **Tragus reconstruction with a Burow cheek advancement (see also p. 219).**
a Banana-shaped excision anterior to the ascending helix and inferior to the base of the earlobe.
b Advancement of the cheek; if necessary, conchal cartilage can be used as support.

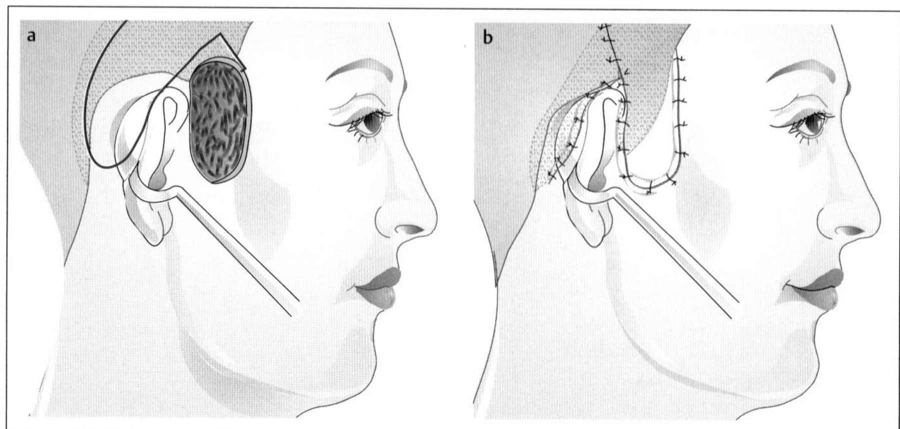

Fig. 4.**116** **Defect with preauricular loss of hair: superiorly based, retroauricular transposition flap.**
a Elevation of the lateral hair-bearing flap.
b Closure of all defects.

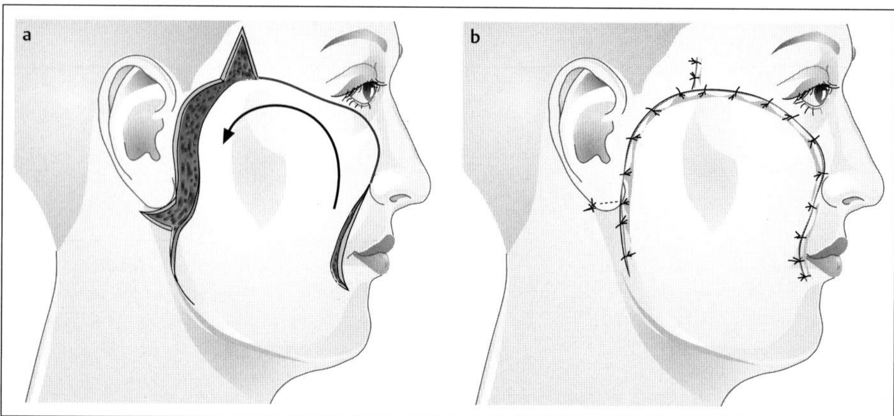

Fig. 4.**117** **Inferiorly based cheek flap rotated in a posterior direction as described by Weerda (1980, 2001).**
a Crescent-shaped excision in the nasolabial fold and dissection of the cheek skin within the subcutaneous fat, as with the traditional Esser cheek rotation flap.
b Closure of all defects.

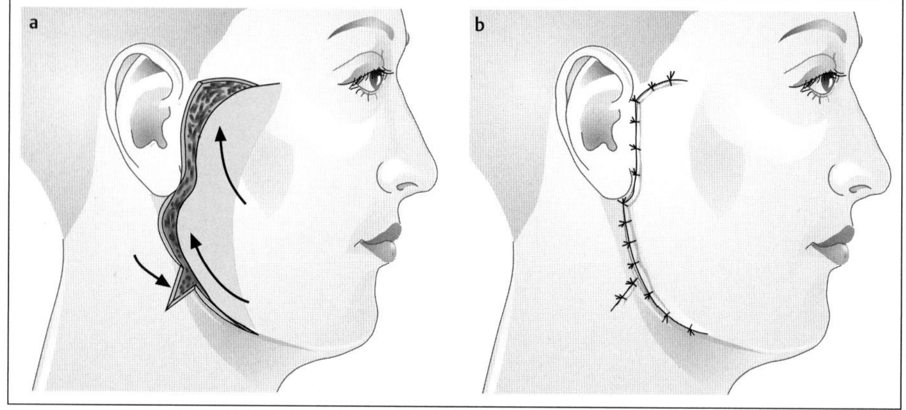

Fig. 4.**118** **Superior preauricular defect.**
a, b Cheek rotation with skin advancement from the submandibular region.

Larger Preauricular Defects

Superiorly Based Retroauricular Flap for Cases with Preauricular Hair Loss

(Fig. 4.**116**)
A larger preauricular defect with hair loss in the temporal region can be closed with a **superiorly based retroauricular flap** (Fig. 4.**116 a**), which also transposes hair from the superior portion into the defect (Fig. 4.**116 b**).

Weerda's Inferiorly Based Lateral Cheek Rotation Flap

(Fig. 4.**117**; Weerda 1984 c)
An inferiorly based cheek flap rotated posteriorly (Fig. 4.**117 a, b**) is also a possibility. The majority of the wound margins come to lie more favorably in the wrinkles and RSTLs. A crescent-shaped segment of skin is excised from the nasolabial fold.

Flaps from the cheek should be dissected within the fatty layer in order to protect branches of the facial nerve, especially the frontal branch.

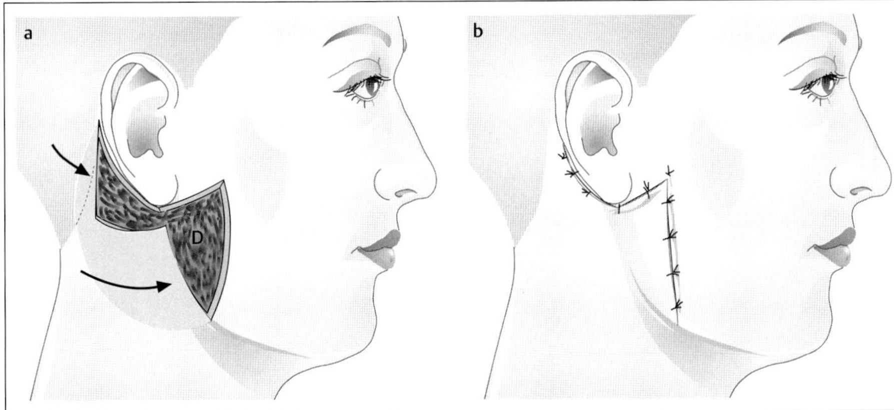

Fig. 4.**119** **Burow advancement flap.**
a Wedge-shaped defect (D) with superior base, excision of a retroauricular Burow's triangle.
b Closure of all defects.

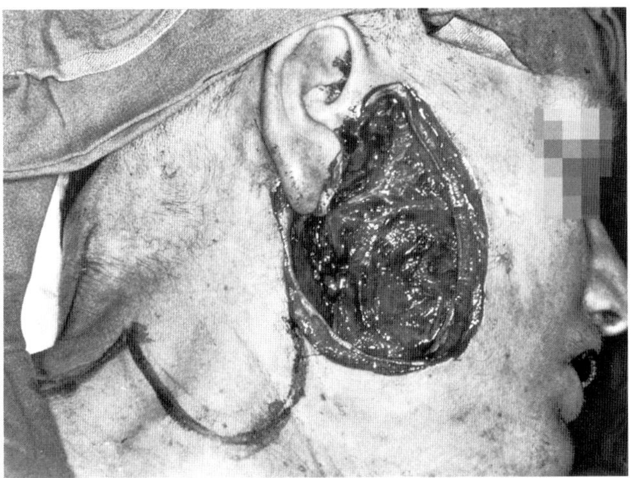

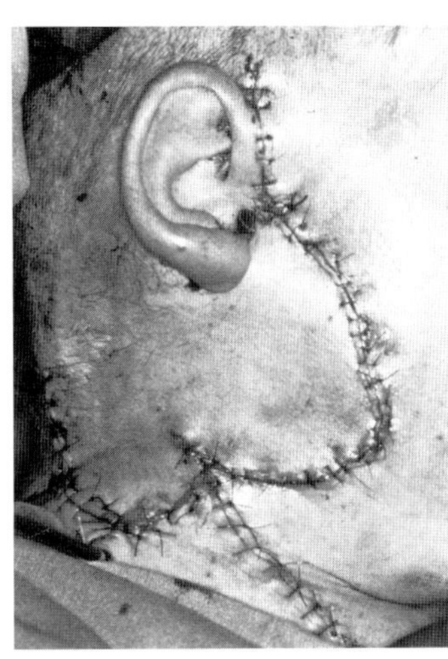

a b

Fig. 4.**120** **Posteriorly or superiorly based bilobed flap to cover a preauricular defect in the region of the lower cheek.**
a Elevation of the superiorly based bilobed flap.
b Closure of all defects.

Upper Preauricular Defect: Skin Advancement from the Subauricular Region
(Fig. 4.**118**)

Burow Flap Advancement for Lower Preauricular Defect
(Fig. 4.**119**)

Closure with a Bilobed Flap from the Neck and Cheek Mobilization
(Fig. 4.**120**)

Preauricular Defects with Partial Loss of the Auricle

If large defects have resulted from tumor excision and if auricular reconstruction is not required in an elderly patient, then the defects are covered with flaps anastomosed using microvascular technique or with larger local flaps.

Large Bilobed Flap
(Fig. 4.**121**; Weerda 1978 b, 1980 c)
For further flaps see Weerda (2001).

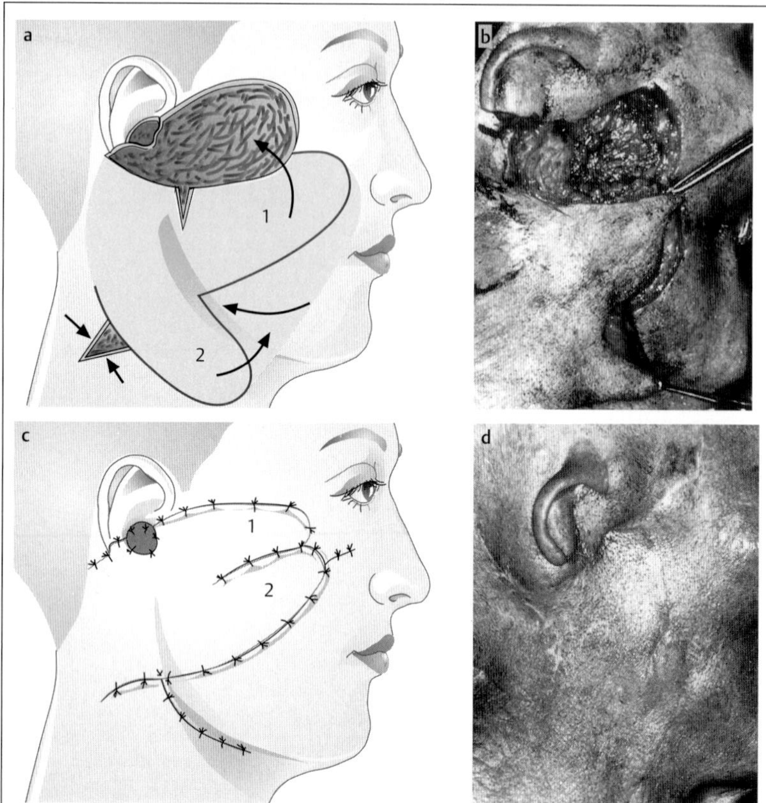

Fig. 4.**121** **Posteriorly based Weerda bilobed flap of the cheek and the submandibular region (1978 b, 1980 c).**

a, b Large defect in the region of the superior posterior cheek, large defect in the region of the ear; 1: flap below the defect; 2: flap in the submandibular region. Burow's triangles used to close the secondary defects.
c Appearance after closure of all defects.
d Result.

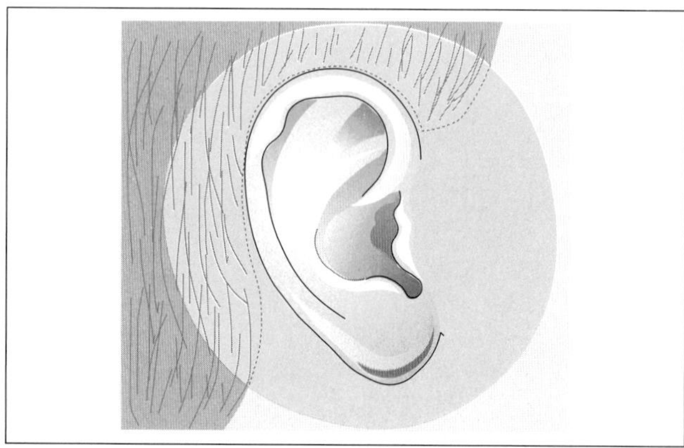

Fig. 4.**122** **Auricular region.**

4.2.9 Reconstruction of Defects of the Auricular Region after Partial or Total Amputation (Fig. 4.122)

If, after amputation or any other loss of the auricle and skin of the auricular region, the intention is merely to reconstruct the defect, then, depending on the size of the defect, free skin grafts (Fig. 4.**123 a, b**), local skin (Figs. 4.**124 a–e**,. 4.**125**), myocutaneous island flaps (Figs. 4.**126 a, b**, 4.**127 a, b**) or, **nowadays, flaps anastomosed using microvascular technique** (Figs. 4.**128**, 4.**129 a–d**) can be used for coverage.

Free Skin Graft
(see Fig. 4.**123**)
When the skin is exhausted, in multimorbid or very old patients, we still occasionally use free, thick split-thickness skin grafts after conditioning the wound bed for the graft.

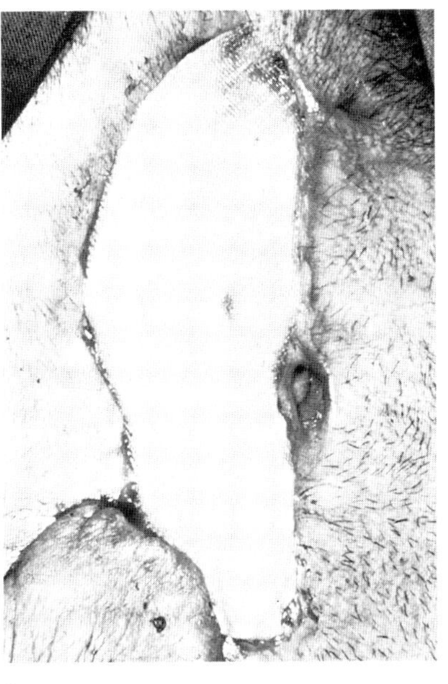

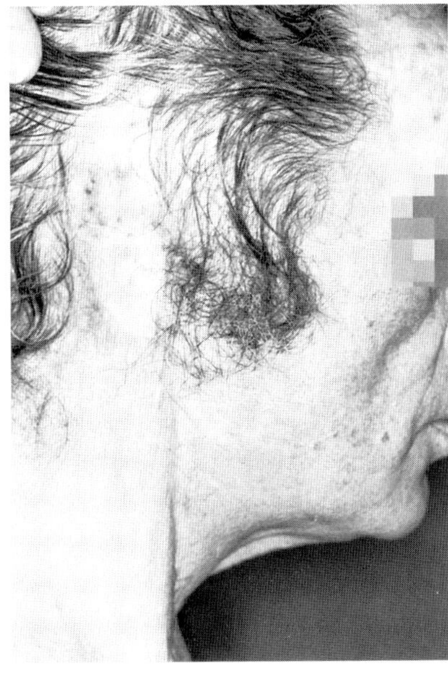

a b

Fig. 4.**123** **Defects resulting from tumors of the auricular region. Coverage with split skin.**

a After tumor removal, a split-thickness skin graft from the thigh (or preferably the gluteal region) is glued with fibrin adhesive onto the defect of the auricular region.

b Appearance about 1 year after reconstruction.

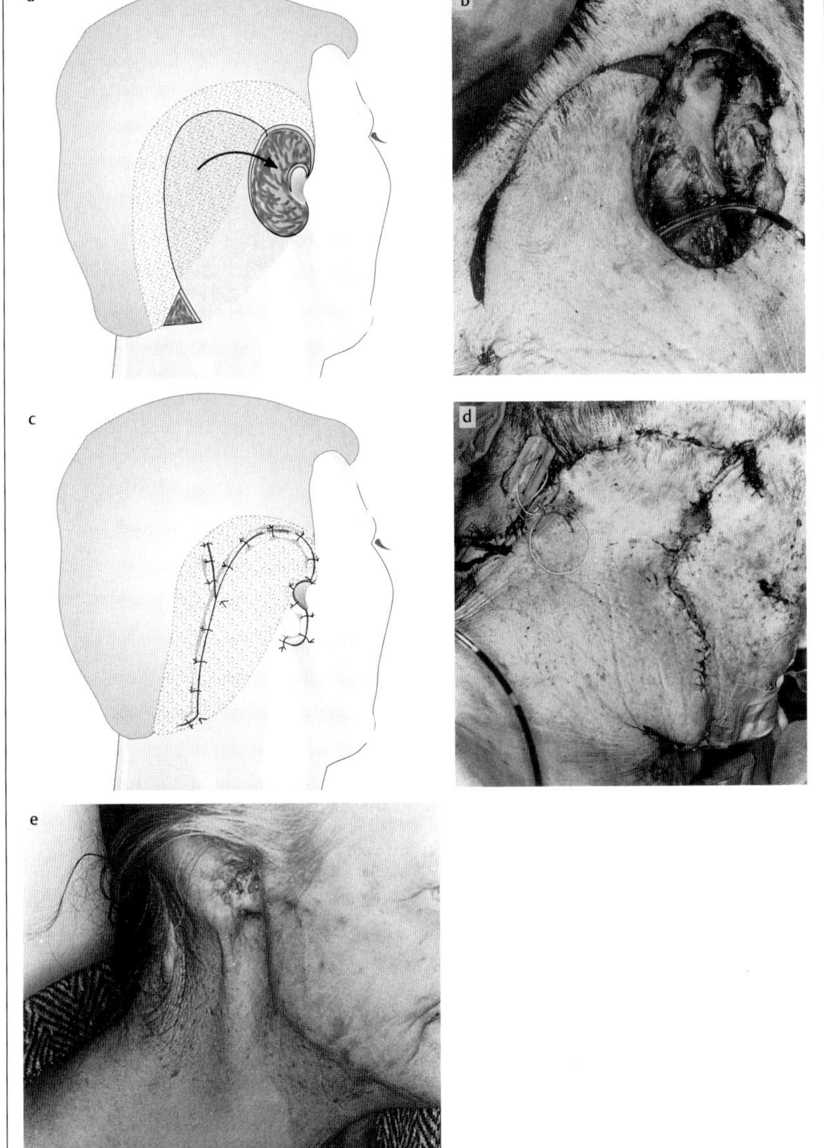

Fig. 4.**124** **Reconstruction with an inferiorly and posteriorly based transposition flap.**

a, b Incision of the flap.

c, d Closure of the defects (submandibular incision for neck dissection).

e Result.

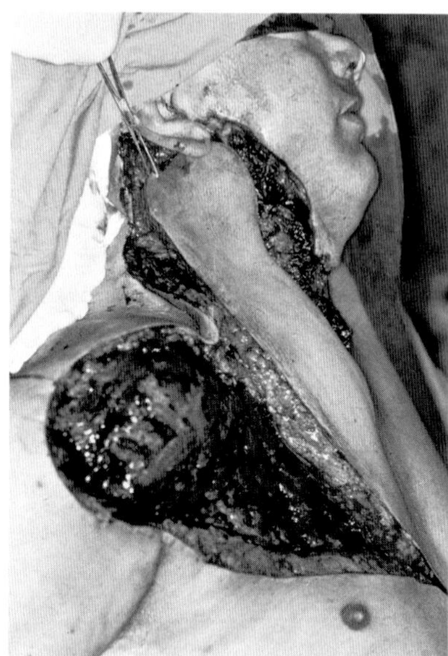

Fig. 4.**125** **Deltopectoral flap.**
Single-stage transposition of the flap into the inferior region of the ear and into the region the neck (rarely used nowadays).

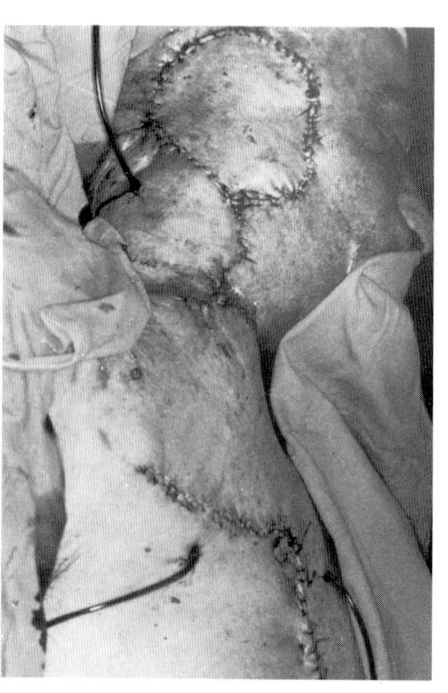

a

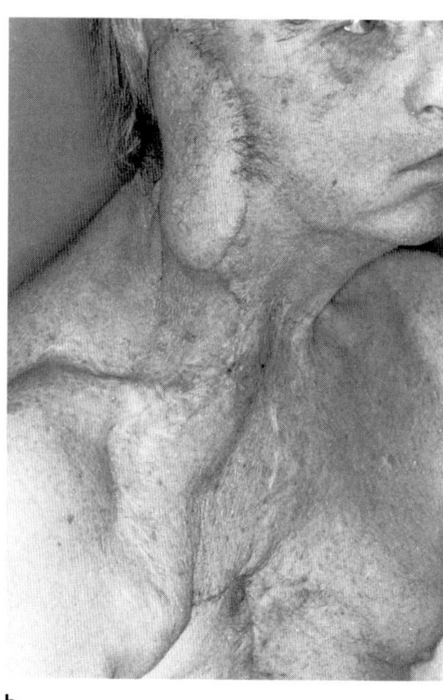

b

Fig. 4.**126** **Myocutaneous pectoralis major muscle island flap.**
a Coverage with a myocutaneous pectoralis major muscle flap following petrosectomy and neck dissection.
b Result.

Deltopectoral Flaps

(see Fig. 4.**125**)
These flaps are hardly ever used today, but could be employed primarily after failure of a myocutaneous pectoralis major muscle flap.

Myocutaneous Pectoralis Major Muscle Island Flap After Petrosectomy

(see Fig. 4.**126**)
It is beyond the scope of this book to provide an exact description of the technique for harvesting this flap (see Weerda 1999 a, 2001), which is used for large lateral defects. It is incised in such a manner that the deltopectoral flap can still be used should it fail.

Myocutaneous Latissimus Dorsi Muscle Island Flap

(see Fig. 4.**127**)
This flap can be readily used for very large defects.

Myocutaneous Scapula and Parascapula Flaps

Similarly, scapula and parascapula island flaps can also be used.

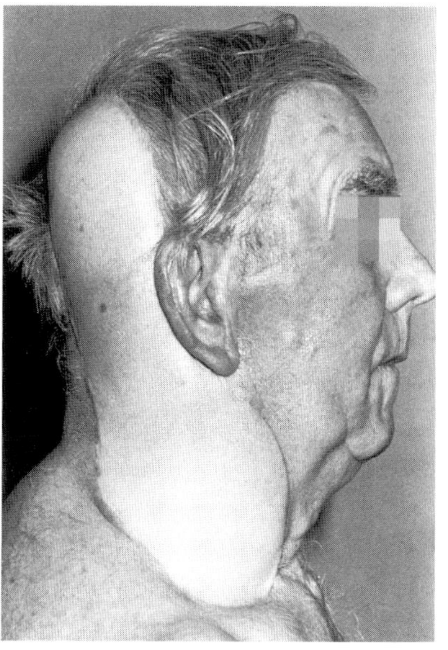

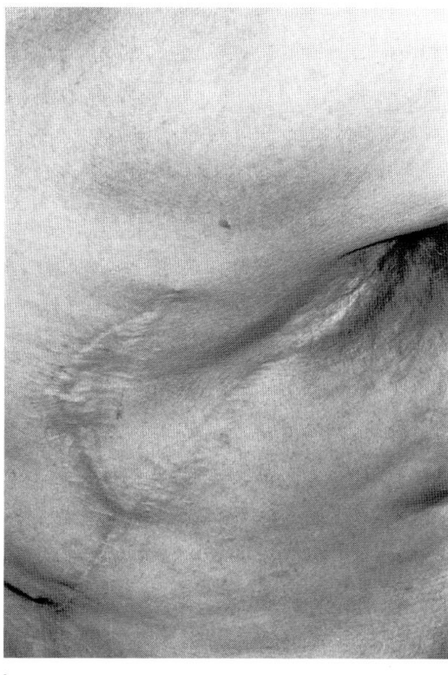

a b

Fig. 4.**127** **Myocutaneous latissimus dorsi muscle island flap.**
a Coverage of the scalp, postauricular region and neck with a latissimus dorsi island muscle flap following melanoma resection.
b Donor site after completion of healing (surgeon: S. Remmert).

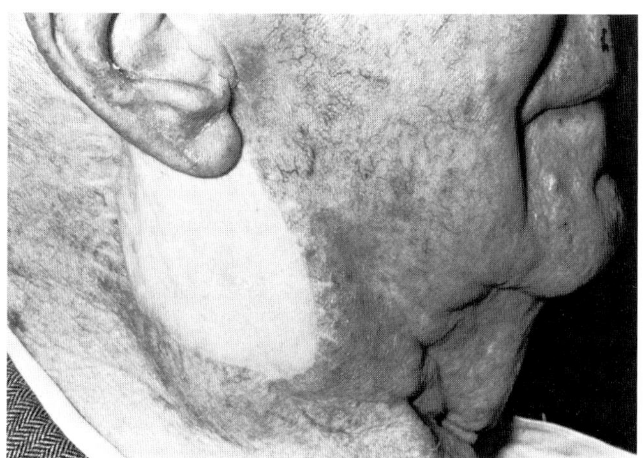

Fig. 4.**128** **Coverage with a radial artery forearm flap anastomosed using microvascular technique (surgeon: S. Remmert).**

Transplants Anastomosed Using Microvascular Technique (see Figs. 4.**128**, 4.**129**)

These are, for example, the free latissimus dorsi flap, the radial artery forearm flap (see Fig. 4.**128**), the parascapular flap (Fig. 4.**129**), or the lateral upper arm flap.

Free transplants anastomosed on the superficial temporal artery and vein, the facial artery and vein, or other vessels are well suited to cover defects of the auricular region (see Fig. 4.**129**) and are now first-choice techniques (Weerda 2001).

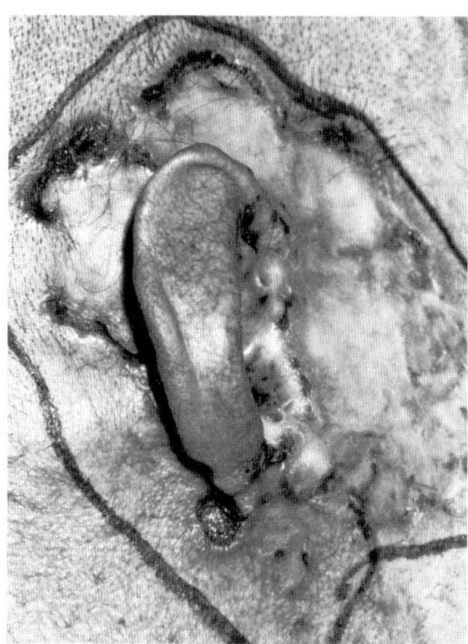

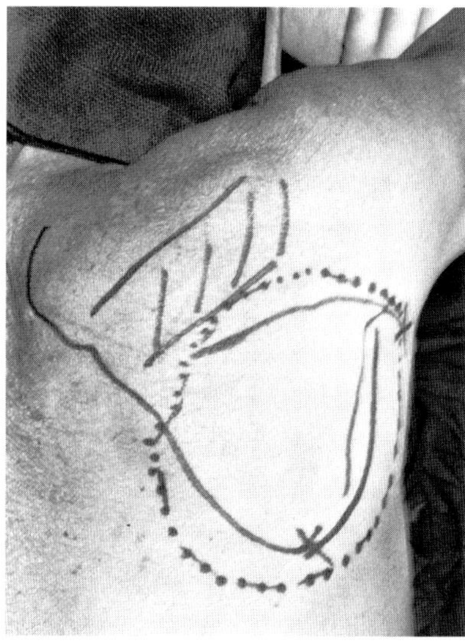

a b

Fig. 4.**129** **Coverage of the auricular region with a free parascapula flap anastomosed using microvascular technique.**
a Tumor recurrence of the auricular region after repeated radiotherapy.
b Parascapula flap, size (dotted line) and scapula outlined.
c Flap anastomosed on the temporal vessels and inset.
d Result after 4 weeks (the edema will settle with time) (surgeon: S. Remmert).

Fig. 4.**129 c, d** ▷

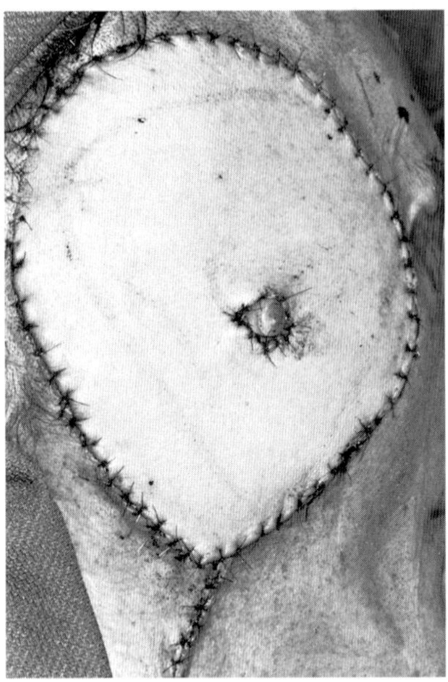

c

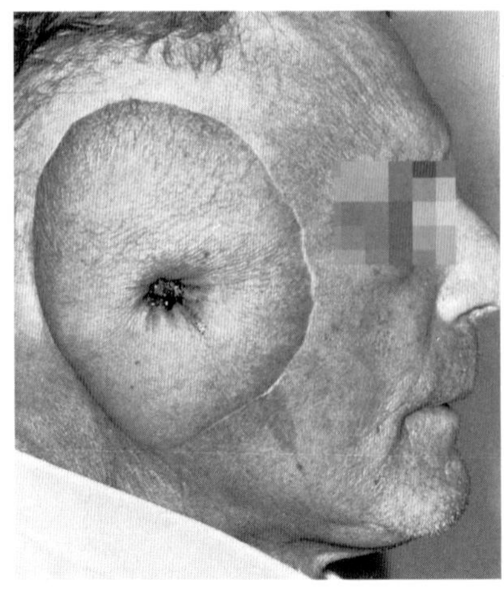

d

Fig. 4.**129 c, d**

4.2.10 Auricular Burns

The different degrees of severity of burns and their management are dealt with in Chapter 3, pp. 24 ff. The resulting defects are reconstructed according to their sites.

Methods of Reconstruction

Converse and Brent's Reconstructive Technique

(Fig. 4.**130**; Converse and Brent 1977)
Since contracture often occurs, the suggestions made by Converse and Brent (1977) are adhered to and the auricle is reconstructed according to the size of the undamaged ear.

First-stage operation. If the mastoid skin is intact, we fashion a template (see pp. 64) and outline the size of the auricle (Fig. 4.**130 b**). An incision is made on the postauricular surface, according to the amount of skin required (Fig. 4.**130 c**), and the skin is dissected anteriorly around the helix (Fig. 4.**130 d**).

The incision of the mastoid skin corresponds to the height of the auricle and is continued somewhat inferiorly (Fig. 4.**130 c, e**). The inferior wound margins are adapted with a 5–0 monofilament suture and, depending on the amount of residual cartilage, a cartilaginous framework is harvested from costal cartilage (see pp. 64, 65, pp. 70–72) or from contralateral conchal cartilage (see p. 59, Fig. 4.**39** and Fig. 4.**130 f**) and attached to the residual cartilage framework with a 5–0 braided suture.

Next, scars from the auricular framework are dissected in such a manner as to achieve a sufficiently good form, and a narrow strip of cartilage is sutured onto the antihelical crura and the antihelix (see Fig. 4.**130 f**). The skin of the anterior surface is then sutured to the upper margin of the mastoid incision (Fig. 4.**130 g**).

Second-stage operation. Six weeks at the earliest after the first operation, following Nagata's suggestions (1994; pp. 215, 216), a full-thickness skin graft is dissected above the hair follicles about 1 cm superior to the upper helical margin using a size 15 blade. This flap remains pedicled on the upper helical rim and is draped over the cartilage framework after exteriorizing the auricle (while leaving a sufficient layer of connective tissue) (Fig. 4.**130 h, i**).

The residual posterior auricular surface is covered with a thick split-thickness skin flap, as is the residual defect over the mastoid (Fig. 4.**130 i**; see also Fig. 5.**172 g–l**, p. 215).

Results are not always satisfactory because of previous damage to the skin (Fig. 4.**130 a, j**), so a fan flap is preferred (see below).

Reconstruction with a Temporoparietal Flap (Fan Flap)

The possibilities of reconstruction using a fan flap are discussed in detail on pages 74 and 93.

Microvascular Transplantation Technique

The possibilities of reconstruction with temporoparietal fascia of the contralateral side, anastomosed using a microvascular technique, or antebrachial fascia, are discussed on p. 95.

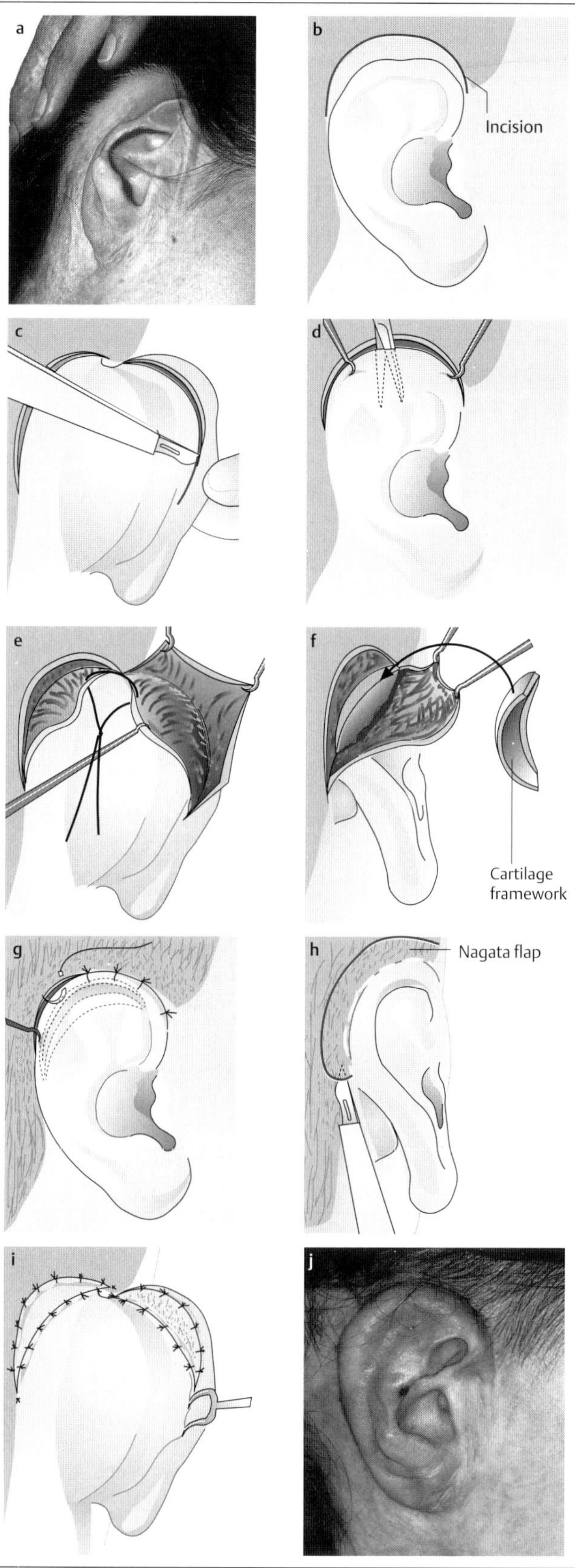

Fig. 4.**130** **Reconstruction of a burned auricle as described by Converse and Brent (1977).**

a Appearance after burn injury.

First stage:

b, c Mastoid incision over the auricle along the hairline designed from a template of the healthy ear. Additional postauricular incision.

d, e Dissection of the skin and suture of the inferior skin margins.

f Insertion and fixation of the cartilage framework onto the stump with 4–0 or 5–0 braided suture.

g Suture of the superior skin margins.

Second stage:

h Elevation of a full-thickness skin flap as described by Nagata (1994 a–d; see Fig. 4.**66 d–f**; see p. 72).

i Coverage of the residual defects (see text) with split skin.

j Result.

5 Abnormalities

5.1 Epidemiology

H. Weerda

About 2–4% of all neonates suffer from a severe deformity; about 1% have a chromosomal aberration. About half of all ENT malformations are to be found in the region of the ear. Brent (1999a) reports one auricular malformation in 6000 neonates. One severe deformity is reported for 10000–20000 neonates (Weerda 1994). Inheritance is a known factor, especially for syndromes such as Franceschetti syndrome or Goldenhar syndrome (Fig. 5.**1 a, b**; Rogers 1968; Weerda 1994). A statistical analysis of 1823244 live births between 1952 and 1962, conducted by Conway and Wagner (1965), revealed approximately one auricular malformation in every 6830 neonates and one severe malformation or aplasia of the auricle for around every 17500 live births. In this analysis 58% of the neonates with a severe malformation were male and 42% female.

Exogenous factors are presumed to be the cause of the malformation in about 10% of cases (thalidomide, rubella embryopathy, other viral infections, alcoholism, etc.; Jörgensen 1972; Eavey 1995).

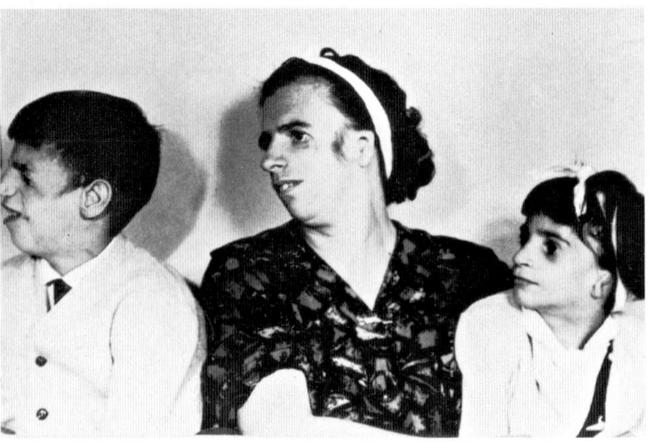

a

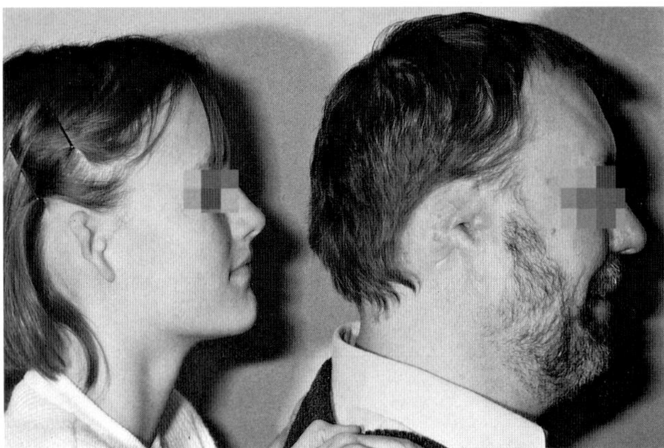

b

Fig. 5.**1 a** Mother with daughter and son with Treacher Collins (Franceschetti) syndrome.
b Father and daughter with right-sided grade III dysplasia; father previously operated.

5.2 Embryology and Classification of Auricular Malformations

H. Weerda

A circumscribed ectodermal swelling appears in the region of the ear between days 21 and 22 of gestation. On day 28 a pit forms in the surface ectoderm (otic vesicle; Uysal et al. 1990).

The auricle develops around the first branchial cleft, with the mesenchymal hillocks 1, 2, and 3 arising from the first branchial arch (the mandibular arch) and the posterior part of the auricle developing from the mesenchymal hillocks 4, 5, and 6 of the second branchial arch (the hyoid arch). Concha and auditory canal arise from the first branchial cleft (Fig. 5.**2 a–d**; Weerda 1994e).

In the course of embryonic development, the auricle forms, enlarges, and migrates from an anterior-caudal to a posterior-cranial position (Fig. 5.**3**; Leiber 1972). While the mandibular and hyoid mesenchyme of the external ear develops between days 40 and 44 of embryonic development, the mandibular mesenchyme regresses during weeks 7 and 8 and later on in the fetal phase; about 85% of the fully grown ear is formed by the hyoid branchial arch (Davis 1987). Over the years, various authors, such as His (1885), Streeter (1922), and Davis (1987), have interpreted the assignment of the different parts of the mesenchymal hillocks to the developed ear in very different ways (Park 1999). My inclination is to endorse the view of Davis (1987) that tragus and helical crus develop from the mandibular arch, while the rest of the auricle is formed by the hyoid arch. The tragus, which initially develops as a two-lobed structure, can sometimes persist in that form.

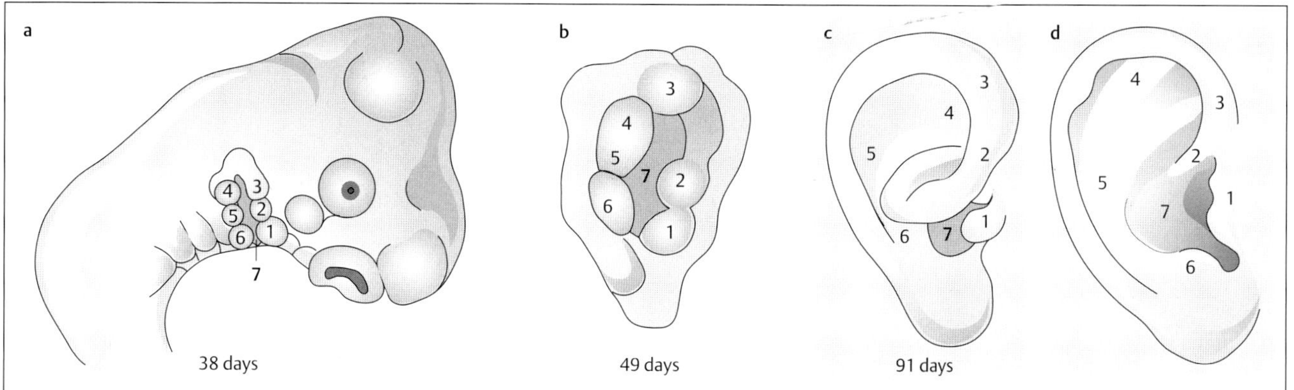

Fig. 5.2 **Development of the auricle from six mesenchymal buds (hillocks):** hillocks 1–3 arise from the first branchial arch; hillocks 4–6 from the second branchial arch; concha and external auditory canal from the first branchial cleft (7) (in Uysal et al. 1990; Weerda 1994 e).

a Location of the six mesenchymal hillocks on day 38 of embryonic development.
b Location of the hillocks on day 49.
c Location of the hillocks on day 91.
d Contribution of the hillocks and first branchial cleft towards the fully developed auricle.

5.2.1 Development of Malformations

Arrested development or failures of differentiation of parts of the auricular primordium or the branchial cleft can result in various types of malformation of the external ear with differing degrees of severity, in addition to overgrowth, such as auricular appendages, and to the formation of sinuses or fistulae in the region of the external ear (see section 5.3, p. 113). The most varied dysplasias of the auricle are encountered (Otto 1979, 1983). This chapter deals in more detail with some typical malformations associated with embryonic development and embryologic maldevelopment, following suggestions put forward by Davis (1987).

Deformities Involving Individual Mesenchymal Hillocks

Malformation of Hillock 3 (Fig. 5.4)

According to Davis, the anterior helical fold, the triangular fossa, and the inferior antihelical crus are formed by hillock 3. In the presence of hillock 3 malformations (Fig. 5.4 **a–c**) there is an absence of the anterior helical portions and we see Tanzer's type I and type II cup-ear deformities (Tanzer 1975; see also Fig. 5.26 **b**, **c**; p. 170).

Malformation of Hillocks (2)–3 (Fig. 5.5)

Apart from malformations of the upper helix, here there is also an absence of the helical crus. It may also be associated with stenosis or atresia of the auditory canal. As an additional contribution by hillock 3, absence of the triangular fossa may also be encountered (Fig. 5.5 **a**, **b**; see Fig. 5.26 **c**).

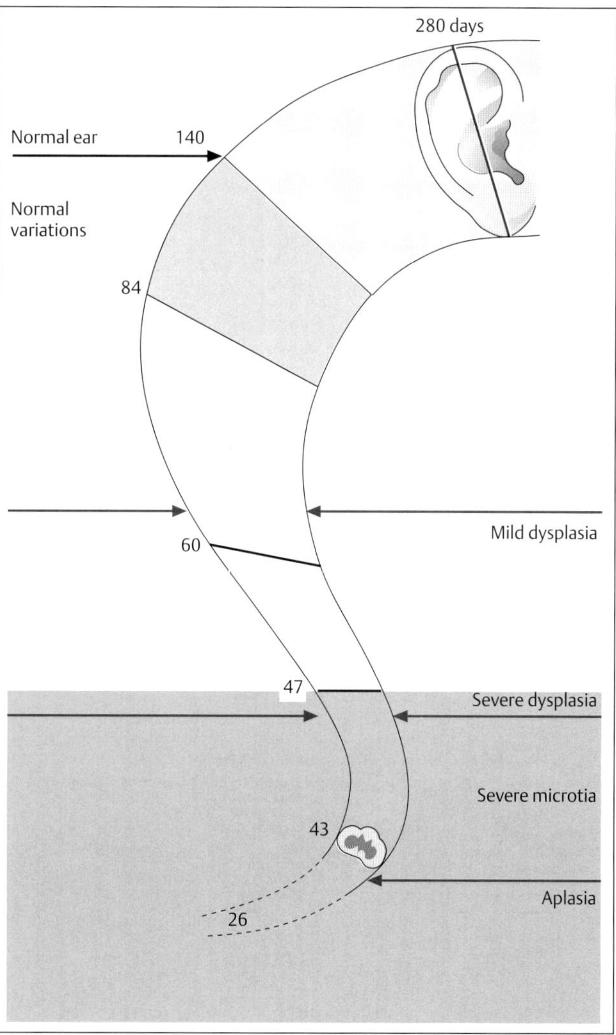

Fig. 5.3 **Changes in the developing auricle as it migrates in the course of embryonic development, as described by Leiber** (1972; from Weerda 1994 e).

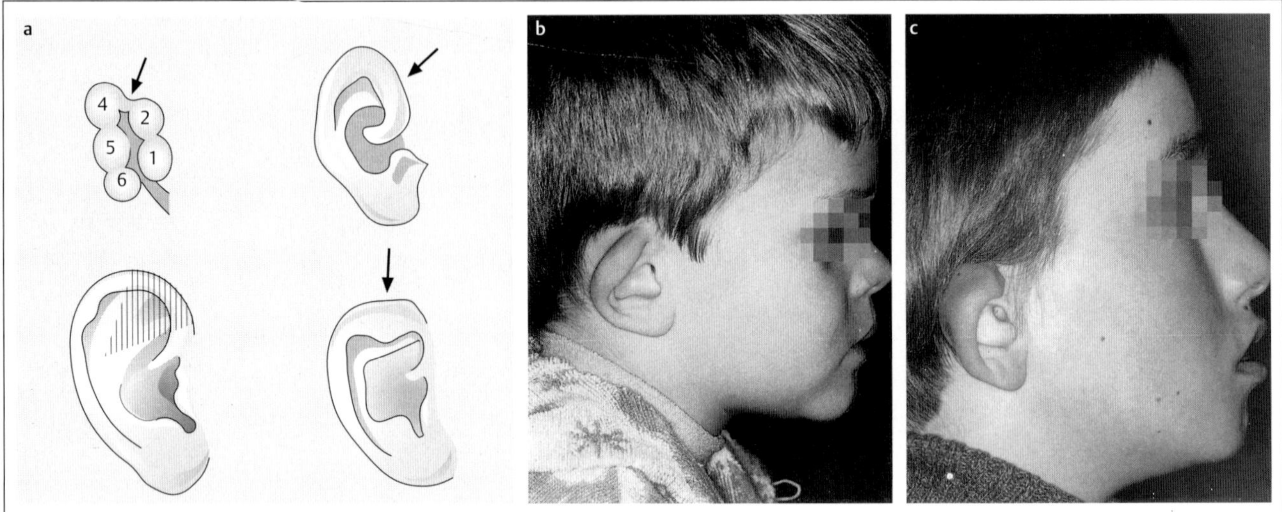

Fig. 5.**4** **Malformations of hillock 3.**
a Hillock 3 malformation: absent anterior helical components, Tanzer's cup-ear deformities (Tanzer 1975; in Davis 1987):
b Type I cup-ear deformity.
c Type II cup-ear deformity.

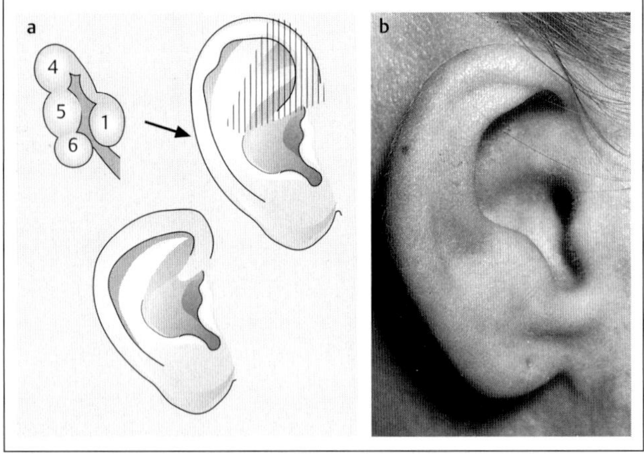

Fig. 5.**5** **Malformations of hillocks (2)–3.**
a Hillocks (2)+3 malformation: as in Fig. 5.**4,** deformed upper helix, absent inferior antihelical crus, absent triangular fossa, additional absence of the helical crus. Occasional deformation of the tragus, external auditory canal stenosis, or atresia.
b Typical deformation with absent helical crus, absent fossa, reduced auricular height: grade II dysplasia (mini-ear), narrowing of external auditory canal.

Cleft of Hillocks 3–4 (Fig. 5.6)

Depending on its severity, this malformation can range from a 3–4 cleft formation to a conical-shaped irregularity of the helix or even severe deformities of the superior helix (Fig. 5.**6 a, b**).

Absence of the Upper Helix due to Hillock 4 Deformity (Fig. 5.7)

Hillock 4 forms the helical dome and the upper part of the descending helix, as well as the adjacent scapha (Fig. 5.**7 a**). Mild deformities result in a **scaphoid ear** (Fig. 5.**7 b**; surgical correction see p. 160).

More severe malformations are associated with absence of the upper helix and scapha, resulting in some cases in an elongation of the helix in the anterior superior region, which is known as **satyr ear** (Fig. 5.**7 c**; p. 163).

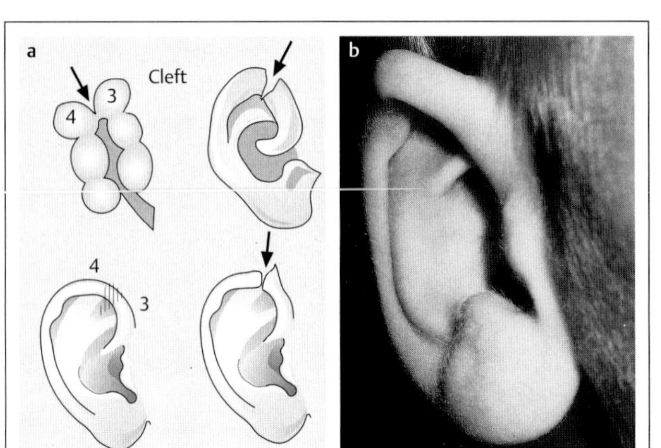

◁ Fig. 5.**6** **Cleft of hillocks 3–4.**
a 3–4 cleft, even to the extent of severe deformities of the upper helical region, depending on degree of fusion and malformation (in Davis 1987).
b Cleft with mild deformity of the helix.

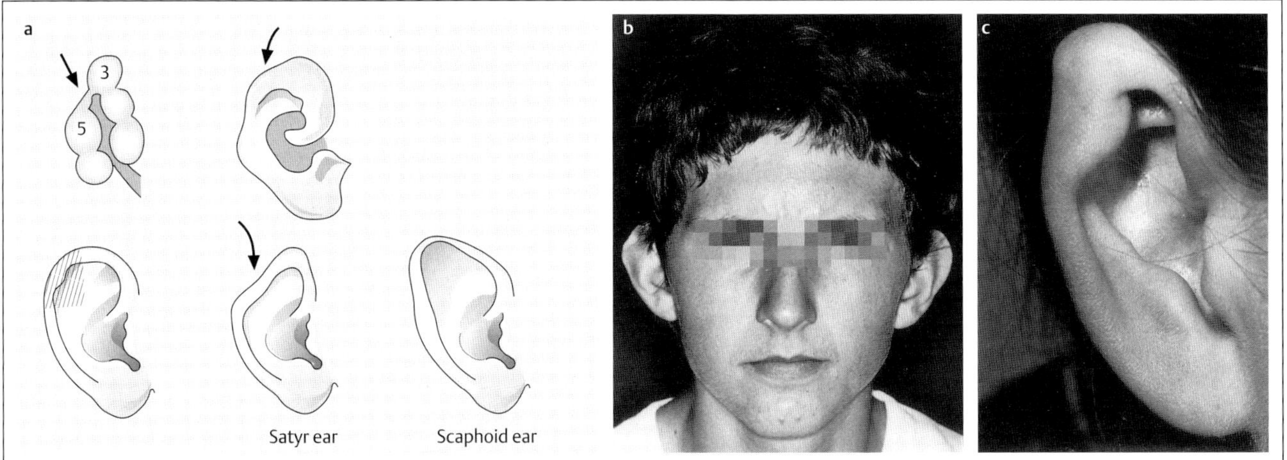

Fig. 5.7 **Malformations of hillock 4.**
a Helical dome, upper and descending helix are affected: angulation of the superior region, absent upper helix, absent scapha (in Davis 1987).
b Scaphoid ear.
c Satyr ear.
(Grade I dysplasia).

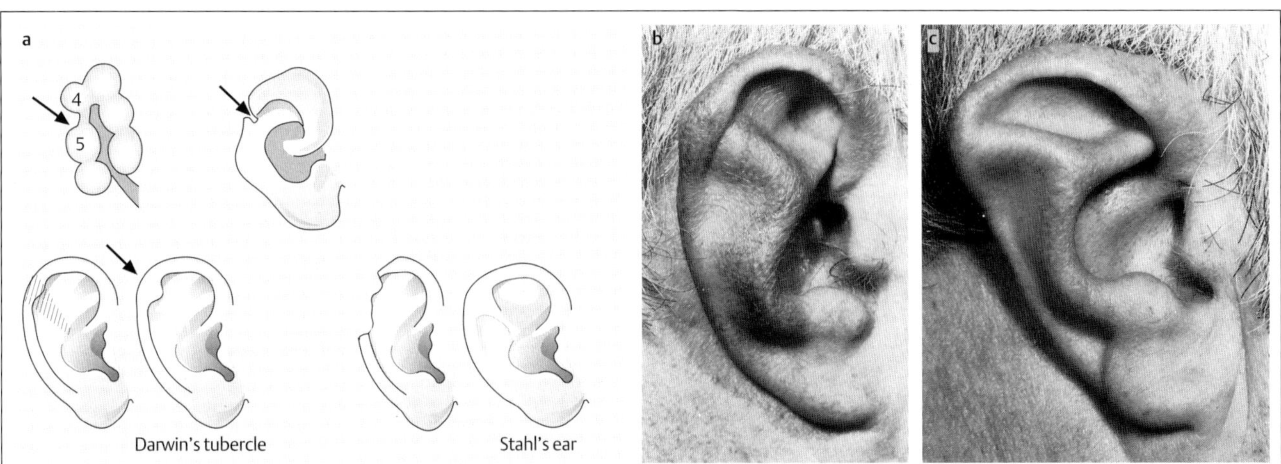

Fig. 5.8 **Cleft of hillocks 4–5.**
a Tubercle, Stahl's ear (additional folds), absent descending helix, absent helix associated with an additional fold (in Davis 1987).
b Darwin's tubercle and additional fold (Stahl's ear).
c Typical Stahl's ear.

Malformation of Hillocks 4–5 (4–5 Cleft) (Fig. 5.8)

Malformations between hillock 4 and hillock 5 can result in a 4–5 cleft, a Darwinian tubercle (p. 164), or an additional fold which, in the form of a third crus, is referred to as **Stahl's ear** (Fig. 5.8 **a–c**; p. 161). In addition, the helix can be absent in this region, or may be prominent. Individual malformations can be found in combination.

Malformation of Hillock 5 (Fig. 5.9)

Davis (1987) ascribes particular importance to hillock 5, given that it forms the descending helix and the lower scapha as well as the floor of the concha. Malformations of the auditory canal and the tympanum can occur. The mildest malformation encountered here is the absence of the lower helix, and the most severe form described is the **mini-ear** (Fig. 5.9 **a–c**; see pp. 183 ff).

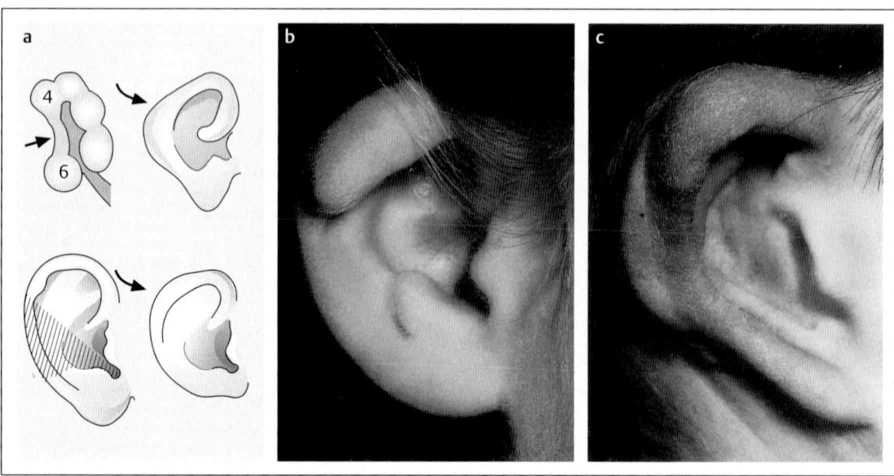

Fig. 5.9 **Malformations of hillock 5.**
a Hillock 5 forms the descending helix, scapha, and the floor of the concha. Occasionally the external auditory canal and tympanum are also involved (**a** in Davis 1987).
b, c Malformations: absent helix and scapha, mini-ear, auricular atresia (**b**: grade I dysplasia; **c**: grade II dysplasia).

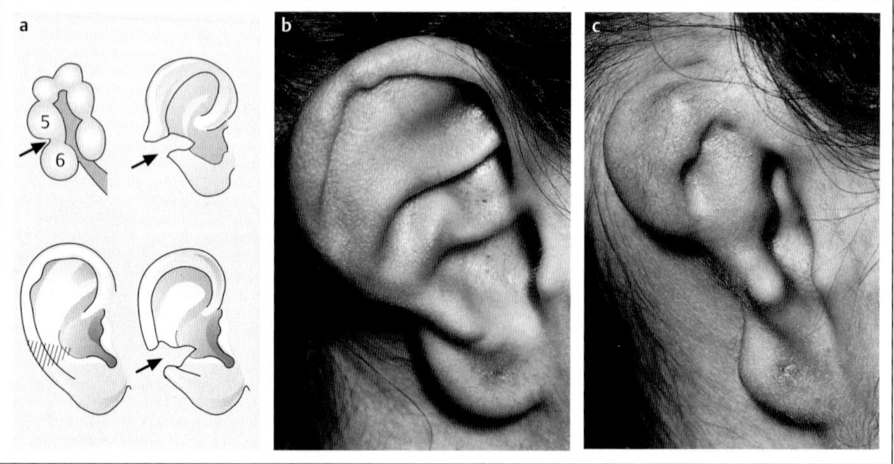

Fig. 5.10 **Cleft of hillocks 5–6.**
a The cleft does not reach the external auditory canal: cleft auricle (grade I dysplasia), occasional additional fold (rarity) and combination with an atypical Stahl's ear (in Davis 1987).
b, c Clefts of increasing severity (**c**: grade II–III dysplasia).

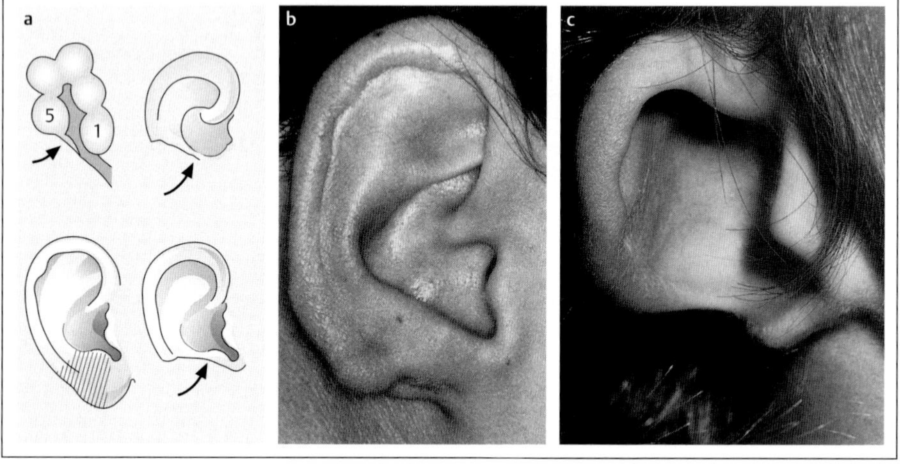

Fig. 5.11 **Malformations of hillock 6.**
a Dysplastic or absent earlobe (in Davis 1987).
b Mild dysplasia of the lower auricle.
c Absent lower auricle (bilateral; grade II dysplasia; mini-ear).

Cleft Between Hillocks 5 and 6 (Fig. 5.10)

Cleft formation between hillocks 5 and 6 does not reach the auditory canal (Fig. 5.**10**) and is referred to as a **coloboma** or **cleft ear** (**question-mark ear** according to Cosman 1984). For surgical correction see pp. 157 ff.

Malformations of Hillock 6 (Fig. 5.11)

Malformations of hillock 6 result in deformities of the earlobe (Fig. 5.**11 a, b**) or even aplasia of the earlobe (Fig. 5.**11 c**; see p. 193).

Cleft Between Hillocks 6 and 1 (Fig. 5.12)

Hillocks 1 and 6 lie very close together (Fig. 5.12 **a**), which can result in the formation of a cleft between the two. This becomes noticeable in the form of a double earlobe, the so-called **bifid** or **tag and cleft** type earlobe (Fig. 5.12 **b**). According to Fumiiri and Hyakusoku (1983; see pp. 168–170), there is an anterior cleft form, a posterior cleft form, and the tag and cleft type.

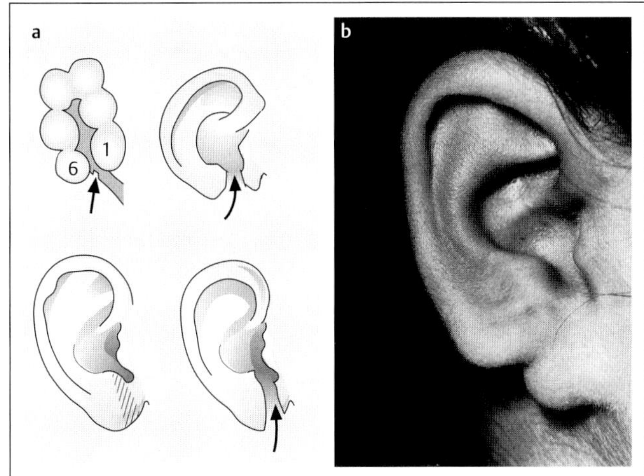

Fig. 5.**12** **Cleft of hillocks 6–1: double or bifid earlobe (in Davis 1987).**

Malformations and Clefts of Hillocks 1 and 2, Hillock 1+2 Malformation (Fig. 5.13)

Malformations of hillock 1 (Fig. 5.13 **a**) result in an **anterior bifid earlobe** (see p. 168), occasionally associated with displacement of the lobular portion onto the cheek (Fig. 5.13 **d**). This malformation can extend into an additional malformation of hillock 2 (Fig. 5.13 **b**), demonstrating a malformed or absent tragus (Fig. 5.13 **c**), absent intertragic notch, separate second tubercle of the tragus (tubercle of His), poor-to-absent tragus development, and occasionally an atresia of the ear in the presence of a helical crus.

Combined Deformities Involving Several Hillocks

Malformation of Hillocks 3–4 (Fig. 5.14)

In malformations of hillocks 3–4 the lower two thirds of the auricle are more or less well developed, with deficits in the superior and superoposterior region (Fig. 5.14 **a**, **b**). Davis has coined the term **snail shell ear** for this type of ear. The typical **type III cup-ear deformity** (grade II dysplasia) belongs to this group of malformations (Fig. 5.14 **c**). Figure 5.14 **b** shows a typical 3–4 deformity with mild involvement of hillock 2, documented by the absence of a helical crus. Figure 5.14 **c** shows a typical type III cup-ear deformity as an example of a malformation of hillocks 3–4. Nagata (1994 b) refers to it as a second-degree dysplasia (see pp. 186 ff).

Malformation of Hillocks 2–3–4 (Fig. 5.15)

Malformations of hillocks 2, 3, and 4 involve the upper half of the auricle and are referred to by Davis (1987) as a **canoe ear**. There is a mere implication of a concha and an auditory canal is also present, but frequently stenosis of the auditory canal or an aural atresia is encountered (Fig. 5.15 **a**, **b**).

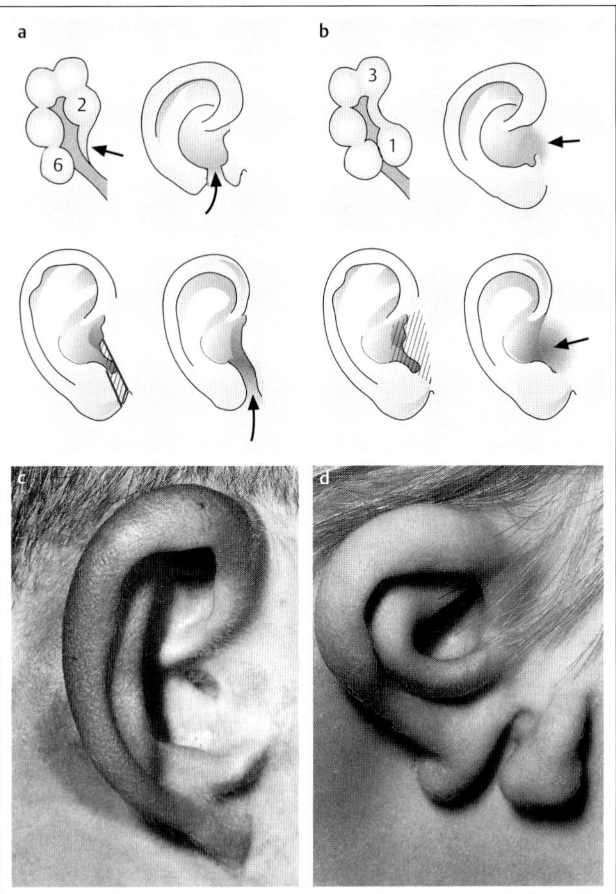

Fig. 5.**13**

a Hillock 1 malformation: anterior bifid earlobe, possible dislocation of the earlobe towards the cheek (**d**), occasionally associated with absent tragus and atresia (in Davis 1987).

b Hillock 2 malformations: anomalies of the intertragic notch, possible supratragal second tubercle = tubercle of His, poor tragal formation = middle-ear defects, absent tragus, and atresia.

c Hillock 2 deformity with absent tragus.

d Hillocks 6–1 cleft with hillocks 2–3 deformity: bifid earlobe with dislocation of the anterior earlobe towards the cheek and absent tragus.

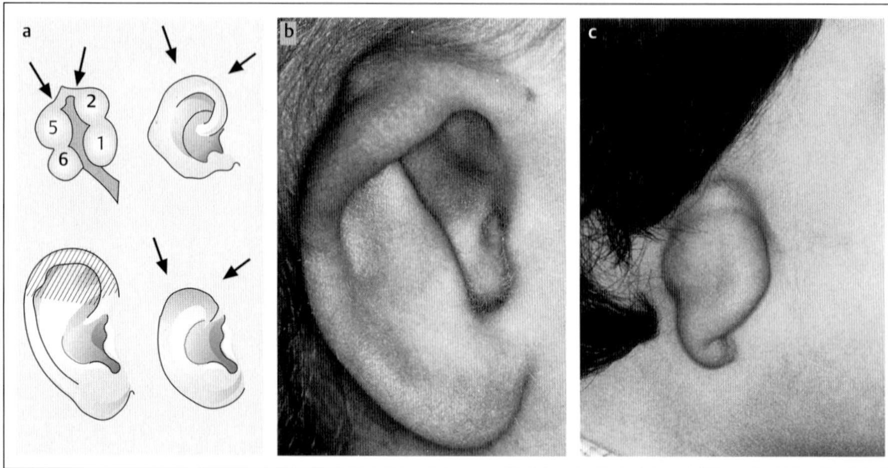

Fig. 5.**14 Combined deformities.**
a Hillocks 3–4 malformations are malformations of the upper auricle. They are referred to as "shell ear" (mini-ear, see p. 183), often associated with a reduced diameter of the external auditory canal with a small tympanum and normal middle ear. Davis (1987) refers to this as "snail shell ear" (**a** in Davis 1987).
b Grade II dysplasia with overhang of the upper auricle.
c Grade II dysplasia, Tanzer's type III cup ear (Tanzer 1974 d); surgery see pp. 185 ff; Nagata's "concha type microtia").

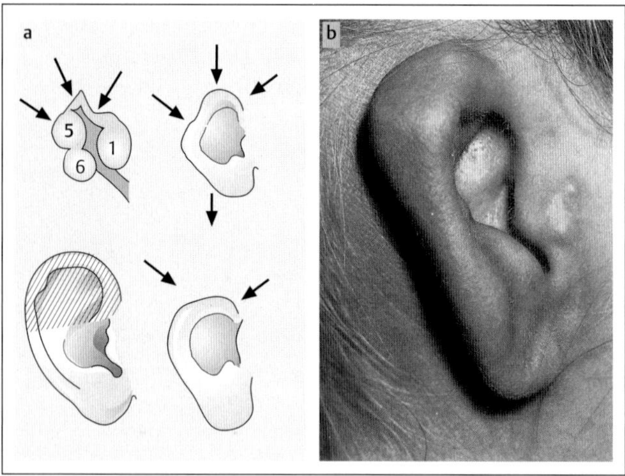

Fig. 5.**15**
a Hillocks 2–3–4 malformation: half ear malformation, referred to by Davis (1987) as "canoe ear" (in Davis 1987).
b Grade III dysplasia with absence of the upper auricle, while tragus, external auditory canal, and tympanum are present (surgery see p. 202, Nagata's "small concha type microtia").

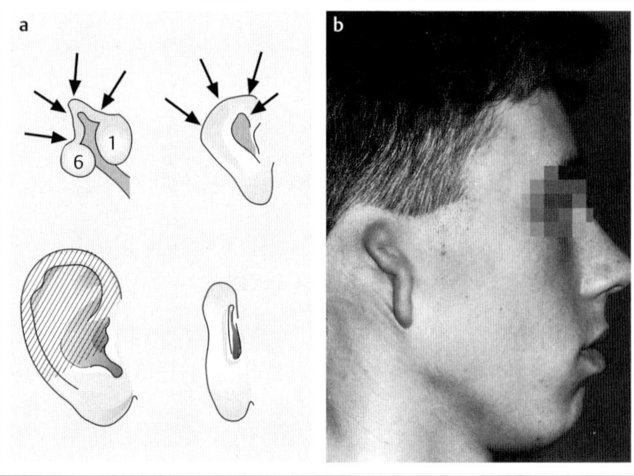

Fig. 5.**16 a, b Malformation of hillocks 2–5: grade III dysplasia (microtia).** Davis (1987) refers to it as a "peanut ear" (2/3 ear deformity), Nagata (1994 a–d) refers to it as "lobule type microtia."

Malformation of Hillocks 2-3-4-5 (Fig. 5.16)

Here we find the typical rudimentary remnant of the severest type of malformation, which we describe as **grade III microtia or dysplasia.** The rudimentary remnant of the lower auricle is present, and Davis (1987) refers to it as a **peanut ear** or a **two-thirds ear deformity** (Fig. 5.**16 a, b**). In this typical example of grade III dysplasia, only a rudimentary earlobe is available for corrective surgery (see p. 207). Nagata (1994 a) refers to the last two forms as **"lobule type microtia"** (for surgical correction, see pp. 209 ff).

Malformation of Hillocks 1–6 (Fig. 5.17)

Complete absence of a rudimentary auricular remnant is referred to as **anotia** (Fig. 5.**17 a–c**).

As well as these rather well-defined malformations, there is also a wealth of variations and deviations. Often malformations of the auricle are associated with other malformations of the face (microsomia) or with clefts and malformations of the hands, feet, or internal organs (e. g., in the form of thalidomide malformations).

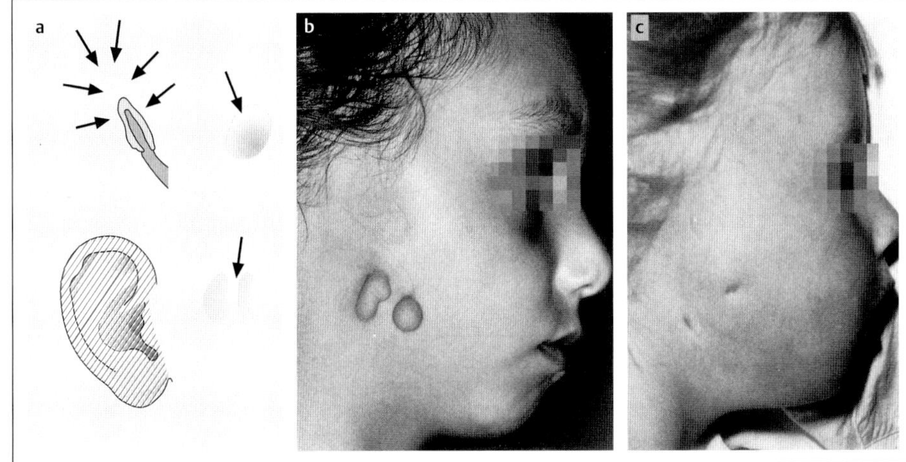

Fig. 5.**17**
a Malformation of hillocks 1–6: **anotia**.
b Malformation of hillocks 1–5, a mere suggestion of an earlobe with auricular appendage.
c Complete anotia with depression in the region of the external auditory canal and low hairline.

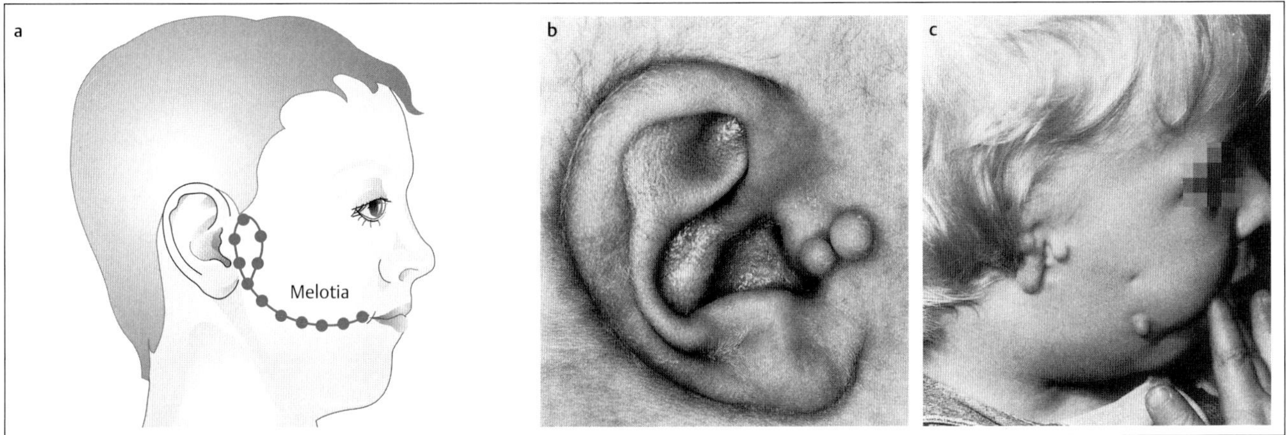

Fig. 5.**18**
a Location of preauricular appendages as described by Otto (1979; in Weerda 1994 e).
b Preauricular appendages associated with a normally developed ear.
c Preauricular appendages, pit associated with grade III microtia.

5.3 Classification and Surgery of Auricular Overgrowth

H. Weerda

Classification. Differing degrees of arrested development or differentiation of the different parts of the auricular primordium or the branchial cleft result in various degrees and types of malformation of the external ear, including overgrowths such as auricular appendages, the formation of sinuses and fistulae in the region of the ear, and dysplasias of various degrees (Otto 1979, 1983).

5.3.1 Auricular Appendages (Fig. 5.18)

These are understood to be excess mandibular formations along the edge of the first branchial cleft. Otto (1979) suggests that they are dispersed hyoidal ectodermal cells above the hyomandibular border (Fig. 5.**18 a**—border between the first and second branchial arch). They appear during the first half of week 6 of gestation, when the first branchial cleft becomes obliterated by fusion. As the face grows, the border shifts towards the cheek; these preauricular appendages are genuine choristomas (Fig. 5.**18 b**, **c**).

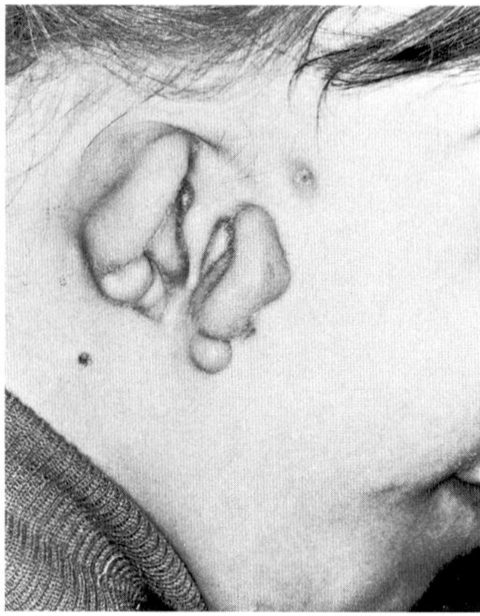

Fig. 5.**19** **Multiple preauricular appendages with rudimentary auricle, referred to as "polyotia."**

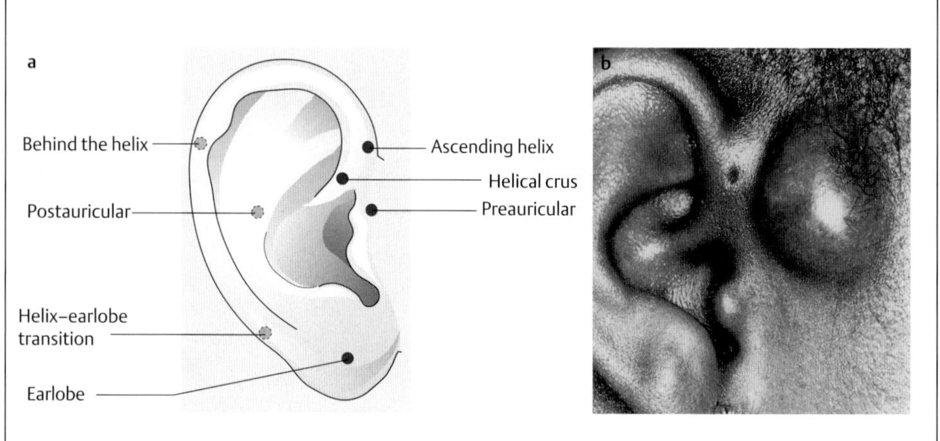

Fig. 5.**20** **Fistulae and sinuses of the auricle.**
a Location of fistulae in the region of the ear as depicted by Gohary et al. (1983; in Weerda 1994 e).
b Infected congenital preauricular sinus, with opening.

Melotia and Polyotia (Fig. 5.19)

Otto (1979, 1983) was able to show that **melotia** (ears located on the cheek) and so-called **supernumary auricles** (**polyotia**; Fig. 5.**19**) are just unusually large auricular appendages. Previously the appearance of such additional "ears" in the region of auricular rudiments or on the cheek was often considered to represent duplicate ears (Blass and Bartholomé 1976). Genuine duplications of the auricle are extremely rare.

Auricular appendages can also appear in combination with more extensive malformations such as hemifacial microsomia, Goldenhar syndrome, or auricular dysplasias (Otto 1979, 1983). Familial clusters are reported, as are malformations of the middle and inner ear (Blass and Bartholomé 1976).

Treatment

In the presence of a normally developed ear, auricular appendages are excised by cutting along the skin tension lines, and the skin is closed using fine monofilament suture material, with due respect to plastic reconstructive principles (see Fig. 5.**18**). If additional auricular malformations are present, then the auricular appendages should not be removed because the skin can be used for further reconstructive measures (Weerda 1984 a).

Audiometric examinations should be conducted to exclude disturbances of hearing.

5.3.2 Fistulae and Sinuses of the Ear (Figs. 5.20–5.22)

Congenital auricular fistulae, preauricular fistulae, and sinuses are entrapped remnants of epithelium found in similar locations to those described for auricular appendages (see Fig. 5.**18**). They usually end blindly and are lined with squamous and/or respiratory epithelium. They are most frequently observed in the preauricular region and around the helical crus (Fig. 5.**20 a**, Fig. 5.**21**). They are not

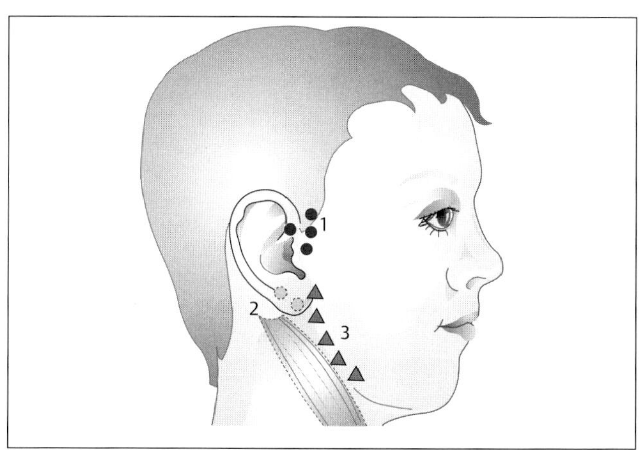

Fig. 5.21 **Location of fistula openings in the region of the ear and neck as described by Otto (1983);** 1: anterior auricular surface: group comprising congenital, preauricular fistulae; 2: postauricular surface: group comprising fistulae of the neck and ear region, also referred to as a "duplication of the external auditory canal" (see also Fig. 5.**22**); 3: proximal group of lateral cervical fistulae (from Weerda 1994 e).

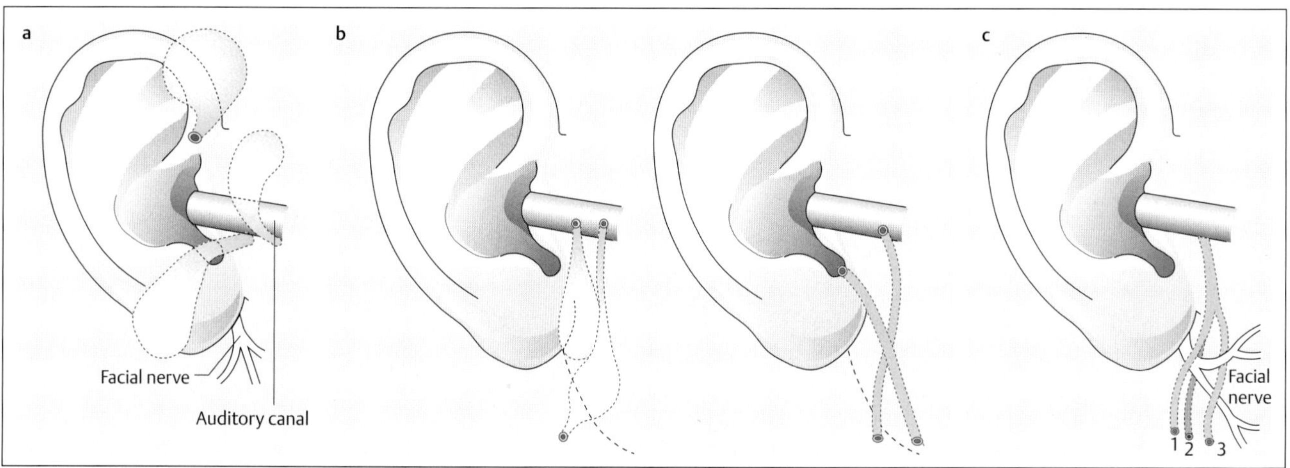

Fig. 5.**22** **Auricular fistulae (from Weerda 1994 e).**
a Location of type I fistulae and type I sinuses of the neck and ear region (in Belenky and Medina 1980).
b Location of type II fistulae, so-called "duplication of the external auditory canal" (in Belenky and Medina 1980).
c Relationship of the facial nerve to type II fistulae of the neck and ear region (in Belenky and Medina 1980; Otto 1983); 1: fistulae passing over the facial nerve; 2,3: fistulae passing beneath the facial nerve.

infrequently bilateral or multiple (Gohary et al. 1983; Otto 1983), and are often subject to inflammatory exacerbations (Fig. 5.**20 b**). Sinuses and fistulae should be removed completely in order to avoid recurrences (see p. 116).

Fistulae of the upper neck and ear region are regarded as duplications of the external auditory canal (Fig. 5.**22** and see Fig. 5.**21**; Hammond 1987; Otto 1983) and are also referred to as **first branchial cleft anomalies** (Belenky and Medina 1980). They are subdivided into two types:

- **Type I** (Fig. 5.**22 a**), which is ectodermal in origin and usually contains skin, is referred to as a duplication of the external auditory canal.
- **Type II** (Fig. 5.**22 b, c**) is ectodermal or mesodermal in origin and, apart from skin, usually also contains cartilage.

The classification depends on clinical rather than histological criteria because cartilage (ectodermal and mesodermal structures) is not always found alongside squamous epithelium (Otto 1983). These fistulae often end blindly in the transitional region between the cartilaginous and bony auditory canal, and have an opening anterior to the sternocleidomastoid muscle (see Fig. 5.**21**). They frequently do not become clinically apparent until they are infected or form abscesses in adulthood. They cross over or under the facial nerve (see Fig. 5.**22**) and for removal they therefore need to be approached by exposing the facial nerve, as in surgery of the parotid (see treatment). Staining the fistulous tract with methylene blue has proved helpful.

A number of fistulae drain in a retroauricular location and are regarded as a proximal group of lateral cervical fistulae

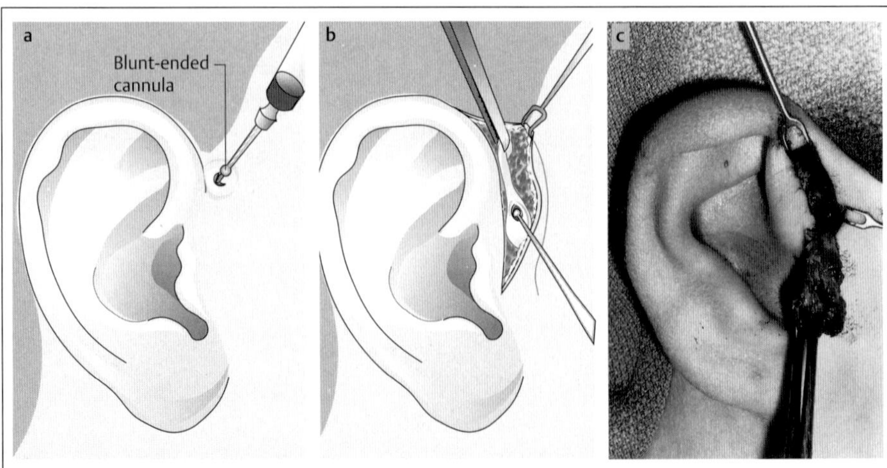

Fig. 5.**23** **Excision of a preauricular fistula after staining with methylene blue using a blunt-ended probe.**
a Staining of the fistula (sinus) with methylene blue using a blunt-ended cannula.
b, c Elliptical excision within the preauricular fold and dissection of the stained fistulous tract (sinus) over a blunt-ended probe.

(see Fig. 5.**21**, 3). These are found in combination with middle-ear and inner-ear malformations. A familial cluster has been reported (Mündnich and Terrahe 1979).

Treatment

Excision of Preauricular Fistulae and Sinuses

Preauricular fistulae that have no tendency to recurrent inflammation do not require surgery.

Pretherapeutic measures. We use general anesthesia for children and local anesthesia for adults. Generally speaking, surgery should not be undertaken during an inflammatory exacerbation. Intraoperatively, before dissection, the tract is stained with methylene blue via an olive-tip probe which is inserted into, and firmly closes, the excretory duct to provide enough pressure to achieve adequate filling and staining of the fistula or sinus. The fistulae usually end blindly at or under the cartilage of the ascending helix. Occasionally the length of the tract can be gauged with the aid of the probe (Fig. 5.**23 a**). A fistulogram using an aqueous contrast agent is an alternative.

It should be excluded before surgery that the fistula lies in the auditory canal, or has penetrated as far as the middle ear (Chami and Apesos 1989; Prasad et al. 1990; Joseph and Jacobsen 1995; Gurr et al. 1998; Lam et al. 2001).

Surgical approach. Incision is around the fistula (Fig. 5.**23 b, c**). We generally use loupes or a microscope for better magnification. After excision around the stained tracts and insertion of the probe, the fistula is identified and excised together with the perichondrium of the helical crus, followed by closure in layers with 5–0 braided sutures or 6–0 monofilament.

The high recurrence rates of between 5 and 32 % (Lam et al. 2001) prompted Prasad et al. (1990) to develop the so-called **supra-auricular excision**, according to which dissection follows a posterosuperior to anterior direction. With this technique the recurrence rate of the standard procedure was reduced from 32 to 3.7 % ($p \geq 0.01$; Lam et al. 2001). Prasad et al. themselves report a reduction in recurrences from 42 to 5 % using this method. They achieved the significantly lowest recurrence rate by staining the tract and excising it over the probe. Based on their experience gained with the excision of 165 fistulae and sinuses, they recommend staining the fistula or sinus and insertion of a probe, more aggressive excision with more tissue around the fistulae and sinuses, and excision of a part of the cartilage.

Surgical Repair of "Duplication of the External Auditory Canal"

As previously described (see p. 115), fistulae of the upper neck and ear region are sometimes regarded as duplications of the auditory canal (Chila and Miehlke 1984; Strutz and Mann 1989; Weerda 1994 e). The so-called "duplication of the external auditory canal" refers to an anomaly of the first branchial cleft. Belenky and Medina (1980) accordingly refer to the type I anomaly as a **preauricular cyst** or **draining sinus** (see Fig. 5.**22 a**). This anomaly is more frequently found in a postauricular location, but is occasionally preauricular, and occurs in young or middle-aged adults. It usually does not become clinically apparent until infected. The fistulous tract courses parallel to the auditory canal and always ends blindly, lateral or superior to the facial nerve.

Genuine duplicate auditory canals are type II fistulae and sinuses (Aronsohn et al. 1976; Fig. 5.**24 a**).

Surgical approach. Positioning is as for surgery of the parotid. The affected half of the face must remain uncovered; **neuromonitoring** for the facial nerve is mandatory. The incision is the same as for type I—pre- or postauricular,

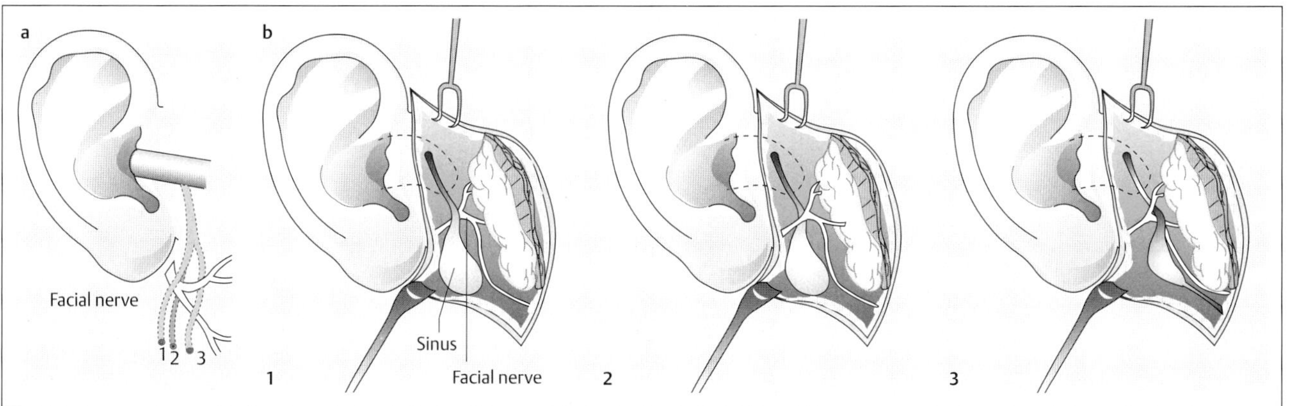

Fig. 5.24 **Location and surgery of type II fistulae (sinuses), so-called "duplication of the external auditory canal," which begins in the neck (see Fig. 5.22, in Weerda 1994e).**

a Schematic illustration; 1: fistula passing over the facial nerve; 2, 3: fistulae passing beneath the facial nerve.

b As with surgery of the parotid, preauricular incision, the main trunk of the facial nerve is always identified. Dissection as far as the cartilaginous auditory canal. Operative site as shown in the schematic diagrams; 1: course of the fistula (sinus) anterior to the facial nerve; 2: course posterior to the facial nerve; 3: course between cranial and distal segments of facial nerve.

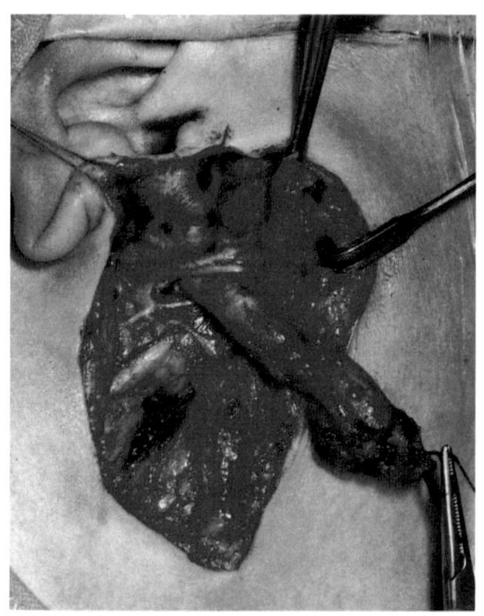

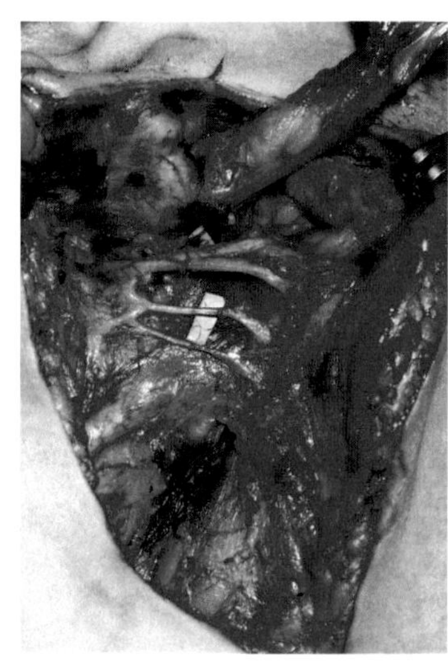

a b

Fig. 5.25 **Type II fistula of the neck and ear region (see Fig. 5.22, 3 and Fig. 5.24, 3).**

a Identification of the main trunk of the facial nerve and the individual nerve branches. Dissection of the fistula (stained with methylene blue).

b Removal of the fistula at the transition between the cartilaginous and bony auditory canal (surgeon: S. Remmert).

depending on location—or for type II fistulae and sinuses, according to surgery for the parotid (Fig. 5.25a, b), preauricular around the earlobe and in an anterior direction down through the cervical soft tissues following the relaxed skin tension lines. Then the main trunk of the facial nerve must be identified. Depending on whether the duplicate auditory canal is located anterior to, posterior to, or between the facial nerve branches, it must be dissected as far as the transition between the cartilaginous and bony auditory canal (Fig. 5.24b, 1–3) where the tract ends blindly (see Fig. 5.21, 1–3). Meticulous hemostasis, closure in layers, a small drain, and a dressing with mild compression are required. The sutures are removed on the 6th or 7th postoperative day.

5.4 Classification and Surgery of Auricular Dysplasias

H. Weerda

Interest in auricular malformations has increased considerably with the development of plastic surgery. Subsequently it has emerged that conventional terminologies and attempts at standardization do not allow a comprehensive presentation of the various different malformations.

A number of authors classify defects according to embryonic development, ranging from the severest form of anotia and grade III microtia to the mildest forms and prominent ears (Streeter 1922; Rogers 1968, 1974). The classification

Table 5.1 Tanzer's classification of auricular malformations (Tanzer 1977)

I	**Anotia**
II	**Complete hypoplasia (microtia):** • With congenital auricular atresia • Without congenital auricular atresia
III	**Hypoplasia of the middle third of the auricle**
IV	**Hypoplasia of the upper third of the auricle:** • Constricted ear, cup and lop ear • Cryptotia • Hyperplasia in the presence of a complete upper auricle
V	**Prominent auricle**

recommended by Tanzer (1977) is presented in Table 5.1. In contrast, Marx (1926) and Altmann (1951, 1965) have developed classifications based on the increasing severity of the malformations. Thus Altmann (1965) classifies macrotia and microtia according to size and position. Marx (1926) suggested classifying microtias into three groups: first-degree microtia, second-degree microtia, and third-degree microtia with anotia. Following Marx's recommendations and taking into account the suggestions of other authors, we have attempted to produce a classification of all dysplasias which allows a useful overview based on increasing severity of the malformation and the time and effort required for surgical repair (Table 5.2; Weerda 1981, 1982, 1994 e, 1999 a, 2001, Weerda and Siegert 1995 a).

Table 5.2 Weerda's classification of auricular malformations arranged in increasing severity of the malformation (Weerda 1981, 1994 e)

Degree of dysplasia	Definition	Subgroup
I: Low-grade malformations (Fig. 5.**26 a–c**)	**General:** most of the structures of a normal auricle are present **Surgical:** additional skin and cartilage are only occasionally required for reconstruction	• Prominent auricle • Macrotia • Cryptotia (pocket ear) • Cleft ear (transverse cleft) • Scaphoid ear • Stahl's ear • Satyr ear • Small deformities – Very pronounced Darwin's tubercle – Absent helical crus – Hyperplasia of the helical crus – Tragus deformities – Antitragus deformities • Lobule deformities – Adherent earlobe – Macrolobule – Cleft earlobe – Microlobule – Aplasia of the lobule • Tanzer's type I, IIA, and IIB cup-ear deformities
II: Grade II microtia; moderate malformations (Fig. 5.**27 a–c**)	**General:** the auricle still displays some structures of a normal auricle **Surgical:** additional skin and cartilage required for partial reconstruction	• Tanzer's type III cup-ear deformity (Tanzer 1977) • Mini ear (Nagata's concha type microtia, Nagata 1994 b): – Hypoplasia of the upper auricle – Hypoplasia of the middle third of the auricle – Hypoplasia (aplasia) of the lower auricle
III: Grade III microtia with anotia; severe malformations (Fig. 5.**28 a–c**)	**General:** structures of a normal auricle no longer present **Surgical:** additional skin and cartilage required for total reconstruction	• Unilateral grade III microtia (Nagata's lobule type microtia) • Bilateral grade III microtia • Anotia • Normally congenital aural atresia will be found; see pp. 245 and 255

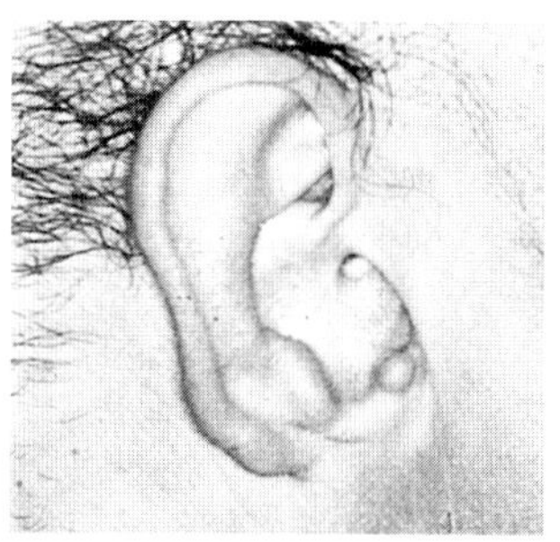
a

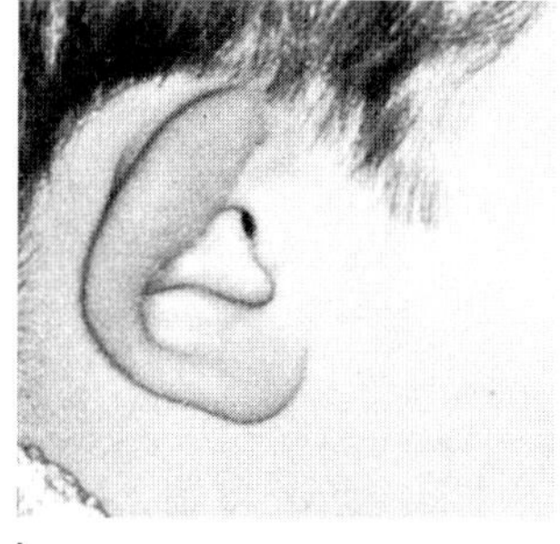
b

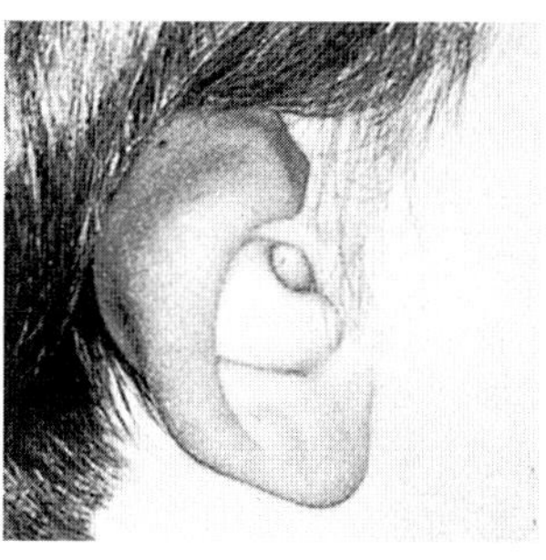
c

Fig. 5.**26** **Grade I dysplasias (from Weerda 1994 e).**
a Aplasia of the earlobe: malformation of hillocks 1–(2) (see p. 107).
b Type I cup-ear deformity (see text): malformation of hillock 3 (see p. 108).
c Type II cup-ear deformity (see text): malformation of hillocks 2–3 (see p. 108).

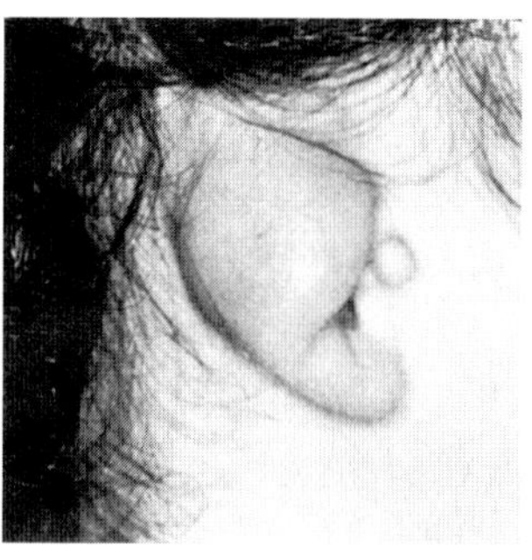
a

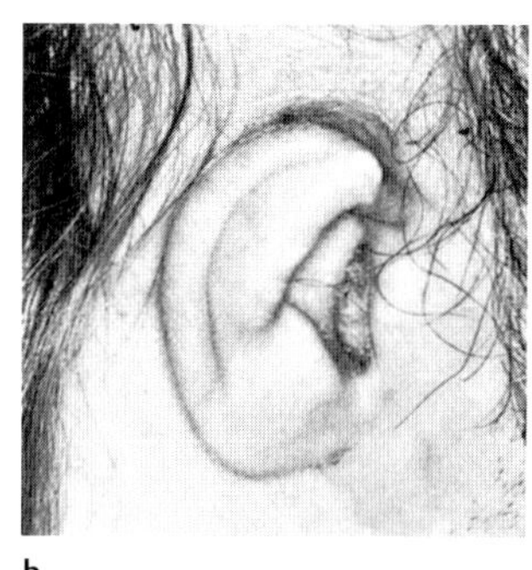
b

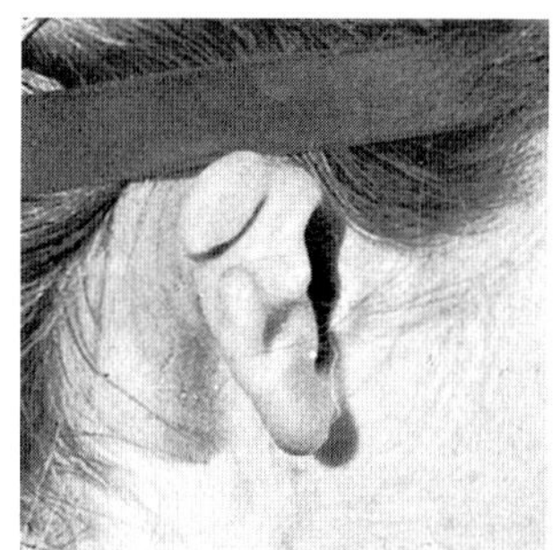
c

Fig. 5.**27** **Grade II dysplasias (grade II microtias; from Weerda 1994 e; Nagata's concha type microtia, Nagata 1994 b).**
a Severe type III cup-ear deformity with dystopia: malformation of hillocks 3–4 (see p. 112).
b Mini-ear with a longitudinal axis length of 4 cm: malformation of hillocks 2–3–(4) (see p. 112, Fig. 5.**15**).
c Mini-ear with absence of the upper auricular segment and reduction of auricular longitudinal and transverse axes (transitional form to grade III dysplasia: malformation of hillocks 2–4; see p. 112, Fig. 5.**15**).

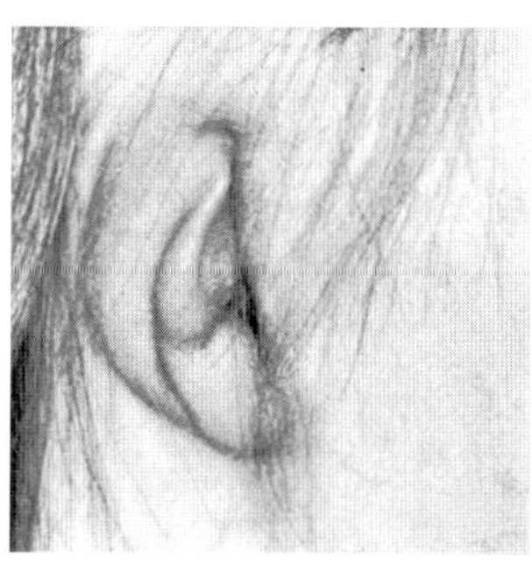
a

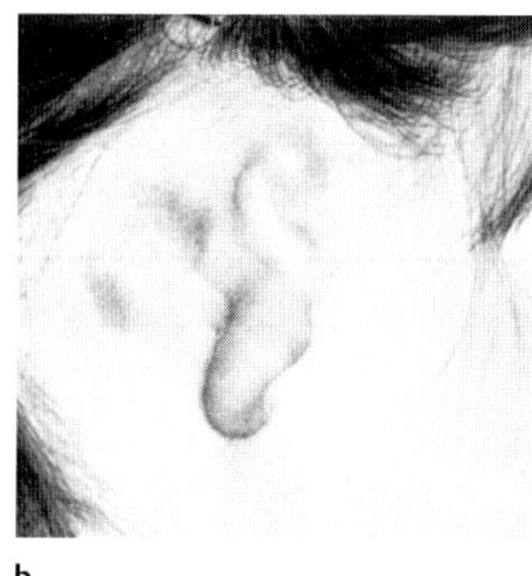
b

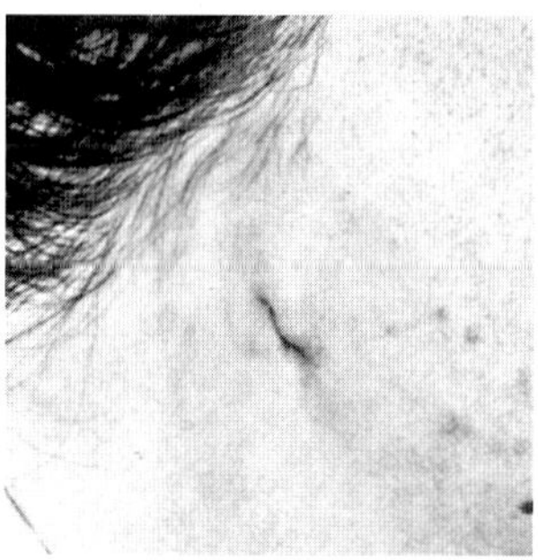
c

Fig. 5.**28** **Grade III dysplasias (grade III microtias with anotia; from Weerda 1994 e).**
a Grade III microtia with preformed auditory canal: malformation of hillocks 2–4 (see p. 112, Fig. 5.**15**).
b Grade III microtia with typical rudiment and congenital aural atresia: malformation of hillocks 2–5 (see p. 112, Fig. 5.**16**, Nagata's lobule type microtia, Nagata 1994 b).
c Anotia with blind-ending fistula: malformation of hillocks 1–6 (see p. 113, Fig. 5.**17**).

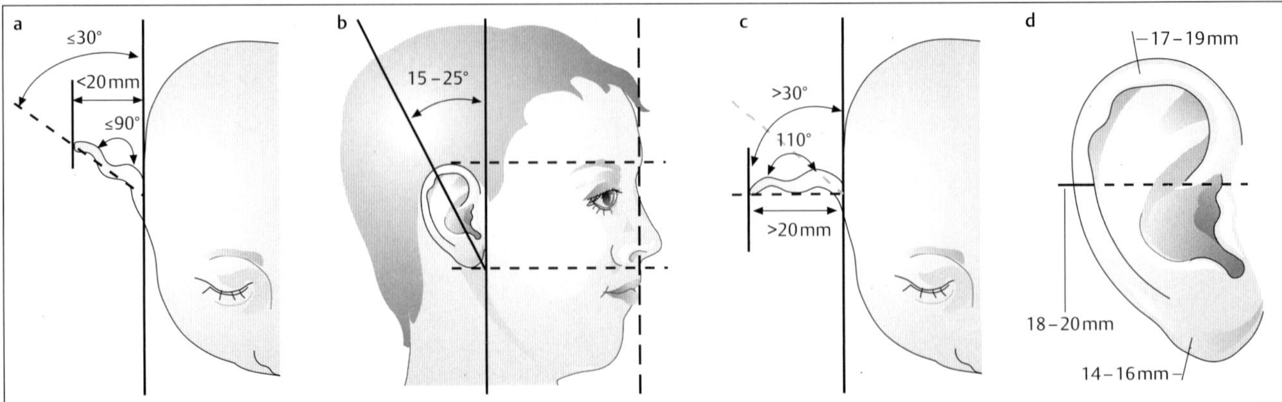

Fig. 5.**29** **Measurements of the normal and the prominent auricle.**
a In the normal ear the angle between ear and mastoid plane is about 30° and the distance between the anterior helical rim and the mastoid is less than 20 mm. The scaphoconchal angle is less than 90°.
b The axis of the ear is angled 15–25° posteriorly relative to the profile axis.
c Prominent auricle with an angle between ear and mastoid plane of about 90°; anterior helical rim–mastoid distance is significantly larger than 20 mm; the scaphoconchal angle is 110° (or more than 90°).
d Average distances of the anterior helical rim to the mastoid at the upper, middle, and lower auricle (always measured before and after ear setback operations).

It is advisable to deal with deformities of the earlobe at the end (p. 165), together with grade I dysplasias (p. 170).

Although it may not always appear appropriate, we have nevertheless decided to honor R.C. Tanzer, one of the most important pioneers of auricular surgery, and adhere to his classification by dividing cup-ear deformities into three grades of severity and inserting them as a block at the end of grade I dysplasias, before the grade II dysplasias (p. 170).

We furthermore distinguish between the following forms of dysplasias:

- Differences in relief definition
- Differences of size and form
- Dystopias with differences in insertion and position on the head

5.4.1 Grade I Dysplasias

Synonym: mild malformations (see Fig. 5.**26**).

Prominent Ear

Synonyms: protruding ear, bat ear, apostasis otum, otapostasis.

Operation. Otoplasty; synonyms: corrective otoplasty (Tanzer 1977), otopexy, antihelix reconstruction, otoclisis, otorthoclisis (Joseph 1912, 1931), pinnaplasty, setback otoplasty, ear pinning.

Causes. As previously mentioned under embryology (see p. 107), this is a hereditary malformation which, according to Maniglia and Maniglia (1981), has a dominant pattern of inheritance. There is known familial clustering. There are certainly exogenic as well as unknown causes of unilateral and bilateral prominent ears. From the third month of embryonic development, the auricle undergoes increasing protrusion while it migrates from an anterocaudal to a posterocranial position. The development of the helical form and the formation of the antihelical furl occur at about the sixth month of gestation (see Fig. 5.**3**, p. 107). A disturbance of normal evolution subsequently results in protrusion of the ear (Tanzer 1977).

Standard Measurements. For a normal auricle, there is an angle of about 30° between the auricular axis and the mastoid plane, a helix-to-mastoid distance of less than 20 mm, and a scapho-conchal angle of less than 90° (Fig. 5.**29 a**).

With the prominent ear we find:

- An angle between the auricular axis and the mastoid plane of more than 30°
- A helix-to-mastoid distance of more than than 20 mm
- A scapho-conchal angle of more than 90° (Fig. 5.**29 c**)

The average distances from the mastoid plane are 17–19 mm in the upper auricle, 18–20 mm in the middle auricular region, and 14–16 mm in the lobular region (Pellnitz 1958; Wodak 1967; Kaesemann 1991; Weerda and Siegert 1995 a; Siegert and Weerda 1998 a; Fig. 5.**29 d**).

The characteristics of the external ear are also altered: there is flattening of the antihelix, even to the extent of an absent antihelix with flattening in the region of the inferior crus or both crura.

Definition. A pseudoconchal hyperplasia is observed, although true enlargement of the concha tends to be rare. Jayes (1951) classifies the prominent ear according to decreasing prominence of the antihelical fold and increasing widening of the scapho-conchal angle.

Quite different forms of prominent ears are possible. Some typical examples are (Weerda 1985 a):

- Poorly developed superior crus
- Flattening of antihelix and superior crus
- Severe hyperplasia of the entire concha, including both antihelical crura
- Prominence of the auricle mainly in its upper region
- Prominence of the middle region only
- Prominence of the lower region only

A number of other malformations can also be included in this category:

- Excessively high antihelix
- Prominent auricle with absent formation of the helix (scaphoid ear; see also p. 160)
- Prominent ear with an excessively long earlobe
- Differences between the left and right ear
- Various additional anomalies such as prominent tragus, prominent antitragus, and other similar malformations

Because the ear grows only very little after the sixth year of life (see Chapter 1, section on anthropometry, p. 4), we operate on children with the stigma of "prominent ears" during their fifth year of life, before they start school.

Although the size of the auricle does not appreciably increase after this time, the elasticity and thickness of the cartilage change with increasing age, and the consistency of the cartilage has an influence on the operative technique used (Weerda 1985 a; see Chapter 1, section on anthropometry, p. 4).

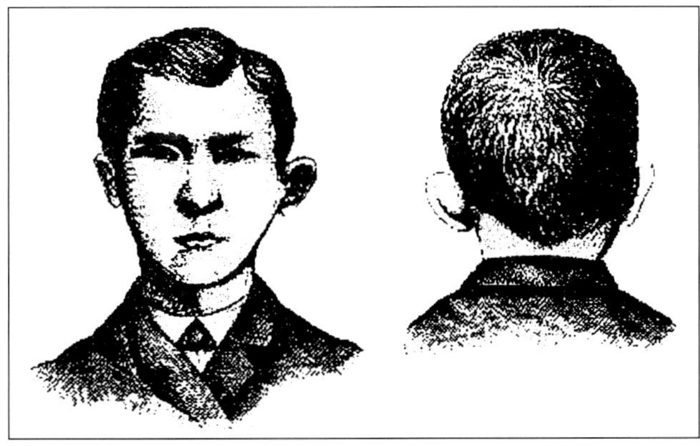

Fig. 5.**30** **One of Ely's patients after corrective surgery of the right ear for bilateral prominent ear (apostasis otum; from Roosa 1881).**

Historical Review. Since Ely described the first setback otoplasties in 1881 (Fig. 5.**30**), almost 100 options, and thus a large variety of techniques, have been reported in the literature. The first setback otoplasty, as cited in the Anglo-American literature, is generally ascribed to Dieffenbach (1845), but this is based on a translation error. He used the term "otoplasty" for all his operations on the external ear, and the literal translation of the word led to this misunderstanding (Schmidt 2000). Dieffenbach in fact only described partial reconstructions of the auricle. Ely (1881) was really the first to describe a setback otoplasty.

Schmidt (2000) examined all the literature currently available and attempted to systematize the operative techniques described in the literature (Table 5.**3**). There are too many different procedures to be described here, and in this chapter only a few of the important operative techniques are described.

Table 5.**3** The surgical techniques of otoplasty, their originators, and further developers; overview of the surgical steps performed by each author (from Schmidt 2000)

Author	**Year**	**Approach**	**Incision/ suture technique**	**Scoring technique**	**Suture technique**	**Skin excision**	**Skin excision ear and mastoid**	**Skin–cartilage excision and mastoid fixation**	**Skin–cartilage incision or excision and anchoring**	**Cup-ear surgery**	**Special forms**
Ely	1881	Posterior				+					+
Stetter	1884	Posterior							+	+	
Keen	1889	Posterior	+								
Monks	1891	Posterior				+					
Schwartze	1892	Posterior				+					
Schwartze	1892	Posterior					+				+

Table 5.3 (Continued)

Author	Year	Approach	Incision/ suture technique	Scoring technique	Suture technique	Skin excision	Skin excision ear and mastoid	Skin–cartilage excision and mastoid fixation	Skin–cartilage incision or excision and anchoring	Cup-ear surgery	Special forms
Haug	1894	Posterior					+		+		
Haug	1894	Posterior					+				
Joseph	1896	Posterior						+			
Joseph	1896	Posterior					+	+			
Weinlechner	1898	Posterior					+	+			
Morestin	1903	Posterior			+						
Gersuny	1903	Posterior	+								
Payr	1906	Posterior							+		
Goldstein 1	1908	Posterior	+			+					
Goldstein 2	1908	Posterior							+		
Ruttin	1910	Posterior					+				
Luckett	1910	Posterior	+								
Streit	1914	Posterior					+				
Eckstein	1912	Posterior	+								
Eitner	1922	Posterior						+			
Hofer & Leidler	1923	Posterior									+
Gersuny	1924	Posterior						+			
Alexander	1928	Posterior	+								
Alexander	1928	Posterior							+		
Schlander	1930	Posterior							+	+	
Lüthi	1930	Posterior							+		
Demel & Feigl	1931	Posterior							+		
Goodyear	1933	Posterior					+				
Wolfe	1936	Posterior						+			
Eitner	1937	Posterior						+			
Davis & Kitlowski	1937	Posterior	+								
Barsky	1938	Posterior									+
Ehrenfeld	1938	Posterior						+			
New & Reich	1940	Posterior	+								
Young	1944	Posterior	+								
Seeley	1946	Posterior	+								
Weaver	1947	Posterior	+								
McEvitt	1947	Posterior	+								
Becker	1949	Posterior	+								
Dufourmentel	1950	Posterior						+			

Table 5.**3** (Continued)

Author	Year	Approach	Incision/ suture technique	Scoring tech-nique	Suture tech-nique	Skin ex-cision	Skin ex-cision ear and mastoid	Skin–cartilage excision and mastoid fixation	Skin–car-tilage in-cision or excision and an-choring	Cup-ear surgery	Special forms
Jayes & Dale	1951	Posterior	+								
Sercer	1951	Posterior									+
Gonzales–Ulloa	1952	Anterior	+								
Borges	1953	Posterior		+							
Seltzer	1954	Posterior						+			
Converse	1955	Posterior	+								
Schütze	1956	Posterior						+			
Walter	1958	Posterior	+								
Friedmann	1959	Posterior	+								
Tamerin	1959	Posterior	+								
Lehnhardt	1959	Anterior	+								
Mustardé	1960	Posterior			+						
Goulian	1960	Posterior	+								+
Vogl	1961	Posterior					+				
Cloutier	1961	Posterior		+							
Tanzer	1962	Posterior	+								
Pitanguy	1962	Posterior	+								
Stark & Saunders	1962	Posterior	+		+						
Reichert	1963	Posterior		+							
Converse	1963	Posterior	+								
Chongchet	1963	Posterior		+							
Stenström	1963	Posterior		+							
Ju & Crikelair	1963	Anterior		+							
Crikelair	1964	Posterior		+							
Reichert	1965	Posterior		+							+
Kaye	1967	Anterior		+							
McDowell	1968	Posterior	+								
Furnas	1968	Posterior			+		+				
Furnas	1968	Posterior					+				
Webster	1969	Posterior	+								+
Spira	1969	Posterior			+			+			
Wieland	1971	Posterior		+							
Tolhurst	1972	Posterior		+							
Stenström	1973	Posterior		+							
Batisse	1973	Posterior		+							

Table 5.3 (Continued)

Author	Year	Approach	Incision/ suture technique	Scoring tech-nique	Suture tech-nique	Skin ex-cision	Skin ex-cision ear and mastoid	Skin–cartilage excision and mastoid fixation	Skin–car-tilage in-cision or excision and an-choring	Cup-ear surgery	Special forms
Bruck	1976	Posterior			+						
Krüger	1979	Posterior			+						
Weerda	1979	Posterior	+		+						+
Vecchione	1979	Anterior		+							
Psillakis	1979	Posterior			+			+			
Smith	1979	Posterior	+								+
Beernick	1979	Posterior			+			+			+
Welsh	1980	Posterior	+	+	+			+			
Schröder	1980	Posterior	+					+			
Staindl	1980	Anterior		+							
Ohlsen	1980	Posterior			+						
Rhys Evans	1981	Posterior		+							
Kastenbauer	1983	Posterior		+							
Stal & Spira	1985	Posterior		+	+				+		
J. Ely	1988	Anterior		+							
Elliot	1991	Anterior		+	+			+			
Stark	1991	Anterior	+		+						+
Romo	1994	Anterior			+			+			
Fritsch	1995	Posterior			+						

Rotation of the Ear without Reconstruction of the Antihelical Fold

Excisions of Skin or Skin and Cartilage Between 1881 and 1910

Skin Excision

The oldest method was the elliptical or crescent-shape excision of skin from the anterior and/or posterior auricular surface with suturing of the excisional margins (Ely 1881; Monks 1891; Schwartze 1892). This method was then expanded to include excision of skin on the postauricular surface and on the mastoid (Haug 1894; Joseph 1896; Ruttin 1910; Goodyear 1933; Vogl 1961; Furnas 1968 among others; Fig. 5.31 a, b).

Skin and Cartilage Excision

In older patients, and in the presence of rigid cartilage in particular, cartilage was excised in addition to the removal

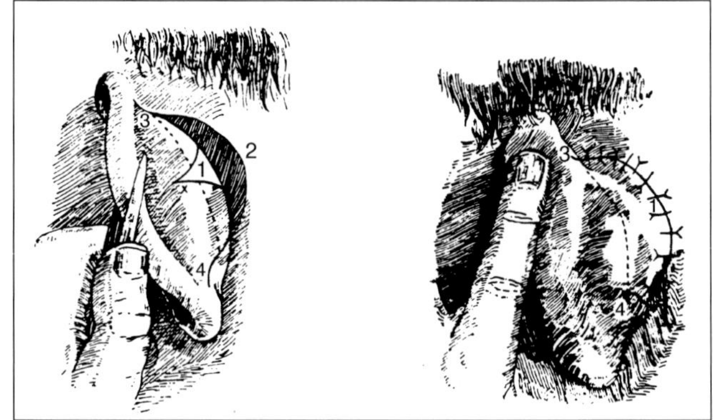

Fig. 5.31 **Posterior skin excision (Ely 1881, Monks 1891; in Schmidt 2000).**

a Crescent-shaped skin excision over the auricle and the mastoid.

b Margin of the wound pulled posteriorly and sutured as described by Haug (1894).

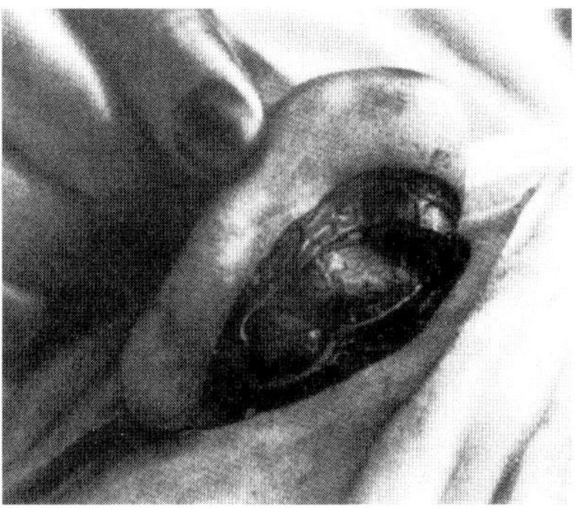

a

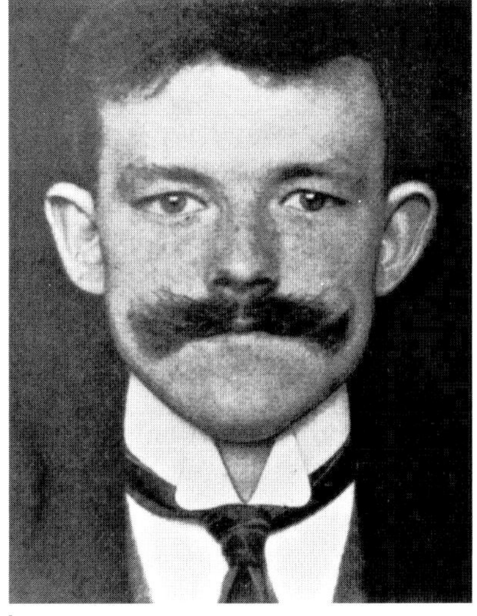

b

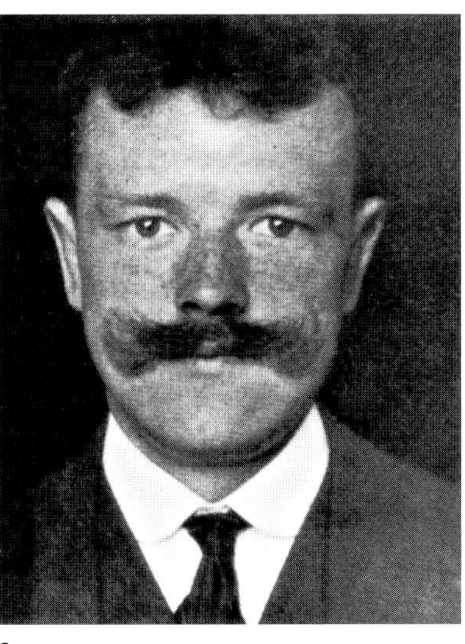

c

Fig. 5.32 **Skin–cartilage excisions.**
a Skin–cartilage excision in the presence of rigid cartilaginous conditions (Joseph 1896, 1912, 1931).
b, c Appearance before and after this form of otoplasty. From: Joseph J. Ohrdefekte (Otoneoplastik). In Joseph J. Nasenplastik und sonstige Gesichtsplastik. 3. Abteilung. Leipzig: C. Kabitzsch (1931: 717–736; c,d). [Ear defects (Otoneoplasty). In Joseph J. Rhinoplasty and other plastic surgery of the face.]

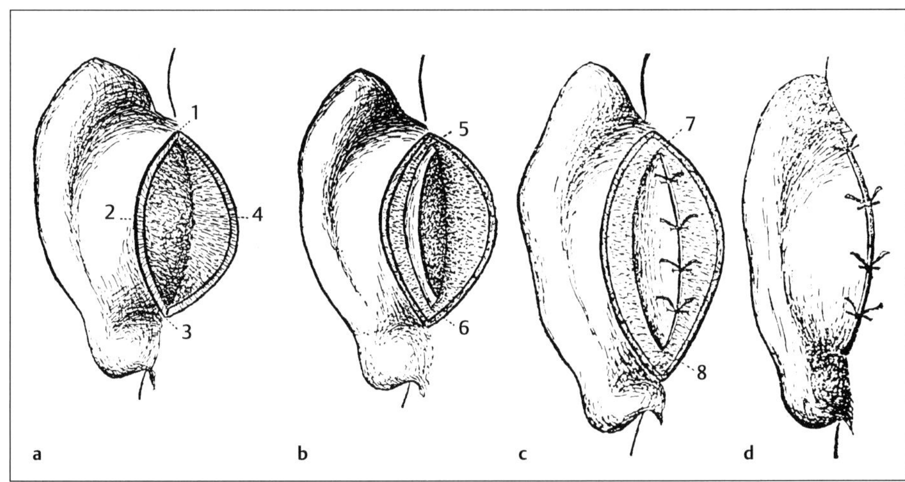

Fig. 5.33 **Otoplasty for prominent ear (apostasis otum; in Goldstein 1908).**
a Excision of skin from the postauricular surface and the mastoid.
b Excision of a vertical strip of cartilage.
c, d Suture of the medial cartilaginous segment to the mastoid periosteum and skin closure with the auricle set back.

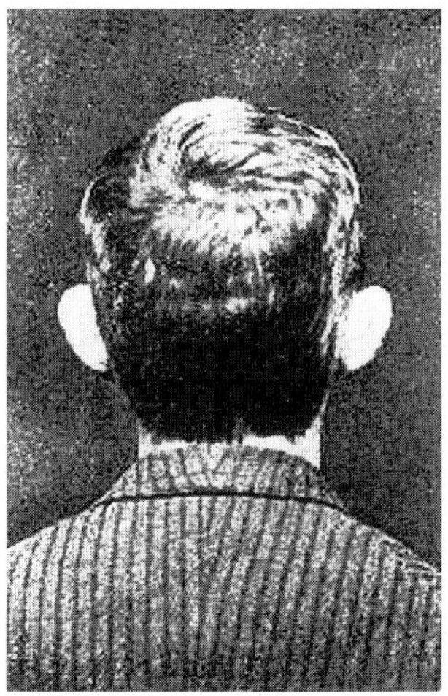

a

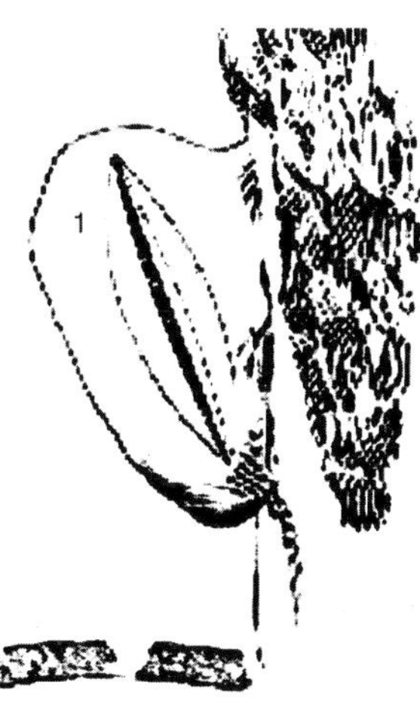

b

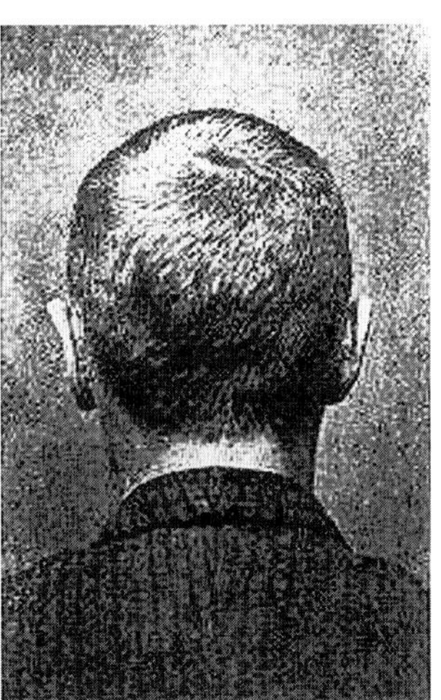

c

Fig. 5.34 **Surgical procedure for skin–cartilage excision (in Keen 1890).**
a Patient.
b Appearance of the left ear with skin and cartilage excision. Care should be taken to make the skin incision wider and longer than the cartilage excision. Transverse section through the cartilage to demonstrate the amount of cartilage excised.
c Result.

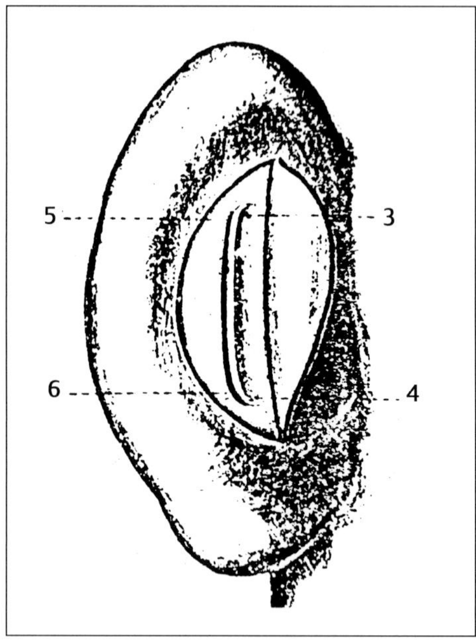

a

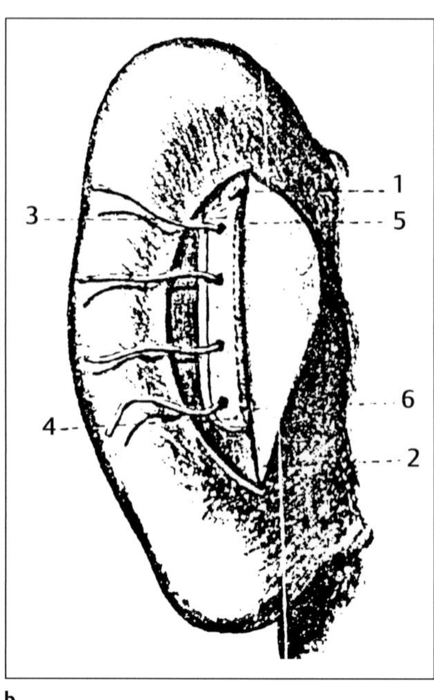

b

Fig. 5.**35** **Surgical technique for reduction of height and improved position (in Goldstein 1908).**
a Vertical skin and cartilage incision from a posterior approach.
b Dorsal suture of the medial cartilaginous segment to the lateral segment to reconstruct the antihelix which is visible from the front.

of skin (Ely 1881; Joseph 1896, 1931; Goldstein 1908; Eitner 1937; Dufourmentel 1950; Psillakis 1979; Welsh 1980 among others; Fig. 5.**32 a–c**). In order to avoid visible anterior cartilage ridging, Joseph (1931) undermined the anterior skin. Between 1886 and 1902, Joseph reported on 12 setback otoplasties.

An interesting variation was described by Keen in 1890 (see Fig. 5.**34**).

Skin Excision and Conchal Setback

In 1908 Goldstein reported on his method of setback otoplasty: he excised skin on the posterior auricular surface and on the mastoid plane (Fig. 5.**33 a**) made a curvilinear incision over the cartilage which he dissected away from the anterior skin (Fig. 5.**33 b**). The cartilage was then sutured to the periosteum of the mastoid plane and the ear subsequently set back with closure of the skin wound (Fig. 5.**33 c, d**).

Since this time, this so-called "conchal setback" ("conchal rotation" or even "cavum rotation") has formed a part of the armamentarium of setback otoplasty and is wrongly attributed to Furnas (1968).

Antihelix Reconstruction

The discovery of antihelix reconstruction is attributed to Luckett (1910). But as early as 1889, Keen performed an operation from the posterior auricular surface, by which he incised skin and cartilage at about the level of the antihelix and placed three catgut sutures through the cartilage in order to create an antihelix. He then closed the skin wound (Fig. 5.**34**).

Gersuny (1903) is known to have used a surgical technique by which he incised the cartilage on its posterior surface in a criss-cross fashion, excised the postauricular skin and skin over the mastoid region, attached the concha to the mastoid, and then closed the skin. Here too, some form of antihelix reconstruction must have been performed (Biesenberger 1924).

Goldstein (1908) also describes an operative technique in which reconstruction is performed in the region of the antihelix. After a curvilinear incision and skin excision, the posterior cartilage is freed of skin and sutured beneath the anterior cartilage, thus achieving folding of the auricle (Fig. 5.**35 a, b**). Goldstein also described the cause of the auricular deformity: "absence of antihelix, projecting ear, and redundancy of conchal cartilage." He defines a prominent ear as having an angle greater than 45°.

Ears set back experimentally in anatomical studies using this method (Schmidt 2000) demonstrated a reduction of the helix-to-mastoid distance of 6–9 mm and the formation of an antihelix.

Goldstein (1908) had probably consciously performed the first antihelix reconstructions even before Luckett (1910).

Luckett's Technique (Fig. 5.36)

Like Morestin (1903) before him, Lucket (1910) analysed the cause of the prominent ear. He pointed out that the prominence of the auricle was more than just an increase in the auriculocephalic angle. For this reason, operative techniques in which only a skin excision or a skin–cartilage excision was performed did not correct the actual deformity. Luckett made an incision on the posterior surface of the auricle, excised skin and (depending on the extent of the antihelix re-

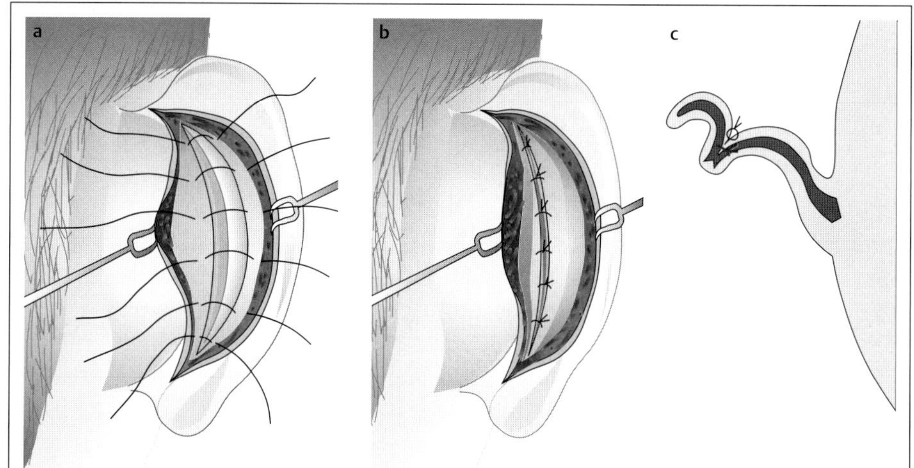

Fig. 5.**36** a–c **Antihelix reconstruction as described by Luckett 1910 (see text).**

construction) cartilage, and sutured the cartilage back-to-back (Fig. 5.**36** a) to create a natural antihelix in the region of the anterior auricular surface (Fig. 5.**36** b, c) and, at the same time, the ear was set back.

Barsky's Technique

Instead of excising the cartilage (Luckett 1910), Barsky (1938) only incised around it and advanced it anteriorly to create an antihelical crest; a method that Pitanguy (1962) and Pitanguay and Flemmings (1976) took up again.

Davis and Kitlowski's Method

Marking of the auricular contours with needles was described by Davis and Kitlowski (1937). These authors were the first to insert needles from anteriorly to mark the antihelix. Brilliant green was used as a marking dye.

Modern Techniques of Antihelix Reconstruction

Techniques used today are defined by their anterior or posterior approach and by the way the cartilage is handled and folded (see Table 5.3).

Incision/Suture Technique (see Fig. 5.45)

Definition. Transection of the cartilage using various techniques and securing the fold of the auricle with sutures.

Becker's Technique

Following a posterior approach, the new antihelix was outlined with needles and methylene blue and the new antihelix incised using the markings (Becker 1949, 1952). Parts of the cartilage were also excised. Skin was then excised and the wound closed, using mattress sutures to create a natural fold in the antihelix. Based on this method, Converse et al. (1955) developed their operative technique which has stood the test of time right up to the present day (see p. 136, Fig. 5.**45**).

Methods using the incision/suture technique with an anterior approach were also developed (Gonzales-Ulloa 1952).

Scoring Technique (see Fig. 5.43)

Definition. Scoring of the anterior cartilage, usually from the posterior aspect. A suture to secure the fold in the cartilage is not necessarily required.

As with the incision/suture technique, most of the operations employing the scoring technique were performed using a posterior approach. It is no easy task to document the initial description of this method.

Borges' Technique

In order to create a well-rounded antihelix, an island of cartilage was incised (Borges 1953), similar to the suggestions made by Barsky (1938). The island of cartilage was then scored anteriorly to obtain a better form.

Cloutier's Technique

The Canadian surgeon Cloutier (1961) referred to the biomechanical studies of cartilage by Gibson and Davis (1958) and incised the cartilage from a posterior approach along the antihelical line. He performed tangential excisions of the cartilage on its anterior surface, causing the two cartilaginous segments to take on an anterior convex fold.

Chongchet's Technique (Fig. 5.41)

Chongchet published his work in September 1963 and reported that he had been performing the scoring technique since 1960, fully aware of Gibson and Davis' (1958) studies on costal cartilage. He made a full-thickness incision through the cartilage from a posterior approach, at about the level of the scapha, undermined the anterior surface and placed superficial parallel incisions along its entire length (see Fig. 5.**41**, p. 133). Crikelair and Cosman reported the same technique in 1964, being aware of the work by Cloutier (1961) and Chongchet (1963).

Stenström's Technique (Figs. 5.42, 5.43)

Stenström's technique (November 1963, 1973; see p. 134, Figs. 5.**42**, 5.**43**) is also based on knowledge of the work by Gibson and Davis on costal cartilage (1958). Stenström made the same experiment regarding the bending of cartilage by studying auricular cartilage, and operated from a small posteroinferior incision. We shall deal with this technique in detail later (see p. 134).

Ju et al.'s Method (Figs. 5.37e, 5.44)

Ju and co-workers recommended an anterior approach within the scapha (December 1963; see Figs. 5.**37e** and 5.**44**); they had previously reported on their method in October 1962 at the meeting of the American Society of Plastic and Reconstructive Surgery (Schmidt 2000).

Reichert (1963), Wieland (1971), Batisse (1973), and Staindl (1980) as well as Rhys-Evans (1981) and Kastenbauer (1983 a) used this method with an anterior or posterior approach.

Suture Technique (see Fig. 5.40)

Definition. Folding the antihelical cartilage without any additional incision techniques.

Posterior approach.

Morestin's Technique

As previously explained, Morestin had recognized in 1903, 7 years before Luckett (1910), that it was the absence of the antihelix which resulted in the auriculocephalic angle being too large. For this reason, Morestin combined a suture technique with a posterior skin excision to create the antihelical fold. This technique was rediscovered 57 years later by Mustardé (1960) and entered the literature as the Mustardé technique. He was not, however, the originator, as stated in most surgical manuals (Schmidt 2000).

Luckett's Technique (Fig. 5.36)

Luckett also stated that reconstruction of the antihelix with thin and flexible cartilage is only possible with sutures (Luckett 1910, p. 126, 127). Similarly, Alexander (1928) also describes creating an antihelical fold with the use of catgut sutures.

Mustardé's Technique (Fig. 5.40)

This is the suture technique from a posterior approach as published by Mustardé (1960, 1963) and imitated many times. So Mustardé is cited as the originator of this method in the literature, although as mentioned above Morestin (1903) as well as Luckett (1910) had reported this technique much earlier. This method has been used and recommended by many authors (Furnas 1968; Spira 1969; Psillakis 1979; Ohlsen 1980; Bull and Mustardé 1985; Romo 1994). The technique is described in detail in the following section on current surgical methods (see p. 131).

Current Methods

General Aspects

Regardless of the technique used, the following requirements should be fulfilled (Davis 1987):

- The operative technique should be applicable to all age groups.
- The ideal age is 5–7 years.
- The operative method should be applicable or adaptable for all types of prominent ears.
- The result must be postoperative symmetry of both ears (measurements made before and after surgery; see p. 120).
- Good auricular proportions must be achieved.
- The helix–earlobe curve should run parallel to the mastoid surface. The distance between the posteromedial helical rim and the mastoid plane should be about 10 mm (Davis 1987), and the distance between the upper helical rim and the mastoid should be about 17 mm, with a maximum of 20 mm.
- The posterior sulcus should be well formed, i. e., skin should be excised very sparingly and only when necessary.
- No sharp ridges should be visible on the anterior surface.
- The earlobe should be set back to the same extent as the rest of the auricle.

Davis (1987) considers blind surgery to be a dangerous technique.

Age of the Patient. We usually operate children on an outpatient basis or with a short hospital stay at the age of 5 years, before they start school. Our oldest patient was 78 years old.

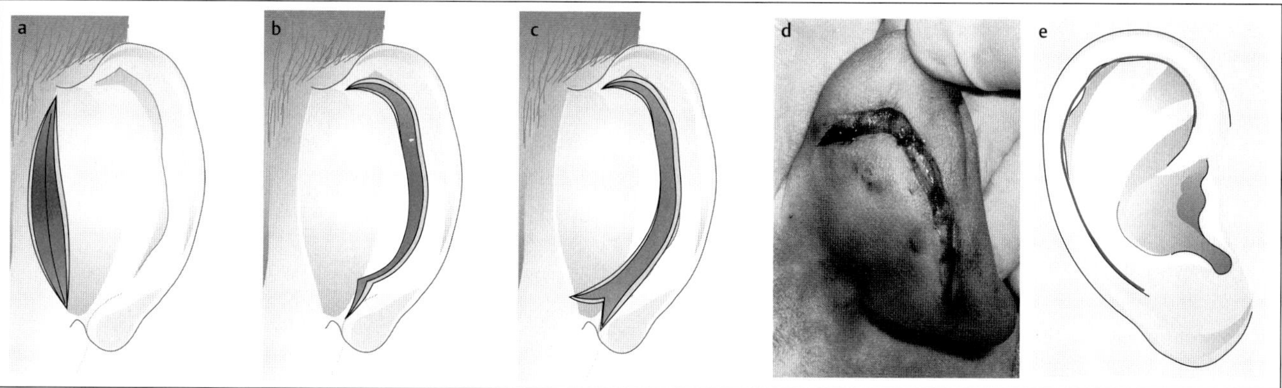

Fig. 5.37 **Operative approaches with skin excision as cited in the literature.**
a Oval resection in the sulcus (Ely 1881; Joseph 1896, 1931; Goldstein 1908; Wolfe 1936; Seltzer 1954; Welsh 1980; Stal and Spira 1985).
b, c Incision and crescent- or banana-shaped excision close to the helix (Keen 1980; Luckett 1910; Lüthi 1930; McEvitt 1947; Converse 1955; Friedmann 1959; Mustardé 1960; Chongchet 1963; Crikelair 1964; Stenström 1973; Weerda 1979 a; Romo 1994).
d An example of our approach.
e Anterior approach: incision in the scapha (e. g. Ju et al. 1963; Fig. 5.**44**, p. 135).

Preparation for Surgery. We use a pre-printed form to document preoperative measurements (see Appendix 1, pp. 301 ff). The patient's hair should be washed on the day before surgery.

Inpatients have their ears and periauricular region washed with an antiseptic solution on the evening before the operation (povidone–iodine solution 1:10) and the ears covered with a sterile dressing.

Positioning and Anesthesia. Unilateral setback otoplasty in an adult can be done under local anesthesia. We prefer to perform bilateral otoplasties and otoplasties in children under general anesthesia. The patient is positioned supine and both ears are left uncovered.

To reduce both pain and bleeding, a local anesthetic with epinephrine 1 : 200 000 is injected into the postauricular surface.

Approaches

The approach is usually a posterior one, the incision coursing parallel to the helix and 1 cm below it (Fig. 5.**37 b**–**d**). Approaches from the sulcus and posteriorly in the scapha have also been reported (Fig. 5.**37 e**).

Posterior approach. After undermining the skin on the postauricular surface towards the helical rim and down to the sulcus, the outer ear is folded back in order to mark with needles or cannulae the position of the new antihelix, together with its transition to the scapha and its transition to the concha (see Fig. 5.**40 a**–**c**). We usually undermine the skin, leaving behind the perichondrium, first in the direction of the sulcus, and then mark the position of the antihelical transitions with needles inserted from the anterior surface, using a marking pen or methylene blue (see Fig. 5.**40 b**, **c**).

The antihelical fold is then created with mattress sutures (see Fig. 5.**40 d**–**f**). We place the plastic tube from a drain or something similar, secured by a long suture, into the lower wound area and, if necessary, resect a narrow strip of skin about 5 mm wide. Finally the wound is closed with a running intracutaneous, or even transcutaneous, suture.

Special points. We like to glue the skin of the posterior auricular surface to the sulcus and the skin of the postauricular surface.

Skin excision and posterior approach. Many authors prefer the elliptical skin excision in the sulcus (Fig. 5.**37 a**), with the amount of resected skin differing widely, even to the extent of subtotal posterior skin resection. Many surgeons, particularly at the beginning of the twentieth century, resected conchal cartilage very generously. There are a number of modifications to these incisions (see history of setback otoplasty, p. 126; Morestin 1903; Davis and Kitlowski 1937; Seltzer 1954; Stark and Saunders 1962; Stenström 1973; Romo 1994).

A posterior incision about 1 cm below the helical rim (Fig. 5.**37 b**, **d**) is preferred by a number of authors, including Converse (1955, 1963), Mustardé (1960), as well as Chongchet (1963), Crikelair (1964), and Stenström (1973; see also Fig. 5.**40 g**).

We recommend being very conservative with the excision of skin.

Anterior approach. An anterior approach is reported by Ju et al. (1963, Fig. 5.**37 e**) as well as by Lehnhardt (1959) in his method of otoplasty adapted from Vogel's operation (1938) to correct macrotia.

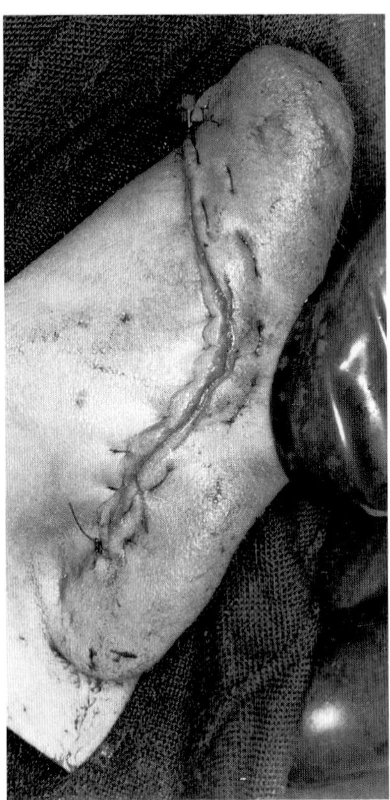

Fig. 5.38 **Continuous suture using 5–0 polydioxanone monofilament.**

Whereas Ju et al. (1963) dissected off the anterior skin as a skin–perichondrium flap, Argamaso and Lewin (1978) extended the incision through the cartilage, exposed the postauricular surface and, after performing an excision at the transition of the antihelix–conchal region, folded the auricle as a modified Converse technique with an anterior approach.

Suture Material

Non-absorbable sutures. Many authors, particularly in earlier years and including Mustardé (1963), recommended silk to create the helical fold. Mustardé (1985) again emphasizes that the success of otoplasty is considerably greater with silk than with other suture material (Bull and Mustardé 1985). Silk is also recommended in 1979 by Smith (1979) and Reichert (1979).

Polyester monofilament. We used to prefer undyed 4–0 braided resorbable sutures, but since the scar does not yet appear to hold the new antihelical fold in position after suture absorption, we saw a number of recurrences. We now prefer a braided white 4–0 polyester suture, which is nonabsorbable and very well tolerated by the tissue. A 3–0 suture of the same material is recommended by Converse (1963), Spira (1969), Welsh (1980), Walter (1994 b) and, for the incisionless otoplasty, by Fritsch (1995).

Braided sutures with a polyamide (nylon) coating are now hardly ever used.

Monofilament stainless steel wire has occasionally been used for otoplasty (Reichert 1979).

Absorbable suture material. We use these only to supplement polyester sutures because of the risk of recurrence.

See Appendix 2 for further details of suture materials.

Skin Closure

Only fine monofilament suture material should be used for skin closure, in the form of interrupted or continuous sutures (Figs. 5.**38**, 5.**40 g**) with several intermediate knots. We recommend 5–0 monofilament sutures for the inconspicuous posterior region and 6–0 or 7–0 monofilament sutures for the anterior region.

If there is no wish to remove the sutures, rapidly absorbable suture material can be used.

Dressing Technique for Otoplasty

It is important to pack the contours of the auricle and support the auricular structures with ointment-soaked fluffed gauze (Fig. 5.**39 a–c**). This is followed by a cover of ointment-soaked cotton, a fenestrated sponge dressing, fenestrated gauze which is covered with a layer of cotton wool (Fig. 5.**39 d, e**), and a circular head bandage (Fig. 5.**39 f**). For medicolegal reasons we give a perioperative prophylactic single-shot dose of antibiotic.

Day 1. Dressing change. The ear is reviewed for hematoma formation, etc., the drain is removed (see Fig. 5.**39 a–c**), the packing of the auricular contours and the rest of the dressing as described above is renewed and the patient is discharged.

Day 4. Review.

Day 8. Removal of sutures and, if necessary, another fenestrated sponge dressing for a few more days. Coverage and circular dressing.

Day 14. Review, if possible. We recommend the wearing of a headband at night for four further weeks.

6 months. Review and renewed documentation of the measurements of the ears (see Figs. 5.**29**, 5.**40 h**), renewed photo documentation.

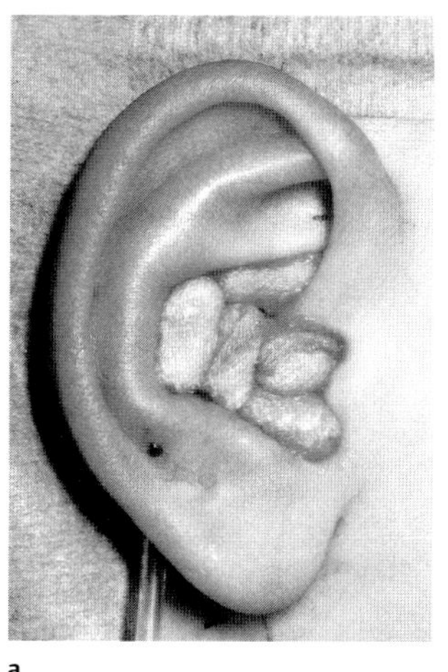
a

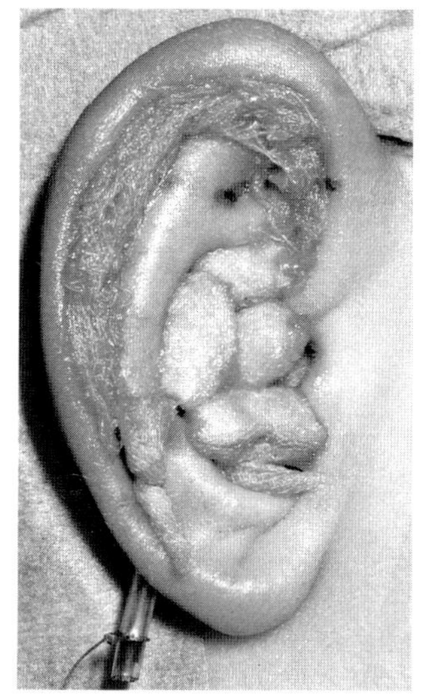
b

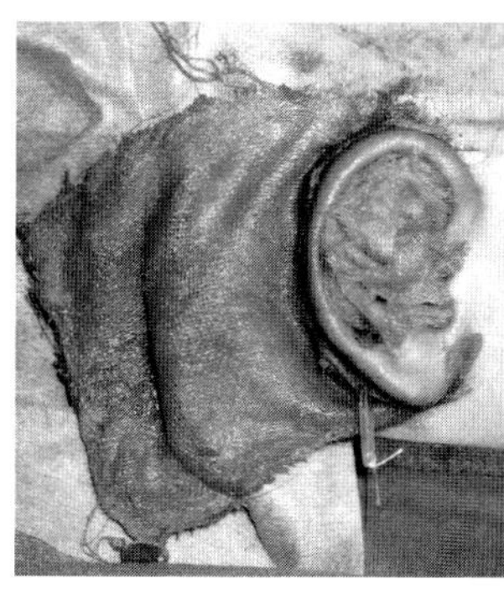
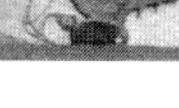
c

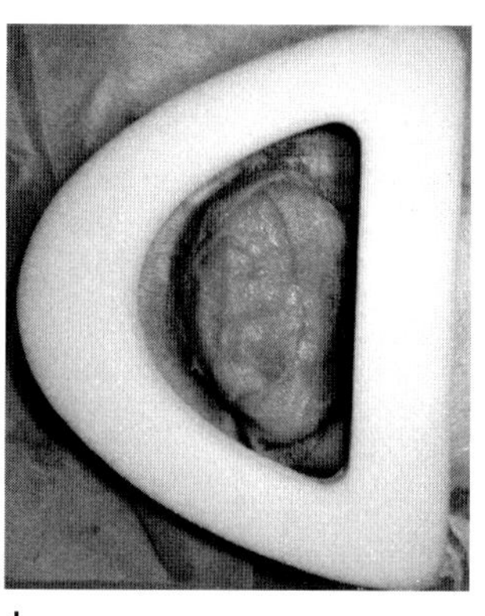
d

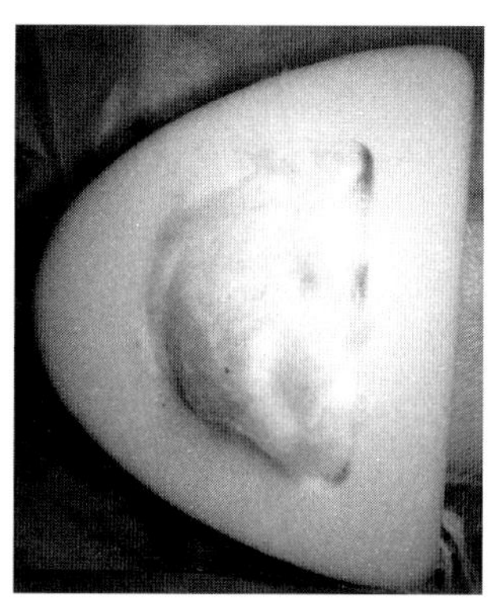
e

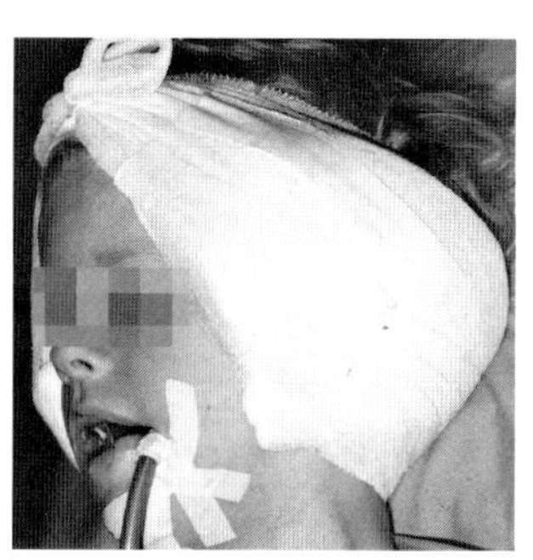
f

Fig. 5.39 **Dressing for otoplasty.**
a Support for the concha using small ointment-soaked pledget swabs (e. g., ointment containing a mixture of petroleum jelly and povidone–iodine).
b Additional support for the scapha and fossa.
c Dressing for the anterior and posterior surfaces, small drain.
d Fenestrated sponge.
e Coverage with cotton wool or sponge (fenestrated sponge).
f Circular or tubular dressing.

Operative Techniques

Suture Technique

Mustardé's Technique

(Fig. 5.40)
In 1960 Mustardé first published the technique that he had been using since 1957 (Mustardé 1960, 1963). We present this technique here in a slightly modified form; it should only be used for very thin cartilage.

Operation. Posterior skin incision, about 1 cm below and parallel to the helical rim and dissection of the cartilage of the entire postauricular surface. The perichondrium is left untouched (Fig. 5.40 **a**, **c**).

The intended antihelical fold in the scapha (Fig. 5.40 **b**, scaphal line; see also Fig. 4.45 **b**, **c**), in the concha–antihelical transitional area (Fig. 5.40 **b**, conchal line) and the triangular fossa (Fig. 5.40 **b**, fossa) is marked with needles or cannulae and highlighted on the perichondrium of the posterior surface with methylene blue (Fig. 5.40 **c**, red dots). The auricular fold is created with mattress sutures (4–0 white polyester monofilament; Fig. 5.40 **d–f**). If required, a conchal setback can also be performed (see p. 136, Fig. 5.45 **p** and p. 137).

We insert a drain for 1 day; the wound is closed using interrupted sutures, mattress sutures, or a continuous suture (Fig. 5.40 **g**). We like to glue the skin with fibrin adhesive, which allows the sulcus to be well formed.

Aftercare. The drain is removed on the first postoperative day and the sutures on day 8.

Dressing. 8–10 days. A headband is worn at night for about 4 weeks.

Critique. If the helix is included when creating the antihelical fold, especially with a rigid cartilage, the helix frequently disappears behind the antihelix when observed from a frontal perspective (Fig. 5.40 **f**, **j**).

When creating the scaphal fold with this suture technique, especially with soft cartilage, a somewhat wavy, uneven scaphal line can result (Fig. 5.40 **i**).

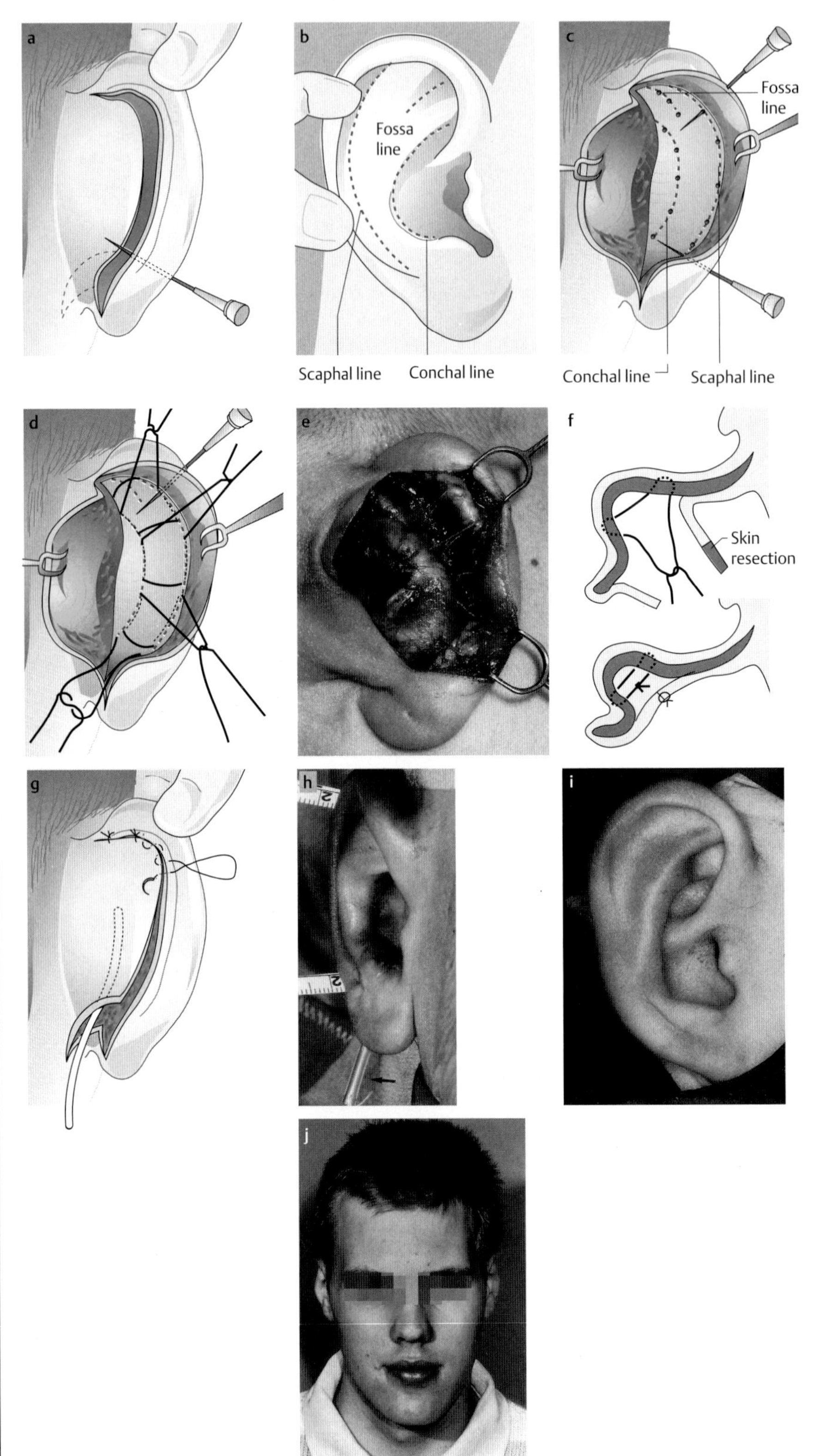

Fig. 5.**40** **Mustardé technique.**

a Incision (excision of a narrow strip of skin) approximately 1 cm below and behind the helix. Additional plasty to set back the earlobe as described by Wood-Smith (1973; broken line). Dissection of the posterior skin towards the helix and as far as the sulcus.

b After elevating the posterior skin, markings are made with needles dipped in ink to indicate the position of the folds.

c The marked lines are transferred to the postauricular surface.

d–f 4–0 white braided polyester sutures are placed and tied. Figure **f** demonstrates a helix which has been positioned too far posteriorly (disappearing helix; see **j**).

g Skin suture (interrupted or continuous) with intermediate knots, drain.

h Postoperative outcome, measurement of the mastoid–superior helical rim distance; arrow: drain.

i Complication: somewhat indistinct, curved scaphal line.

j Helical contour disappears behind the antihelix.

Figures **i** and **j** demonstrate **typical complications** of this technique (see p. 143).

Anterior Scoring Technique

Chongchet's Technique

(Fig. 5.**41**)
An anterior scoring technique using a posterior approach was described by Chongchet (September 1963) and Crikelair (1964). Gorge (1953, cited in Schmidt 2000) had reported this method even before knowledge of the biomechanical properties of superficially scored cartilage, as had been demonstrated by Gibson and Davis (1958) on costal cartilage.

Most authors have opted for a posterior approach, in order to avoid leaving conspicuous scars over the anterior region.

Preparation for surgery. See pp. 129 ff.
As Gibson and Davis (1958) have demonstrated on costal cartilage and Stenström (1963) on elastic auricular cartilage, when one surface is scored cartilage folds towards the other, unscored surface (Fig. 5.**42 a**).

Operative technique. Operation under general anesthesia or local infiltration anesthesia. Incision approximately 1 cm parallel to the antihelix on the posterior surface (see Fig. 5.**40 a**) and dissection of the skin off the posterior cartilage down to the perichondrium (see Fig. 5.**40 a, d**; Rhys-Evans 1981).

Marking the antihelix. As previously described for the Mustardé technique (see Fig. 5.**40 b, c**), the transition of the scapha to the antihelix as well as that of the antihelix to the concha are marked with needles and the markings transferred to the posterior auricular surface.

For this purpose, methylene blue is applied to the inserted tip of the needle which is then withdrawn. Thus both the skin and the anterior surface of the cartilage are marked.

Rhys-Evans (1985) referred to this method as the **anterior scoring technique**. He incises the already marked scaphal line (Fig. 5.**41 a**), as previously reported by Chongchet (September 1963), goes through the cartilage in an anterior direction and dissects the skin off the cartilage together with the perichondrium of the anterior surface down to the floor of the concha (Fig. 5.**41 a–c**), and scores along the entire marked surface of the antihelix, until the form of the antihelix develops spontaneously (Fig. 5.**41 d**). **The depth of the scoring should not exceed half to two-thirds of the thickness of the cartilage.**

The skin is then redraped and the helix folded back, and the wound is closed (see Figs. 5.**40 g**, 5.**41 d**). We recommend additional gluing with fibrin adhesive.

Chongchet (1963) and Crikelair (1964) also excise a narrow strip of skin posteriorly (see Fig. 5.**40 f**).

In addition, we insert a small drain, as previously mentioned (see p. 132; see Fig. 5.**40 h**).

Dressing technique. See p. 131.

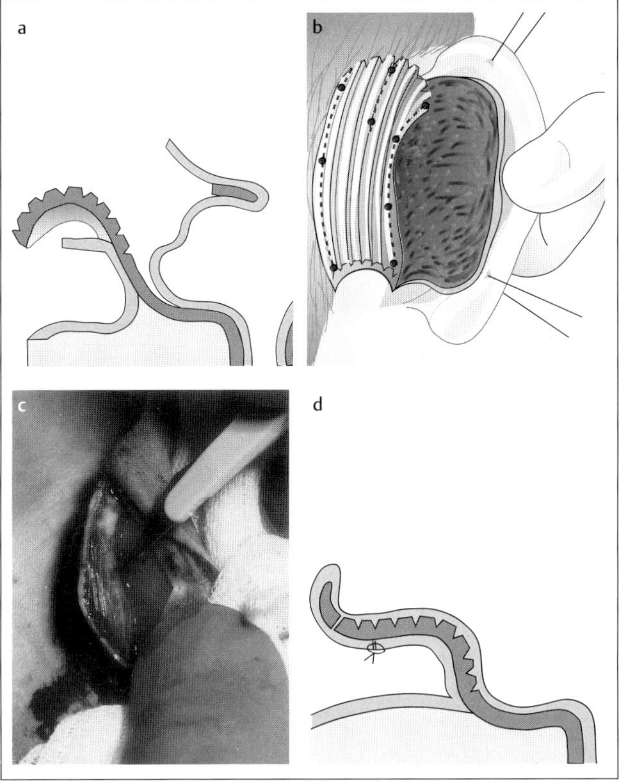

Fig. 5.**41** **Anterior scoring technique using a posterior approach as described by Chongchet (1963) and Crikelair (1964).**
a Posterior skin incision (exposure of the posterior surface and marking of the folds; see Fig. 5.**40 a–c**) and incision of the cartilage through the scapha.
b, c Anterior dissection of the skin–perichondrium flap. Cartilage incision in the scapha, subperichondrial exposure of the anterior cartilaginous surface and scoring (to no more than one-half of the thickness of the cartilage) of the new antihelix with a size 15 or even size 11 blade (the latter is more difficult to control). The folds are marked with ink (ret dots).
d The antihelix spontaneously folds back into position. We glue the skin of the anterior and posterior surfaces with fibrin adhesive. Skin closure using interrupted or continuous sutures (see Fig. 5.**40 g, h**) after measuring the height of the helix (see p. 120). If necessary, skin excision. Additional use of 4–0 white braided polyester sutures to produce the fold is an option.

Postoperative care. See p. 130.

Advantages. Particularly suited for thick, less pliable cartilage: produces elegantly proportioned auricular contours.

Disadvantages.
- Conspicuous cartilage ridging develops if scoring is too deep or the anterior auricular perichondrium is breached— this can even result in severe deformities (see also section on complications, p. 150).
- Not suitable for older patients because of the limited elasticity of the cartilage.

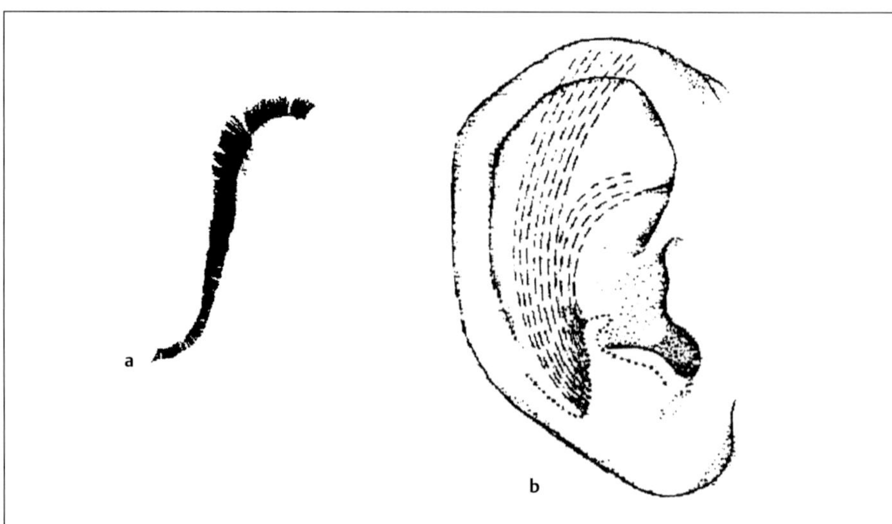

Fig. 5.**42** **Anterior scoring technique using a posterior approach as described by Stenström (1963).**
a Experimental study of the auricular cartilage: after incision, the cartilage folds towards the intact surface.
b Incision of the posterior skin and removal of a strip of skin, incision of the cartilage in the region of the tail of the helix, dissection of the anterior skin and blind rasping of the antihelix and crura with special rasps (see Fig. 5.**43**).

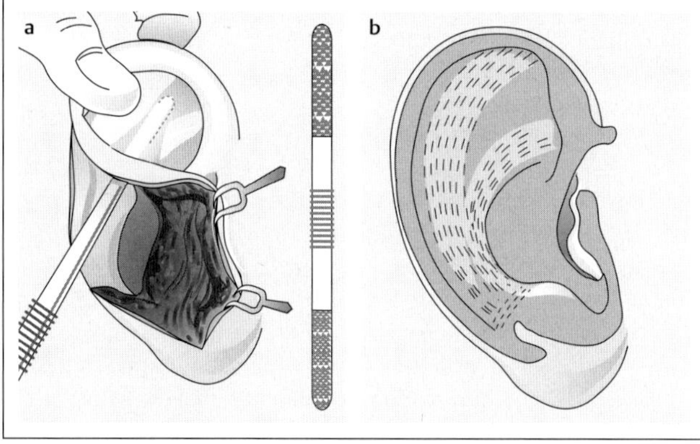

Fig. 5.**43** **Modification of Stenström's technique (Stenström 1973).**
a Extended posterior approach through the scapha. Elevation of the anterior perichondrium–skin flap.
b The marked region is rasped with an otoabrader, which has surfaces of varying degrees of coarseness.

- Suture-related complications.
- The technique is somewhat more difficult and therefore not so well suited for novices: revision surgery after failure is difficult, unlike the Mustardé technique (see p. 142).

As well as Rhys-Evans (1981, 1985), Kastenbauer (1983 a), Elliot (1991) and Nolst-Trenite (1994) have used this technique in recent years. An additional conchal setback (p. 137) is performed as required.

Stenström's Technique
(Figs. 5.**42**, 5.**43**)

The anterior scoring technique from a posterior approach was described by Stenström (1963, 1973). As mentioned above, Stenström (1963) proved that, after scoring, the elastic cartilage bends to the opposite side in a convex manner (Fig. 5.**42 a**).

Preparation and positioning. See p. 129 ff.

Operation. Stenström (1963) first made an incision on the postauricular surface in the form of an elliptical skin excision in the usual manner (see p. 132, Fig. 5.**40 a**). Next, an incision is made around the tail of the helix and, from this cartilage incision, skin perichondrium is raised in the anterior antihelical region and the cartilage of the antihelix, superior crus, and inferior crus (Fig. 5.**42 b**) is rasped blindly. Stenström developed special instruments for this.

Stenström (1973) slightly modified this method by creating a wider posterior approach to the anterior antihelix via the scapha and blindly rasping only the upper part of the antihelix and both crura (Fig. 5.**43 a**). Furthermore, an otoabrader bearing surfaces of varying fine roughness is described (Fig. 5.**43 b**). At the end of the operation a narrow strip of skin was excised on the posterior surface as required and the wound closed (see p. 132, Fig. 5.**40 f**).

Stenström stated that, when rasping, the cartilage should be pushed anteriorly from the posterior surface, thus keeping the pressure of the rasp under control. Only the superficial structures of the cartilage should be rasped. An additional conchal setback can be done as required (see p. 137).

Critique. Since blind rasping is exceptionally dangerous and, despite much experience, cannot always be controlled because the entire posterior skin has been incised in the usual manner, the advantage over an incision across the entire scapha as with Chongchet's technique is not very great (1963, see p. 133; Fig. 5.**41**). Complications and risks are discussed on pp. 141 ff.

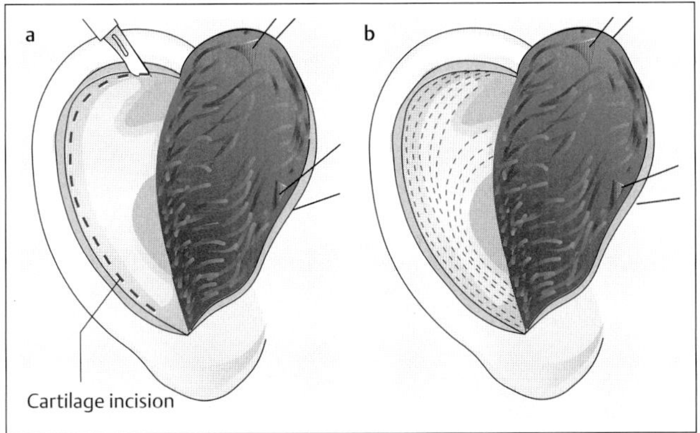

Fig. 5.**44** **Anterior approach and scoring technique as described by Ju et al. (1963), modified.**
a Skin incision in the scapha and dissection of the skin–perichondrium flap.
b Scoring of the cartilage about one-half of the thickness of the cartilage (see also Fig. 5.**41**).

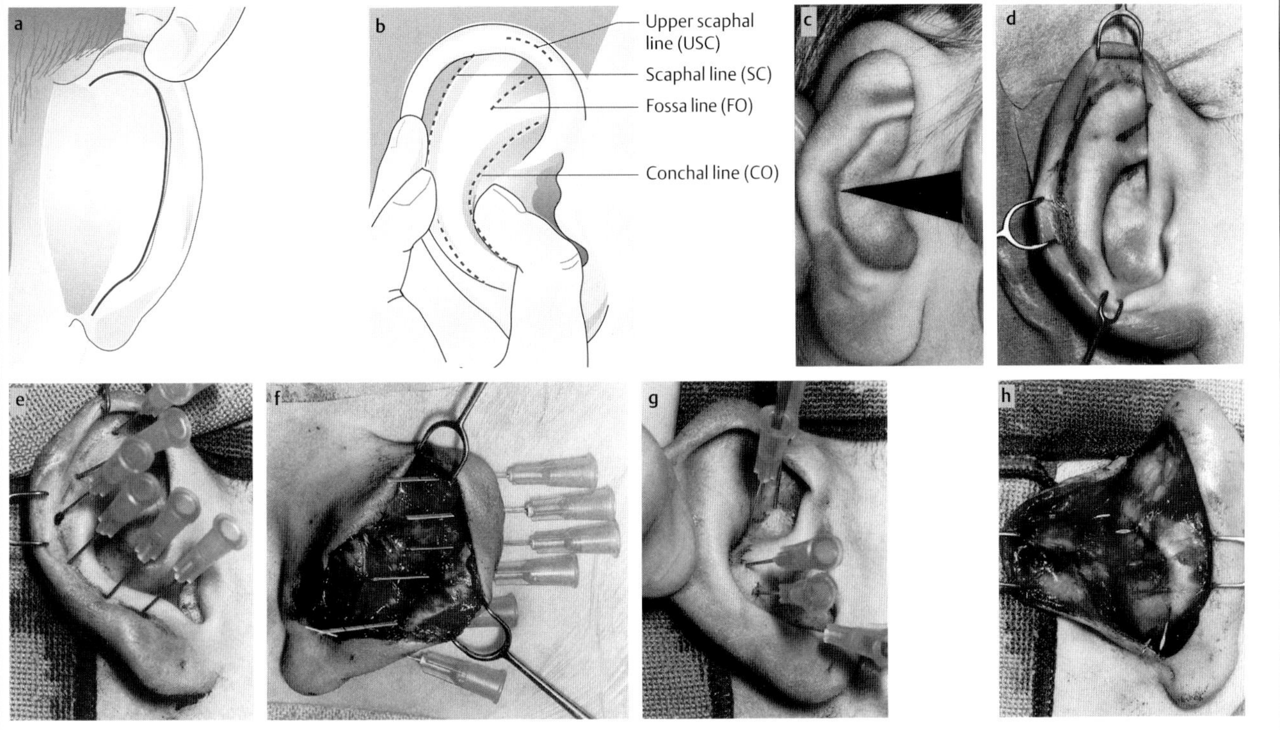

Fig. 5.**45** **Incision/suture technique as described by Converse et al. (1955, 1963, 1977).**
a Posterior skin incision and dissection of the cartilage (see Fig. 5.**40 c**).
b–d Demonstration of the antihelix (arrow in **c**) and marking of the lines on the anterior surface (red broken line), the later cartilage incisions on the posterior surface (see **i**; see Fig. 5.**40**).
e, f Needles in the scaphal line: anterior (**e**), posterior (**f**).
g, h Needles in the conchal line: anterior (**g**), posterior (**h**).

Fig. 5.**45 i–t** ▷

Ju et al.'s Anterior Scoring from an Anterior Approach
(Fig. 5.**44**)

Ju et al. (1963) describe the anterior skin incisions in the scapha, extending from the inferior crus down to the helical tail (Fig. **5.44 a, b**; see also p. 129, Fig. 5.**37 e**). A conchal setback can only be accomplished with great difficulty.

Incision–Suture Technique

Converse's Technique
(Fig. 5.**45**)

Probably the most commonly used method of otoplasty is the incision–suture technique as described by Converse (1955, 1963). This involves creation of the absent antihelical fold and superior crus and, if required, reduction and setback of the concha (see p. 137).

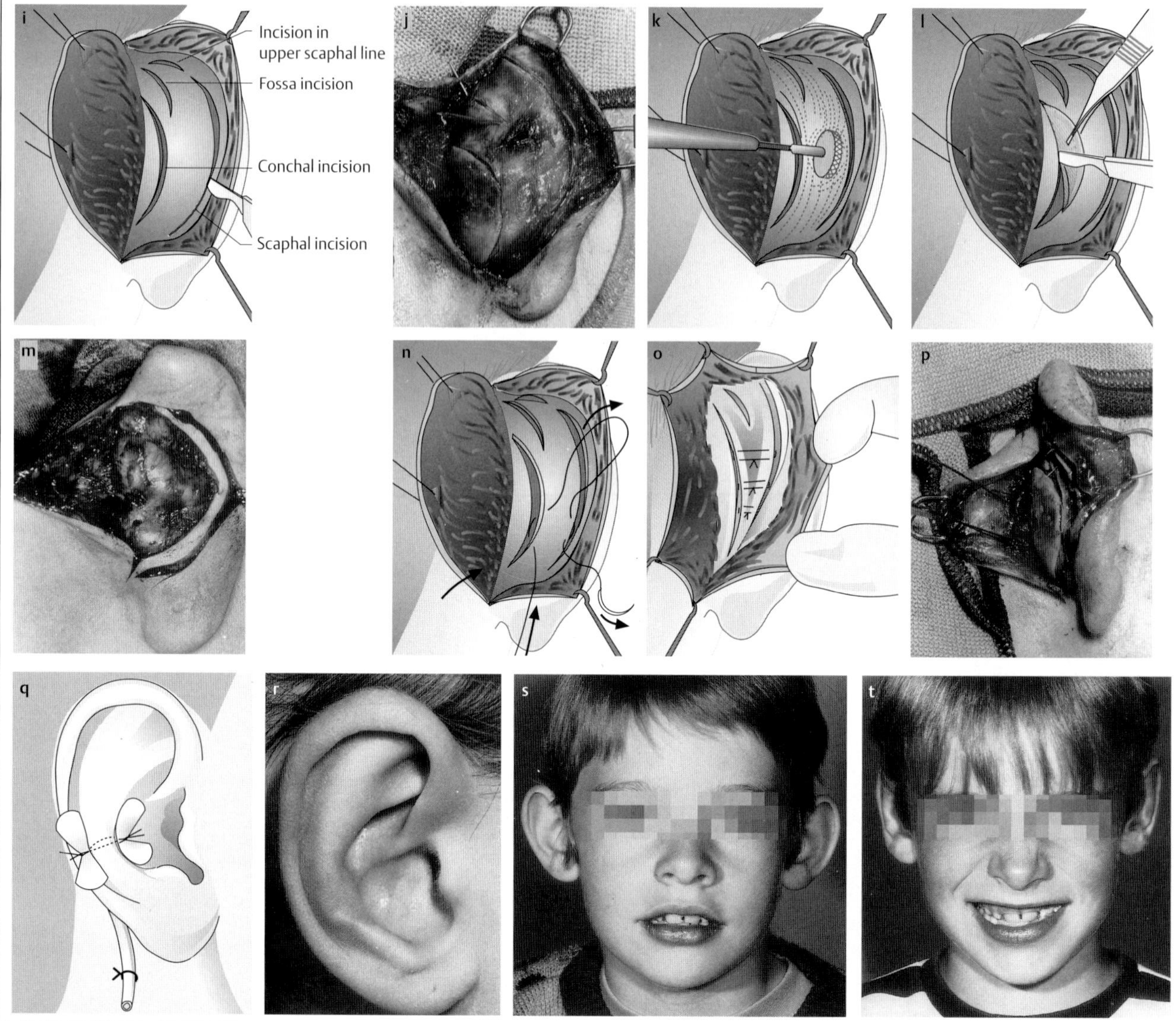

Fig. 5.**45 i–t**

i, j Incisions; in **j** the fossa line is marked with needles.

k The antihelix is slightly thinned out with a diamond burr or brush if the cartilage is thick.

l If necessary, excision of the conchal cartilage with dissection of the anterior skin as far as the external auditory canal (prophylaxis against folds).

m Excision of a strip of skin.

n, o Suture and creation of the antihelical fold with 4–0 white polyester monofilament.

p If required, additional setback of the concha (cavum/conchal rotation; black 3–0 polyester monofilament sutures; see Fig. 5.**46**).

q Posterior continuous suture (see Fig. 5.**38** and Fig. 5.**40** g) or interrupted sutures, small drain secured with polyester monofilament, if necessary an anterior mattress suture for one week (monofilament suture, e. g. 5–0 Prolene, PS 3 needle).

r Outcome.

s, t Pre- and postoperative appearance.

Based on the ideas of Becker (1949, 1952), Converse sharply divides the cartilage of those regions requiring folding (Fig. 5.**45 i**). This allows him to bring the new helix into a good position slightly above the antihelical contour after folding (Fig. 5.**45 p**). This step also clearly defines the transitions in the region of the scapha and the transition of the concha to the antihelix.

Preparation. Preparation, supine positioning, draping, anesthesia, and posterior approach are as previously described (see pp. 129 ff).

Surgical approach. After administering some local anesthetic with epinephrine 1 : 200 000 in the region of the posterior skin and in the mastoid region, an incision is made 1 cm below and parallel to the helical rim (Fig. 5.**45 a**). The cartilage is identified from the helix to the sulcus; while leaving the perichondrium, the muscles of the sulcus are divided and meticulous hemostasis is ensured.

Manual pressure is exerted in a medial direction on the helix to form the new antihelical fold and the intended posterior incisions on the anterior auricular surface are marked

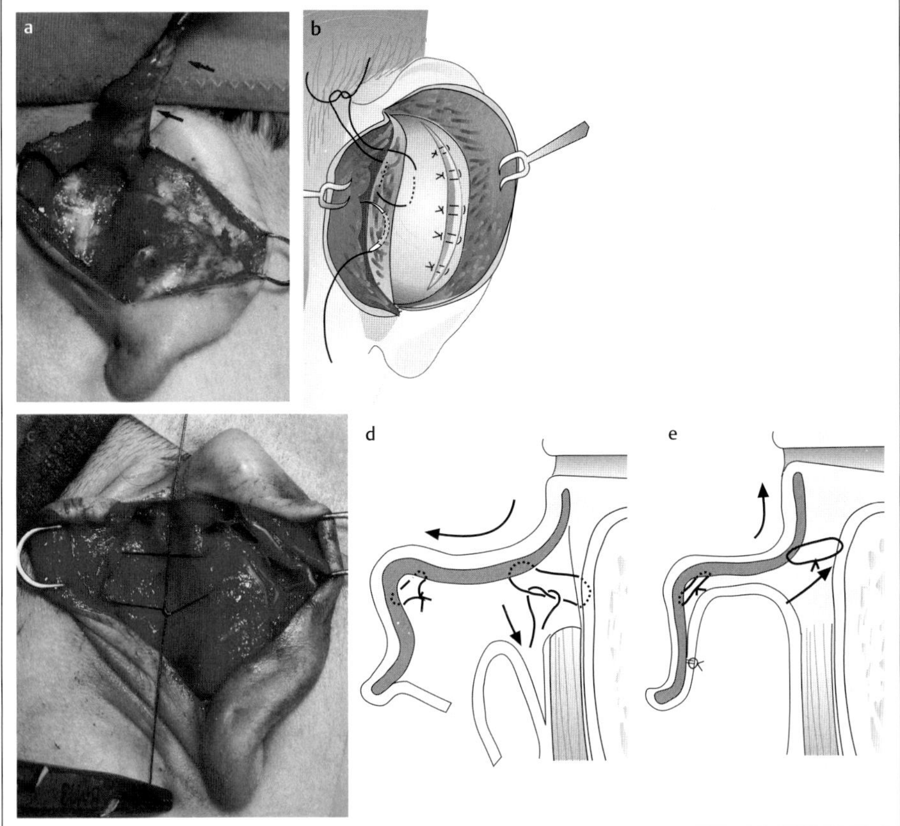

Fig. 5.**46** **Conchal setback (cavum/conchal rotation) without cartilage incision in the concha.**
a Resection of muscle and soft-tissue (arrows) from the post-auricular sulcus.
b, c Sutures (2–0; 3–0 black polyester monofilament and FS or FS1 needle) through the mastoid periosteum with a corresponding suture through the conchal cartilage.
d, e When the sutures are tied, the traction is applied in a slightly posterior direction (arrows in **d**) to prevent narrowing the auditory canal (arrows in **e**) (**e**; see complications, pp. 141 ff, Fig. 5.**55**).

(Fig. 5.**45 b–d**): the conchal line extending under the inferior crus, scaphal line reaching under the inferior crus, fossa line, and upper scaphal incision.

When incising the upper scaphal line (Fig. 5.**45 n**), there must be no connection with the other incisions in order to avoid sharp ridges in this region. Each incision lies at the base of the new antihelix; transection of the anterior perichondrium must be avoided. This incision prevents the superior helix from flattening off when creating the new antihelical fold.

Dressing. See p. 131; see also Fig. 5.**39**.

Critique. The technique is applicable for the majority of prominent ears and, with carefully planned incisions, the cosmetic results are good (Fig. 5.**45 r, t**).

Occasionally an additional conchal setback must be performed to achieve a helix–mastoid distance of less than 20 mm (Fig. 5.**45 p**, Fig. 5.**46**).

Crescent-shaped cartilage incisions require dissection of the anterior skin as far as the auditory canal to avoid anterior cutaneous folds (Fig. 5.**45 l**).

Suture. See Fig. 5.**40 g**.

Advantages

- Unlike the Mustardé technique, good positioning of the helix over the antihelix is achieved (Heppt and Trautmann 1999).
- Natural contours of the cartilage are achieved, as well as a smooth fold in the transition areas between antihelix and helix and antihelix and concha.
- The procedure is also suitable for less experienced surgeons.
- Revision surgery is unproblematic.

Disadvantages

- Conspicuous cartilaginous ridging if the anterior perichondrium is breached.
- If incisions are placed incorrectly, risk of recurrence after suture dehiscence, risk of exaggerated folding, and subsequent narrowing of the auricle.

Additional Measures

Conchal Setback without Incision

(Fig. 5.**46**)

Even pioneers such as Ely (1881), Monks (1891), and Joseph (1896) had excised the sulcus, sutured the skin and postauricular surface to the mastoid, and thus achieved setback otoplasty through conchal setback and reduction of the auriculocephalic angle (see also Fig. 5.**45**).

Operative technique. If the auricle is not set back enough by otoplasty, i. e., the mastoid–helical distances are too great (see p. 120), then a conchal setback is performed in addition.

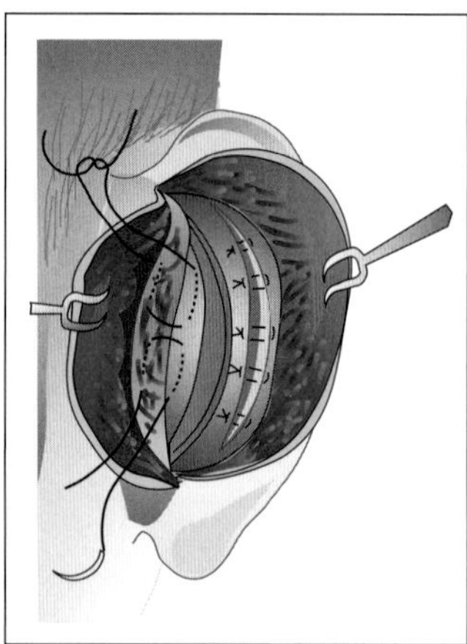

Fig. 5.47 **Conchal setback (cavum/conchal rotation) with incision or cartilage excision. Dissection of the anterior perichondrium–skin flap as far as the auditory canal to prevent a skin fold (see Fig. 5.46 c; Feuerstein 1985).**

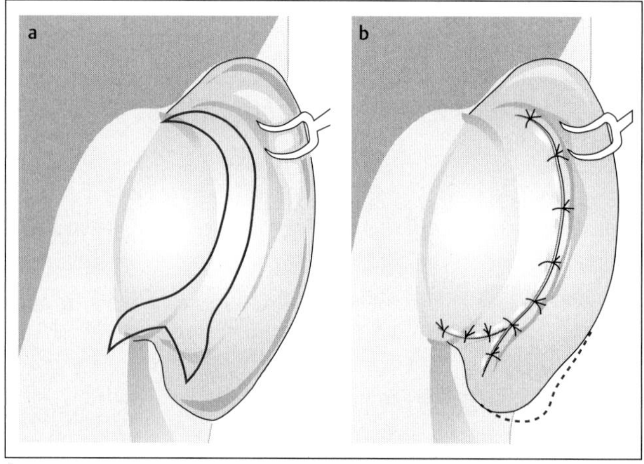

Fig. 5.48 **Skin excision for setback of the earlobe.**
a Y-shaped excision
b Suture

We dissect the skin down to the mastoid and in a posterior direction, excising muscles and fibrous tissue while protecting the temporalis fascia (Fig. 5.**46 a**). Two polyester monofilament sutures (2–0 with FS needle or 3–0 with FS1 needle) are passed through the periosteum of the mastoid and, after slightly setting back the auricle, through the appropriate place on the conchal cartilage (Fig. 5.**46 b, c**). The two knots are tied after bringing the ear back towards the mastoid, and the skin closed (Fig. 5.**46 d**). If there is narrowing of the auditory canal, skin and cartilage are appropriately excised (Fig. 5.**46 e**; see also p. 142).

Furnas (1968) reintroduced this method after World War II and used it together with the Mustardé technique (Wood-Smith 1973).

Conchal Setback with Cartilage Excision
(Fig. 5.**47**)

Feuerstein (1985) recommends an additional crescent-shaped excision for conchal reduction (Fig. 5.**47**). The anterior skin should then be undermined as far as the auditory canal in order to avoid wrinkles.

Earlobe Setback
(Figs. 5.**48**, 5.**49**)

To achieve a concomitant correction of the earlobe, the cauda should be made pliable by scoring or should be separated. However, the earlobe often remains prominent after simple otoplasty because the cartilage-free end of the auricle does not always adequately follow the transposition and folding of the cartilage.

Simple techniques of posterior earlobe-skin excisions (Fig. 5.**48 a, b**):

- **Y-shaped or fishtail excisions** (see also pp. 129 and 140, Fig. 5.**40 g**). When describing the Mustardé technique, we showed a Y-shaped or fishtail excision to set the earlobe back slightly with the aid of the mastoid skin suture.

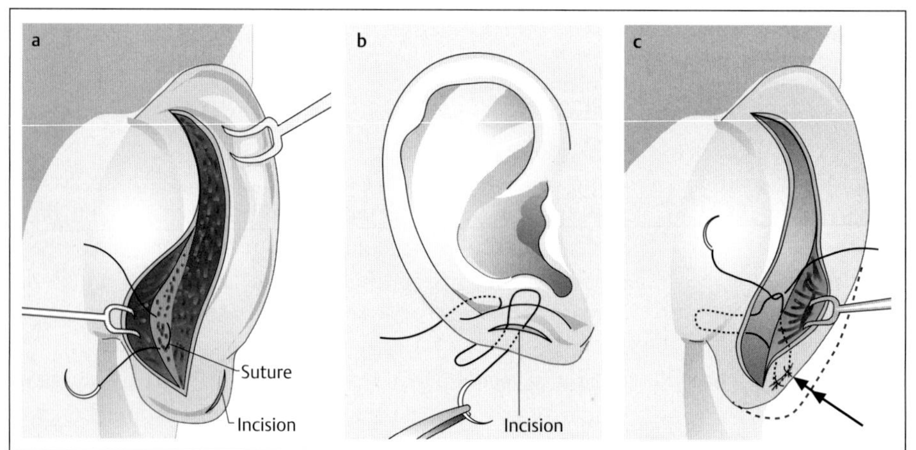

Fig. 5.**49** **Adaptation of the earlobe with a suture.**
a After setting back the auricle, the suture (4–0 white polyester monofilament) is anchored to the connective tissue of the posterior concha.
b The needle is inserted as far as the posterior, superior margin of the earlobe where an incision is made using a size 11 blade with the needle still in place, then the needle is brought back through the incision (see **a**).
c The suture is knotted, thus lowering the earlobe.

- **Lobule suture.** Dissection towards the periosteum of the mastoid from the earlobe end of the retroauricular incision (Fig. 5.**49 a**). The 4–0 white polyester monofilament suture, armed with a PS2 needle, is secured in the depth of the wound and brought back out through the fat of the earlobe near the lobular margin (Fig. 5.**49 b**). With the needle still in place, a small incision is made in the earlobe. The needle is brought out through this incision and passed back, parallel to the first suture strand, through the earlobe, and tied to the other end of the suture which lies in the connective tissue of the posterior surface of the concha. The knot is tied slowly and carefully, to avoid creating a hollow in the anterior region of the incision and to draw the earlobe gently toward the mastoid. The incision is closed with a 7–0 monofilament suture (Fig. 5.**49 c**).

Synopsis of Otoplasty (Tab. 5.4)

If the cartilage is very soft, one can use the Mustardé technique (see p. 131, 132) to correct the protruding ear. In most cases, we use the Converse technique (see pp. 135–138). Only in a few cases, i. e., if the cartilage is very sturdy, we incise through the scapha, mobilize the anterior surface, and score it (see pp. 133–135). In addition, we can reduce the height of the antihelix by a cavum rotation (see pp. 137, 138).

To correct the position of the earlobe, a skin incision can be used (see p. 138, 139), or one can adapt the earlobe with a special suture technique (see Fig. 5.**49**).

Other techniques (Chongchet 1963, p. 133; Stentström 1963, 1973, p. 134; Ju et al. 1963, p. 135; Weerda's technique, p. 140; or incisionless techniques, pp. 139, 140) should only be used by experienced surgeons.

Special Forms of Otoplasty

Folding Techniques without a Long Incision

Kaye's Technique

(Fig. 5.**50**)

Kaye (1967) makes a posterior incision at the caudal end of the auricle in the region of the new antihelix (Fig. 5.**50 a**), raises the anterior skin and blindly scores the antihelical and crural regions, as in the method described by Stenström (1963).

He then makes small incisions in the skin along the conchal line and in the scaphal line (Fig. 5.**50 a, b**; four incisions) and inserts sutures from the concha to the scapha by passing them though these incisions beneath the antihelix (Fig. 5.**50 b**). The needle is inserted beneath the skin of the scapha (Fig. 5.**50 c**), from where it is brought back into the first incision in the concha (Fig. 5.**50 d**). In all, three of these mattress sutures are knotted (Fig. 5.**50 e**), the skin surrounding the area of the incisions is undermined, the ends of the knots are buried, and the incisions closed using 7–0 monofilament sutures (Fig. 5.**50 f**).

Vecchione (1979) used a cannula with a bent tip to score the auricular cartilage and was therefore able to fold the ear by anterior scoring, but without any specific incision.

Tramier (1995) describes a similar procedure to that of Kaye (1967). He writes that he had been using this method for 20 years. He uses monofilament suture material for his mattress sutures and knots them in the incisions in the scapha. His scoring instrument is the arm of a pair of toothed forceps which he introduces through an incision in the conchal line and the scaphal line.

Fritsch's Incisionless Technique

(Fig. 5.**51**)

Fritsch (1995) reported a much-reduced Mustardé technique in which he places multiple sutures beneath the skin via small incisions (Fig. 5.**51**). He recommends 3–0 polyester as a suture material, introducing the needle in a posterior to anterior direction. Here too, the knots are buried beneath the skin, which is then closed. Fritsch used 6–0 catgut to close the incisions. He also uses a small incision to carry out a concha–mastoid fixation.

Merck (2000: personal communication) also prefers mattress sutures, which are used in a similar manner to that of Fritsch (1995) and inserted via anterior or posterior stab incisions to create the antihelical fold.

Critique. On the assumption that, in all operative techniques using a wide anterior or posterior approach, the auricle is held in the intended form and position by a broad scar after the auricular wound has healed, then after these minimized Stenström and Mustardé techniques with a minimized approach, the ears are held merely by the tension of the new antihelix and the inserted sutures. There is no broad scar formation. The tearing out of sutures as a result of any kind of violent force—during sports or in an accident, for ex-

Table 5.**4** Synopsis of Otoplasty for Protruding Ears (Siegert 2004)

Malformation	Characteristics	Technique
Antihelix hypoplasia	Very soft cartilage Average cartilage Strong cartilage	Suture (Mustardé; pp. 131 ff) Sutures and posterior scoring (Converse; pp. 135–138) Sutures and anterior scoring (Crikelair modif.; pp. 133–135)
Conchal hyperplasia	High antihelix	Cavum rotation (p. 137)
Protruding earlobe	Prominent helix Soft tissue tension	Scoring Mattress suture and slight skin resection (s. p. 138)

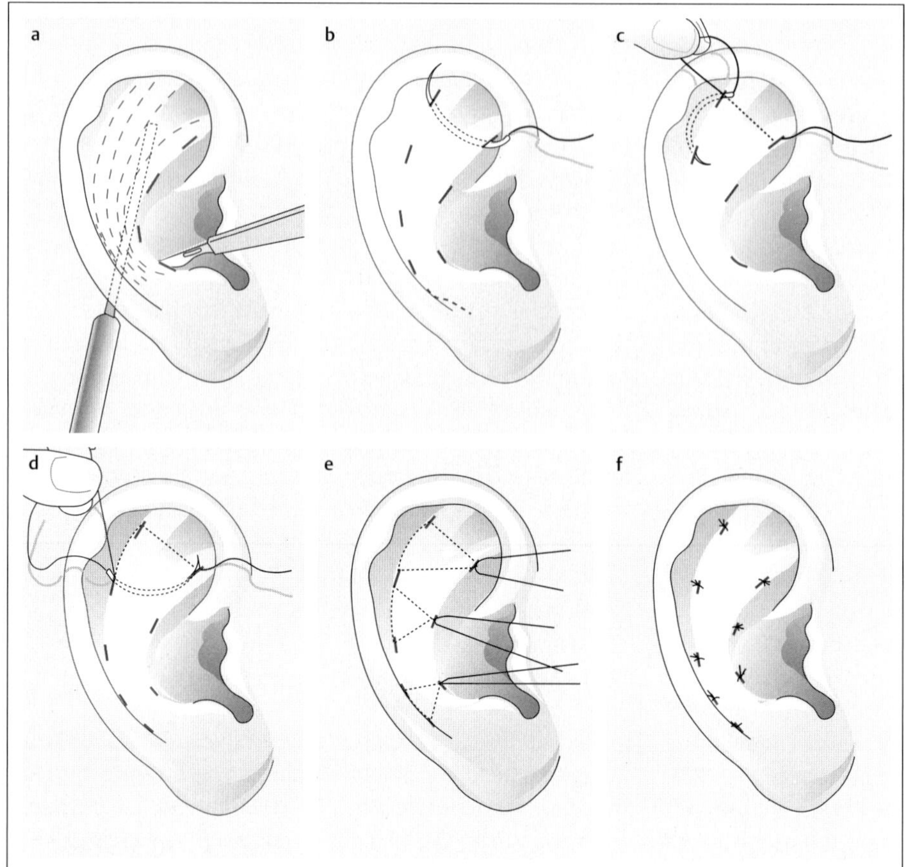

Fig. 5.**50** **Incisionless otoplasty: technique for inserting internal mattress sutures as described by Kaye (1967) and Tramier (1995)**
a The antihelix is striated via a caudal incision.
b, c Stab incisions for placement of subcutaneous 4–0 white polyester monofilament sutures.
d, e Sutures are tied and the knots buried subcutaneously.
f Skin incisions are closed with 6–0 (7–0) monofilament suture material.

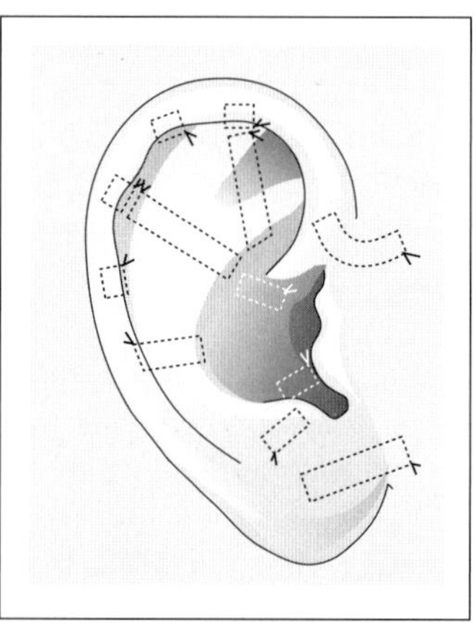

Fig. 5.**51** **Technique described by Fritsch (1995) with the partially posterior placement of retention suture knots.**

ample—will result in a deterioration of the primary result, even after years. Furthermore, suture granulomas and, with monofilament suture material, knot slipping are frequently observed (see Fig. 5.**56**, p. 145). There have been no reports on long-term results.

Weerda's Technique

(Fig 5.**52**)

In the late 1970s we developed a method which we particularly liked to use for grade I dysplasias, especially for type I and type IIA cup-ear deformities, and which lies between the Converse (1963) and the Mustardé (1963) techniques (Weerda 1979).

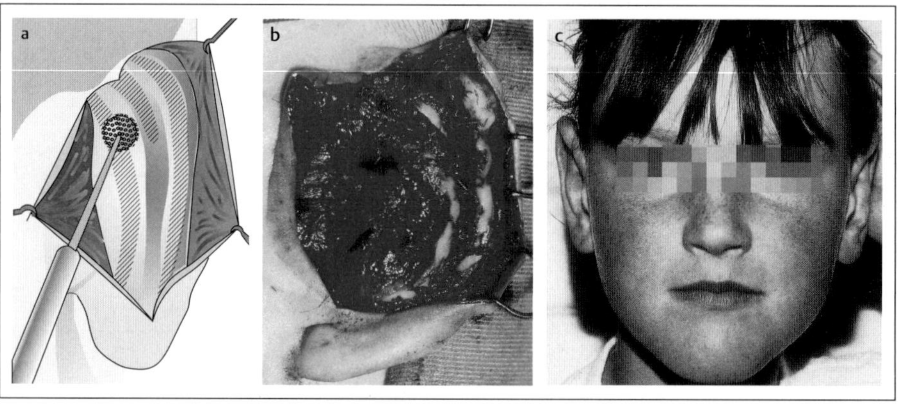

Fig. 5.**52** **Otoplasty as described by Weerda (1979).**
a The posterior surface of the cartilage is abraded with a round-headed diamond burr or "Mercedes star," instead of being incised as in the Converse (1955, 1963) technique (see Fig. 5.**45**).
b Creation of the antihelical fold.
c Result.

At the sites where Converse incises, we abrade a furrow of about half the thickness of the cartilage, using a round-head or diamond burr (Fig. 5.**52 a**). This allows some degree of variation in the folding of the antihelix, according to the size of the concha (Fig. 5.**52 b**), and conchal setback is also possible.

Advantages. With this technique it is possible to vary the degree of antihelical folding. The antihelix can be brought nearer to the helix or to the concha. Parts of the "hyperplastic concha" can be transferred somewhat more beneath the antihelix without having to excise cartilage, allowing the successful treatment of a large number of different grade I dysplasias, ranging from the prominent ear to type I and type IIA cup-ear deformities (see Fig. 5.**117**, p. 175). Otherwise the advantages of the Converse technique still apply, and we also have the advantages of the Mustardé technique without its disadvantages (see p. 132, Fig. 5.**40 f, j**).

Suture material. See p. 130.

Dressing technique. See p. 131.

Conservative, Noninvasive Otoplasty Techniques

At the time of the early attempts at otoplasty, Monks (1891, Fig. 5.**53**) reported a case for which he, with the aid of his father, had constructed an apparatus held by metal springs, not dissimilar to ear muffs, which he had his patient wear to provide compression on the prominent ears. He was unable to observe any success with this technique.

In 1984 Matsuo et al. published their studies on conservative splint therapy in 150 neonates with minor auricular deformities. The relief definition of the auricle was lined with gutta-percha and the position additionally held with adhesive tape. Matsuo et al. (1984) and Muraoka et al. (1985) conducted experiments to examine the possibility of creating an antihelical fold in mild deformities. Millay et al. (1990) reported that good long-term results could be achieved for the prominent ears of neonates 48 hours after birth and with a treatment duration of 13 days (Matsuo and Hirose 1989, 1991; Matsuo 1990). As previously described, Krummel (1986) reported on 36 auricles, while Matsuo et al. (1984) reported on over 140 patients. Over the next few years, further articles on this subject appeared (Millay et al. 1990; Tan et al. 1994; Sudhoff 1996; Yotsuyanagi et al. 1998). We have no personal experience with this method, allowing us only to state the cited successes from the literature.

Critique. On the whole, it can be deduced from the literature that some success can be achieved immediately after birth by creating an auricular fold with the aid of splints or dental molds and a longer-lasting treatment. There are varying assertions regarding the age until which these techniques are possible. Matsuo et al. (1984, 1989, 1991), for example, demand treatment in the first 72 hours of life, whereas Muraoka et al. (1984, 1985) still recommend plaster fixation treatment even in patients of 5 years of age. There certainly appears to be good reason for a systematic evaluation of this type of therapy.

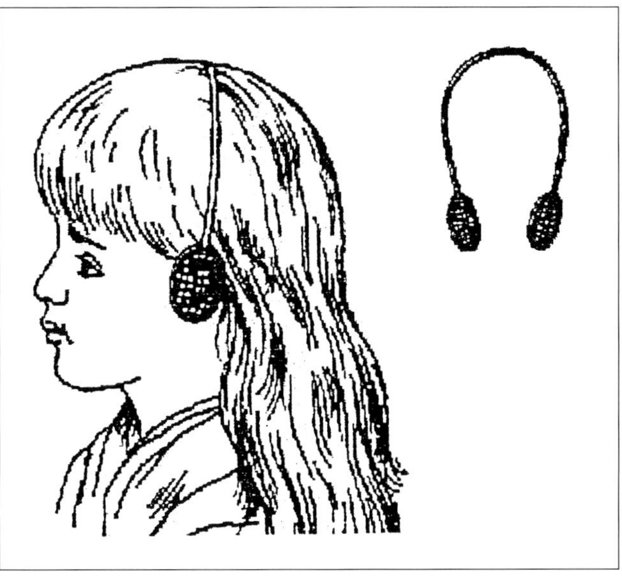

Fig. 5.**53** **Ear muff for prominent ears (in Monks 1891).**

Additional Measures

- Deformities of the helix (see pp. 156 ff)
- Hyperplasia of the helical crus (see pp. 164 ff)
- Correction of the tragus (see p. 164)
- Correction of the antitragus (see p. 164)

Results and Complications of Otoplasty Procedures

Complications need to be classified into those caused by the operating surgeon and those that arise despite a faultless operation. It seems likely that many complications are of iatrogenic origin.

Iatrogenic Errors

In 1978 Nagel writes that errors can occur from an ill-defined indication, faulty operative technique, incorrect dressing technique, or faulty aftercare.

Ill-defined Indication

An exact analysis and documentation of the form of auricular malformation must be conducted before any operation, including measurement of distances, quality of the cartilage and skin, hypertrophic scars on the body, etc. (see Appendix 1, p. 301).

Table 5.5 Early complications: up to 14 days after surgery (meta-analysis)

Complication	Literature synopsis	Cause	Treatment
Hypersensitivity: Pain, pressure, cold			
Bleeding Hematoma	11/712 = 1.5%		Hemostasis, drainage
Allergic reactions		Disinfectant, ointment, suture material	Elimination of the irritant
Infection: Local defects (perichondritis) Pressure sores (pressure necrosis)	22/593 = 3.6%	Type of dressing	Antibiotics, fenestrated gauze dressings
Auditory canal stenosis		Rotation of the concha	Cartilage excision
Narrow, high-riding auriculocephalic sulcus Ear set back too far		Excessive removal of postauricular skin	Skin graft
Defects Residuals Recurrence Partial or total asymmetry		Infection, iatrogenic cause, surgical error	Re-operation and reconstruction

Faulty Operative Technique

Proficient ear surgeons can certainly set back the various types of prominent ears using their preferred operative techniques. They must also produce an esthetically pleasing form of the ear by using additional measures such as conchal setback, reduction of the antitragus, reduction of the earlobe, narrowing of the helix, etc.

Faulty Dressing Technique

Even though the auricle has been correctly set back, incorrect dressing technique can put the result at risk. Additional compression of the ear, packing it with cotton soaked in a solution which then results in a very coarse cotton dressing, the use of adherent dressings, or even dressings with compressive bandages, can all cause complications (Simo and Jones 1994, and see p. 131).

We have suggested the use of a fenestrated sponge, under which the ear lies in a hollow (see p. 131, Fig. 5.**39**). In addition we support the concha and form the auricular folds with an ointment-soaked dressing (see Fig. 5.**39 b**).

Faulty Aftercare

There is always the risk that dressing changes, etc. are undertaken too late, and a hematoma, infection, or other complication is missed. This is especially so in the case of patients operated on an outpatient basis who live some distance from the hospital.

Complications of Surgical Techniques

We have attempted to list the results of the various techniques and their complications, based on the literature available to us and supplemented by our own results and experience (Tables 5.**5**, 5.**6**).

Suture Technique

Mustardé technique and Mustardé technique plus conchal setback; see pp. 131 and 137.

Between 1979 and 1991, a 7.7% recurrence rate (164 of 2136 ears) was observed by various authors, keloids in 1.2% (5 of 410 ears), hematomas in 1.3% (7 of 560 ears), long-lasting hypesthesias, hypersensitivity, and other disturbances of sensation in 5.2% (15 of 291 ears), and suture fistula formation in 3.6% (50 of 1381 ears) of cases, with one article citing polyester (Mersilene) monofilament as the cause in 8% of cases and recommending PTFE (Gore-tex) sutures (Mustardé 1967; Bruck and Gisel 1976; Martin 1976; Minderjahn et al. 1979, 1980; Moser and Wespi 1991; Andes and Koch 1991; Fissette and Nizet 1992; Messner and Crysdale 1996). We personally have been using Mersilene 4–0 for over 25 years and have never seen a tendency for suture fistula formation.

Scoring Technique

Methods as described by Stenström (1963), Ju et al. (1963), and Crikelair (1964) (see Fig. 5.**41**, p. 133; Fig. 5.**43**, p. 134).

Nielson et al. (1985) in particular reported on their results using the Stenström technique in 162 patients. They found results were good in 57% of cases, satisfactory in 39%, and poor in 4%. There was overcorrection or undercorrection in 12% of cases, and sharp irregular ridges in the antihelical region in 12% of cases. The helix was positioned behind the antihelix in the frontal view in 6% of cases.

Rhys-Evans (1985) praises this technique, but the results he demonstrated were not particularly satisfactory.

Severe deformations and ridge formation can arise from deep scoring, supplementary sutures for folding, and exaggerated skin excisions (see pp. 150 ff).

Table 5.6 Late complications

Complication	Literature synopsis	Cause	Treatment
Hypersensitivity: Pain, pressure, cold	7/213 = 3.3%	Disappears after 6–12 months	None needed
Suture fistulae, granulomas	53/533 = 9.9%		Remove suture material
Obstructed sebaceous cyst (rare)		Everted suture	
Hypertrophic scar formation Keloids	14/775 = 1.8%		Steroid, excision, skin graft (full thickness), silicone gel sheet, pressure dressing, radiotherapy (up to 20 Gy)
Deformation of the ear: Asymmetry Overcorrection (pinned back, flat ears) Telephone ear deformity (upper and lower auricle projecting too far), reverse telephone ear deformity (inadequate medialization of the central portion of the auricle) Formation of sharp ridges "Catastrophic ear" as described by Staindl (1986; destroyed cartilage, deformation in every plane)	255/3100 = 8.2%	Wrong technique, excessive scoring, excessive skin excision, infection	**Re-operation,** skin graft, revision, reconstruction with skin flaps, with fascia, with cartilage; **Limitation of damage by corrective surgery** (see pp. 147 ff)

Mustardé 1967; Maniglia et al. 1977; Draf 1979; Minderjahn et al. 1979; Rigg 1979; Steuer 1979; Ohlsen 1980; Rasinger et al. 1983; Adamson 1991; Andes and Koch 1991; Fisette and Nizet 1992

Incision/Suture Technique

Converse's method (see Fig. 5.45). Although Converse's is the most frequently used otoplasty technique, there are not many reports on results. The recurrence rate is cited at 10.5% (85 of 812 ears), keloid formation was found in 2.3% (5 of 213 ears), and hypersensitivity (hyperesthesia or hypesthesia, cold intolerance, etc.) in 3.3% (7 of 213 ears) of cases.

We can subdivide the complications of otoplasty into early complications, i. e., until 2 weeks after surgery (Table 5.5), and late complications, i. e., those which occur later than 2 weeks after the operation (Table 5.6). In addition, deformities of the auricle can also develop.

Early Complications (Table 5.5)

It is in the first few days that the typical postoperative complaints are encountered.

Pain, Hypersensitivity to Pressure and Cold

Complications related to the operative technique.

Hematoma Formation

In collective statistics covering all operative techniques, we found 11 of 712 cases, or 1.5%, with hematoma formation. They usually appear up to the third day after surgery.

Therapy. Meticulous intraoperative hemostasis and drainage for 1 day. Postoperative: open up the wound under sterile conditions, hemostasis, drainage, and mild compression.

Allergic Reactions

We occasionally see allergic reactions to disinfectants, to the ointments applied (e. g., iodine allergy) or, very infrequently, to suture materials.

Therapy. Elimination of the irritant.

Infections

In a synopsis of the literature we found infections in 3.6% of cases (22 of 593 ears).

Local infections. Administration of broad-spectrum antibiotics and, if possible, elimination of the local causes to prevent perichondritis. A wound swab is obligatory. An incipient perichondritis responds well to appropriate antibiotics and local measures. The causative pathogen is most frequently ***Pseudomonas aeruginosa*** (see p. 27).

Pressure ulcers and necrosis (Fig. 5.54 a, b). As previously discussed, pressure on the set-back auricle is avoided by packing the auricle and applying a fenestrated sponge dressing (see p. 131, Fig. 5.39 e).

Stenosis of the Auditory Canal (Fig. 5.55)

Traction in the direction of the auditory canal, particularly from conchal setback (see Fig. 5.46 d, e, p. 137), can result in stenosis of the auditory canal.

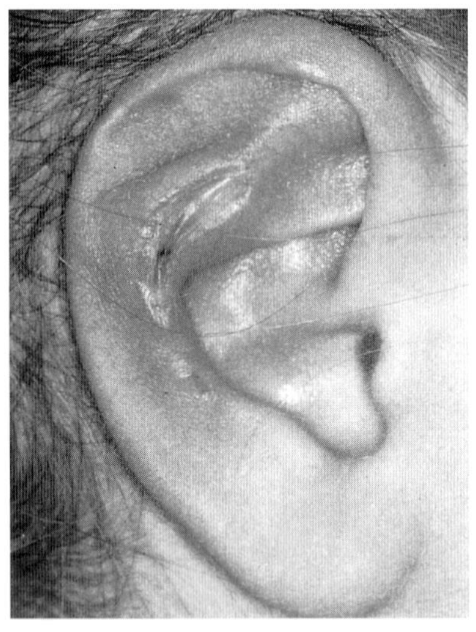

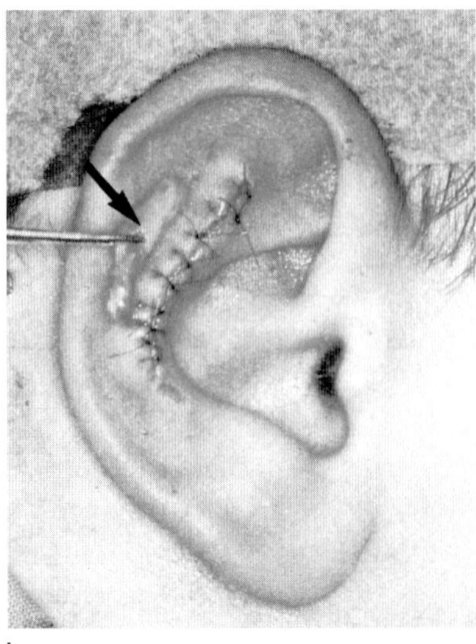

a b

Fig. 5.**54** **Necroses.**
a Pressure necrosis due to an excessively tight dressing.
b Excision of the necrosis and suture; arrow: excised cartilage.

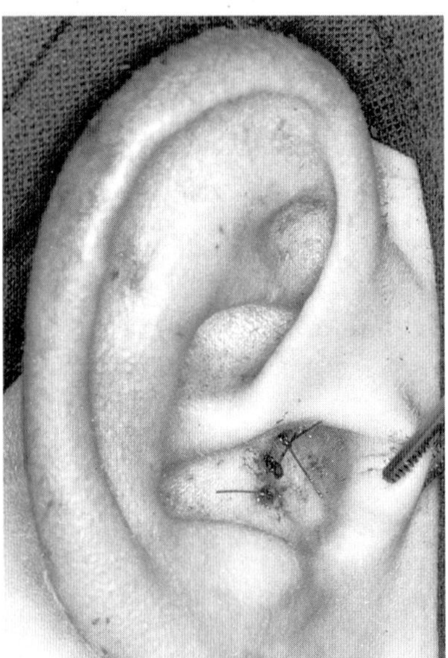

Fig. 5.**55** **Stenosis of the auditory canal following conchal setback: excision of surplus cartilage from the auditory canal and wound closure (see Fig. 5.46 e).**

Therapy. Excision of the cartilage from an incision within the auditory canal. If the posterior access is still open, the cartilage can be exposed from that direction and excised.

Ear Set Back Too Far, High-riding Auriculocephalic Sulcus
(see Figs. 5.**60**, 5.**61**)

Errors. Skin excision too extensive, ears set back too far, poor formation of the sulcus.

Therapy. Intraoperative gluing of the skin in the sulcus (fibrin glue; see late complications, p. 148; see Fig. 5.**61**).

Defects, Residuals, Recurrence, Partial or Total Asymmetry
See also late complications.

Causes. Infections, iatrogenic operative errors.

Therapy. Revision and reconstruction (see pp. 147 ff).

Late Complications (Table 5.6)
Late complications are those that occur more than 14 days after the operation (Staindl 1986; Weerda and Siegert 1994 a, b, 1997).

Pain, Hypersensitivity to Pressure and Cold
We find longer-lasting hypersensitivity, paresthesias, painful sensations to pressure and cold, and similar complaints particularly frequently after a posterior approach. In a synopsis of the literature we found such sensations in 3.3 % of cases (7 of 213 patients).

Therapy. Treatment is not necessary; these sensations usually disappear within the first postoperative year.

Suture Fistulae and Granuloma (Fig. 5.56)
In a search of the literature we found suture fistulae in 9.9 % of cases (53 of 533 ears).

Cause. Hypersensitivity to suture material, suture material, or knots placed too close to the surface of the skin (Fig. 5.**56**), suture ends left too long. Reaction to braided polyester sutures is said to be greater than to other suture materials (Adamson et al, 1991), although we were unable to confirm this after using them for many years. The use of monofilament sutures is risky because knot slippage occurs easily. Monofilament PTFE (Gore-tex) sutures have been recommended in recent years.

Hypertrophic Scars and Keloids
(Figs 5.**57**, 5.**58**)
In a summary of the literature we found keloid formation in 1.8 % of cases (14 of 775 auricles).

Hypertrophic scars (Fig. 5.57) are limited to the area of the wound and can be treated by corticosteroid infiltration. For this purpose 10 mg triamcinolone acetonide diluted in 2 ml Ringer's solution is used. Steroids may also be introduced into the scar by needleless injection (Dermojet).

Unlike keloids, hypertrophic scar formations are limited to the original scar region and should regress over the course of several years. A consensus conference (Lemmen 1995) reiterated that although the hypertrophic scar is indeed raised and bulging, it remains confined to the scar area and may spontaneously regress within 1–2 years. Watchful waiting is recommended.

Keloids, on the other hand, encroach on healthy skin (Fig. 5.58 a–d). They are referred to as intradermal neoplasms; but fibroblasts in keloids demonstrate no histological difference from normal fibroblasts or those in hyperplastic scars. The collagen filaments form a network of atypical nodules and whirls (Kischer et al. 1982). Kischer et al. subsequently developed the so-called "ischemia therapy." Many authors consider increased wound tension to be the cause of increased collagen synthesis (Langrana et al. 1983). Furthermore, an abnormal rise in melanocyte-stimulating hormone (MSH) is presumed, which could explain the increased frequency of keloids in dark-skinned individuals (Koonin 1964).

The keloid proliferates, like cancer, beyond the boundaries of the wound; it develops after about 1–2 months and practically never regresses spontaneously. A number of causes have been cited, including immune deficiency, medications, smoking, hormone abnormalities, connective-tissue diseases, age, skin color, and inheritance. Patient-independent factors are the location of the wound and operative technique.

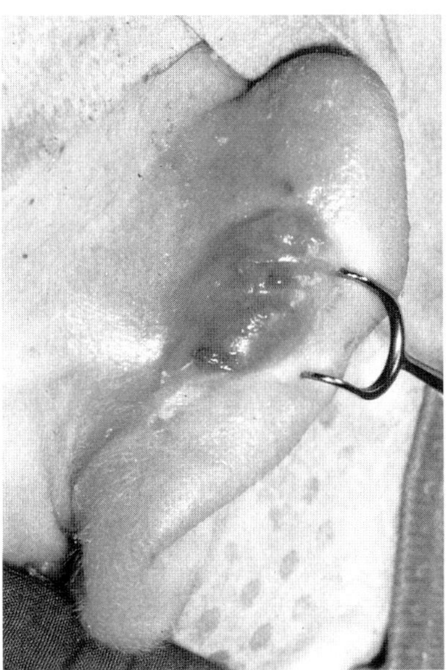

Fig. 5.56 **Suture fistula and granuloma, approximately 4 weeks after surgery using the so-called incisionless technique (see pp. 139, 140).**

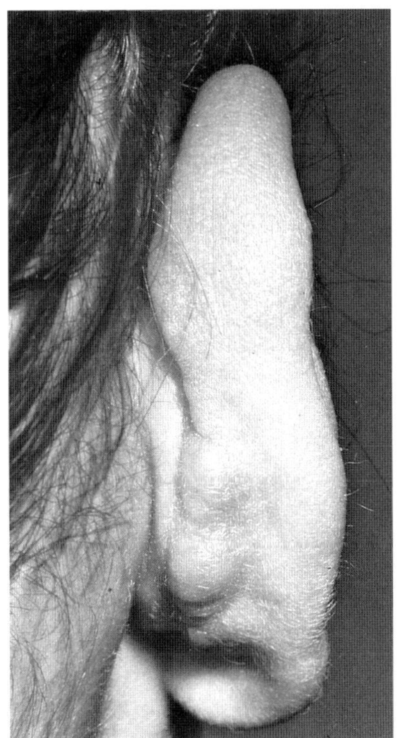

Fig. 5.57 **Scar hypertrophy.**

Therapy. Any kind of ischemia or tension on the wound must be avoided. Wound treatment, suture techniques, suture material, and incision have to take this into consideration. The consensus conference (Lemmen 1995) also makes mention of the use of superfluous disinfectants and the timely removal of sutures. Patients at risk should receive treatment with topical agents and compression dressings (see above). Silicone gel sheets are recommended to prevent recurrences.

It is important to emphasize that keloids should only be excised in exceptional cases, because of the high risk of recurrence.

Surgical excision of keloids. Excision is reported to have a recurrence rate of as high as 60 % (Cosman et al. 1961; Stern and Lucente 1989; Tilkorn et al. 1990). Removal with the aid of cryotherapy techniques or with lasers of various types appears to demonstrate no further reduction in the recurrence rate; long-term observations are still lacking.

Lawrence (1997) registered recurrences in just under 13 % of 111 cases which had undergone keloid excision of the earlobe and had received aftercare with steroids in some cases and radiotherapy in others.

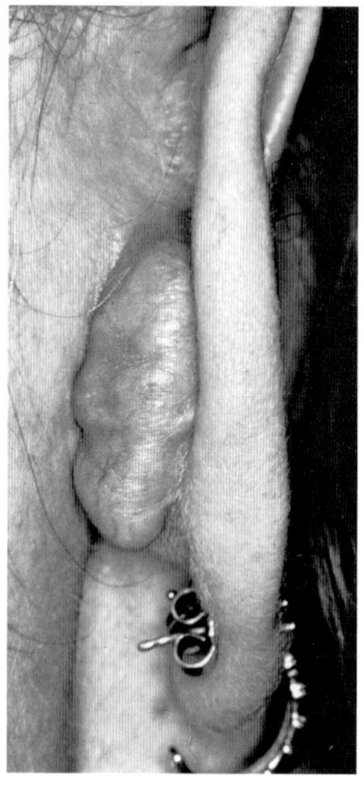

a

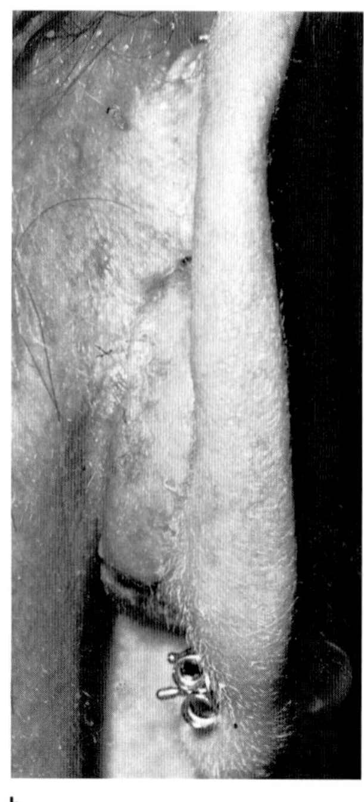

b

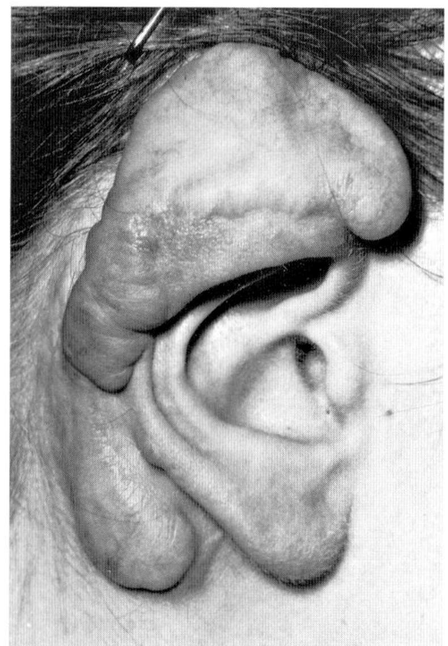

c

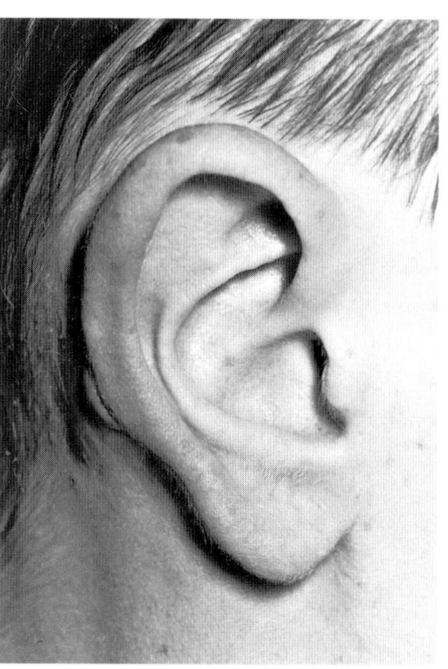

d

Fig. 5.**58** **Keloid formation.**
a Small keloid in the scar.
b Appearance 2 years after excision and coverage with a full-thickness skin graft taken from the mastoid region.
c Large keloid of the postauricular region.
d Appearance 1 year after excision, coverage with full-thickness skin and radiotherapy (see below).

We excise keloids, and with small defects we try to close the wound without tension or to resurface it with full-thickness skin (see Fig. 5.**58**). Occasionally freely mobile skin over the keloid is used to cover the resulting defect.

Aftercare. We always apply intraoperative steroid infiltrations into the scar area, and if necessary later, occasionally using Dermo-jet. We had as high as a 100% recurrence rate in 25 patients in whom no additional therapy was done after excision. In our 14 most recent patients radiotherapy was performed (by the Department for Radiotherapy and Nuclear Medicine of the Medical University of Lübeck, Germany, Director Professor E. Richter, MD), initially using 5–6 MeV radiation electron therapy with tissue-equivalent bolus material in order to concentrate the maximum dose on the skin surface. On 3 days per week, a dose of 1.5 Gy per day is applied. A total dose of 16–20 Gy is administered because a preliminary study on 7 patients using 10 Gy had resulted in a success rate of only 60% (3 recurrences in 7 patients). We saw no more recurrences in 7 further patients in a review conducted 10 months after postoperative radiation therapy using 20 Gy (see Fig. 5.**58**).

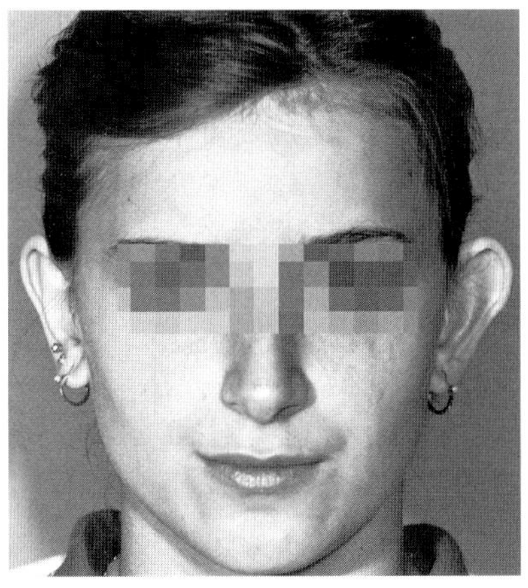
a

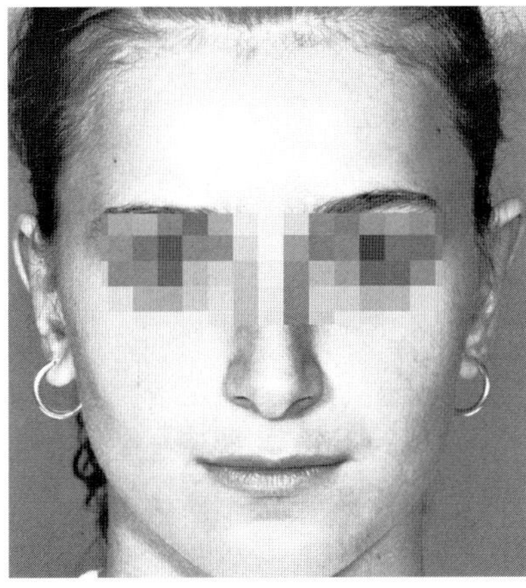
b

Fig. 5.**59** **Postoperative asymmetry.**
a Asymmetry after otoplasty.
b Result after revision surgery.

Many authors recommend radiotherapy at various doses and with the use of various emitters (Ernst et al. 1979; Norris 1995). In a search of the literature, Lawrence (1991) reported that the success rate in 248 patients who had received various forms of therapy lay between 7 and 55%, with the average success rate being just short of 26%. It is worth mentioning that 91% of the patients were suffering from keloids of the auricle.

In those studies that reported good results (Ernst et al. 1979), there was no strict distinction between keloid and hypertrophic scar formation, so the spontaneous remission of the hypertrophic scars probably falsified the results to a considerable degree. A further problem is that the studies reported on all keloids occurring on the body, so that it not certain whether the results also apply to keloids of the ear.

Finally, it should be pointed out that good results can be obtained by applying postoperative pressure, for example with the oyster-splint technique described by Mercer and Studd (1983).

Deformities of the Auricle

Postoperative Asymmetry or Recurrent Prominence
(Fig 5.**59**)

Unequal prominence of the auricles after surgery is usually iatrogenic, a result of omitting to measure the ears before and after surgery (see Fig. 5.**29**, p. 120 and Fig. 5.**40 h**, p. 132). It can also arise from suture breakdown, knot slipping, suture tear-out, etc. (Fig. 5.**59 a**, **b**). For this reason, patients are instructed to wear a headband at night for 4–6 weeks after the operation and to abstain from team sports or any other type of sport that could lead to the sutures being torn out. After a few weeks the scar in the antihelical rim will have become sufficiently strong. Ears that are folded and held only by sutures, using the purely incisionless technique as currently described in the literature (Kaye 1967; Fritsch 1995 and Merck 2000), run the risk of the sutures tearing at any time, as mentioned earlier.

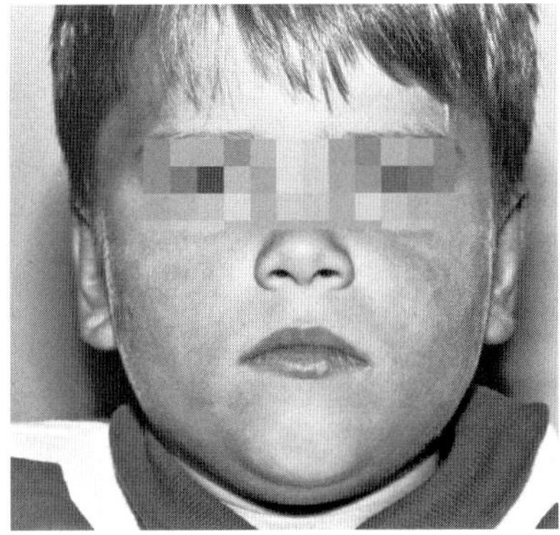

Fig. 5.**60** **Excessive resection of postauricular skin, ears "plastered" to head after surgery.**

Therapy. Revision surgery will be necessary—on either one or both ears—after taking measurements of the ears.

Ears Pinned Back Too Far, Telephone Ear Deformity
(Figs. 5.**60**–5.**62**)

As previously mentioned under early complications, ears pinned backed too far are most frequently seen as a result of extreme skin resection (Fig. 5.**60**); the upper helix lies behind the antihelix when observed from the frontal aspect (Fig. 5.**61 a**). This error is occasionally seen in association with prominence of the superior and inferior part of the ear (**telephone ear deformity**; Fig. 5.**62 a**), or prominence of the middle third with the superior and inferior thirds set back (**reverse telephone ear deformity**). We also find prominence of just the upper part or just the lower part of the auricle (see also Fig. 5.**40 f**, **j**).

Therapy. If possible, an attempt is made to mobilize the auricle and cover the skin defect with an advancement flap (Fig. 5.**61 b**) or with a full-thickness skin graft (Fig. 5.**62 b**, **c**). After an incision or after excising the old scar, careful dissec-

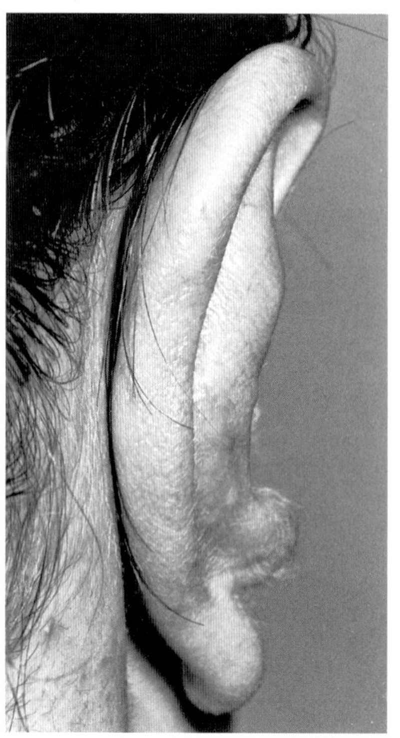
a

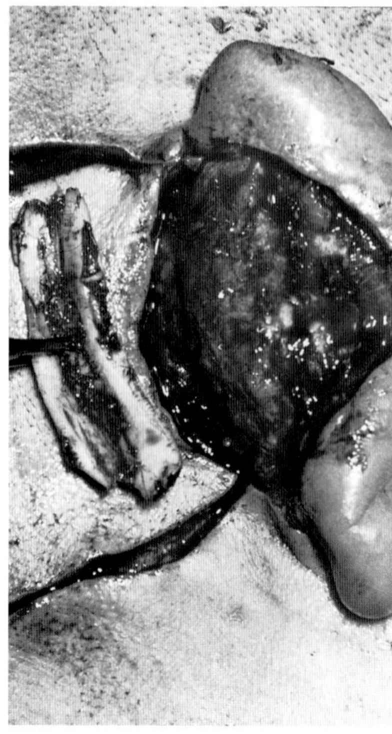
b

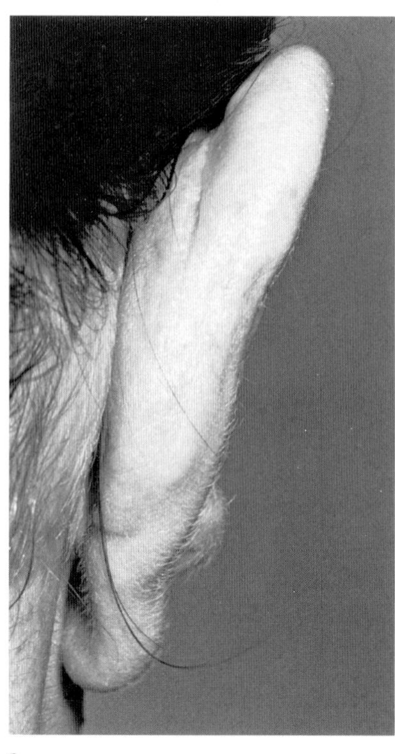
c

Fig. 5.**61** **Ears too tight to head.**
a Ear too tight to head due to extreme overcorrection, destruction of the cartilage, and displacement of the sulcus after excessive skin resection behind the helix.
b Reconstruction of the cartilage after scar revision, using a thin shell of costal cartilage, and resurfacing of the considerable skin deficit with a U-shaped advancement flap (see p. 86, Fig. 4.**95**).
c Outcome.

tion of the skin, careful incision of the scar beneath the antihelix and unfolding of the ear in the part which has been set back too far or exaggeratedly folded is required, followed by setback of the overly prominent parts. An undamaged elastic cartilage is a prerequisite. Here too, careful measuring of the ears (see Figs. 5.**29**, 5.**40 h**) is required before and after the operation. Since skin frequently has to be recruited into the resulting defect, it should be ensured that the cartilage remains covered with well-perfused fibrous tissue (Fig. 5.**61 b, c**).

Should this prove impossible, the defect will require coverage with a U-shaped advancement, a rotation or transposition flap raised over the mastoid. Occasionally cartilage will have to be incorporated to provide additional support (Fig. 5.**61 b**).

Formation of Sharp Ridges
(Figs. 5.**63**, 5.**64**)

The causes of such ridge formations are usually faulty technique, too deep scoring of the antihelix, overgenerous excisions between antihelix and concha, the placement of the incision in the wrong place, or faulty suture techniques, often associated with excessive posterior skin excision (Figs. 5.**63 a**, 5.**64 a**).

Therapy. Treatment of these usually iatrogenic defects is operative. Small ridges in the transitional region between concha and antihelix can be leveled off by an incision in the concha and excision of the ridge. Depending on the extent and prominence of the ridge formation, form of the antihelix or the crura, temporal fascia (Figs. 5.**63 b, c**; 5.**64 b, c**) can also be harvested and drawn in via small incisions in the scapha, antihelix (see Fig. 5.**65 c**) or posteriorly near the helical tail or behind the scapha (see Figs. 5.**63 b**, 5.**64 b**) after undermining the anterior skin. The auricle can also be refolded. Good improvements in the form and position of the ear are possible with these techniques (Figs. 5.**63 d**, 5.**64 d**).

Catastrophic Ear
(Figs. 5.**63**–5.**67**)

This term was coined by Staindl (1986). Parts of the auricle can be destroyed by iatrogenic damage, necrotic infections, or perichondritis (Fig. 5.**65**). We frequently see this type of destruction after exaggerated anterior or posterior scoring of the cartilage, and excessive cartilage excisions or incisions, not infrequently in association with excessive skin excision on the posterior auricular surface (see Fig. 5.**61**).

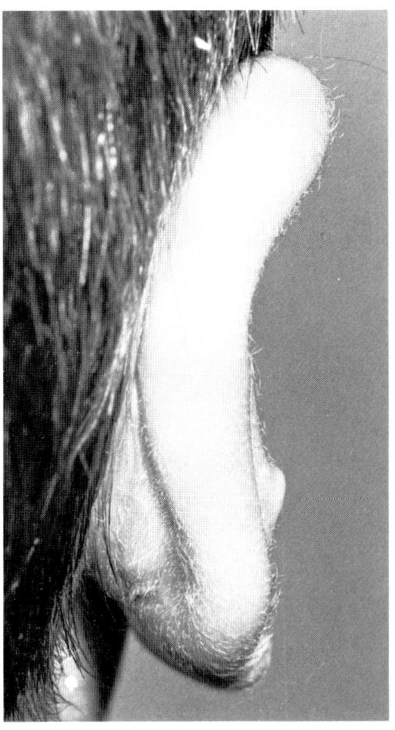

a

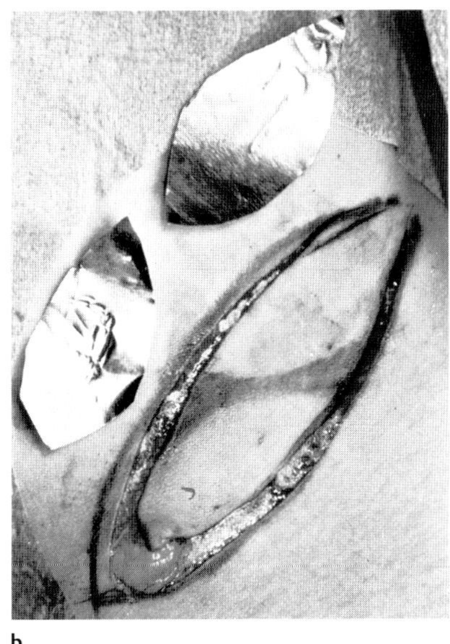

b

Fig. 5.62 **Telephone ear deformity.**
a Bilateral excessive projection of the upper and lower auricle (telephone ear deformity) after previous surgery; excessive skin excision in the middle portion.
b After incision and scar dissection, skin is harvested from the inguinal region with the aid of templates.
c The skin is sutured and glued with fibrin adhesive.
d Result.

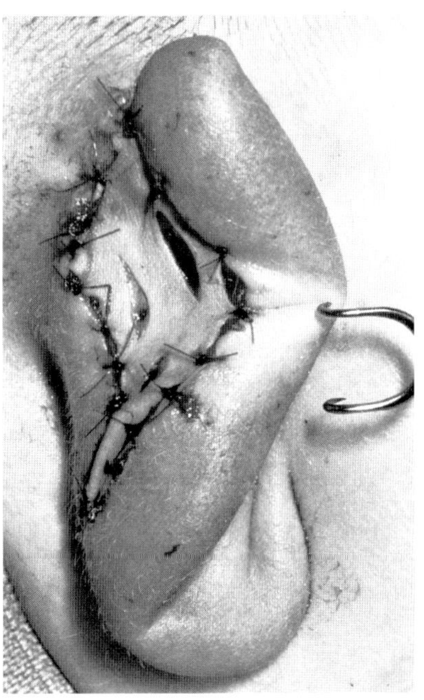

c

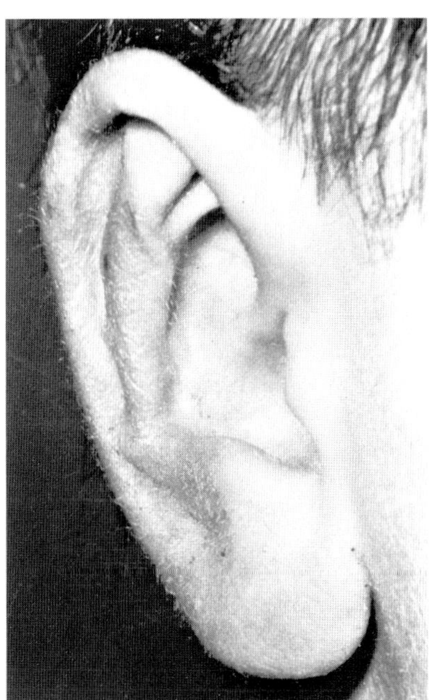

d

Therapy. In cases of severe destruction, attempts are made to reconstruct the auricle according to the defects. However, it is not be possible to restore the auricle completely, only to limit the damage (see also defect surgery, pp. 43 ff).

Defects after repeated surgery. Attempts had been made to set back the ears of a 12-year-old girl with bilateral prominent ears (Fig. 5.**66 a**) in five operations and revisions for each ear. She was referred to us with defects and ears that were still prominent (Fig. 5.**66 b, e**).

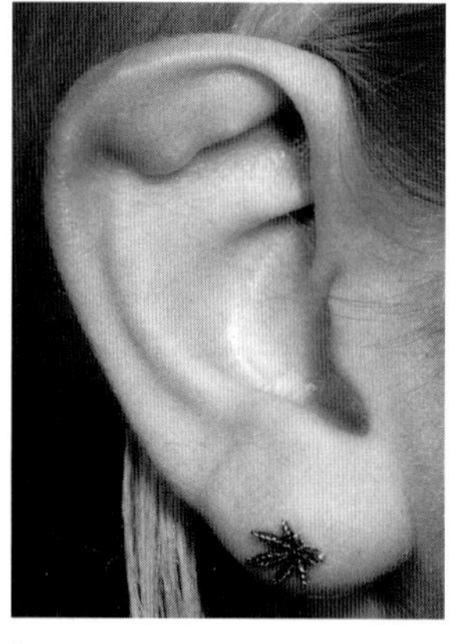
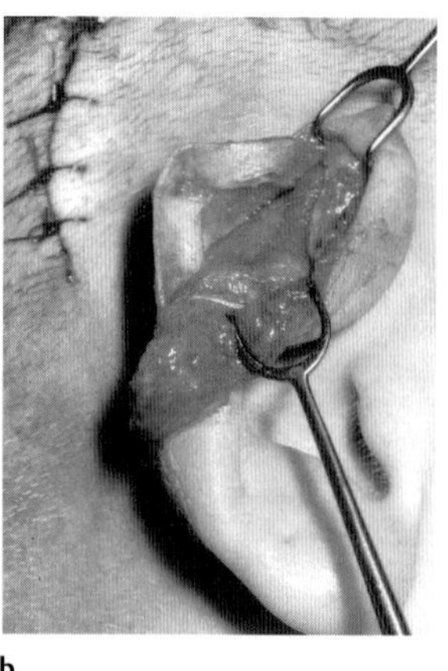
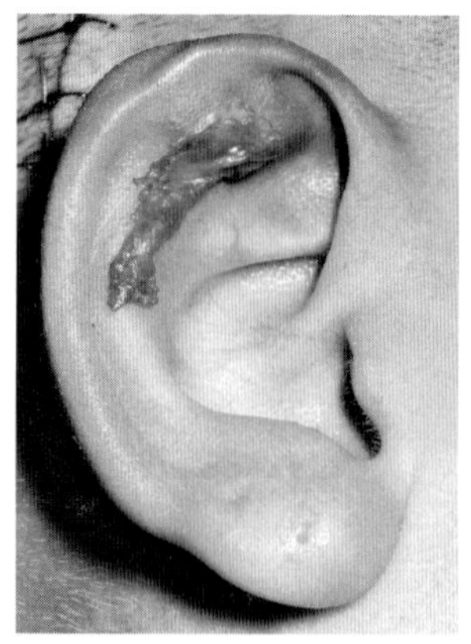
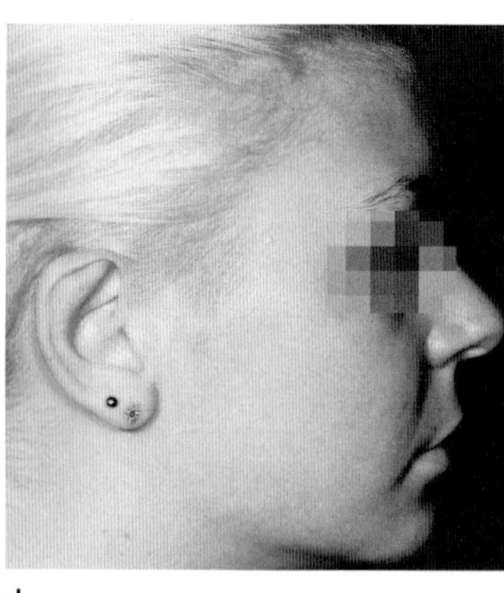

a b c d

Fig. 5.63 **Formation of a sharp ridge in the region of the upper auricle.**
a Deformation.
b Posterior incision and dissection of the skin anteriorly towards the scapha. Antihelix and helix smoothed out and re-folded.
c Additional harvesting and insertion of a strip of temporal fascia.
d Result (surgeon: Ms. S. Klaiber).

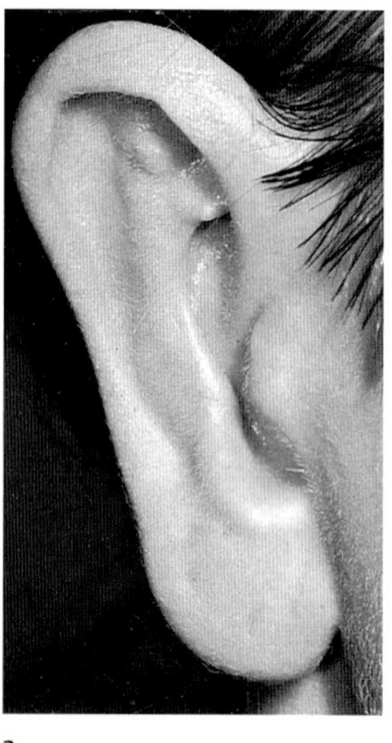
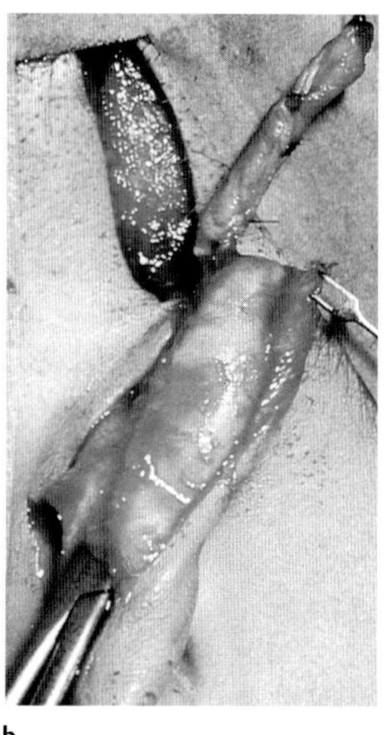
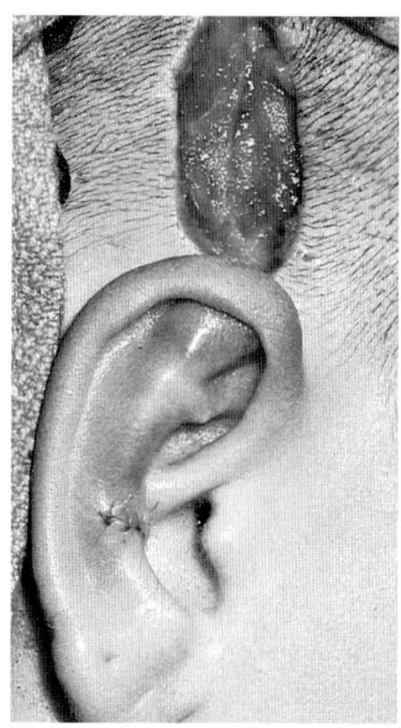
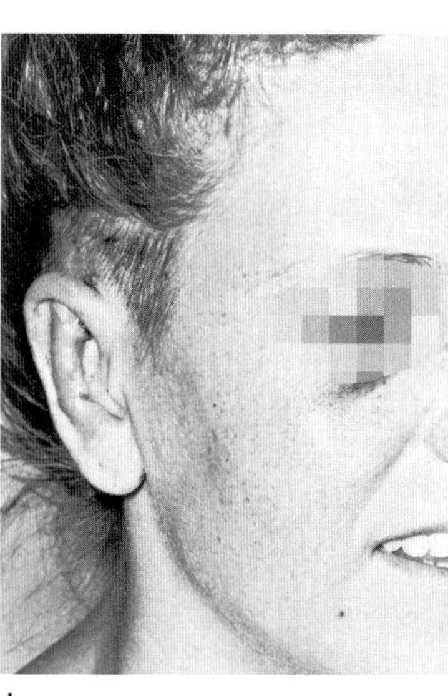

a b c d

Fig. 5.64 **Deformation with formation of a sharp ridge after otoplasty (probably using Stenström's technique).**
a Deformation of the auricle.
b Exposure of the temporal fascia. Insertion of the fascia which is armed with sutures from a posterior or anterior approach, or via several short incisions.
c Several thick strips of fascia armed with sutures are drawn under the skin (the sharp ridges may be smoothed out beforehand and, if necessary, the scars excised).
d Result.

- **Right ear** (Fig. 5.**66 b–d, g**). Reconstruction with costal cartilage and skin from the mastoid and a tube pedicle flap (Fig. 5.**66 f, g**).
- **Left ear** (Fig. 5.**66 e, f, h**). Renewed setback and reconstruction of the upper auricle with conchal cartilage and a rotation flap (Fig. 5.**66 c–e**, see also p. 148).

Infection with necrosis after otoplasty. Reconstruction with a rotation flap and cartilage (Fig. 5.**67 a–d**) in two stages.

Cartilage destruction. In further patients with severe deformation of the auricles after otoplasty, costal cartilage was used for reconstruction (Fig. 5.**68 a–f**).

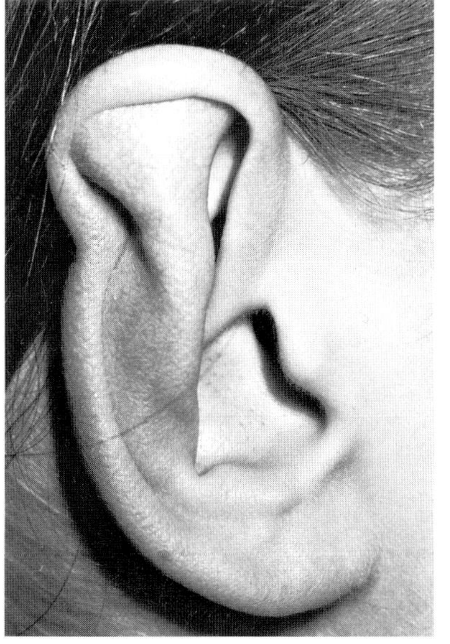

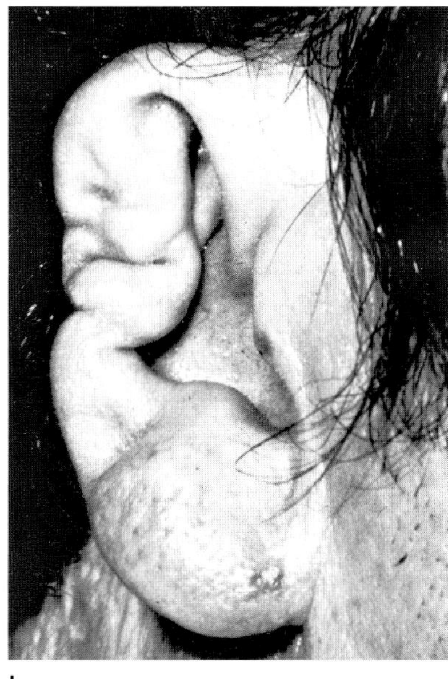

Fig. 5.**65** **Significant deformations of the auricle secondary to otoplasty:**
- **a** **Cartilage destruction by scoring technique (see Fig. 5.68 a).**
- **b** **Perichondritis.**

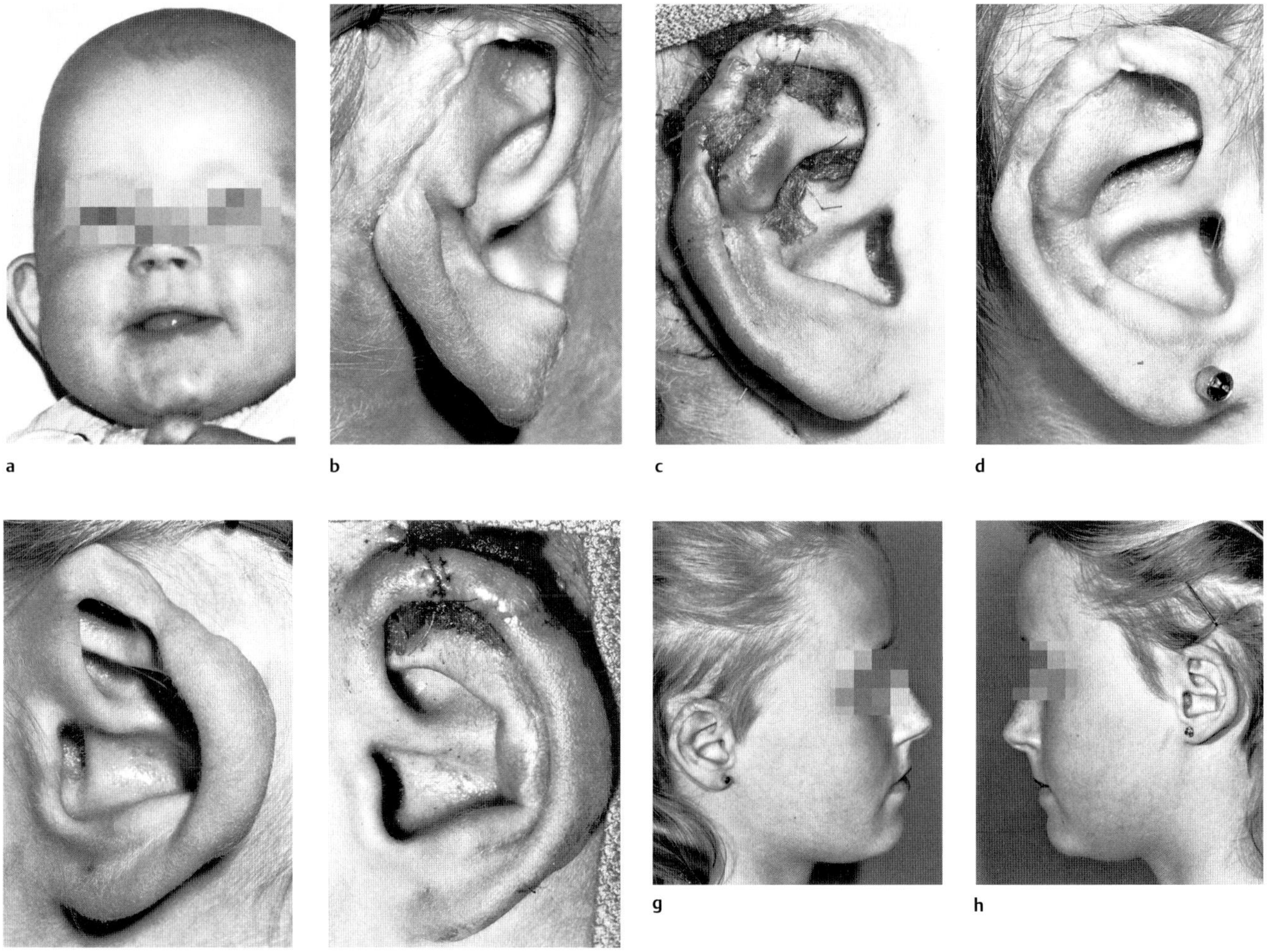

Fig. 5.**66** **Patient referred to us after several attempts at otoplasty demonstrating bilateral auricular destruction.**
- **a** Child before surgery (parents' picture).
- **b, c** Destruction of the right upper auricle with sharp ridge and scar formation. Reconstruction in several stages with costal cartilage and a tube-pedicled flap.
- **d, g** Result.
- **e** Slightly less destruction of the left auricle of the same patient and recurrence of protrusion.
- **f** Reconstruction with a mastoid flap, a conchal cartilage strut and setback otoplasty.
- **g, h** Bilateral result after otoplasty with reconstruction ca. 6 months after surgery.

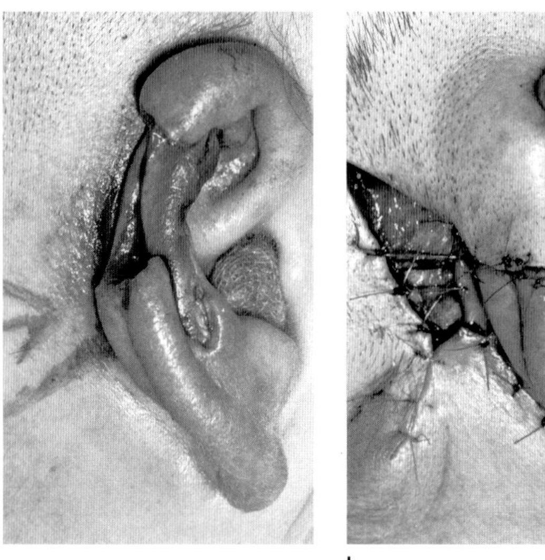
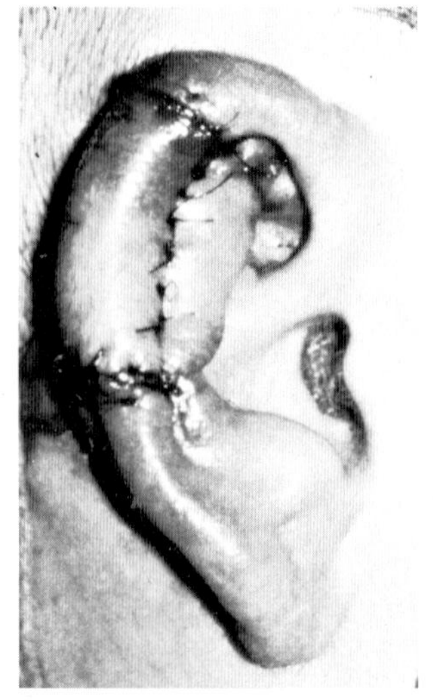
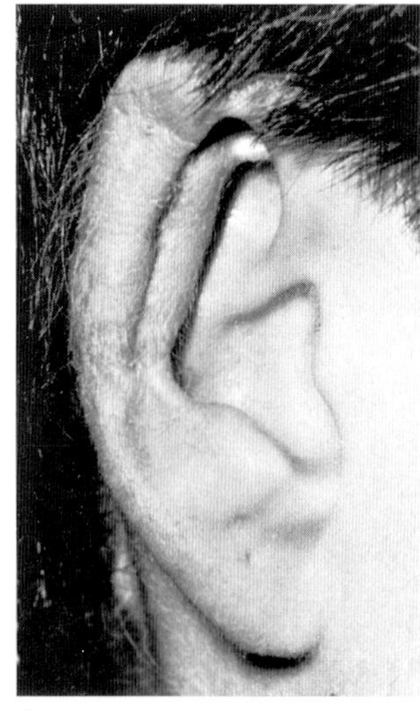

a b c d

Fig. 5.67 **Infection and necrosis secondary to otoplasty.**
First stage:
- **a** Necrosis, rotation flap marked out.
- **b** Flap inset, cartilage strut harvested from the concha.

Second stage:
- **c** Division and inset of the flaps.
- **e** Result (surgeon: R. Siegert).

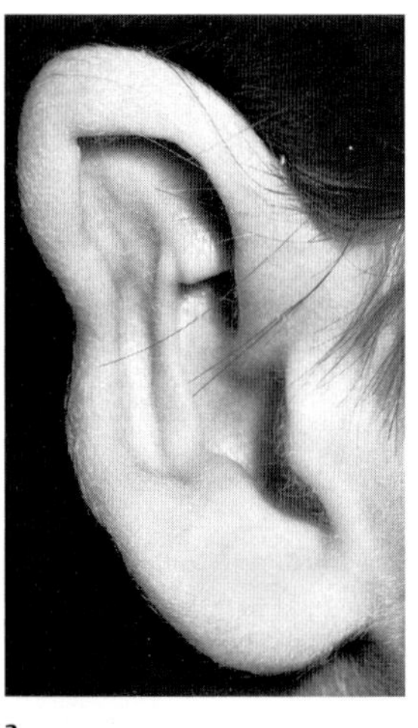
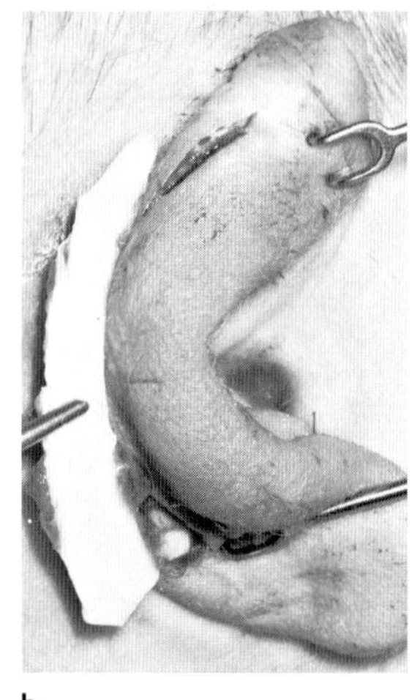
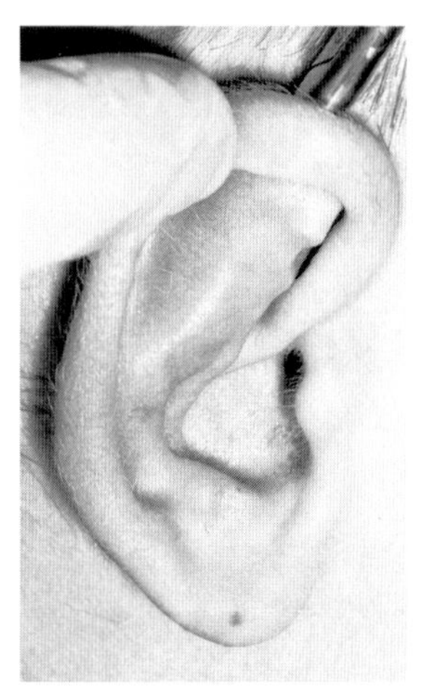
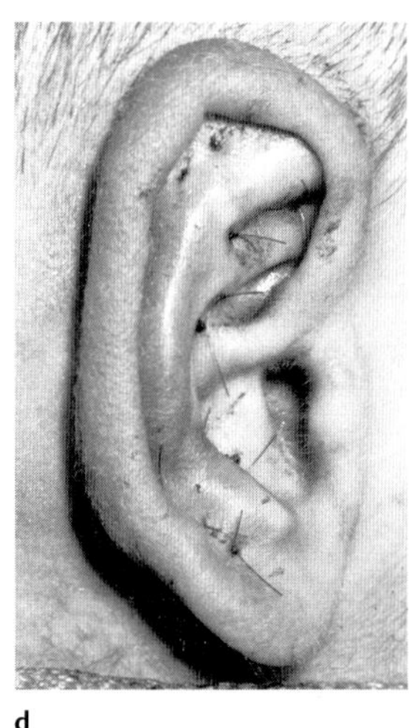

a b c d

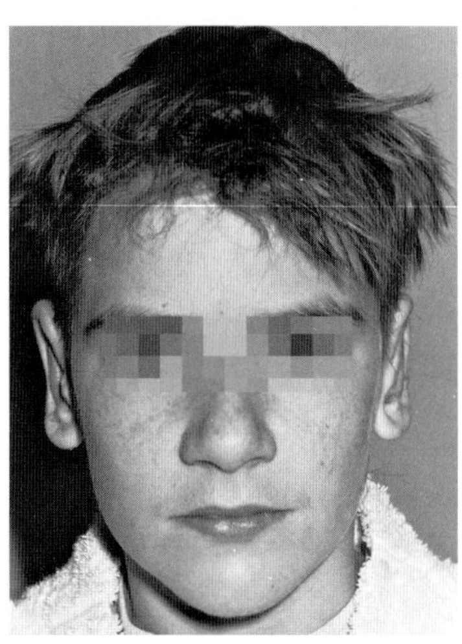

e f

Fig. 5.68 **Cartilage destruction.**
- **a, e** Appearance after otoplasty demonstrating destruction of the cartilaginous structure, with the right ear worse than the left.
- **b** Reconstruction of the auricle with costal cartilage which was fashioned and inserted via posterior incisions.
- **c** Skin and perichondrium are dissected off the cartilage in the region of the antihelix.
- **d** Appearance after insertion of the cartilage, moulding of the form achieved with the aid of a few sutures.
- **e** Appearance before reconstruction.
- **f** Appearance after bilateral reconstruction.

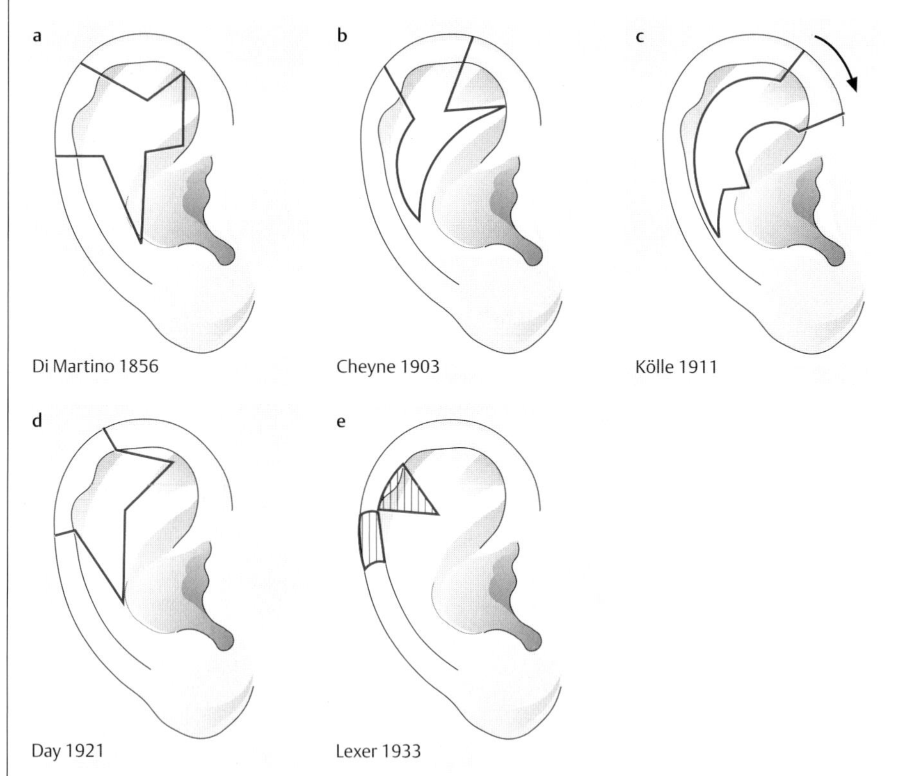

Fig. 5.**69** **Historical overview of various forms of wedge excisions for auricular reduction to correct macrotia (from Sercer and Mündnich 1962; Senechal and Pech 1970).**
a Di Martino (1856).
b Cheyne (1903).
c Kölle (1911).
d Day (1921).
e Lexer (1933).

Macrotia

(see Table 5.**2**; p. 118)

Definition. Macrotia refers to ears that are conspicuously oversized, i. e., an auricular axis length of 65–68 mm in short individuals and more than 70 mm in tall individuals. Normal values are 58–62 mm in women and 62–66 mm in men (s. Table 1.**8**, p. 5).

The **aim** is to reduce the overlarge ear, in both length and width, in such a manner that no additional deformity or scar remains.

Surgery to correct macrotia is discussed in detail under operations for peripheral defects (see pp. 43 ff).

Operative Techniques

Wedge Excisions and Reduction of the Earlobe

(Fig. 5.**69 a–e**)

As early as the nineteenth century, Di Martino (1856) and Cocheril (1895) reported on wedge excisions for auricular reduction (see also p. 53).

Joseph's Wedge Excision with Reduction

(Fig. 5.**70 a, b**; Joseph 1931)

Joseph (1931) took up the reduction techniques as described by Di Martino (1856) and Trendelenburg (1886, cited in Joseph 1931) and in addition performed a reduction of the earlobe (Sercer and Mündnich 1962; Senechal and Pech 1970; Tanzer et al. 1977).

Vogel's Operation

(Fig. 5.**71 a–c**; Vogel 1938)

After incision in the scapha, extending approximately from the superior antihelical crus to the level of the antitragus, the skin is undermined from the anterior surface in the direction of the concha. Based on a previously fashioned template (see Fig. 4.**50**, p. 64), a wedge-shaped excision comprising cartilage and skin is made on the posterior surface (Fig. 5.**71 a**). Then skin closure of the posterior auricular surface is done with 6–0 monofilament suture material, followed by a few cartilage sutures using 5–0 braided sutures and adaptation of the skin of the anterior surface by excision in the region of the scapha (Fig. 5.**71 b**). This is rounded off by closure of the skin wound in the scapha (Fig. 5.**71 c**).

Gersuny's Helical Sliding Flap Technique

(Fig. 5.**72**; see also pp. 54 ff)

After removal of a tumor of the helix, Gersuny (1903) made a full-thickness, crescent-shaped excision from the scapha (Fig. 5.**72**). This resulted in reduction of the auricle (see Fig. 4.**27**). This technique has been modified in many ways over the last 100 years (Jost et al. 1977 a).

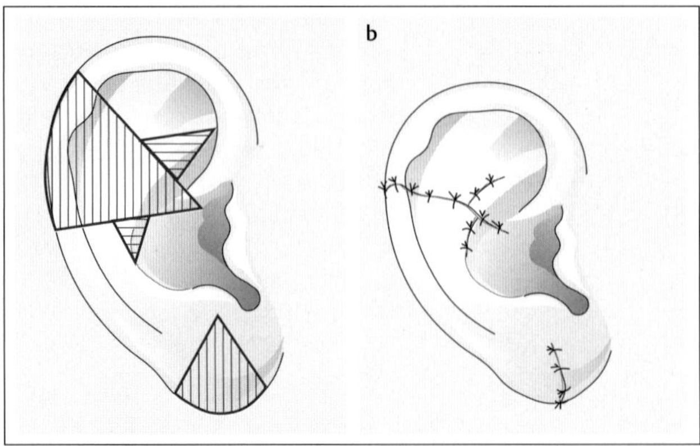

Fig. 5.70 **Wedge-shaped excisions for reduction of the auricle and earlobe as described by Di Martino (1856) and Trendelenburg (1886; cited in Joseph 1931).**
a Suggested excisions.
b Appearance after closure of the wounds.

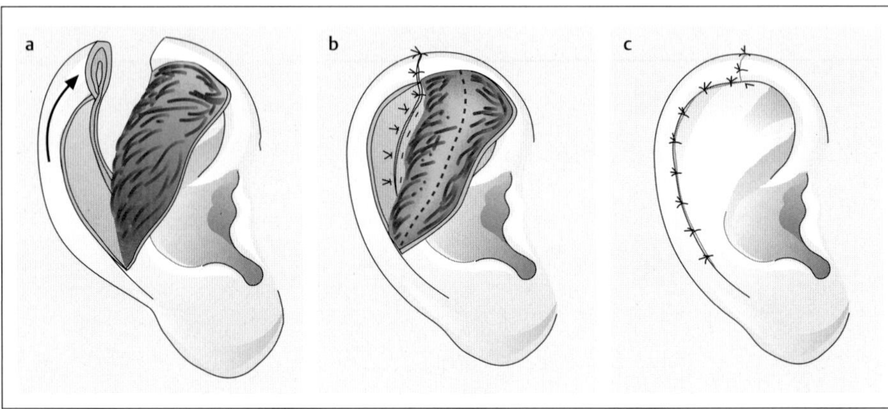

Fig. 5.71 **Operation to reduce auricular size as described by Vogel (1938) and Hinderer et al. (1987) (from Mündnich 1962 a).**
a After incising the scapha, the skin is dissected and cartilage and posterior skin are excised according to a template.
b 6–0 monofilament material for the posterior skin suture, 5–0 braided polyglactic acid for the cartilage suture, resection performed from an anterior approach (red broken line).
c The anterior skin is sutured using 6–0 monofilament material (polydioxanone or polypropylene).

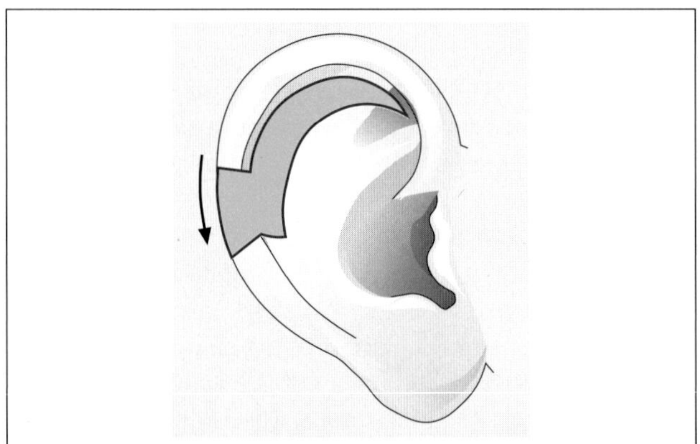

Fig. 5.72 **Auricular reduction using the Gersuny technique (1903); red: full-thickness excision.**

Eisenklam's Technique

(Fig. 5.**73 a, b**; Eisenklam 1930; Meyer and Sieber 1973; Tebetts 1982; Zenteno 1992)

The full-thickness excision was placed at the transition between helix and earlobe, while a two-layer crescent-shaped scaphal excision was performed as described by Meyer and Sieber (s. pp. 54 ff).

Excision in the Anterior Helical Region

(Meyer and Sieber 1973); see also Cavanaugh 1982; Argamaso 1989; Fig. 4.**32**, p. 56)

Gersuny's Technique, as Modified by Meyer

(Fig. 5.**74 a, b**; Meyer and Sieber 1973)

Meyer describes a modified Gersuny technique with transposition of the helical defect into the helical crus. The helix was rotated anteriorly after excision of the crus in order to achieve an inconspicuous scar. At the same time, he also performed a reduction of the earlobe. (Tebbets 1982; Davis 1989; Argamaso 1989.)

Gersuny's Technique, as Modified by Weerda and Zöllner

(Fig. 5.**75 a–g**; Weerda and Zöllner 1986; Weerda 1988, 1999 a)

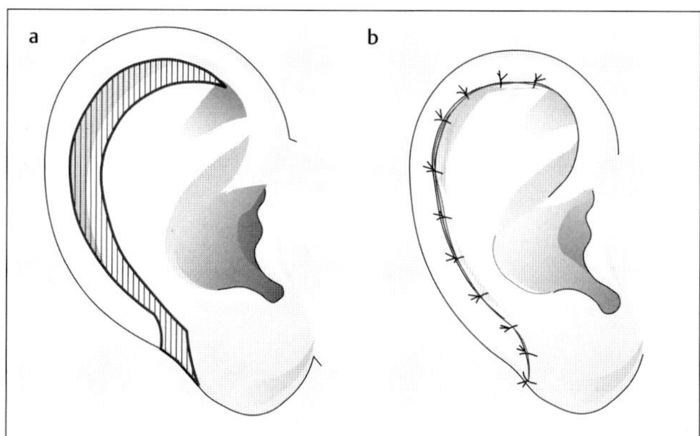

Fig. 5.73 a, b **Extension of the helix excision to the helix–earlobe transition as described by Eisenklam (1930) and Zenteno (1992).**

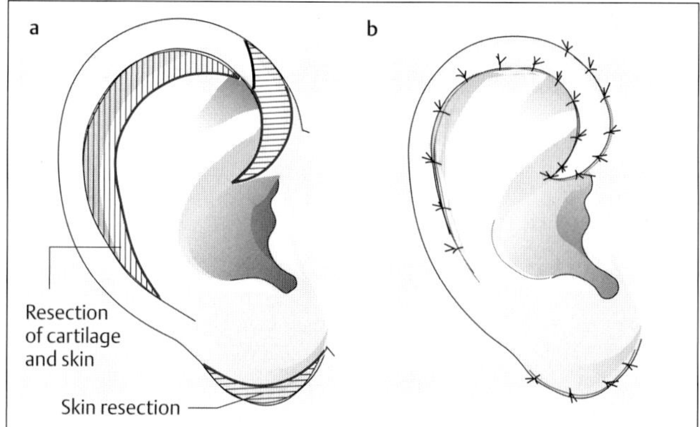

Fig. 5.74 **Auricular reduction by advancing the helix to the helical crus and reduction of the earlobe as described by Meyer and Sieber (1973).**

a Resection of cartilage and skin from the scapha (as described by Gersuny 1903) and excision of the helical crus, resection of skin from the earlobe.
b Closure of all wounds.

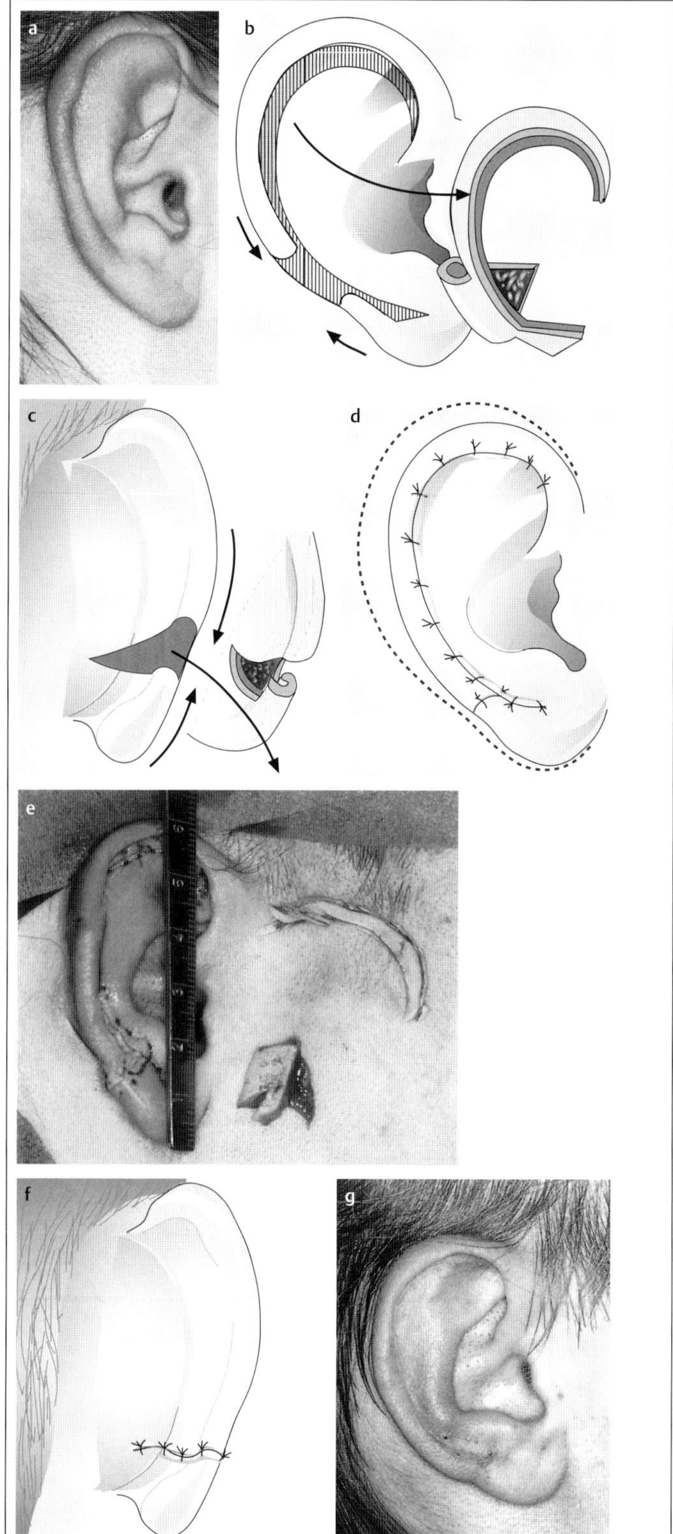

Fig. 5.75 **Auricular reduction using a modified Gersuny technique (1903) and earlobe reduction as described by Weerda and Zöllner (1986).** ▷

a A young woman with macrotia (72 mm).
b Schematic illustration and template to simulate those parts of the scapha to be resected. Two-layered, crescent-shaped resection of skin and cartilage in the scapha, full-thickness excision at the transition of earlobe to helix.
c Excision of the posterior dog-ear.
d, e Closure of all wounds with 6–0 monofilament suture material.
f Closure of the posterior surface.
g Result (62 mm).

A two-layer scaphal resection and a full-thickness excision of the helix at the transition to the earlobe were performed. Reduction of the earlobe is accomplished by a two-layer excision of a Burow's triangle. This technique reduces both the upper and the lower part of the auricle.

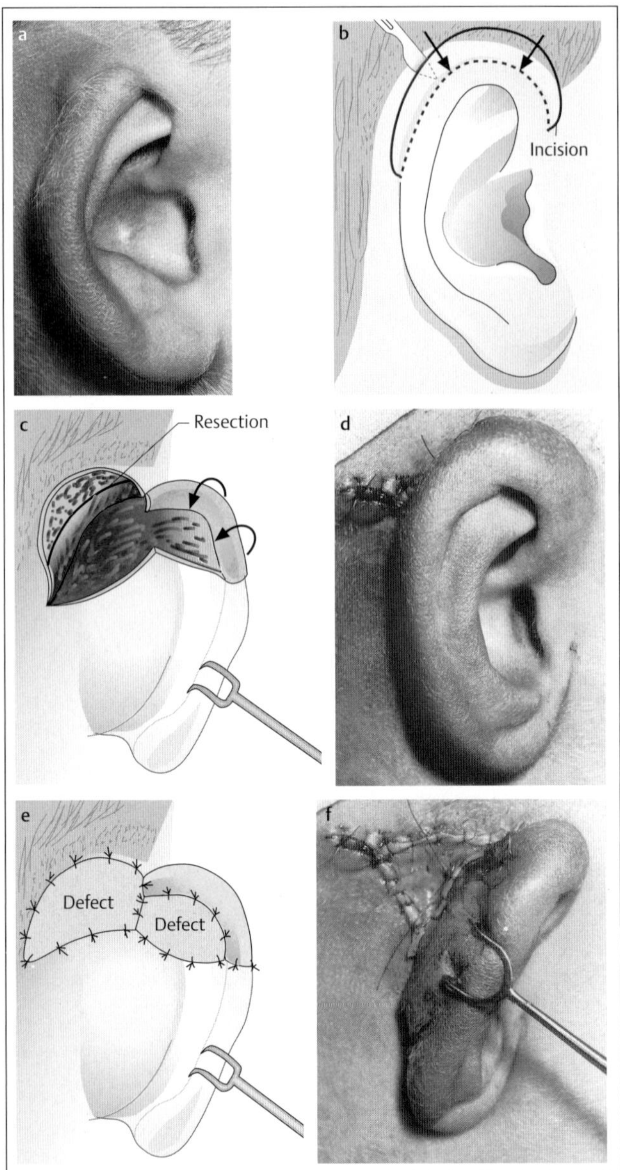

Fig. 5.**76** **Reconstruction for cryptotia (pocket ear) using free skin grafts.**
a, b Incision and flat dissection, above the hair follicles, of a thick split-thickness skin flap based on the superior helical rim.
c, d Elevation of the auricle from the pocket, resection of the full-thickness-skin donor site.
e, f The post- and retroauricular defects are either resurfaced with split-thickness skin or closed primarily by mobilization of the surrounding skin (surgeon: Ms. S. Klaiber).

Cryptotia

Synonym: pocket ear (see Table 5.**2**; p. 118).

Definition. This malformation occurs more frequently in Asians and is rarely seen in Europeans. The upper part of the auricle is adherent and the cartilage is buried under the skin in a pocket. In addition to this malformation, which accounts for one-fourth to one-third of all malformations affecting the upper auricle, other deformities may also be present (Simons 1974): the upper sulcus may be absent, and the scapha and antihelical crura are often underdeveloped (Yano et al. 1994). There is some discussion of familial clustering (Hayashi et al. 1993; see also section on embryology, p. 106).

Yano et al. (1994) undertook a morphometric study involving 45 patients and demonstrated that in the presence of this malformation, which is encountered quite frequently in Japan, the malformed side is significantly narrower in its upper part in comparison with the healthy side. Similarly, they also demonstrated that there was also a shortening of the longitudinal axis when the ear was measured from the intertragic notch upwards.

Cause. An anomaly of the intrinsic oblique and transverse auricular muscles (Hirose et al. 1985).

Treatment. A number of authors suggest early formation of the sulcus with thin, soft tubes, dental mold, or taping of the ear (Muraoka et al. 1984; Matsuo and Hirose 1989; see p. 141).

Surgery. The ear must be released from the pocket, the post- and retroauricular defects resurfaced, and the sulcus reconstructed. If necessary, the form of the ear should be normalized, e. g., by otoplasty for prominence of the auricle.

Recommended Surgical Methods

Coverage with Full-Thickness Skin and Thick Split-Skin Graft — (Fig. 5.**76**)

Along the lines of Nagata's suggestions for the reconstruction of grade III microtia (1994 d; see Fig. 5.**172 a–c**; p. 215), a full-thickness skin flap is raised about 1 cm superior to the upper cartilage margin of the auricle (Fig. 5.**76 b**) with a size 15 blade, keeping above the hair follicles and proceeding towards the helix, after which the auricle is elevated from its bed as in stage 2 of Nagata's reconstruction (see p. 215). A layer of fibrous tissue should be left behind on the cartilage. After dissecting the auricle off the mastoid, the full-thickness flap, pedicled on the helix, is then folded over posteriorly to resurface the helix with a flap similar in texture and color (Fig. 5.**76 c**). The defects on the postauricular surface and on the mastoid are then covered with split skin (Fig. 5.**76 e**). The postoperative result is shown in Figures 5.**76 d** and 5.**77 e**.

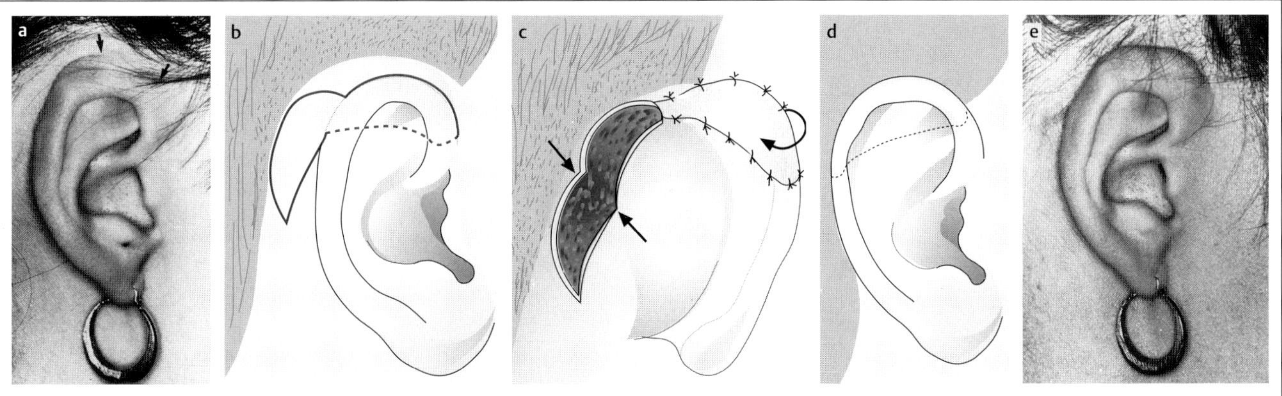

Fig. 5.77 **Coverage with a posteriorly based transposition flap as described by Weerda (1980 b).**
a Cryptotia (pocket ear).
b Incision around the helix and elevation of a patterned flap, which is based on the helix where it is folded over.
c The flap is folded over and sutured to the posterior surface, primary closure of the defect over the mastoid or coverage with a thick split-thickness skin graft (see Fig. 5.**76 e**).
d, e Result.

Coverage of the Postauricular Defect with a Flap Based Posteriorly on the Helix, as Described by Weerda
(Fig. 5.**77**)

The flap extends as far as the hairline and is elevated in a slightly curved manner, according to a template taken after the auricle has been freed from its bed (Fig. 5.**77 b**; see Weerda 1987). The flap is turned back and the postauricular defects are resurfaced (Fig. 5.**77 c**). The skin surrounding the residual defects over the mastoid is mobilized and closed (Fig. 5.**77 d, e**).

Cleft Auricle

Synonym: question-mark ear, coloboma (see Table 5.**2**; p. 118).

Definition. Vincent et al. (1961) were the first to report on this malformation in the literature. Cosman et al. (1970) referred to it as a **question-mark ear**; Park et al. (1998) call it the **malformation between helix and earlobe.** A number of operations have been described for this malformation (see section on embryology, p. 110).

Operative Techniques for Closure of the Defect

Weerda's Z-plasty
(Figs. 5.**78**, Fig. 5.**79**; Weerda 1980, 1982 a, 1999 a, 2001)

The boy depicted here has a right-sided cleft auricle. In addition, we found a mild macrotia and a prominent auricle as well as hyperplasia of the earlobe and dystopia (Fig. 5.**78 b**).

The defect was eliminated by a Z-plasty designed by us (Weerda 1980, 1982 a, 1999 a, 2001) and the earlobe reduced by transposing flap (1) superiorly along the longitudinal axis. A similar procedure was used in Fig. 5.**79 a–c**, supplemented by a Gersuny plasty.

Mobilization of the Posterior Skin in the Form of a VY-plasty
(Fig. 5.**80**; Hall and Stevenson 1988; see also p. 68, Fig. 4.**59**)

A film template is first fashioned from the normal ear (see Fig. 4.**50**, p. 64).

Instead of a full-thickness skin graft, Al-Quattan (1998) imports a two-layer composite graft from the contralateral ear into the defect.

Brodovsky and Westreich (1997) recommend a "mini **Gersuny technique**" (Fig. 5.**79**) with shortening of the axis (Fig. 5.**81 a–c**), similar to our suggestion.

Uysal et al.'s Technique
Uysal and co-workers (1990) treat this malformation like a wedge-shaped defect of the middle third of the ear; they remove the epithelium of the cleft and insert a slightly smaller strut. A large postauricular transposition flap is then used to cover the wedge-shaped defect (Barsky 1950, cited in Mündnich 1962; see Fig. 4.**65**, p. 71).

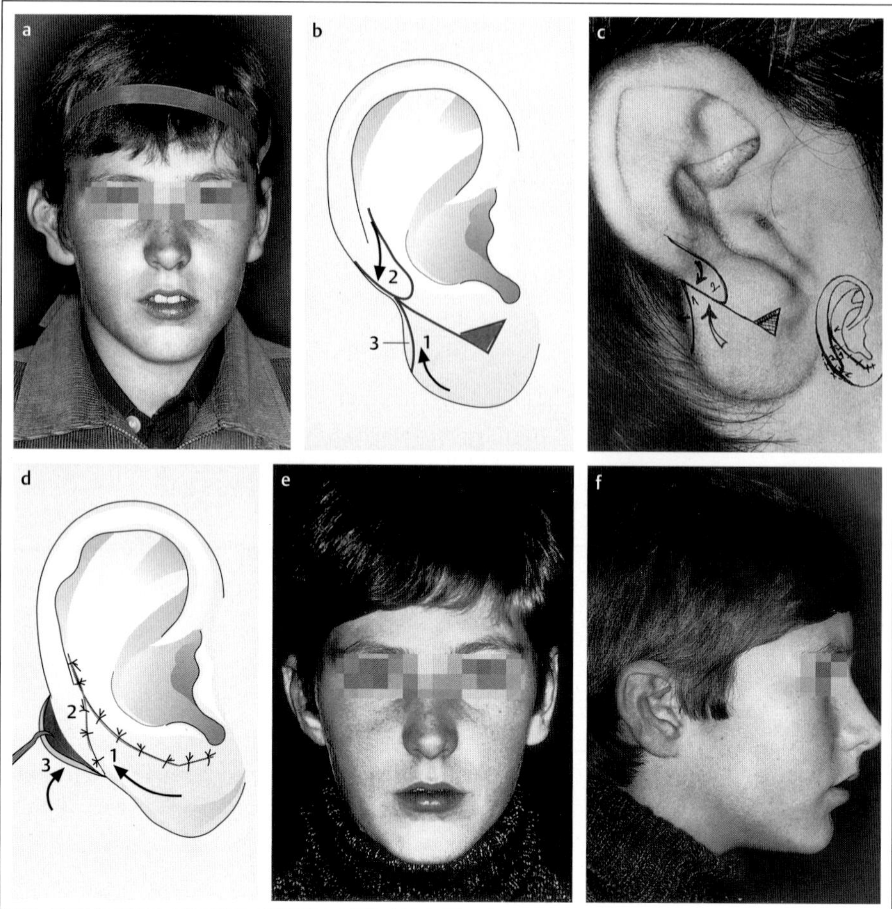

Fig. 5.78 **Operation for cleft auricle using a Z-plasty as described by Weerda (1980 b).**

a Cleft auricle with prominent ear, slight dystopia, macrotia, and hyperplasia of the earlobe.

b, c The Z-plasty is outlined: exchange of flaps 1 and 2 and coverage of the helical rim with the small, broadly based earlobe flap (3).

d Exchange of flaps 1 and 2, thus filling out the defect by reducing the auricle. The auricle is set back by otoplasty as described by Weerda (see Fig. 5.**52**, p. 140).

e, f Result.

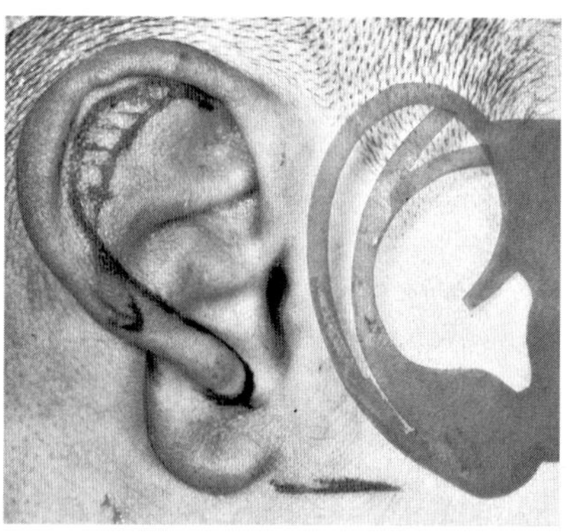

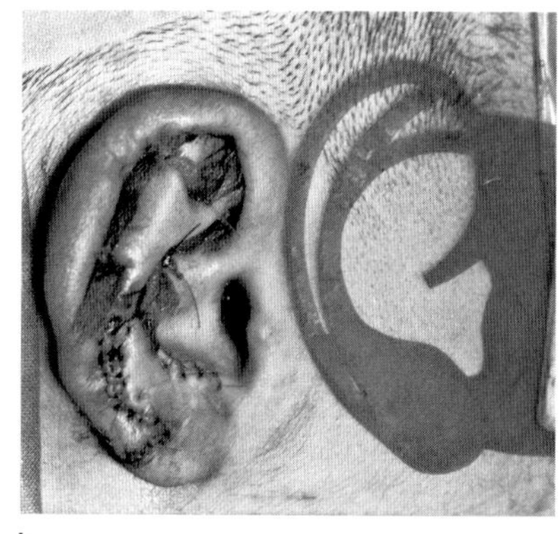

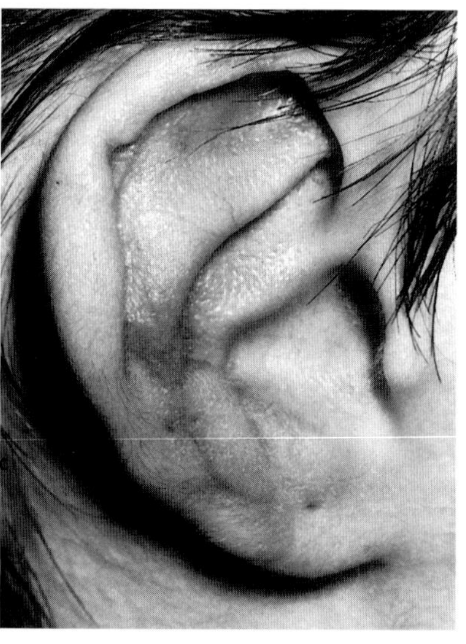

Fig. 5.**79** **Transverse cleft and hyperplasia.**

a Z-plasty with reduction of the auricle in the form of a **Gersuny plasty** (Gersuny 1903 and Weerda Z-plasty, Fig. 5.**78**). The template indicates the intended size.

b Appearance after completion of the operation.

c Result.

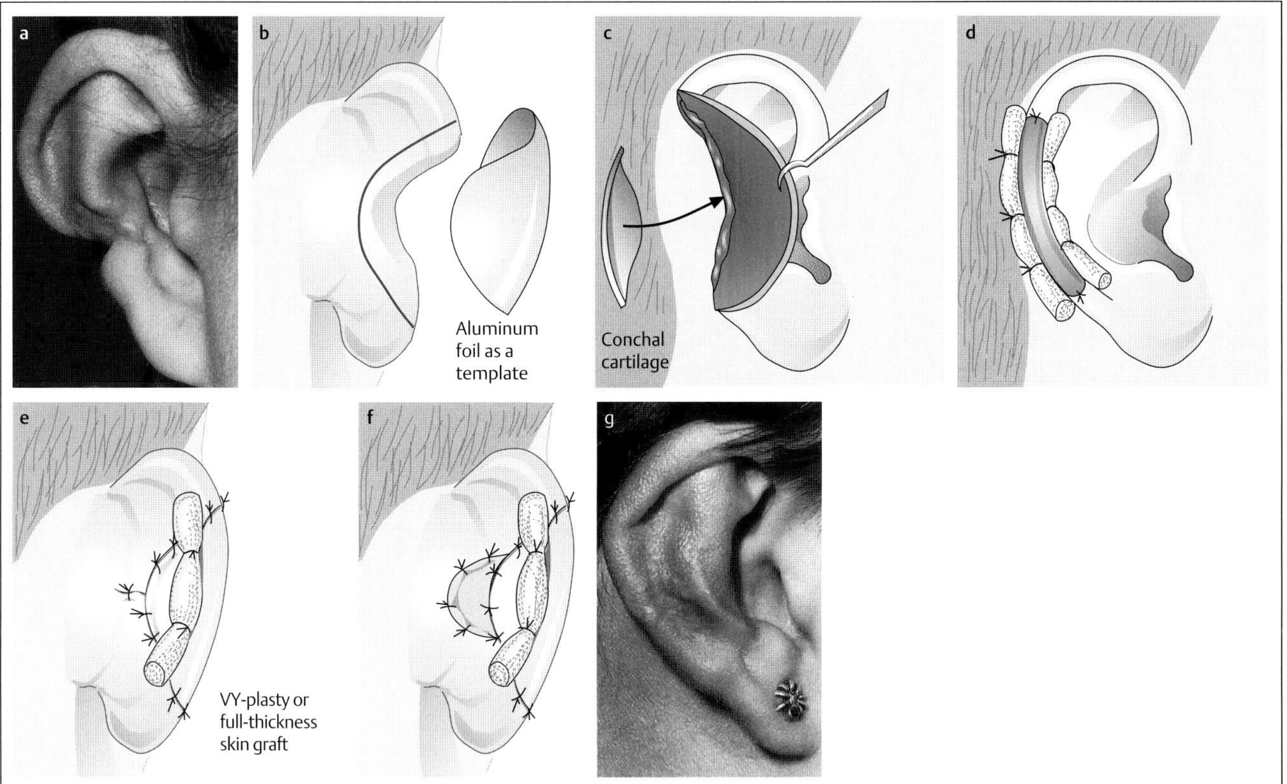

Fig. 5.**80** **VY-advancement as described by Hall and Stevenson (1988; see also section on "Defect surgery," Fig. 4.58, p. 67).**
a Cleft auricle.
b Incision on the postauricular surface and dissection of the skin towards the helix.
c A piece of cartilage is carved out and inserted (harvested from the contralateral concha or rib).
d–f VY-plasty for skin closure (**e**), or even full-thickness or split-thickness skin graft (**f**; Hall and Stevenson 1988; Al-Quattan and Cosman 1998) for the residual defect. Hall and Stevenson (1988) use a composite graft from the contralateral ear for support instead of a full-thickness skin graft.
g Result (surgeon: Ms. S Klaiber).

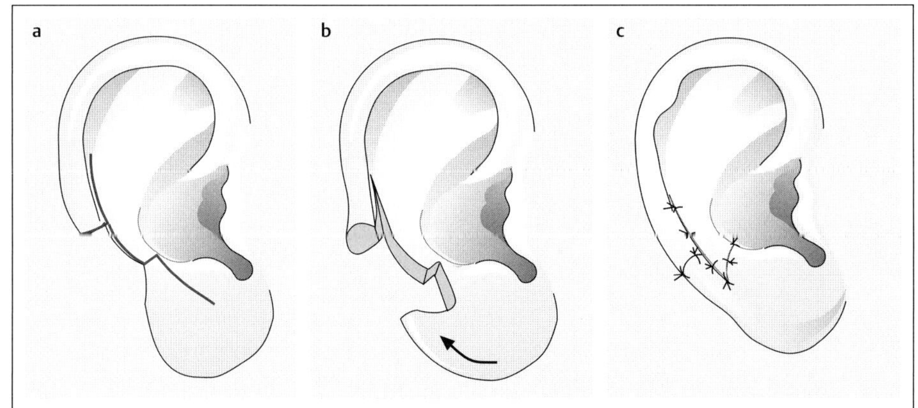

Fig. 5.**81** **Mini-Gersuny technique as described by Brodovsky and Westreich (1996).**
a Plan of the incisions.
b Incisions and cranial advancement of the earlobe into the defect.
c Closure of the defects.

Scaphoid Ear

Term coined by Davis (1987; Fig. 5.**82 a, b**; see Table 5.2; p. 118).

Definition. This type of minor deformity, which is frequently associated with prominence of the auricle (Weerda 1979 a; Davis 1987), involves absence of the scapha, or rather an absent folding of the typical helical contour, so that the concha or the antihelix extend upwards in a flattened manner into the ascending helix. There is a plethora of operations to reconstruct the helical roll.

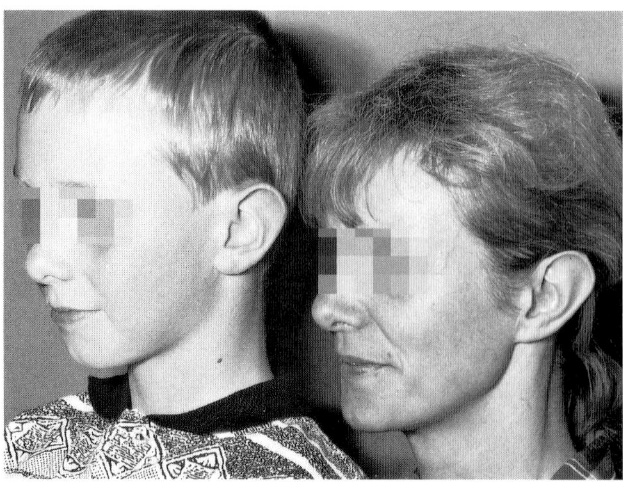

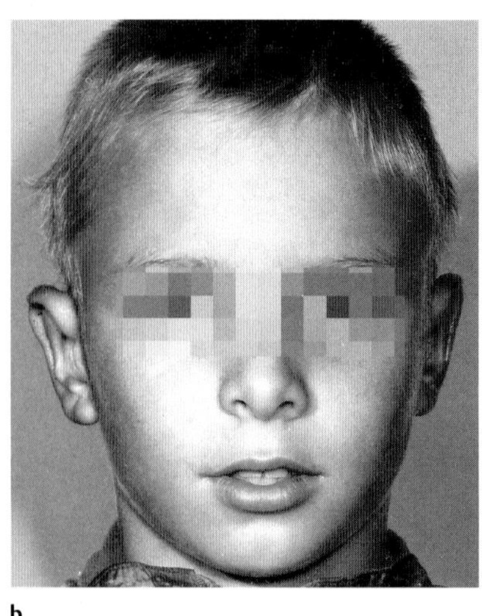

Fig. 5.**82** **Bilateral scaphoid ear.**
a Flattening of the helical rim in a mother and son.
b Appearance after bilateral Becker's procedure (Becker 1952; surgeon: Ms. S. Klaiber).

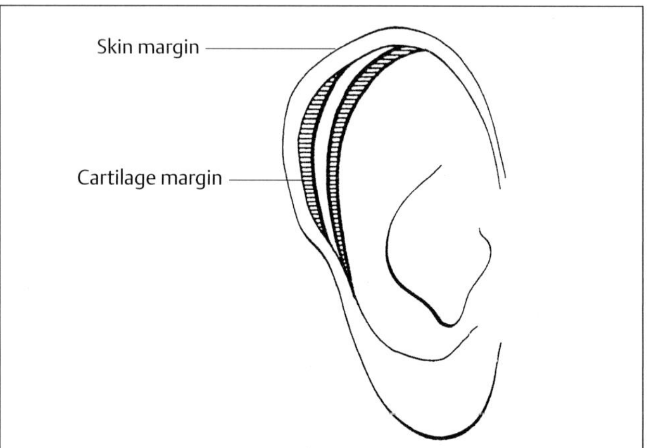

Fig. 5.**83** **Repair of the scaphoid ear as described by Joseph (1912).**
"The shorter hatched strip indicates the marginal excision for reduction, while the longer strip that is situated nearer the concha shows the excision to create the normal fold of the auricular margin" (from Joseph 1931).

Operative Techniques

Joseph's Method

(Fig. 5.**83**; Joseph 1912)

Joseph (1912, 1931) referred to this type of malformation as a "flattening of the auricular margin." He recommends placing an incision on the anterior auricular surface 4 mm from, and parallel to, the ear margin (Fig. 5.**83**). He then excises a 2–3 mm wide strip of cartilage. With overlarge auricles, the skin is undermined to the rim of the helical cartilage and a second strip is excised. The skin is then closed, at times requiring some shortening, and the new helix (white strip) is turned over anteriorly.

Jost et al.'s Method

(Fig. 5.**84**; Jost et al. 1977 a)

These authors proceed in a similar manner to that of Joseph (1912), but also excise a wedge from the scapha and anteriorly from the helix (Fig. 5.**84 a–c**) in order to lend the helix a better form (Fig. 5.**84 d**).

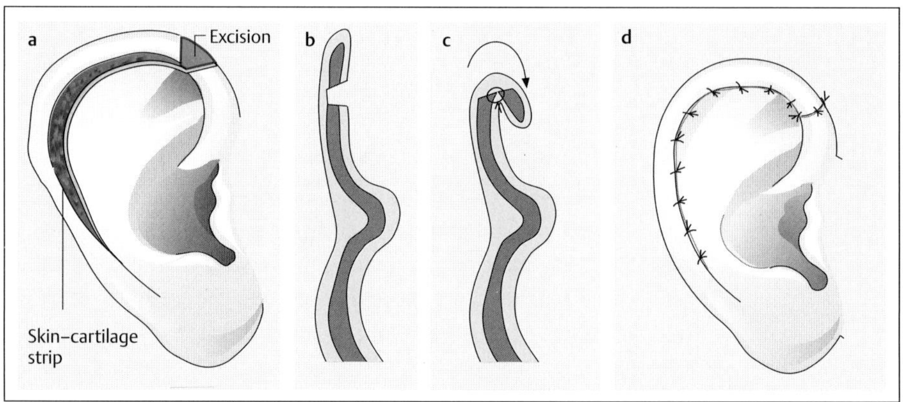

Fig. 5.**84** **Repair of the scaphoid ear as described by Jost et al. (1977).**
a, b Excision of a strip of skin-cartilage and an anterior skin-cartilage wedge.
c, d The margin is folded over and the wounds sutured.

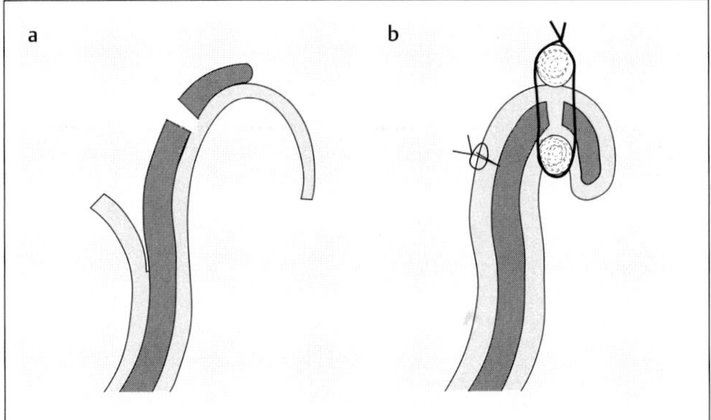

Fig. 5.85 **Becker's technique (Becker 1952).**

a Incision on the postauricular surface and skin dissection to the helical rim, resection of a cartilage wedge.

b The skin is redraped and sutured, and the new scapha is supported by mattress sutures tied over cotton bolsters.

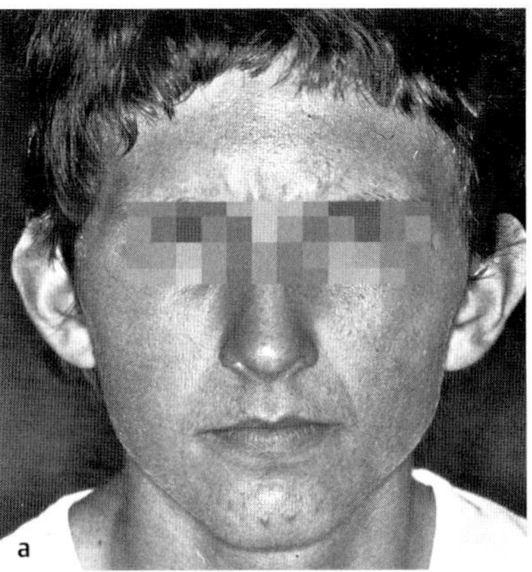

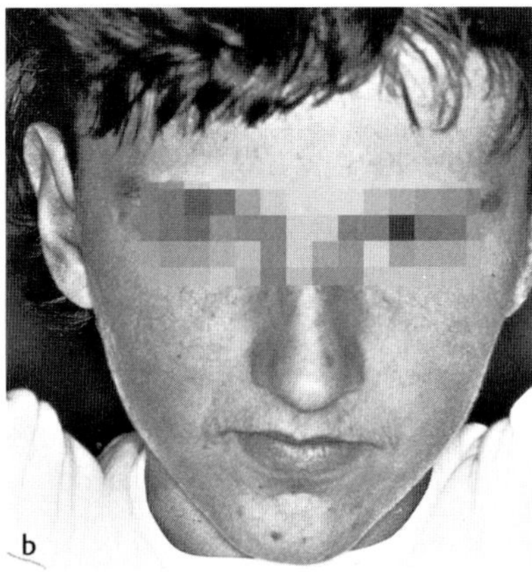

Fig. 5.86 **One of our patients operated on by using the scaphoid operation as described by Becker (1952; see Fig. 5.85).**

a Prominent scaphoid ears before surgery.

b Result.

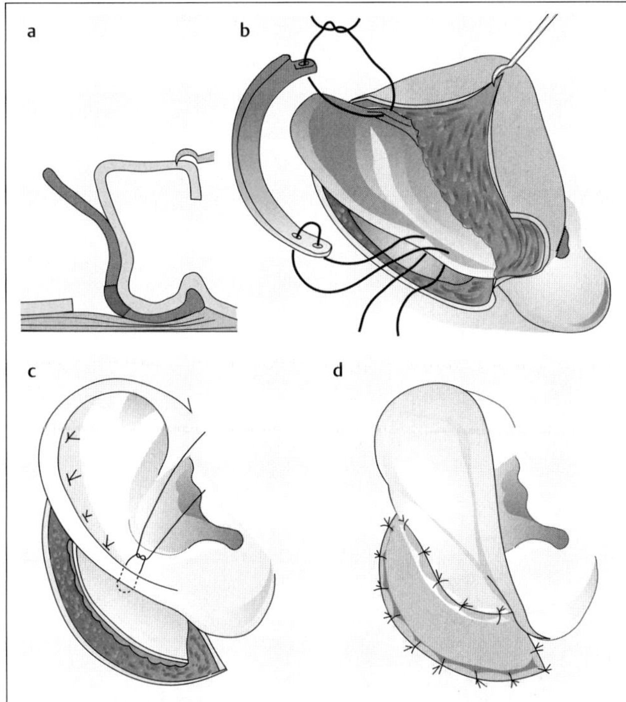

Fig. 5.87 **Reconstruction for cartilage deficit in the region of the helix (scaphoid ear; Converse and Brent 1977).**

a Posterior incision in the sulcus and skin dissection around the helix and anteriorly. Removal of cartilage strip from concha (red).

b The cartilage is sutured onto the scapha.

c The skin is redraped and glued with fibrin adhesive.

d The skin deficit in the sulcus is resurfaced with a free skin graft (pink).

Becker's Method

(Figs. 5.**85**, Fig. 5.**86**; Becker 1952).

Converse and Brent's Method

(Fig. 5.**87**; Brent 1977; similar operation to that described by Zoltan 1968; Bethmann and Zoltan 1968)

Undersized scaphoid ear. Incision over the mastoid and sulcus (Fig. 5.**87 a**). Undermining of the skin over the helical rim and placement and suture fixation of a new helix harvested from the concha (Fig. 5.**87 a**, **b**). The helix is contoured (Fig. 5.**87 c**), the skin redraped, and fibrin glue applied. The skin defect is covered with a free graft (Fig. 5.**87 d**).

Critique. A rather time-consuming operation.

Stahl's Ear

(See Figs. 5.**88**–5.**91**; Table 5.**2**, p. 118.)

Definition. This involves the formation of a third antihelical crus (see Fig. 5.**91**). Occasionally the superior crus is absent, the auricle is frequently prominent and the helix unfurled outwards (Figs. 5.**88**, 5.**89**; combination with a satyr ear deformity; Nakajima et al. 1984), or there is only a mere suggestion of a superior crus. Combinations with a cup-ear deformity have also been reported (Davis 1987), or there is only a superior antihelical crus which is displaced inferiorly.

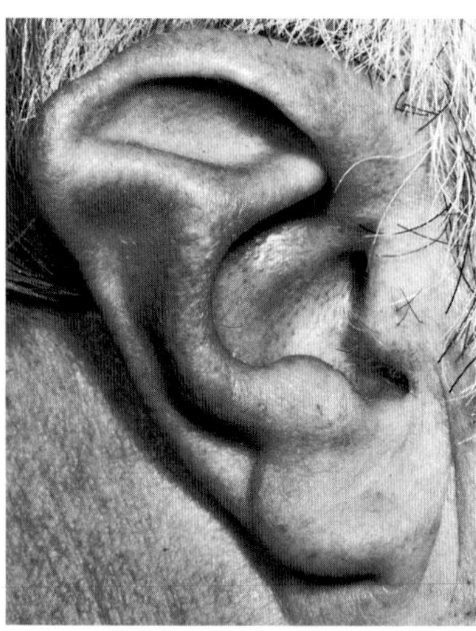

Fig. 5.**88** **Stahl's ear**
Third crus with absent superior crus.

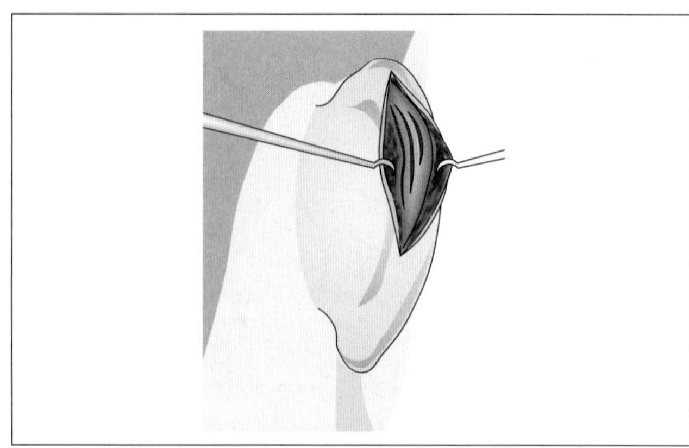

Fig. 5.**89** **Surgical repair of a Stahl's ear using the technique according to Furukawa et al. (1985).**

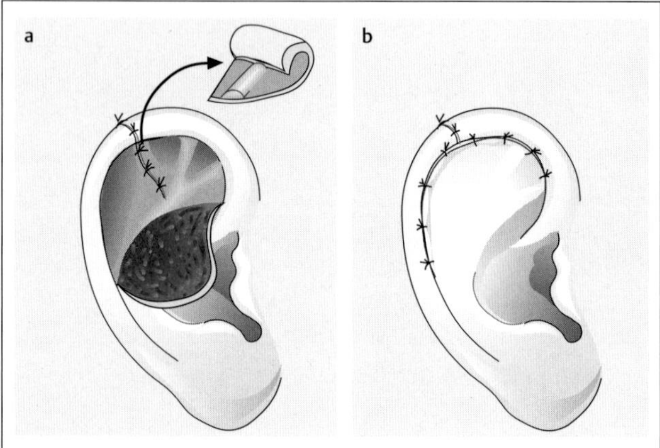

Fig. 5.**90** **Surgical repair of the third crus and satyr ear as described by Kaplan and Hudson (1999).**

a Resection of the crus together with the postauricular skin and wound closure.
b The anterior skin is redraped and sutured.

Operative Techniques

Furukawa et al.'s Method

(Fig. 5.**89**; Furukawa et al. 1985)

To approach the third crus, a skin incision is placed posteriorly about 1 cm below, and parallel to, the helix, and the region of the third crus identified. Parallel scoring incisions are then placed at right angles across the crus to soften up the region for unfurling. After unfurling the crus, the incision is closed.

Kaplan and Hudson's Surgical Correction of a Third Crus and Satyr Ear

(Fig. 5.**90 a, b**; Kaplan and Hudson 1999

Kaplan and Hudson (1999) describe an incision in the scapha (Fig. 5.**90 a**), dissection of the skin inferiorly, and wedge-shaped excision of the crus together with the posterior skin (Fig. 5.**90 b**).

The classic techniques of otoplasty are frequently required in addition, in order to create the necessary fold of the ear (Nakajima et al. 1984).

Full-thickness Excision of the Crus

(See Fig. 5.**91 a–c**)

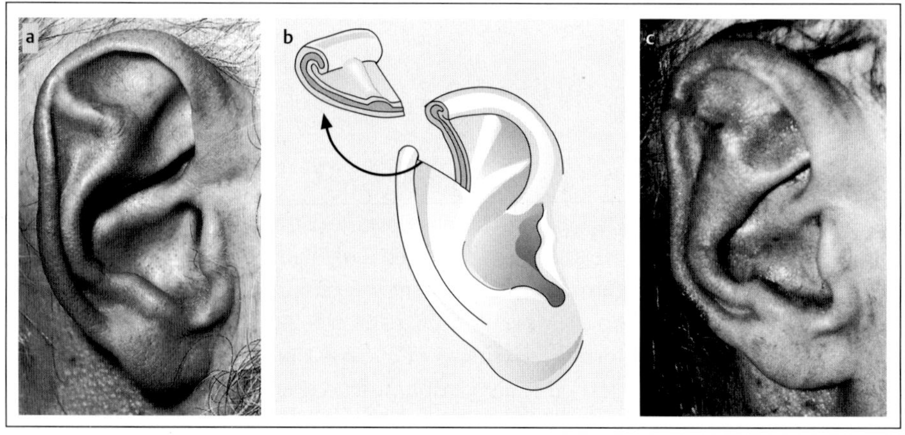

Fig. 5.**91** **Full-thickness excision of the third crus (see also Fig. 5.90).**

a Third crus in the presence of an inferior and superior antihelical crus.
b Skin incision over the crus and dissection. The third crus is excised and the cartilage and skin are sutured.
c Result (Surgeon: R. Siegert; see p. 53, Figs. 4.**25**, 4.**26**).

Satyr Ear

Synonyms: macaque-monkey ear (Marx 1926), Vulcan or Spock ear. (Fig 5.**92**; see Table 5.**2**, p. 118)

Definition. Hillock 4 and 4–5 deformities (Davis 1987; see p. 109).

Like Stahl's ear, the satyr ear has a protrusion and extension of the longitudinal axis with a narrowing of the upper region. The scapha is flattened, the helix bends over sharply or is dented (Davis 1987), occasionally the helix can also be adherent to the scapha. The transition to Stahl's ear is continuous, and there are combinations with conchal hyperplasia, mini-ear forms, or cryptotia (Davis 1987).

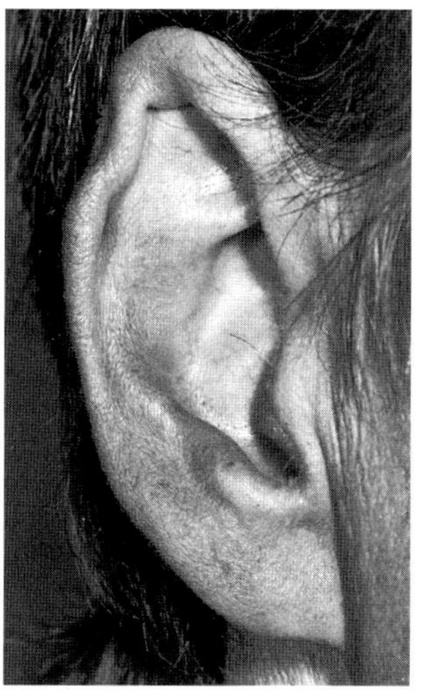

Fig. 5.**92** **Satyr ear.**

Operative Techniques

Fukuda's Method

(Fig. 5.**93**; cited in Davis 1987)

With the aid of a template, cartilage is excised from the concha of the ipsilateral side, inserted into the defect with the concave side showing anteriorly, and secured with 5–0 braided sutures (Fig. 5.**93 c**). The skin wound is closed with 6–0 monofilament suture material and the shape of the auricle formed with mattress sutures tied over cotton bolsters (Fig. 5.**93 d**). The skin defect can be eliminated by advancing the postauricular skin towards the initial defect in the form of a VY-plasty.

Davis's Method

(Fig. 5.**94**; Davis 1987)

Davis (1987) suggests undertaking surgery only in cases of obvious deformity. In mild cases he excises the cartilage overhang (Fig. 5.**94 a**). From an anterior incision, he molds the form of the scapha and helix using retained skin (Fig. 5.**94 b**). Where there is a lack of skin, a free full-thickness skin graft is excised from the sulcus using a template and sutured and glued (with fibrin glue) into the defect in the scapha. Here too, the result is secured with cotton bolsters tied over with transfixion sutures.

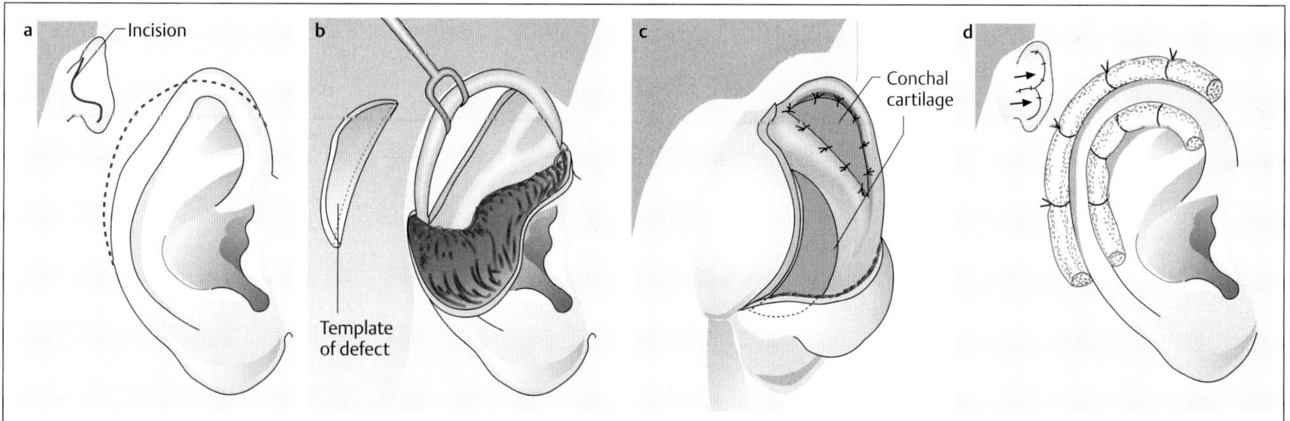

Fig. 5.**93** **Surgical repair of a satyr ear as described by Fukuda (1974, cited in Davis 1987).**

a Deficit in the upper helical region: template is made of the normal ear (see p. 64). Curved posterior incision.

b Dissection of the skin around the helix and anteriorly, incision of the cartilage in the scapha and fashioning of a defect template.

c Posterior view: conchal cartilage is harvested patterned on the defect template and sutured into the defect of the posterior surface to support the helix (5–0 braided polyglactic acid suture).

d The skin is redraped in the manner of a VY-advancement, skin suture and mattress sutures, knotted over bolsters.

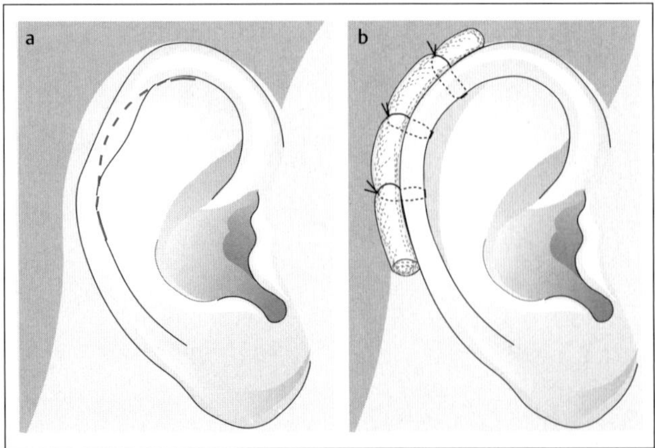

Fig. 5.**94** **Surgical repair of a satyr ear as described by Davis (1987).**
a Adhesions are released and surplus cartilage is resected.
b The scapha is formed using the surplus skin.

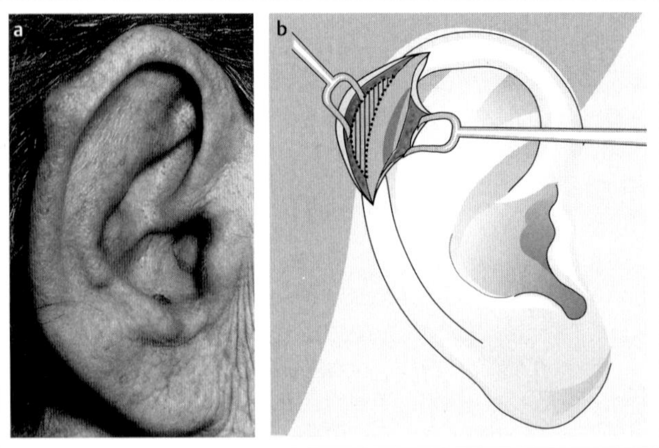

Fig. 5.**95** **Removal of a tubercle.**
a Tubercle.
b Removal via an incision in the scapha as described by Sénéchal and Pech (1970); resection of cartilage shown in red.

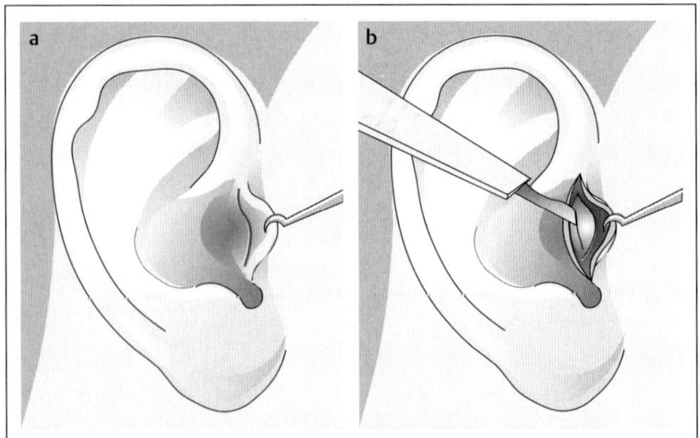

Fig. 5.**96 a, b** **Surgery for deformities of the tragus.**
Access to the tragus (see text; as described by Davis 1987).

Minor Deformities

For details see Table 5.**2**, p. 118.

Operative Techniques

Excision of a Very Pronounced Tubercle

Incision in the scapha, undermining of the skin, resection of the surplus cartilage, and suture in the scapha(Fig. 5.**95 a**, **b**).

The procedure for Darwin's tubercle is similar.

Absent Helical Crus

An absent helical crus is usually inconspicuous and does not require treatment. If necessary, reconstruction with a preauricular flap, pedicled superiorly on the helix, can be undertaken as suggested for tumor excision in this region (see Fig. 4.**20**, p. 51).

Hyperplasia of the Helical Crus

Incision beneath the hyperplastic crus, undermining of the skin in a posterosuperior direction, and excision of the surplus cartilage. The reduced cartilage of the crus can then be thinned out with a diamond burr, cooled with saline. The flap is redraped into place and trimmed off.

Tragus Deformities

The approach to the tragus in cases of hyperplasia and hypoplasia is from behind (Fig. 5.**96 a**). The skin over the tragus is undermined anteriorly and, in cases of hyperplasia, the cartilage is thinned out (Fig. 5.**96 b**; Davis 1987) and the skin redraped.

Augmentation and reconstruction are discussed under grade III dysplasia (see pp. 201 ff).

Antitragus Deformities

Revision or reduction of the antitragus. In cases of hyperplasia or eversion of the antitragus, we make an incision on the inner aspect of the antitragus (Fig. 5.**97 a**), dissect the skin over the antitragus towards the helical rim and fashion, shorten, or transpose the antitragus (Fig. 5.**97 b**). The skin is then trimmed and the wound closed with 7–0 monofilament suture material (Fig. 5.**97 c**).

Davis (1987) suggests a postauricular approach.

Lobular Deformities

Definition. Deformities of the earlobe (see Table 5.2, p. 118) result from malformations in the region of hillock 6 or hillocks 6 and 1 (Davis 1987; see pp. 110 ff).

The height of the earlobe is measured by placing a horizontal line through the fundus of the intertragic notch (width of earlobe), from which a perpendicular is dropped to the lowest point of the earlobe to give the height of the earlobe (Fig. 5.98).

Adherent Earlobe

Synonym: pixie earlobe.

Operative Techniques

Berson's Reconstruction of the Earlobe

(Fig. 5.99; Berson 1948; Rich et al. 1982)

Berson excises the surplus earlobe to achieve the desired lobular curve (Fig. 5.99 a). He mobilizes the skin and closes the defect in the region of the earlobe and its insertion (Fig. 5.99 b).

Weerda's Reconstructive Technique

(Fig. 5.100; Weerda 1982)

Incision on the cheek near the lobular insertion (Fig. 5.100 a) and excision of the posterior skin together with the fatty tissue (Fig. 5.100 b). Skin is excised from the new posterior surface of the earlobe, allowing for the curvature of the earlobe and the newly formed anterior flap, and the anterior flap of the adherent earlobe is turned over

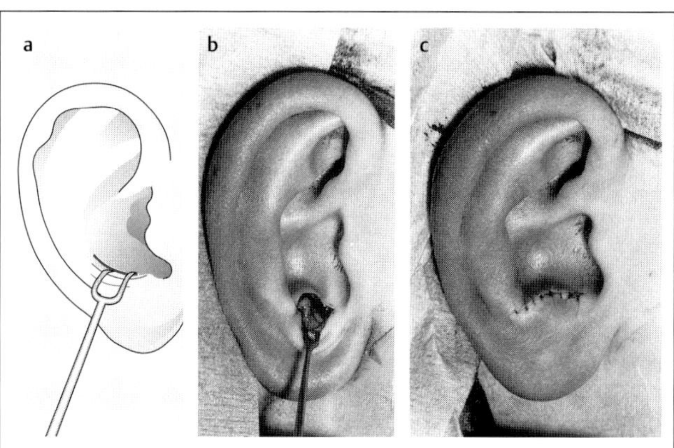

Fig. 5.**97 a–c** **Surgery of the antitragus (see text).** Reduction of the antitragus.

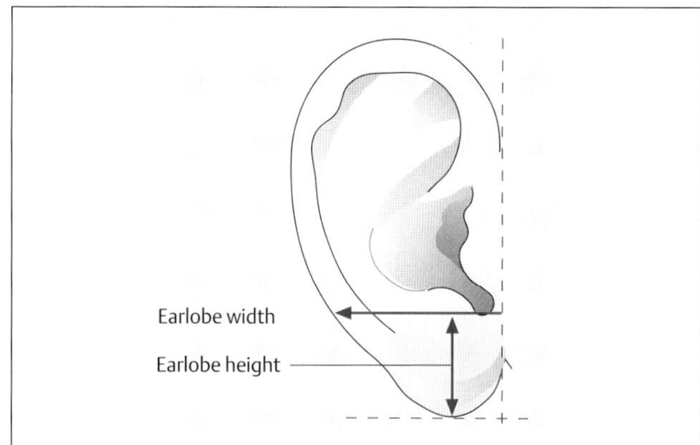

Fig. 5.**98** **Measuring the earlobe.**
Width: horizontal line through the fundus of the intertragic notch; height: vertical line down to the lowest point of the earlobe.

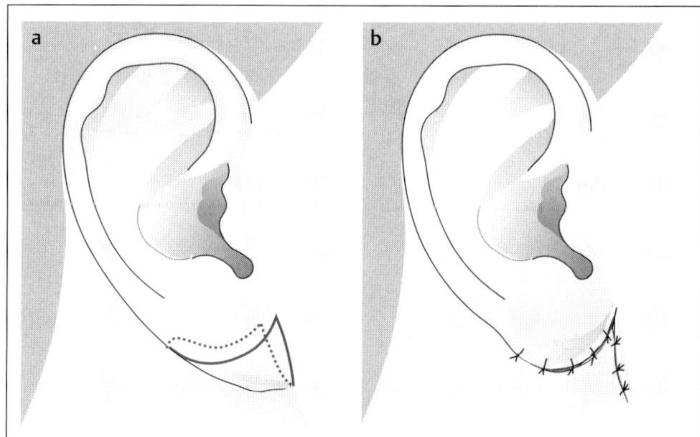

Fig. 5.**99** **Berson's operation for the adherent earlobe (Berson 1948; Rich et al. 1982).**

- **a** The desired curvature is outlined and surplus earlobe is resected.
- **b** Wounds are sutured.

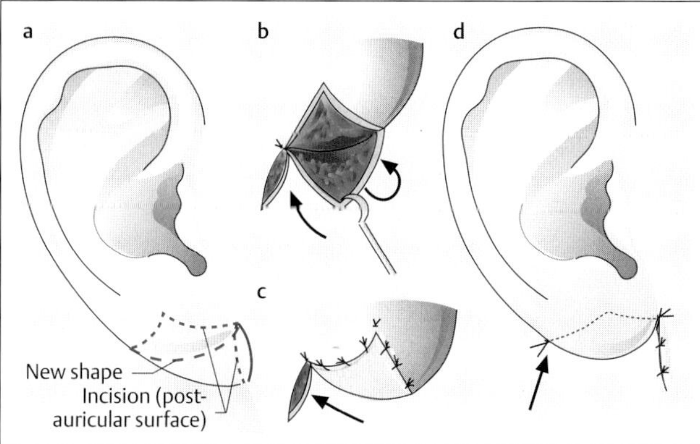

Fig. 5.**100** **Shaping the adherent earlobe (red line) as described by Weerda (1982).**

- **a** Incision of the earlobe on the cheek, V-shaped posterior incision (red dotted lines).
- **b** The earlobe is dissected, after which fat and surplus flap tissue are trimmed.
- **c** Closure of the posterior wound with the anterior skin flap. Closure of the cheek defect after posterior advancement of the skin.
- **d** Result.

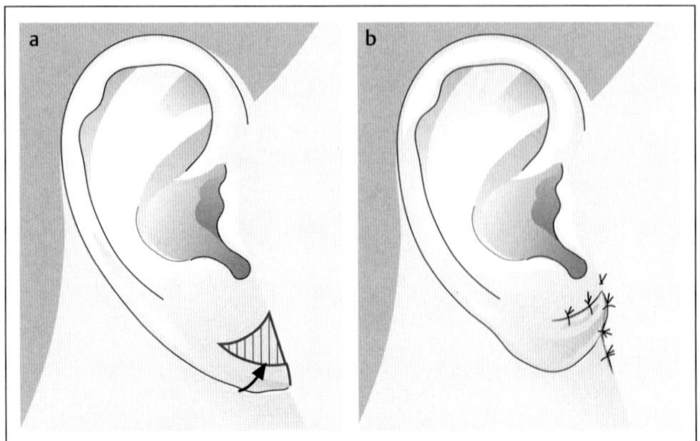

Fig. 5.**101** **Surgical repair of the adherent earlobe as described by Boo-Chai (1985).**
a Incision around the lower earlobe, full-thickness excision in the middle part of the earlobe.
b The lower earlobe is rotated upwards and the wounds closed.

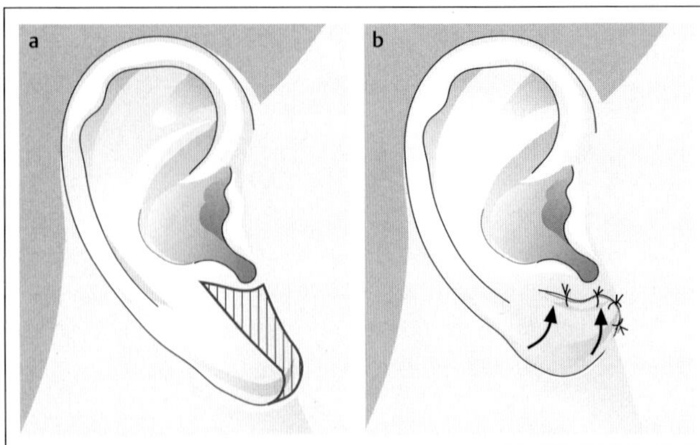

Fig. 5.**103** **Reduction of the earlobe as described by Jost et al. (1977 a).**
a Full-thickness resection.
b Suture.

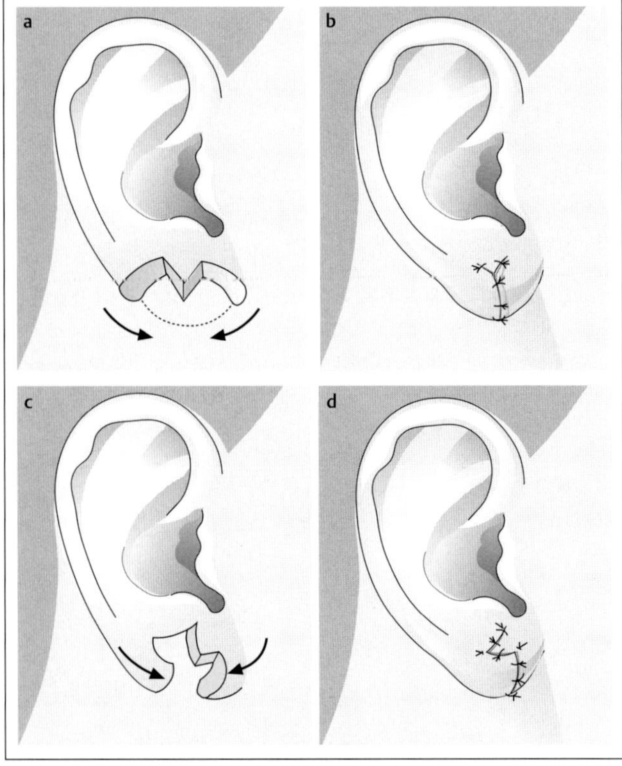

Fig. 5.**102 a–d** **Closure of defects of the earlobe (reduction of the enlarged earlobe; from Weerda 1999 a).**

posteriorly and sutured. The residual defect where the earlobe had inserted onto the cheek is then mobilized, transposed superiorly behind the earlobe and closed with fine monofilament suture material (Fig. 5.**100 c**). This technique allows the curvature of the earlobe to be better formed and the closure comes to lie posteriorly, behind the earlobe.

Boo-Chai's Operation

(Fig. 5.**101**; Boo-Chai 1985)

An incision is made around the insertion of the earlobe, a wedge excised from the middle of the earlobe, and an upper, full-thickness excision is made to produce the curvature of the earlobe (Fig. 5.**101 a**). The defects are closed with fine suture material (Fig. 5.**101 b**).

Macrolobule

Synonym: macro-earlobe, enlarged earlobe, hyperplastic earlobe.

Operative Methods

Senechal and Pech's Operation

(Fig. 5.**102**; Senechal and Pech 1970; Furnas 1974 b; Weerda 1999 a, 2001)

Jost et al.'s Reduction

(Fig. 5.**103**; Jost et al. 1977 a)

Where the macrolobule is a more oblong in form, the posterior crus of the earlobe can be reduced in addition to performing a wedge excision (Fig. 5.**103 a, b**).

Bethmann and Zoltan's Reduction of the Macrolobule at its Cheek Insertion After Face Lifting

(Fig. 5.**104**; Bethmann and Zoltan 1968)

This technique (Bethmann and Zoltan 1968) involves making a wedge-shaped excision with its base in the scar and extending it high up into the intertragic notch. To reduce the length of the earlobe, a wedge is cut from its posterior part (Fig. 5.**104 a, b**; McCollough and Hom 1989).

Weerda's Posterior Reduction

(Fig. 5.**105**; Weerda 2004)

In order to avoid producing a scar in the anterior part of the ear, a wing-shaped excision can be made on the posterior surface according to the desired degree of reduction (Fig. 5.**105 a**). The fat is carefully trimmed and the wounds closed (Fig. 5.**105 b**; Weerda 2004).

Berson's Surgical Correction of an Overly Wide Inferior Auricle and Earlobe

(Fig. 5.**106**; Berson 1948)

If the transition of the helix to the earlobe is too wide, a crescent-shaped excision is made in the scapha, similar to the Gersuny technique, and extended to the earlobe, which is then combined with an excision from the helix (Fig. 5.**106 a**). The wounds are closed with fine suture material (Fig. 5.**106 b, c**).

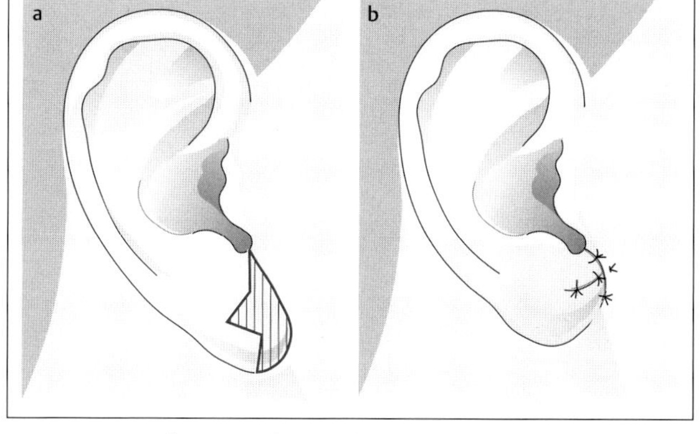

Fig. 5.**104** **Reduction after a facelift as described by Bethmann and Zoltan (1968).**
a Full-thickness excision reaching as far as the intertragic notch.
b Suture.

Cleft Earlobes

Yamada et al. (1976) and Fumiiri and Hyakusoku (1983) distinguish between three types of cleft formation, based on the involvement of mesenchymal hillocks 1 and 6:

- anterior form (Fig. 5.**107 a, b**)
- posterior form (Fig. 5.**107 c, d**)
- bifid earlobe or tag and cleft type (Fig. 5.**107 e, f**).

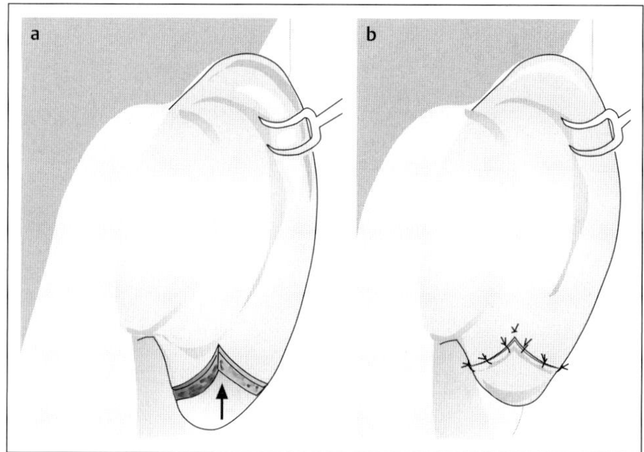

Fig. 5.**105** **Posterior reduction as described by Weerda (2004).**
a Two-layer, wing-shaped posterior excision; the anterior skin remains intact.
b Closure by advancing the skin.

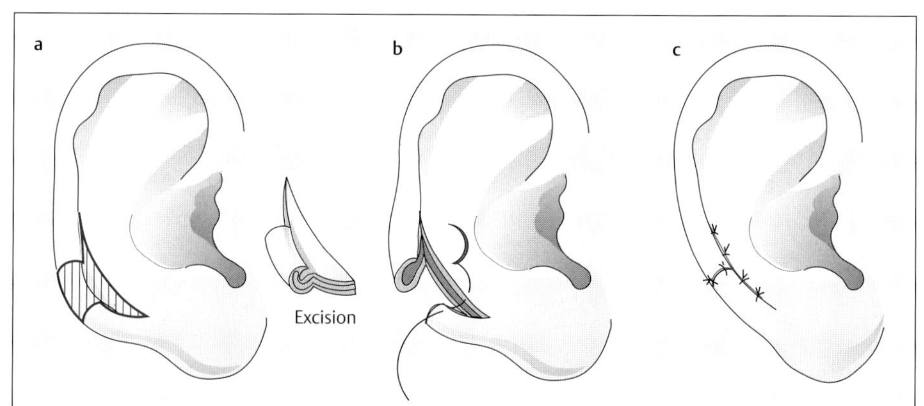

Fig. 5.**106** **Narrowing of the lower auricle as described by Berson (1948; see also Lexer 1933, Fig. 4.30).**
a Full-thickness excision.
b, c Suture.

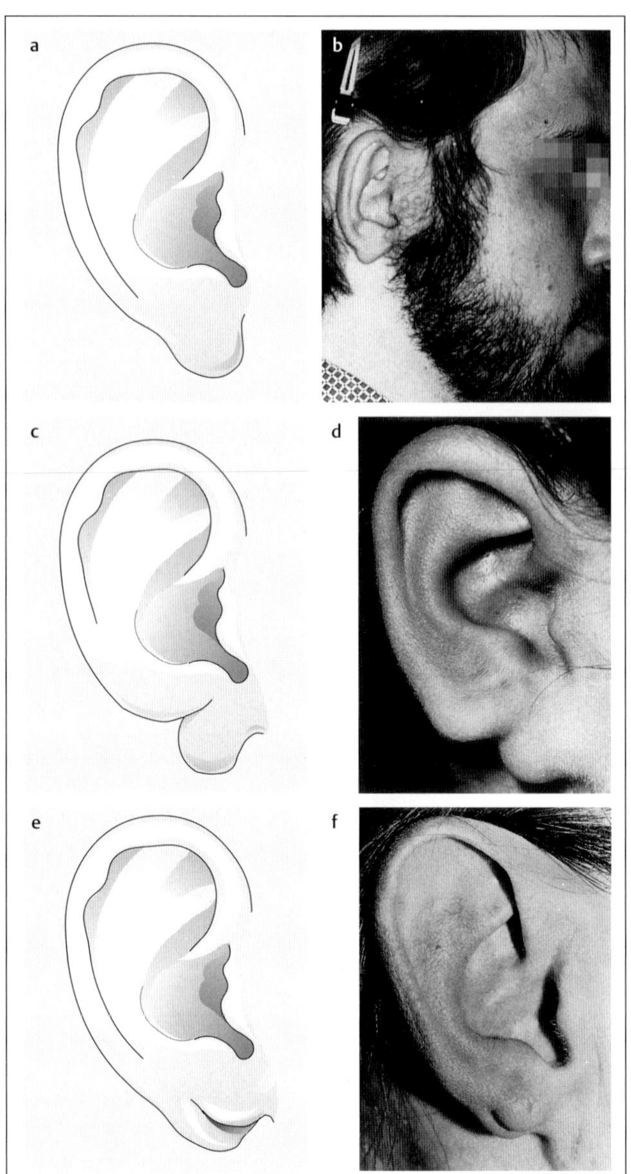

◁ Fig. 5.107 **Classification of cleft earlobe by Yamada et al. (1976) and Fumiiri and Hyakusoku (1983).**
a, b Anterior form.
c, d Posterior form.
e, f Tag and cleft (bifid) type.

Operative Methods for Anterior Cleft Earlobe

Davis's Method

(Fig. 5.**108**; Davis 1987)

Skin is excised at the auricular insertion, and the same is done in the region of the anterior earlobe (Fig. 5.**108 a**). If necessary, some fat may be excised. The earlobe is medialized and the wound closed with a full-thickness suture using fine material (Fig. 5.**108 b, c**).

Yotsuyanagi's Closure of the Anterior Cleft with a Chondrocutaneous Flap

(Fig 5.**109**; Yotsuyanagi 1994; s. Fig. 5.**107 a, b**)

Operative Method for Posterior Cleft Earlobe

Passow's Reconstructive Method

(Fig. 5.**110**; Mündnich 1962 a)

This dates from around 1920.

Operative Methods for the Bifid or Tag and Cleft Earlobe

Park and Roh's Method

(Fig. 5.**111**; Park and Roh 1997)

These authors advance the excess skin and thus fill out the cleft (Fig. 5.**111 a–c**).

Hohan et al.'s Reconstruction with a Preauricular, Inferiorly Based Flap

(Fig. 5.**112**; Hohan et al. 1978)

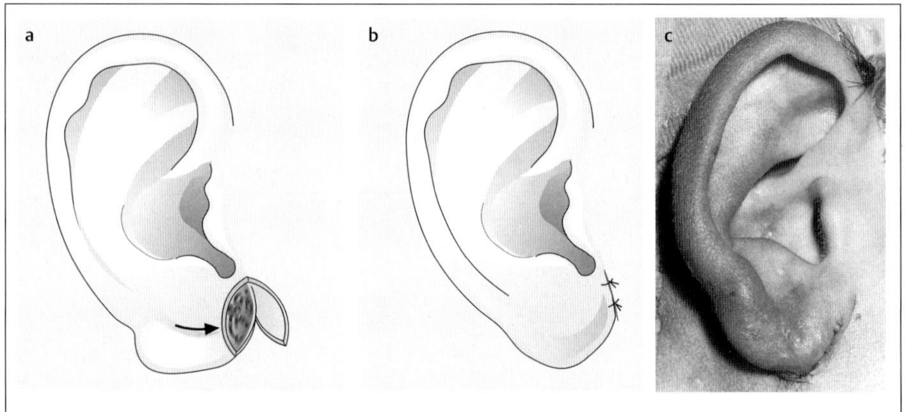

Fig. 5.**108** **Operative repair of the cleft earlobe (see Fig. 5.107 a) as described by Davis (1987).**
a Wedge-shaped symmetrical skin excision.
b Suture.
c Result (surgeon: Ms. S. Kaiber).

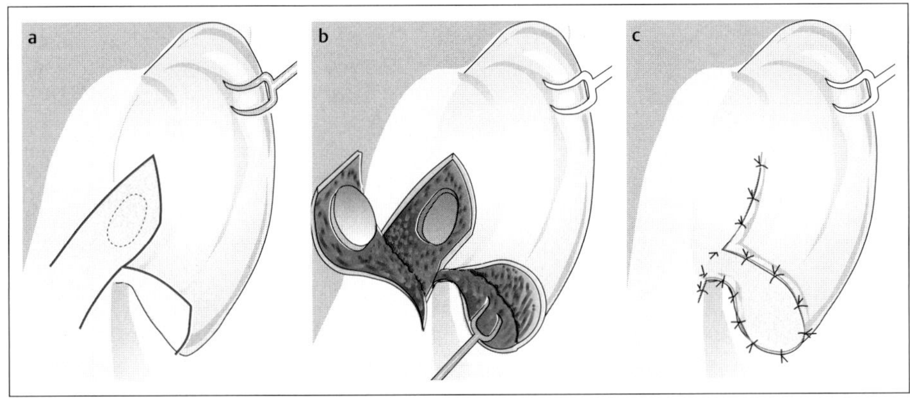

Fig. 5.**109** **Closure of the anterior cleft with a chondrocutaneous flap as described by Yotsuyanagi (1994; s. Fig. 5.107 a, b).**

a A hinge flap is incised on the posterior surface of the earlobe, with a corresponding incision on the cheek. The inferoposteriorly based chondrocutaneous flap is elevated (using a template).

b Dissection and suture of the hinge flap to be used as anterior earlobe skin.

c The chondrocutaneous flap is inset and the wounds closed.

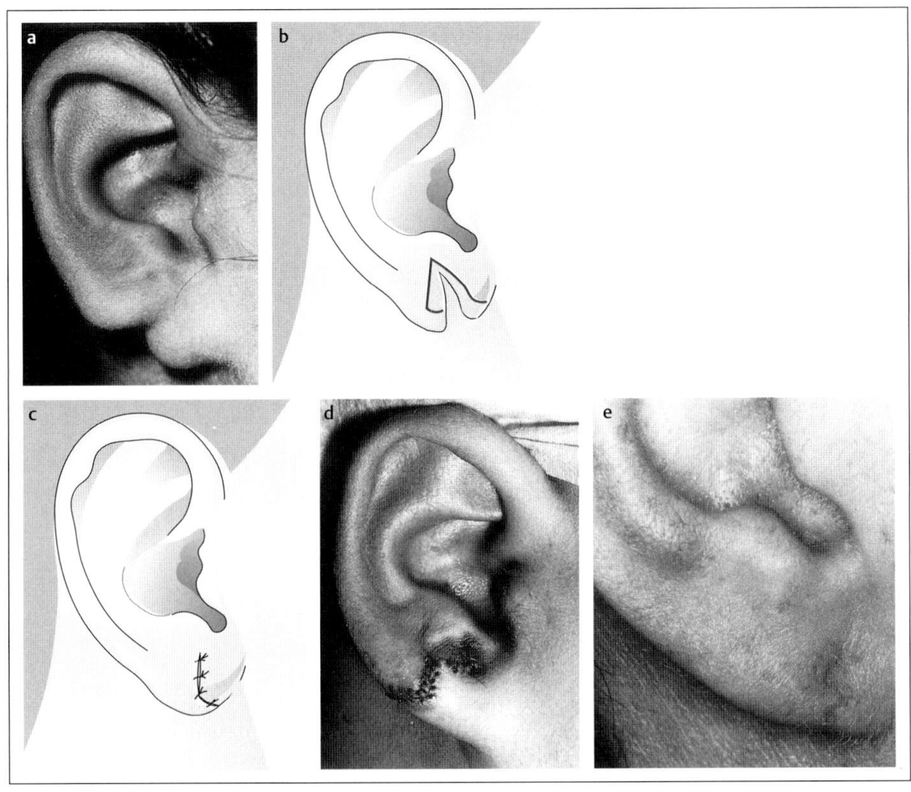

Fig. 5.**110** **Closure of the posterior cleft as described by Passow (cited in Mündnich 1962 a; s. Fig. 5.107 c, d).**

a Posterior cleft; see Fig. 5.**107 c**.

b Excision of the anterior portions.

c, d Closure.

e Result (surgeon: R. Siegert).

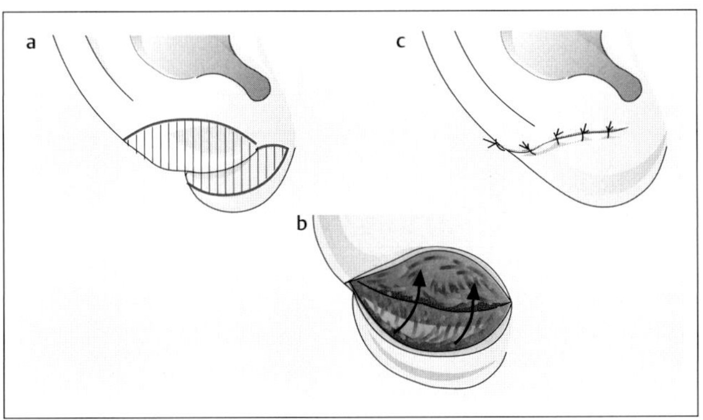

Fig. 5.**111** **Reconstruction of the bifid earlobe as described by Park and Roh (1997), modified (Fig. 5.107 e, f).**

a Excision of the anterior epithelium and preservation of the posterior skin.

b Dissection of the posterior skin (red).

c Anterior advancement of the posterior part of the earlobe onto the anterior part and two-layer suture.

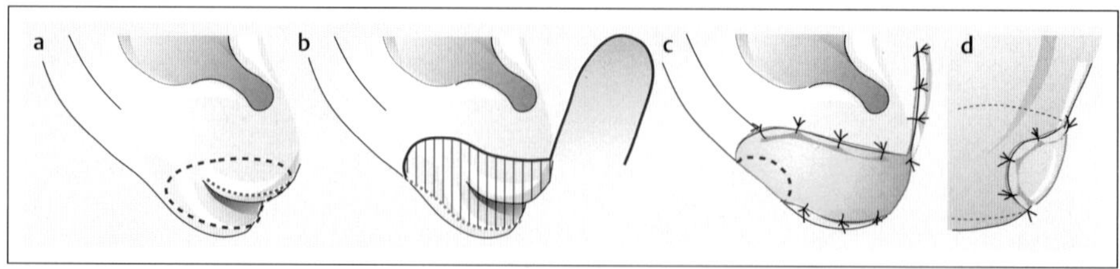

Fig. 5.**112** **Reconstruction of the bifid earlobe with a postauricular flap as described by Hohan et al. (1978; s. Fig. 5.107 e, f).**
a Incision around the anterior and posterior parts of the earlobe.
b Elevation of an inferiorly based preauricular flap according to a template.
c, d Coverage of the defect and filling of the defect (if necessary, the pedicle can be inset in a second stage).

Microlobule

Synonym: hypoplastic earlobe.

For suggestions on the reconstruction of hypoplasia and auricular defects, see pp. 80 ff.

Aplasia of the Earlobe

For suggestions on reconstruction, see avulsion of the earlobe, pp. 80 ff.

Table 5.**7** Cup-ear deformities, according to Tanzer (1975): synonyms

Type/group	Synonyms
I (Fig. 5.**113 a**)	Mild cup-ear deformities (Cosman 1974; Tanzer 1974 b, 1975; Weerda 1982 b) Mild lop ear deformities and mild lops (Davis 1987) Lidding helix, constricted helix (Tanzer 1974 b) Lid-like overhang, ptosis of the helix (Davis 1987) Folded-over helix, flopping over (Musgrave 1966) Snail ear (Mündnich 1962 a) Cat-ear (Marx 1926)
IIA (Fig. 5.**113 b**)	Mild-to-moderate cup-ear deformities (Tanzer 1974 b, 1975; Weerda 1989 b) Moderate cup-ear deformities (Cosman 1974) Minor cupping (Tanzer 1974 b) Moderate lop-ear deformities (Davis 1987)
IIB (Fig. 5.**113 c**)	Moderate-to-severe cup-ear deformities, severe lop-ear deformity (Davis 1987)
III (Fig. 5.**113 d**)	Severe cup-ear deformities (Tanzer 1974 d, 1975; Weerda 1989 b) Grade II dysplasia, grade II microtia (Tanzer 1974 d, 1975; Weerda 1985 a) Severe lop-ear deformities (Cosman 1974; Davis 1987) Folding ear (Marx 1926; Mündnich 1962 a) Concha-type microtia (Nagata 1994 b, d)

Cup-ear Deformities

Synonym: lop ear deformities.

Details of cup-ear deformities, as described by Tanzer, can be found in Tables 5.7, 5.**8** and Fig. 5.**113**; see also Table 5.2, p. 118.

Cause. These deformities represent a malformation of hillock 3 and, in the case of type III, hillocks 3–4 (Davis 1987; see p. 106). This form of hillock 3 deformity is occasionally associated with other hillock deformities (Davis 1987).

Fregenal et al. (1992) believe that cup ear is an autosomal dominant, inherited malformation with variable expression.

Classification. We prefer to adhere to the classification of the great innovator Tanzer. In 1975 he divided the deformities into three grades of severity, i. e., mild, moderate, and severe cup-ear deformities (Table 5.7):

- Type I (see Fig. 5.**113 a**)
- Type IIA and IIB (see Fig. 5.**113 b, c**)
- Type III (see Fig. 5.**113 d**)

Historical review. This group of malformations has been given a plethora of different names. In German-speaking countries, for instance, it is known as **cat ear** (Marx 1926, 1938; Altmann 1965; Mündnich and Tehrahe 1979).

Type IIB (Tanzer 1975) is referred to by Marx (1938) and also by Mündnich (1962 a) as **folded ear**. In the American literature these ears are known as **lop ears** (Erich 1963), a term which Rogers (1968, 1974) uses for all those malformations we call **cup-ear deformities**. Erich (1965) used the term "cup-shaped," while Tanzer (1974 d) speaks of a "constricted helix" and suggests the term "cup ear."

Davis (1974 b, 1987) is at pains to make various distinctions under the term lop ear, and speaks of **snail-shell ear** and **canoe ear**, as well as **border-line ears**. He also proposes classifying lop ears into: the mild form, which comprises Tanzer's "constricted" ear, group I; moderate lop ears which

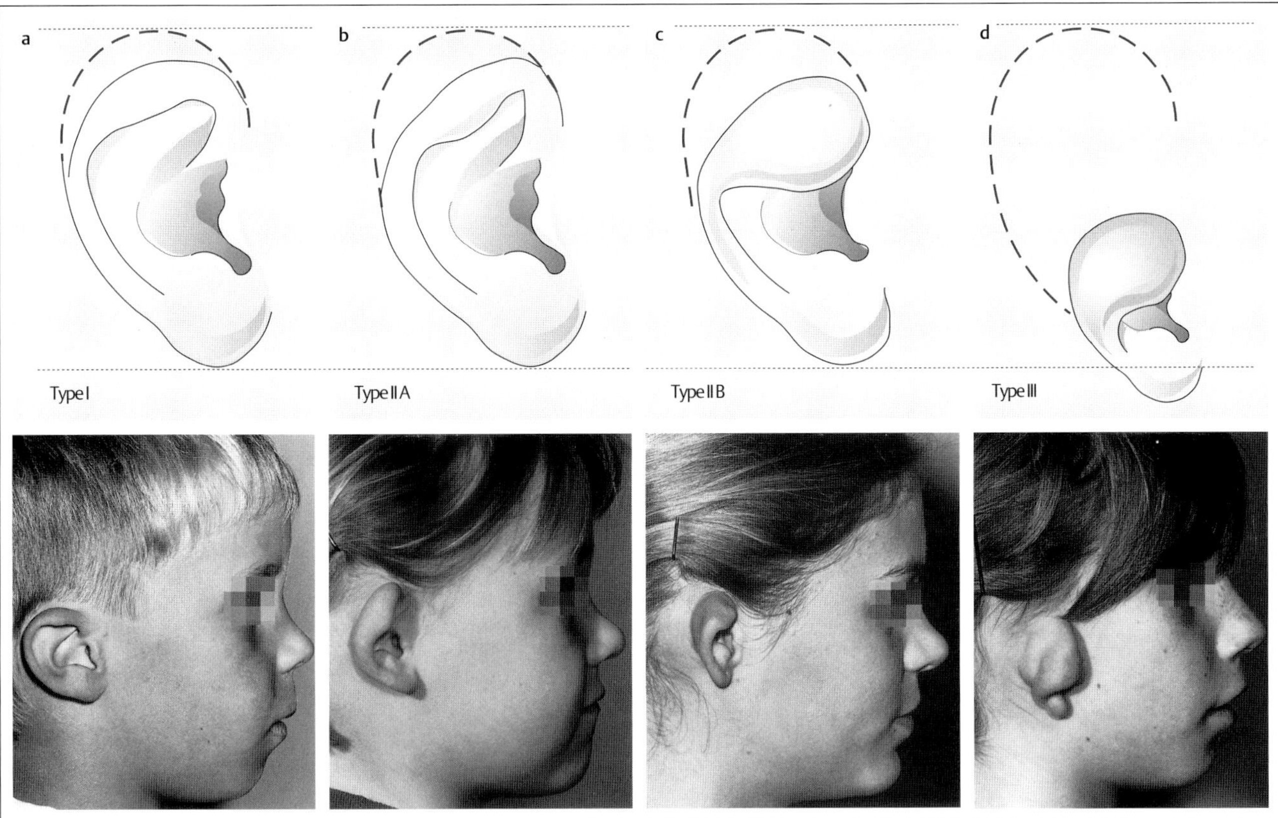

Fig. 5.**113** **Different types of cup-ear deformities (according to Tanzer 1975; see also Tables 5.6, 5.7).**

a **Type I:** Mild deformities: mild helix overhang, inferior crus usually present, long axis slightly shortened.
Therapy: Reconstruction by otoplasty: Mustardé or Weerda technique (see pp. 173–175; Figs. 5.**114**–5.**116**).

b **Type IIA:** Mild to moderate deformities: more pronounced helix overhang, crura usually not present, long axis more shortened.
Therapy: Reconstruction by otoplasty (Figs. 5.**114**–5.**117**).

c **Type IIB:** Moderate to severe deformities: even more pronounced helix overhang, antihelical crura missing, large deficits in long and transverse axes.
Therapy: Reconstruction with various incisions and flaps, if necessary cartilage replacement (Figs. 5.**119**–5.**131**).

d **Type III:** Severe deformity with microtia, severe cupping and dystopia.
Therapy: Total reconstruction (see Figs. 5.**132**–5.**139** and pp. 183–197)

consist of Tanzer's moderate "constricted" ears, group IIA; and severe lop ears or Tanzer's "constricted" ear, group IIB.

Mündnich (1962 a) speaks of **snail ear** and regards Tanzer's type IIB and type III as severe forms. He uses a similar classification as Tanzer.

Cosman (1974), like Tanzer (1975), describes various grades of severity for cup-ear deformities. He suggests using this term on account of the different surgical operations, and disregards embryonic development.

Classification (see Fig. 5.**113**, Tables 5.**7**, 5.**8**). Table 5.**8** shows the classification of cup-ear deformities according to Tanzer (1975; Weerda 1994e). It is apparent that the severity of the malformation increases from type I through type III, and this is associated with an increase in the surgical time and effort required for reconstruction. Variation is great, even within the individual types. Mixed forms with other deformities are encountered, depending on the number of involved mesenchymal hillocks of the first and second branchial arch (Cosman 1974; Davis 1987). In particular, additional alterations are seen in the tragus–antitragus and lobular regions (Davis 1987).

Type I Cup-ear Deformity

Synonyms: see Tables 5.**7**, 5.**8** and Fig. 5.**113 a**.

Definition. Tanzer (1977) describes this as a malformation where helix and scapha overhang like a lid, and antihelix and crura are flattened to varying degrees. One has the impression that the rim of the helix is constricted.

Only the helix is involved in this mild deformity of the upper auricle (lop ear), as it hangs down relatively wide over the scapha (lidding) where it is sometimes affixed.

Table 5.8 Cup-ear deformities (Tanzer 1974 d, 1975, modified; Weerda 1985 a, 1991 b, 2004): description and interventions

Description	Operation
Type I: mild deformity (see Fig. 5.113 a)	
Mild overhang Antihelix and helix present Reduction in auricular height Frequently associated with prominent auricle	1. Excision of the overhang and/or 2. Expansion by otoplasty (Black 1971; Weerda 1979 a, 1982 b)
Type IIA: mild-to-moderate deformity (see Fig. 5.113 b)	
More severe overhang Helix and scapha are often associated with prominent auricle Reduction in auricular height plus: flattened helical crus, absent superior antihelical crus, prominent inferior crus	Surgical correction without addition of skin: 1. Expansion of the auricle 2. Elongation of the helix, if necessary 3. Otoplasty (Musgrave 1966; Tanzer 1975; Moore 1977; Millard et al. 1988; Brent 1975; Ono et al. 1993; Weerda 1982 b, 2004)
Type IIB: moderate-to-severe deformity (see Fig. 5.113 c)	
Upper auricle is affected Upper auricle overhangs the middle auricle Antihelical crura absent Greater reductions in auricular height and upper auricular width Prominent auricle	Surgical correction with addition of skin (possibly also of cartilage): 1. Reconstruction with elongation of the helix, cartilaginous deficit, often too soft, additional skin deficit, skin and cartilage 2. Otoplasty (Alexander 1926, cited in Marx 1926; Tanzer 1974 a; Weerda 1979 a, 1982 a; Barsky 1950, cited in Mündnich 1962 a; Luckett 1963, cited in Cosman 1974; Stenström 1968; Senechal and Pech 1970; Tanzer 1975; Davis 1987; Mavili 1996; Horlock et al. 1998)
Type III: severe deformity (grade II dysplasia) (see Fig. 5.113 d)	
Microtia with extreme cupping; reduction in height and width of the entire auricle dystopia, occasionally low hairline, occasional congenital atresia of the external auditory canal	Surgical correction: total reconstruction with skin and costal cartilage: ipsilateral or contralateral side (Brent 1974, 1980, 1981; Nagata 1994 a–d ; Weerda 1982 a, 1989 b, 2004)

The cartilage is soft, the auricle is shortened in its longitudinal axis, and there is reduction in height of the upper third, while the remaining parts of the auricle are usually normal in their development. Of all anomalies of the ear, 10% are cup-ear deformities, and 2% of cup-ear deformities are type I (Cosman 1974).

A characteristic of type I is that only the helix is deformed.

Operative Techniques

Resection of the Overhang

(Fig. 5.**114**)

If the height of the ear is acceptable and there is no more than a 3 mm difference between the height of the healthy ear (template) and the height of the malformed ear, then resection of the overhang to achieve a normalization in helical width is acceptable (Fig. 5.**114 a–d**).

Weerda's Expansion of Type I Cup-ear Deformity

(Fig. 5.**115**; Weerda 1979 a, 1982 b)

Preparation for the operation. Photographic documentation, fashioning of a template of the normal ear or, in cases of bilateral cup-ear deformity, to the desired height. The possibility of expanding the auricle with simple setback otoplasty is tested by raising the overhanging part of the ear over the antihelix with a double skin hook (Fig. 5.**115 b**).

The degree of remaining prominence of the ear is registered by measuring the distance between helix and mastoid (Fig. 5.**115 c**).

The auricle and the overhanging helix are expanded (Fig. 5.**115 d**) by using Mustardé's technique or one of our modified setback otoplasties, via a posterior incision (see p. 140, Fig. 5.**52**; Fig. 5.**115 d**).

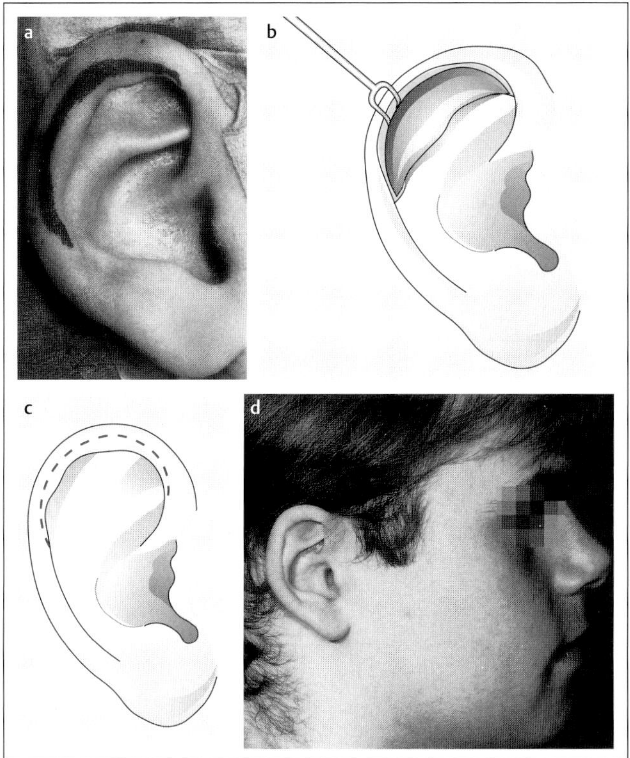

Fig. 5.**114** **Excision of the overhang (superior antihelical crus is present).**
a The line for excision is marked.
b The overhang is lifted and the underside of the helix is incised, dissection is continued around the cartilage to the anterior surface and the cartilage resected.
c The skin is adapted and sutured (broken red line).
d Result.

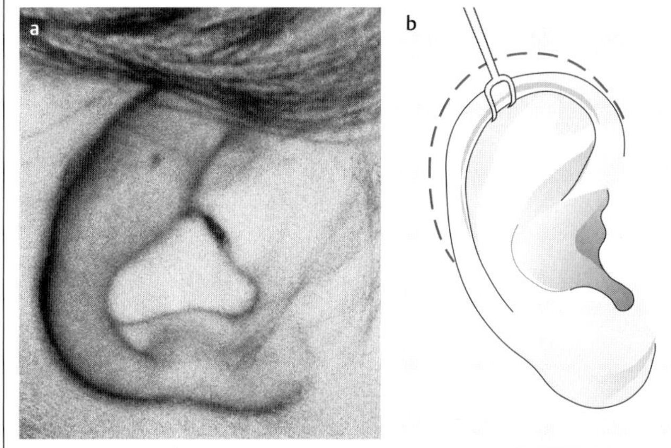

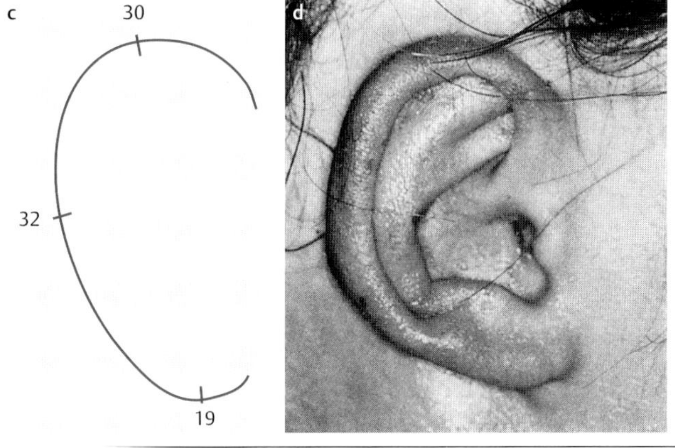

Fig. 5.**115** **Surgical correction of type I cup-ear deformity (absent superior antihelical crus).**
a Type I cup-ear deformity and prominent ear.
b The auricle is displaced upward using a double skin hook (normal size: broken red line).
c The distance from the upper helical margin to the mastoid is measured.
d Appearance after expanding the auricle using the otoplasty technique described by Weerda (1979 a; see p. 140). Residual shortening of the longitudinal axis and slight reduction in the height of the upper part of the ear.

Black's Expansion of the Overhang
(modified, Fig. 5.**116**; Black 1971)

Approach from posterior is possible (see Figs. 5.**119 c**, 5.**123 b**).

Type II Cup-ear Deformities
Synonyms: group IIA and IIB cup-ear deformities (Tanzer 1975), moderate cup-ear deformity (Cosman 1974), moderate lop ear deformity (Davis 1987).

Group II (type IIA and type IIB according to Tanzer 1975; see Fig. 5.**113 b**, **c**, Tables 5.**7**, 5.**8**; Weerda 1985 a, 1988 a, 1994 c, 1997 a) includes a considerable variation of cup-ear deformities. Apart from the more pronounced overhang of the upper auricle, we see a flattening of the superior crus which can be either incomplete or absent. The helical margin forms a hood over the concha. A reduction of the longitudinal axis is noticeable when the auricle is expanded, and we also frequently find a narrowing in the region of the upper auricle as well as auricular prominence (see Fig. 5.**117**).

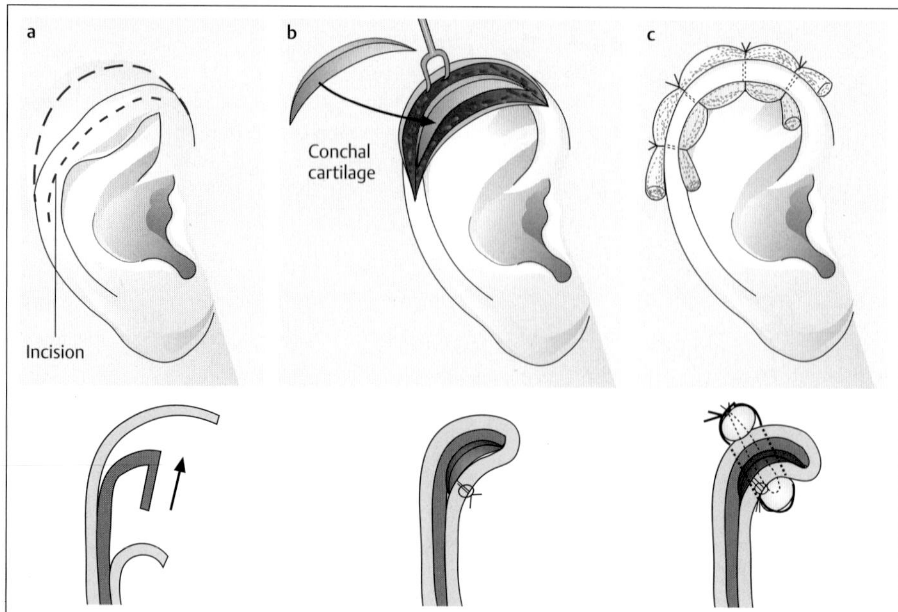

Fig. 5.**116** **Surgical expansion of type I cup-ear deformity using conchal cartilage as described by Black (1971), modified.**

a The height is marked according to a template (broken line), the scapha is incised and the skin dissected.

b The cartilage of the overhang, which is usually very thin, is dissected off and supported (if necessary excised), and/or expansion of the upper auricle with the aid of conchal cartilage from the ipsilateral or contralateral ear.

c The skin is sutured and the result secured with mattress sutures tied over cotton bolsters.

Definition. Mild deformity of helix and scapha with increasing hood-like overhang, insufficient cartilage with usually adequate skin in type IIA and skin deficit in type IIB, associated with a prominent auricle. The depth of the concha is increased. Increase in the underdevelopment of antihelix and crura. This malformation can occur both unilaterally and bilaterally. It is characteristic of type II that both helix and scapha are deformed (see Fig. 5.**113 b, c**).

Operative planning. As with type I malformation, a template is first fashioned (see pp. 64, 202, 203, Fig. 5.**119 h**). As a rule, with type IIB an improvement in form is not possible without expansion of the helix.

Type IIA Cup-ear Deformity

In the case of this deformity, in contrast to type I, helix and antihelix as well as superior crus are involved (see Fig. 5.**113 b** and Tables 5.**7**, 5.**8**). The auricle is prominent. Skin defects are rare.

Operative Techniques

The imprecise definition of type IIA does not always allow the operative methods described below to be assigned exactly to the different types.

Preparation. Fashioning of a template, expansion of the auricle with a double skin hook, or a similar instrument (see Fig. 5.**115 b**), and measurement of the helix-to-mastoid distance for each ear (see Fig. 5.**29**, p. 120).

Weerda's Method

(Fig. 5.**117**; Weerda 1979 a, 1982 b, 1984 a)

As previously described for type I (see Fig. 5.**115**), the auricle with a mild deformity can be expanded using Mustardé's otoplasty technique (see Fig. 5.**40**, p. 132) or Weerda's method (Weerda 1979 a, 1984 a; see Fig. 5.**52**, p. 140). The absent superior antihelical crus is also restored by these methods (Fig. 5.**117 a, b**).

Ono et al.'s Expansion of the Upper Auricle

(Fig. 5.**118**; Ono et al 1993)

An incision for setback otoplasty is placed on the postauricular surface, parallel to the helix. The incisions correspond to those for Converse's otoplasty (see Fig. 5.**45**). A new antihelix is created by suturing the scapha to the concha. Next, a strip of cartilage is excised via an anterior incision (Fig. 5.**118 a**) and this piece of cartilage is spliced to the posterior surface of the cartilage to expand the overhang (Fig. 5.**118 b–d**). The skin incisions are then closed. Ono et al. (1993) demonstrate good results with their four examples. Elsahy (1990) inserts an anterior cartilaginous strut.

Type IIB Cup-ear Deformity

Helix and scapha are deformed, there is shortening of the helical dome (constriction) and an obvious shortage of skin when the helix is expanded. There is a further increase in the hood-like overhang, and usually a shortening of the longitudinal axis and a narrowing in width of the ear. Antihelix and crura are flattened or absent (see Fig. 5.**119 a, b**). The addition of skin is generally required. See Fig. 5.**113 c**, p. 171 and Tables 5.**7**, 5.**8** for further details of these deformities.

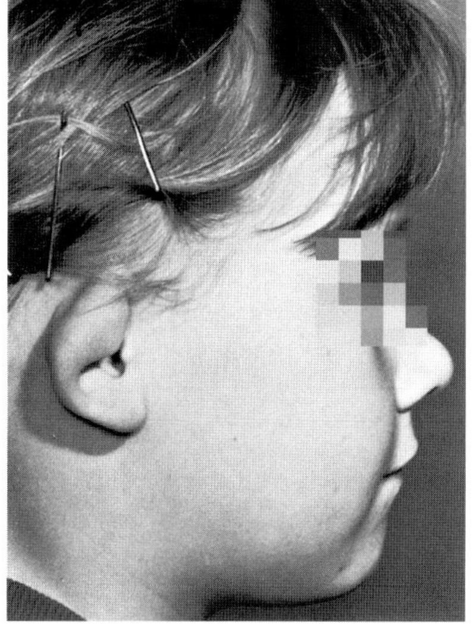

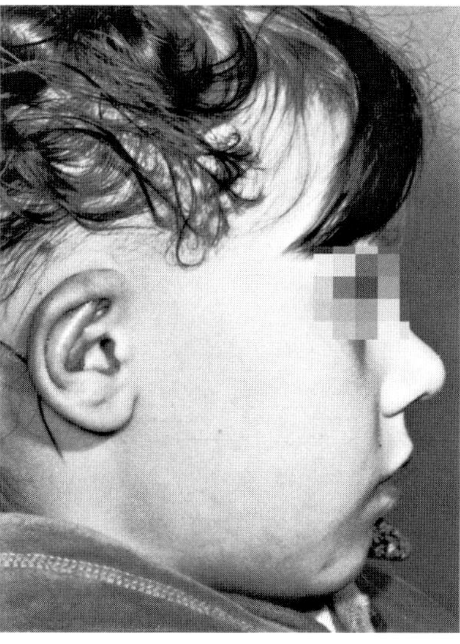

Fig. 5.**117** **Weerda's operation (1982 b).**
a Tanzer's type IIA cup-ear deformity (Tanzer 1975).
b Appearance after otoplasty with expansion of the auricle as described by Weerda (1979; see Fig. 5.**52**, p. 140). Obvious shortening of the longitudinal axis (more than in type I, Fig. 5.**115 d**).

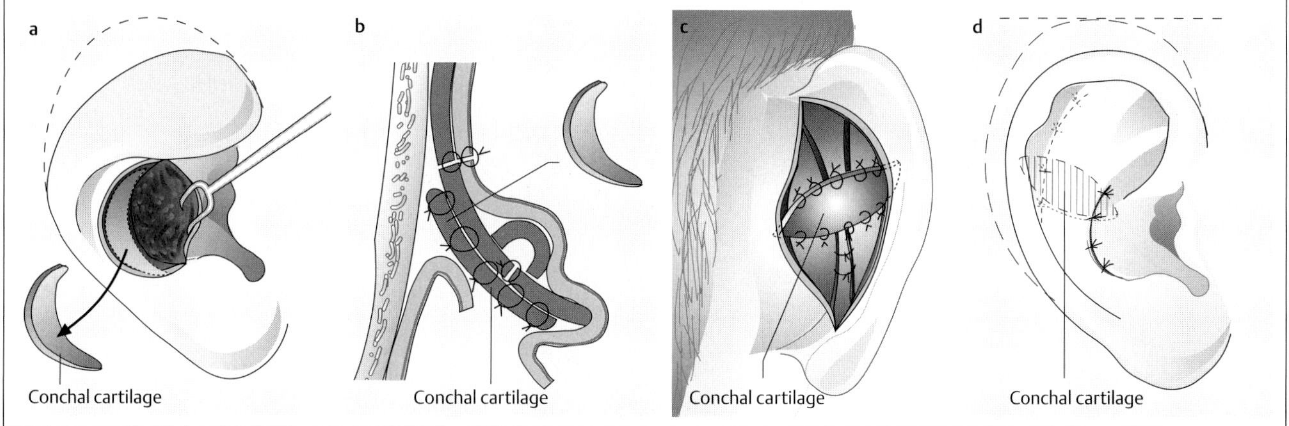

Fig. 5.**118** **Correction of cup-ear deformity (type IIA) as described by Ono et al. (1993).**
a Anterior incision beneath the helix and removal of an approximately 23 mm × 10 mm segment of cartilage from the concha.
b–d Reconstruction of the antihelix and posterior fixation of the cartilage with sutures for support, closure of the incisions.

Operative Techniques—Posterior Approach

The inadequate amount of skin on the too narrow helical dome must be compensated for when the ear is expanded. Expansion of the cartilaginous overhang and any necessary stabilization of the new helical dome are achieved by supporting the upper part of the auricle with additional cartilage.

VY-Advancement of the Helical Crus, Plus Otoplasty

(Fig. 5.**119**; Holmes 1949, Barsky 1950 and Stenström 1968)

Expanding the auricle produces a deficit in the region of the anterior helix which can be compensated for by a VY-advancement of the helical crus (McCoy 1972; Davis 1974 b; Fig. 5.**119 d, g**). The method provides good results and can therefore be recommended (Fig. 5.**119 j**).

Stenström (1968) dissects the antihelical region via an anterior incision using his otoplasty technique, which was published in 1963. He raises the skin and scores the anterior surface of the antihelix (see Fig. 5.**43**, p. 134). This technique of antihelix reconstruction can also be performed using a posterior approach (Millard et al. 1988).

Modification of Barsky's Technique

(Fig. 5.**120**; Dufourmentel and Mouly 1959, Converse and Brent 1977)

Instead of an incision around the helix, a preauricular flap is raised (Fig. 5.**120 a, b**).

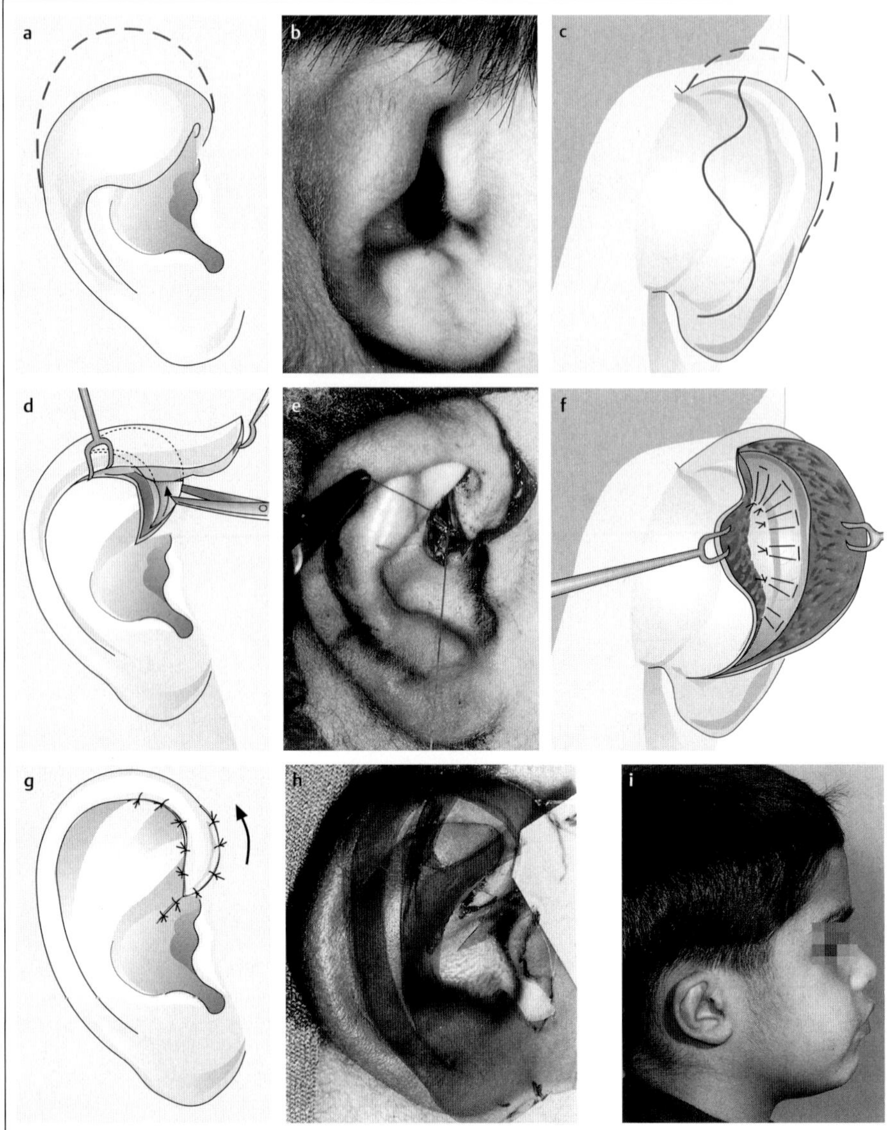

Fig. 5.**119** **VY-advancement of the helical crus for type IIB cup-ear deformity as described by Holmes (1949), Barsky (1950), and others.**

a, b Type IIB cup-ear deformity. The height of the normal ear is marked according to a template (broken red line).
c Posterior incision.
d, e Incision around the helical crus and VY-advancement superiorly.
f Expansion of the ear by otoplasty.
g, h The helical crus is sutured into its new position and the result secured with mattress sutures tied over cotton bolsters (skin closure see Fig. 5.**128 e**).
i Outcome (see **b**).

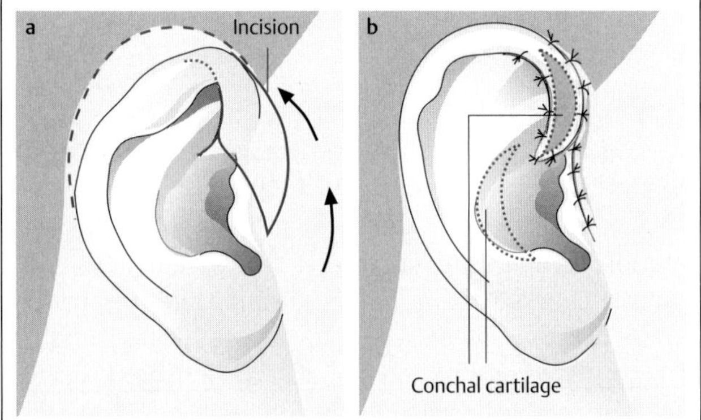

Fig. 5.**120** **Modification of Barsky's method (Holmes 1949; see Fig. 5.119) and the method of Dufourmentel and Mouly (1959) from Converse and Brent (1977).**

a Incision around the ascending helix, raising of a preauricular flap and expansion from a posterior approach by otoplasty.
b VY advancement. The anterior helix can be augmented by a cartilaginous strut harvested posteriorly from the concha (red).

Davis's Transposition of the Helical Crus

(Fig. 5.**121 a–c**; Davis 1987)

The auricle is expanded by otoplasty and the form of the antihelix is developed. If a Z-plasty does not suffice to raise the height of the antihelix, or the cartilage does not provide enough support, an additional strip of cartilage harvested from the concha can be used to reinforce the scapha (Fig. 5.**121 c**). The interlacing cartilaginous flaps are secured with 5–0 braided sutures.

Alexander's Method

(Fig. 5.**122**; Alexander 1919)

The skin is dissected off via a posterior incision (see Fig. 5.**119 c**) and the overhang is resected (Fig. 5.**122 a**), the cartilage is trimmed straight, rotated through 180° and resutured to the cartilage stump to expand the auricle (Fig. 5.**122 b**). Afterwards, the skin is redraped over the now expanded helix (Fig. 5.**122 c**).

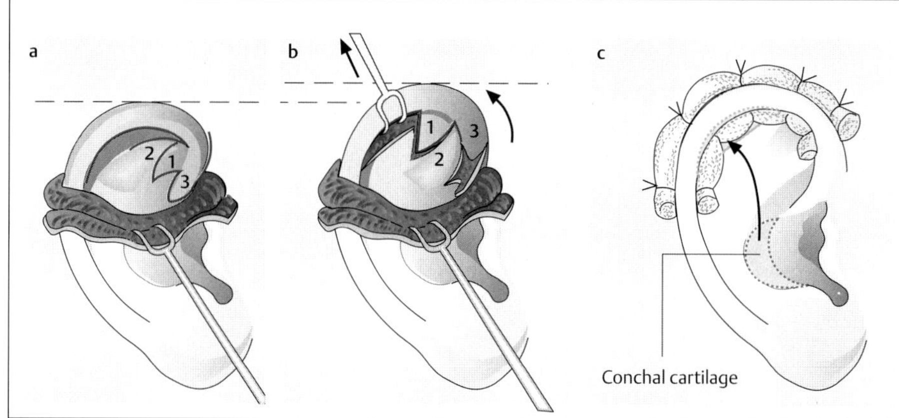

Fig. 5.**121** **Transposition of the helical crus as described by Davis (1987), modified.**

a Posterior incision and dissection of the skin off the helical crus in an anterior direction. Incision around the crus (3), together with a cartilage flap (1) superior to it, followed by incision of the superior antihelical crus (2).

b Otoplasty is performed to expand the auricle, and the cartilage is advanced superiorly (3, 1), with a Z-plasty performed to transpose the superior antihelical crus inferiorly (2).

c Suture and knotting of mattress sutures over cotton bolsters. In addition, conchal cartilage, harvested from a posterior approach, can be used to support the upper auricle. (Not to be recommended).

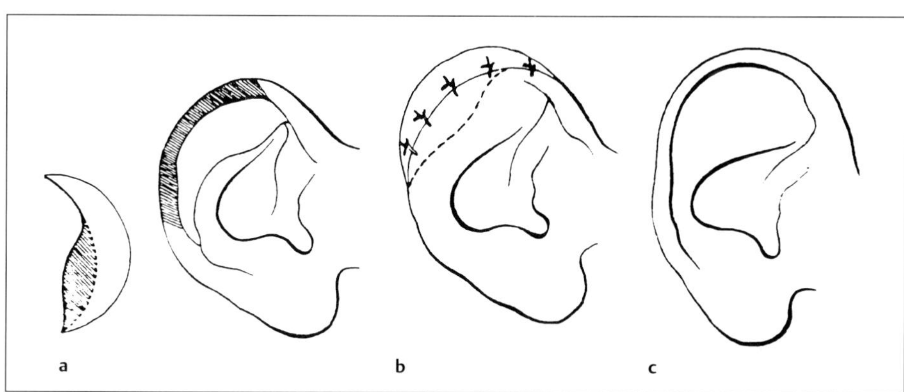

Fig. 5.**122** **Correction of the "cat ear" as described by Alexander (1919; type IIB cup-ear deformity; from Marx 1926; see Fig. 5.123)**

a Excision of the overhang after posterior incision and dissection of the skin off the helix and scapha in an anterior direction (see Fig. 5.**121 a**, Fig. 5.**123 c–e**).

b The overhang is trimmed straight, rotated through 180°, and sutured to the scapha.

c The skin envelope is redraped into position (see Fig. 5.**123**).

This technique, described by Alexander (1919), was later rediscovered by Tanzer (1974 d; see Fig. 5.**124**).

Marx (1926) writes that these operations are only suitable for milder "cat ears."

Modification of Alexander's Method

(Fig. 5.**123**; Weerda 1979 a, 1982 b, 1991 c, 1997 a)

This is a modification of Alexander's method (1919), with expansion of the scapha and Weerda's otoplasty technique.

After placing a curvilinear incision on the postauricular surface (see Fig. 5.**128 a**), we dissect the skin off the auricle in an anterior direction and excise the overhang (Fig. 5.**123 b**, **c**). The auricle is formed using our otoplasty technique (see p. 140, Fig. 5.**52**), the prominent ear is set back and, if necessary, the concha is also set back (see p. 137).

This procedure expands the residual scapha (Fig. 5.**123 c**). The previously dissected piece of cartilage is rotated through 180° and sutured to the new scapha (Fig. 5.**123 c**, **d**, **e**, arrow). The skin is then redraped into position, if necessary advanced superiorly on its postauricular surface with the aid of a VY-plasty (see Fig. 5.**128 e**) to gain as much skin as required. After suturing, the auricle is supported for 1 week by mattress sutures tied over cotton bolsters (Fig. 5.**123 f**).

The purpose of rotating the cartilage overhang through 180° is to retain a small helical margin to support the new helix. Tanzer (1974 d) regretted that, with his technique, the helix consisted only of duplicated skin.

Should the cartilage be too soft, or the new auricle not of sufficient height, then we use cartilage harvested from the concha of the ipsilateral or contralateral ear, or even costal cartilage, to expand and support the auricle (Fig. 5.**123 h**; Weerda 1982 b).

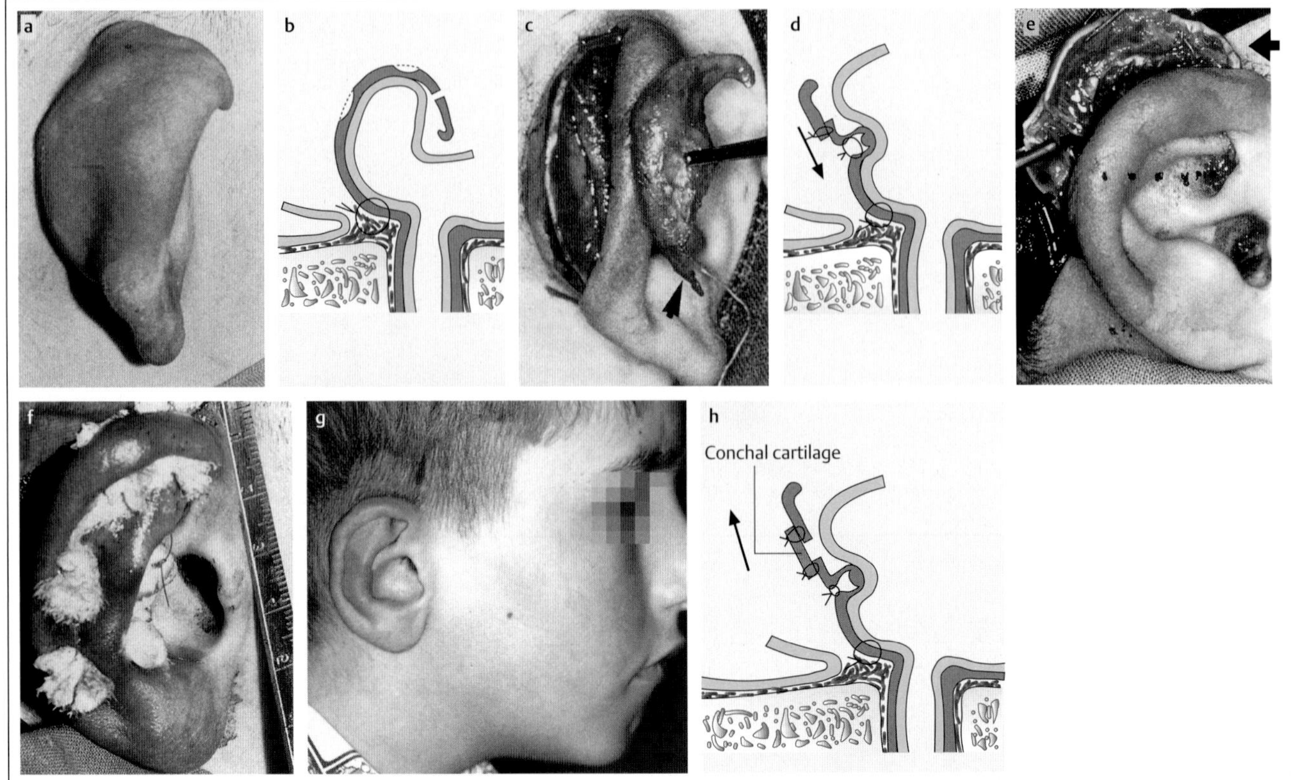

Fig. 5.**123** **Alexander's extended method (Alexander 1919) with expansion of the auricle as described by Weerda (1979 a, type IIB).**

a Type IIB cup-ear deformity.

b, c Posterior incision and dissection of the skin in an anterior direction. Excision of the helical overhang (**c**, arrow). Otoplasty as described by Weerda (see p. 140; additional conchal setback).

d, e Rotation of the overhang through 180°, with the round contour providing the helix (**e**, arrow; see **c**, arrow).

f The skin envelope is returned to its original position and supported with mattress sutures tied over cotton bolsters.

g Outcome.

h Costal or conchal cartilage can be interposed if the cartilage is too soft or there is reduced auricular height.

Tanzer's Banner Flap

(Fig. 5.**124**; Tanzer 1974 d, 1975)

This is a modification of Alexander's method for type IIB cup-ear deformity (Fig. 5.**124 a–j**). Tanzer, like Alexander, also recommends the use of cartilage as a free graft if necessary.

Brent's Procedure

(Fig. 5.**125**; Brent 1980)

In a manner very similar to that of Alexander (1919), Tanzer (1974 d), or Weerda (1982 b), Brent (1980) incises the cartilage in the scapha from a posterior approach after expanding the auricle (Fig. 5.**125 a–c**). The useful part of this resected overhang, supplemented by cartilage taken from the concha of the contralateral side using a template, is placed on top to expand and reinforce the upper part of the auricle and give it shape (Fig. 5.**125 d,e**). The incision in the scapha is then closed (Fig. 5.**125 f–h**).

Tanzer's Modification of Müsebeck's Double Banner Flap

(Fig. 5.**126**; Müsebeck 1970, Tanzer 1974 d, 1975)

Like Müsebeck before him, Tanzer recommends incising the cartilage as an anteriorly and inferiorly pedicled double flap for cases with more pronounced overhang (Fig. 5.**126 a**, 1 and 2).

Modifications were also reported by Hinderer (1972), Hinderer et al. (1987 a), Fregenal et al. (1992), and Tateshita and Ono (1999).

Horlock et al.'s Expansion of the Auricle

(Fig. 5.**127**; Horlock et al. 1998)

This modification uses the double banner flap with transposition of the helical crus.

Musgrave's Method

(Fig. 5.**128**; Musgrave 1966)

A modification of Musgrave's (1966) method is shown in Fig. 5.**128 a–e**. Usually an additional otoplasty is required. This method is based on operations by Ragnell (1951) and Stephenson (1960).

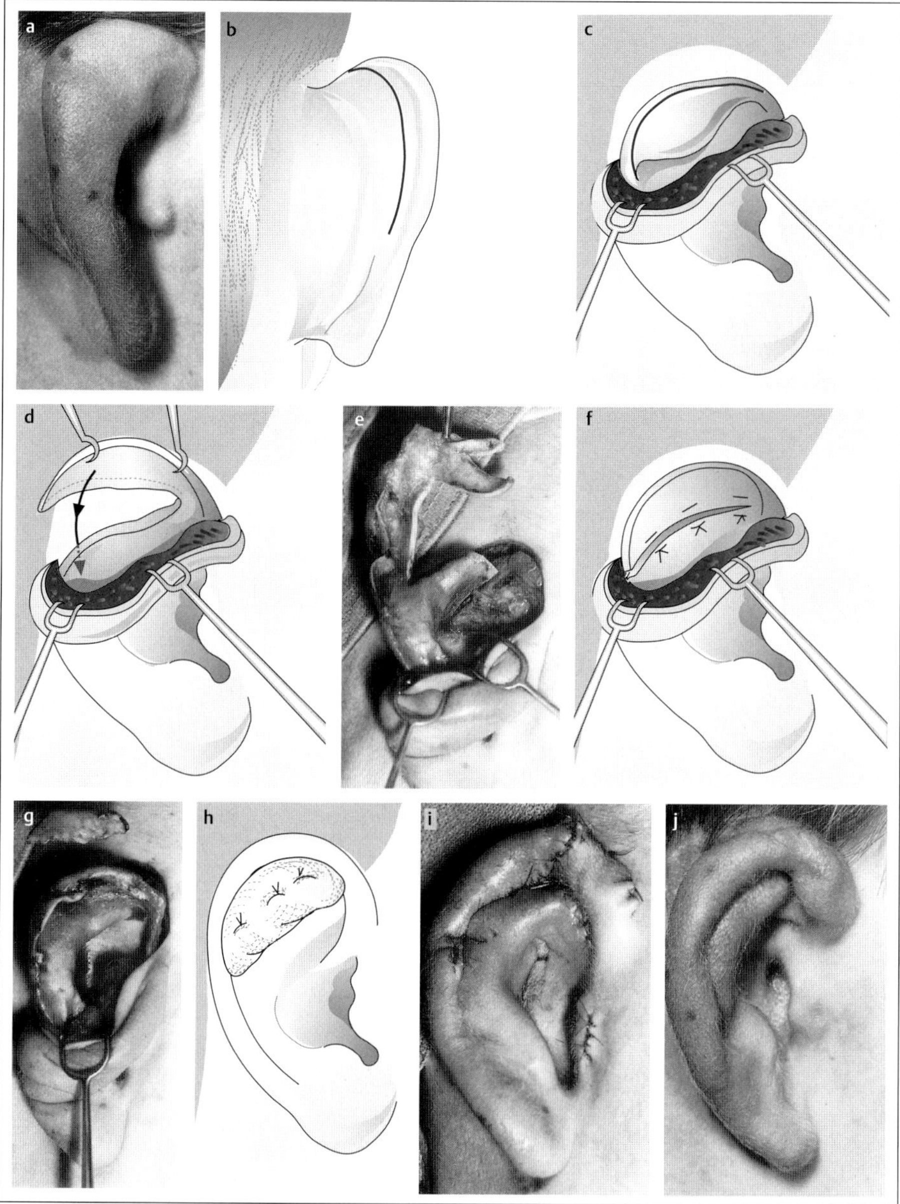

Fig. 5.**124** **Tanzer's banner flap (Tanzer 1977) for type IIB cup-ear deformity.**
a Type IIB cup-ear deformity.
b, c Posterior incision and dissection of the skin in an anterior direction, incision of the cartilaginous overhang with an anterior pedicle (or even a posterior pedicle or as a free graft).
d Banner flap with anterior pedicle.
e Posterior pedicle.
f The banner flap is secured behind the cartilage of the scapha with 5–0 braided polyglactic acid sutures.
g Additional small cartilaginous strut from the concha.
h The skin envelope is returned to its position and supported with mattress sutures tied over cotton bolsters.
i **Second stage refinements:** here, skin sutures in the scapha and the tragus after trimming.
j Outcome.

Less Popular Operative Techniques—Reconstruction with Additional Skin Flaps

Posterior Flap Used for the Anterior Expansion of the Auricle — Here too, reconstruction is governed by the severity of the deformity so that, apart from small incisions and skin additions, larger skin flaps are required, even in cases of more severe type IIB malformations.

Smith's Preauricular Tube Pedicle Flaps

(Fig. 5.**129**; Smith 1950)

Stephenson's Method

(Fig. 5.**130**; Stephenson 1960)

After a postauricular incision, Stephenson (1960) expanded the auricle using a method similar to that of Luckett (1910) for his setback otoplasty (Fig. 5.**130 a**). An incision is made over the insertion of the anterior helix, the foreshortened helix is expanded, and the skin defect is resurfaced with a skin flap raised superior to the incision (Fig. 5.**130 b–d**).

Luckett's Method

(Luckett 1963, cited in Cosman 1974)

The helix is expanded with the aid of a Z-plasty. Additional reconstruction of the antihelix is performed via a posterior approach.

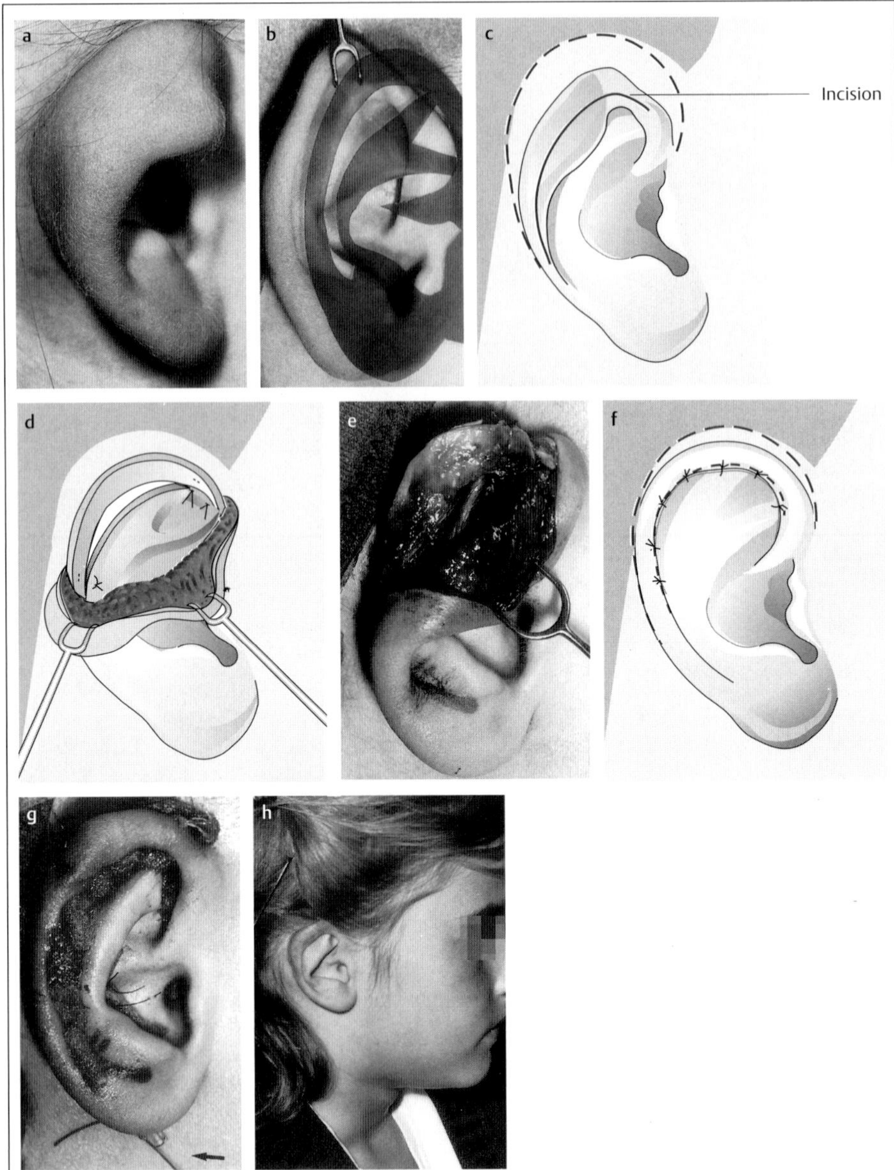

Fig. 5.**125** **Brent's technique (Brent 1980, II) to expand type IIB cup-ear deformity (moderately constricted ear).**

a–c Type IIB cup-ear deformity. The normal height is marked using a template of the healthy ear (or marked with the ear displaced upwards: **b**). Anterior incision in the scapha (Brent) or even posterior incision (Weerda: see **e**) and dissection of the skin (degloving incision).

d, e The conchal cartilage harvested from the contralateral ear is affixed by sutures.

f, g Suture and support by mattress sutures tied over cotton bolsters, drain shown in **g** (arrow).

h Result.

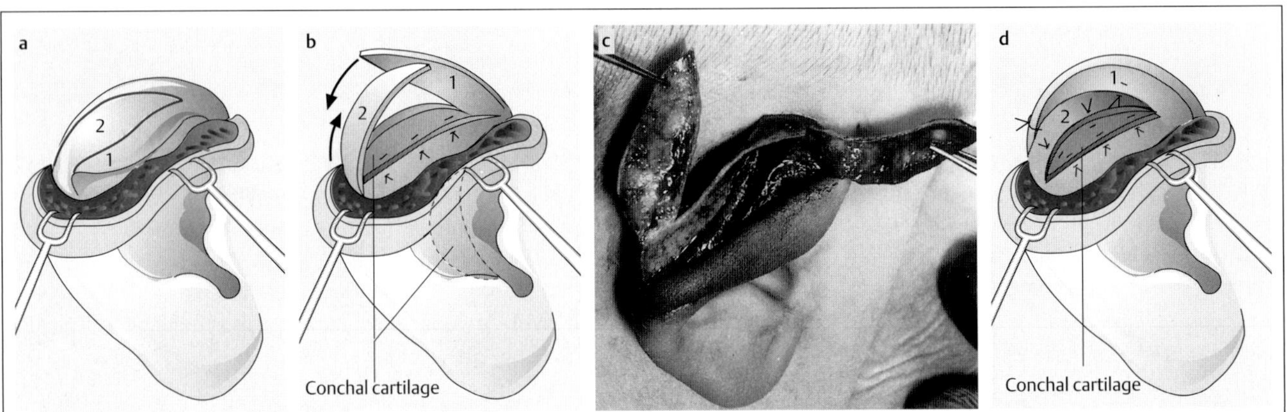

Fig. 5.**126** **Double cartilage flap as described by Müsebeck (1970; according to Tanzer 1974 a, 1975; double banner flap).**

a, b Type IIB cup-ear deformity after postauricular incision (see Fig. 5.**124 b**). Skin dissection and elevation of an anteriorly and posteriorly pedicled cartilage flap (1 and 2). An additional crescent-shaped cartilage segment is harvested from the concha and inset.

c, d The two cartilage flaps (1 and 2) are sutured together to expand the upper auricle according to a previously prepared template. The crescent-shaped conchal cartilage (**d**: red) has been inserted for stability and a supplementary otoplasty has been performed (see Fig. 5.**123**).

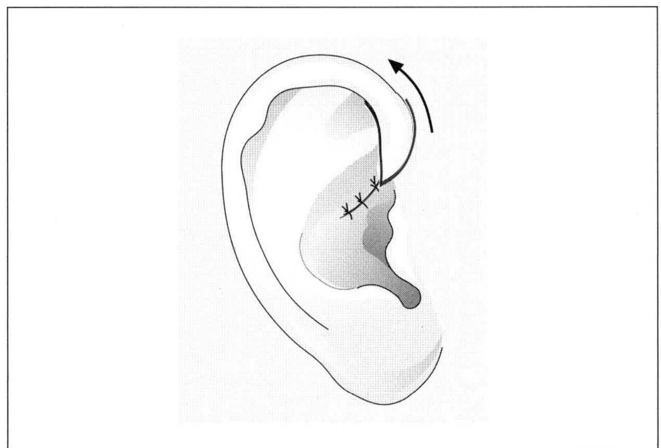

Fig. 5.**127** **Double banner flap (see Fig. 5.126) with additional VY-advancement of the helical crus (see also p. 176, Fig. 5.119).**

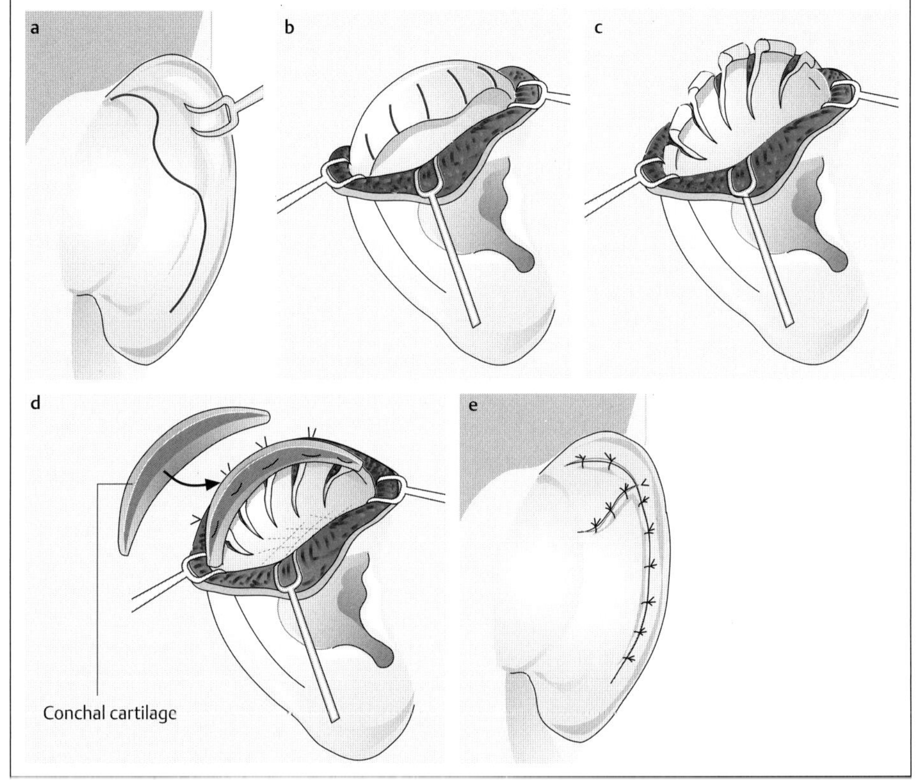

Fig. 5.**128** **Method according to Musgrave (1966), modified.**

- **a** Posterior curvilinear incision, extended in its superior portion concave towards the sulcus.
- **b** Skin dissection in an anterior direction (see also Figs. 5.**119 c**, 5.**124**).
- **c** Radial incision of the cartilage overhang.
- **d** Cartilage is harvested from the concha of the ipsilateral or contralateral ear in the transitional region to the antihelix, according to a template, and sutured posterior or anterior to the overhang.
- **e** Closure of the skin defect using a posterior VY-advancement.

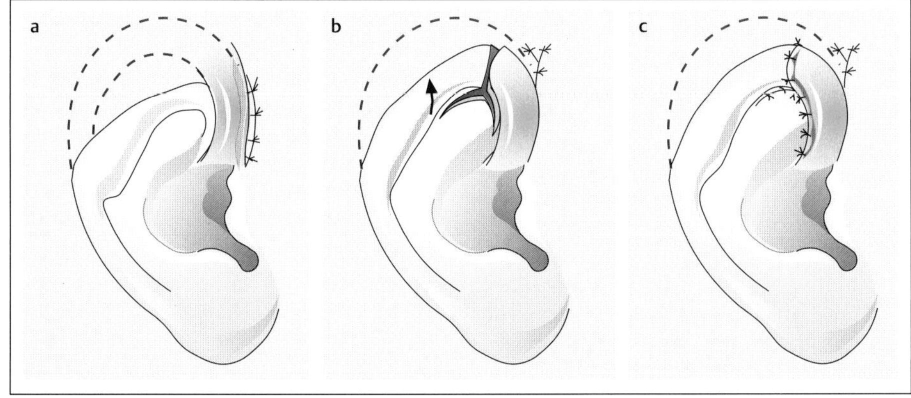

Fig. 5.**129** **Preauricular tube pedicle flap as described by Smith (1950; according to Cosman 1974).**

- **a** First stage: Design of a tube pedicle flap with its base pedicled inferiorly on the root of the helical crus.
- **b** Second stage: Superior separation of the tube pedicle flap after about 3 weeks, expansion of the auricle using setback otoplasty and expansion of the excessively short helical dome using the tube pedicle flap.
- **c** Appearance after surgery.

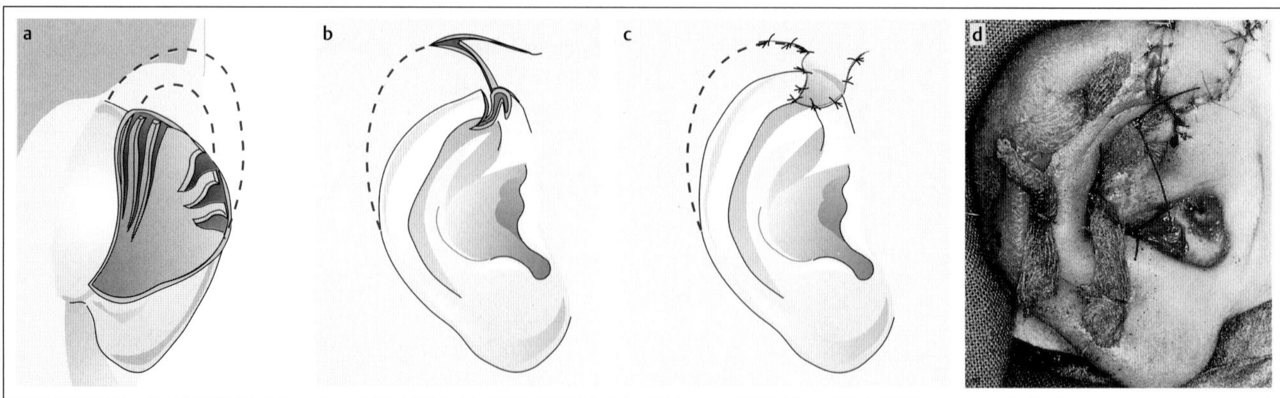

Fig. 5.**130** **Stephenson's operation (1960; according to Cosman 1974).**

a Posterior incision, radial incision of the overhang and expansion of the auricle, support with costal cartilage strut (see also Fig. 5.**128 d**).

b–d The helical dome is expanded with the aid of an anteriorly pedicled flap.

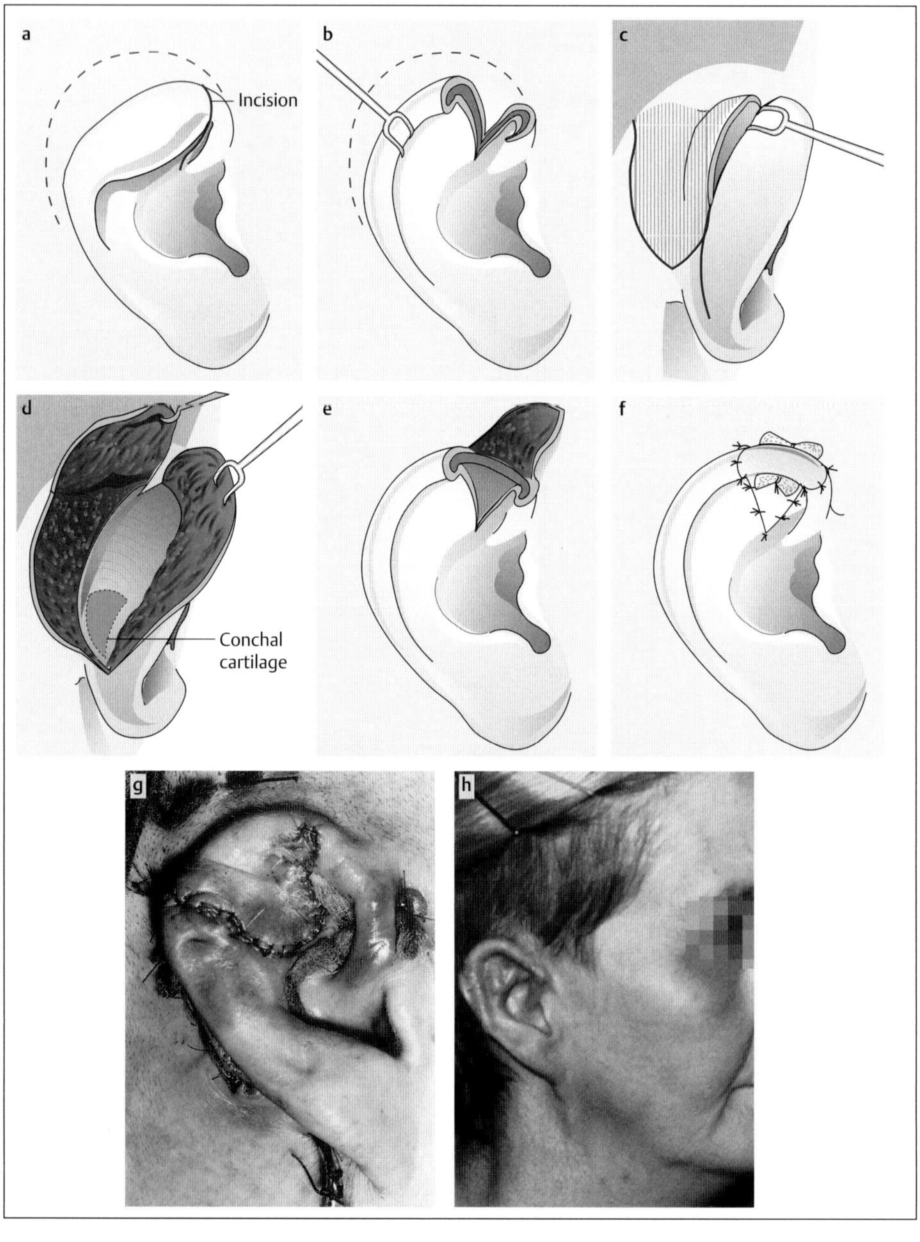

Fig. 5.**131** **Expansion of the upper auricle (type IIB cup-ear deformity) with a posterior, anterosuperiorly pedicled flap as described by Fischer (1926, cited in Marx 1926; Becker 1952 and others; according to Converse and Brent 1977).**

a, b Marking of the normal auricular height (broken red line) according to a template (see Fig. 5.**125 b**) and elevation with a double skin hook and full-thickness incision. A template is fashioned for the required flap.

c Posterior elevation of the flap and incision for the setback otoplasty.

d Conchal cartilage is harvested according to a template (or taken from more stable costal cartilage).

e The cartilage is inserted using 5–0 braided polyglactic acid suture material.

f, g The flap is inset, anteriorly and posteriorly. The form of the helix is moulded, drainage.

h Primary result, corrective surgery for helix and earlobe is planned (surgeon: Ms. S. Klaiber; **see also p. 192**, Fig. 5.**139**).

Reconstruction with a Superiorly Pedicled Posterior Flap ——— (Fig. 5.**131**; Fischer 1926, cited in Marx 1926; Becker 1952, and others)

This method is recommended by a number of other authors (Grotting 1958; Barsky 1964; Kislov 1971; Converse and Brent 1977; Mavili et al. 1996).

The techniques of Ragnell (1951) and Cosman (1974) are not to be recommended.

Type III Cup-ear Deformities

According to Tanzer (1974d, 1975; Cosman 1974), type III cup-ear deformity (see Tables 5.7 and 5.8, Fig. 5.**113 d**) belongs, together with the mini-ear, to the **grade II dysplasias (microtias)**; i. e., reconstruction of these auricles requires considerable time and effort, including the harvesting of costal cartilage. In addition, we also commonly find dystopias associated with this type of auricular malformation.

For this reason, reconstructive surgery for this class of malformations is discussed in the next section, together with the reconstruction of mini-ears (see pp. 188 ff).

Summary

Type I Cup-ear Deformity

In cases with mild overhang and an axis reduced by less than 3–4 mm, the overhang can be shortened by an incision in the upper scapha.

With somewhat more severe overhangs, expansion of the usually prominent auricles can be undertaken from an anterior or posterior incision and thus the shape of the overhang can be formed (by using the anterior approach, reconstruction of the antihelix can be performed using Stenström's technique (1963; see p. 134).

Type IIA Cup-ear Deformity

Here we already find obvious constriction of the helical dome with increasing overhang. Apart from an otoplasty from an anterior or posterior approach, elongation of the helix by incising around the helical crus, followed by a V-Y-plasty in a superior direction, has proved effective (see Figs. 5.**117**, 5.**118**).

Type IIB Cup-ear Deformity

In addition to reconstruction of the superior auricle using the cartilage of the overhang, this type requires replacement of the skin deficit by transposing skin or skin flaps from the posterior surface (see Figs. 5.**119**–5.**125**) and expanding the constricted helical dome using additional cartilage from the ipsilateral concha or the concha of the contralateral auricle, or occasionally even costal cartilage.

5.4.2 Grade II Dysplasias

Synonyms: Grade II microtia, concha-type microtia (Nagata 1994b), moderate auricular malformations, cup-ear deformity type III (Tanzer 1974, 1975), mini-ear.

The severe forms of cup-ear deformity (type III) and mini-ears are reconstructed by using the same operative techniques.

- **General definition.** The ear still displays some structures of a normal auricle.
- **Surgical definition.** Additional skin and cartilage are required for reconstruction (Weerda 1987, 1988 a, b, 1994 e, 2004).

This class comprises two forms of malformation, which are both malformations of hillocks 3–4 (see pp. 110, 112):

- **Type III cup-ear deformities.** (see Fig. 5.**132 a, b**; Fig. 5.**113 d**, Tables 5.7, 5.**8**). The upper part hangs far over the lower, antihelix and crura are rarely present, there is often dystopia and occasionally congenital atresia of the auditory canal. These deformities have a large number of variations.
- **Mini-ears.** This ear is reduced in its longitudinal and horizontal axes. It has a good profile and a deformed helix (see Fig. 5.**133**; Davis 1974b). **Depending on the type of malformation, the upper, middle, or lower auricle requires reconstruction.** It is often advisable to reconstruct the entire auricle using Nagata's technique (1994b; concha-type microtia; see Fig. 5.**135**).

Type III Cup-ear Deformities (and Mini-ear with a Deficit in the Superior Region)

Synonyms: group III cup-ear deformity (Tanzer 1974b, 1975), severe lop ear deformity (Rogers 1968), snail-shell ear (Davis 1987), cockleshell ear (Davis 1974b, 1987), severe cup-ear deformity. See Tables 5.7, 5.**8**; Fig 5.**113**, p. 171.

These are deformities of the mesenchymal hillocks 3 and 4 (see p. 109). The severe forms of cup-ear deformities have the following common characteristics (see Fig. 5.**132 b**; p. 185):

- severe underdevelopment of the upper auricle, i. e., the upper helix, scapha, and antihelical crura together with the triangular fossa
- the upper auricular part overhangs the lower
- insertion of the superoanterior auricular portion on the cheek, anterior to the tragal region
- in the majority of cases there is obvious dystopia and an anterior location of the ear (see Fig. 5.**132 a, c**)
- frequently associated with microsomia (see Fig. 5.**194**, p. 229).

Combinations with other hillock malformations are encountered. Stenosis of the auditory canal and narrowing of the tympanic membrane are also seen, but congenital atresia of the auditory canal is a rarity (Davis 1987).

The following characteristics require surgical correction:

- Severe overhang of the auricle
- Considerable shortening of the axes
- In addition, there is frequently dystopia (inferior position and anterior displacement)

Operative Techniques

Weerda's Technique of the Reconstruction of Dystopic Type III Cup-ear Deformity

(Fig. 5.**132**; Weerda 1988 b, 1994 e; Nagata 1994 b; in this context see also pp. 185–188, 193–196)

First operative stage. A template of the normal ear is made (see p. 202) and the position of the auricle is planned, based on the contralateral ear (Fig. 5.**132 a, c**; see also p. 202). Incision is at the base of the rudimentary ascending helix (Fig. 5.**132 e**, A), around the auricle and onto the postauricular surface, approximately 5–8 mm inferior and parallel to the helix, to about 5–8 mm from the inferior margin of the earlobe, continuing across the sulcus and, in a superior direction, to the retroauricular skin of the mastoid (Fig. 5.**132 d**, A′). The incision in the region of the base of the rudimentary ascending helix (Fig. 5.**132 e**, A) is then extended into the concha in order to create a flap (Fig. 5.**132 d**, 1) to form and/or enlarge the rudimentary tragus. The rudimentary tragus is incised over its superior margin and undermined. The helical cartilage at point A is divided down into the concha in the region of flap 1, and the posterior flap (Fig. 5.**132 d, e**, 2) is incised along the red continuous line over the mastoid to develop a pocket superiorly beyond the hairline (red broken line; Fig. 5.**132 f**, AA′).

The auricle is expanded and the base (Fig. 5.**132 e**, A) is transposed to the higher point A′ over the mastoid, while the posterior skin of the auricular vestige is sutured to the inferior wound of the mastoid skin in two layers, subcutaneously (5–0 braided sutures) and cutaneously (5–0 monofilament sutures) (Fig. 5.**132 f**).

A small cartilaginous tragus, fashioned from costal cartilage or from the cartilage remnant, is then inserted into the previously prepared pocket in the rudimentary tragus (Fig. 5.**132 f**) and enveloped by flap (1).

Next, the previously prepared costal cartilage framework (see pp. 187, 203–206, Fig. 5.**135 i, j**) is inserted into the tunneled lower part of the rudimentary cup ear, the upper part placed into the skin pocket, and the incisions closed (Fig. 5.**132 g, h**). The form of the tragus is created by cotton bolsters tied over with small mattress sutures, and the same is done for the helix (see Fig. 5.**125 g**). Before that, a size 6 or size 8 vacuum drain is inserted to adapt the skin to the underlying framework and provide a good contour to the new auricle (Figs. 5.**132 g**, 5.**170 h**).

Second operative stage. See also the method described by Nagata, p. 213. As with complete reconstruction of the auricle, the ear is exteriorized after 6–10 weeks at the earliest (see Fig. 5.**172**). Following the suggestions made by Nagata (1994 b–d) a crescent-shaped disc of cartilage is inserted as a spacer and covered with temporalis fascia. The post- and retroauricular region is then resurfaced with a thick split-thickness or full-thickness skin flap (Fig. 5.**132 i**).

Reconstruction of the Upper Mini-ear

(Fig. 5.**133**; Weerda 1988 b; Nagata 1993, 1994 a–d)

The mini-ear with deficit in the upper region is reconstructed in the same way as the dystopic type III cup-ear deformity (Fig. 5.**133 a–f**).

Brents' Reconstruction of the Mini-ear or Severe Cup-ear Deformities

(Fig. 5.**134**; Brent 1980 II, 1993, 1999 b)

First operative stage. Brent reconstructs severe cup-ear deformities and mini-ears as he does ears with grade III dysplasia (see p. 207, Fig. 5.**160**). With severe dystopic cup-ear deformities he also incises the overhang, then dissects the postauricular skin over the mastoid (Fig. 5.**134 a**) to create a pocket, and inserts the framework (for construction of the framework, see p. 205; operative technique, see also grade III dysplasia, pp. 201 ff).

Second operative stage. In a second session, 8–10 weeks later at the earliest, a part of the lower auricular vestige is affixed to the framework to form the earlobe (Fig. 5.**134 b**), while the rest of the nubbin is used to construct the tragus and the concha (Fig. 5.**134 c**). The auricle is then elevated in a **third stage** (Brent 1980 II; see p. 185, Fig. 5.**132 i, j**; p. 187, Fig. 5.**135**; pp. 214 ff).

Nagata's Reconstruction of Severe Cup-ear Deformities

(Fig. 5.**135**; Nagata 1993, 1994 a–d)

Nagata refers to the group of malformations (Fig. 5.**135 a–c**), in which a concha and also usually a rudimentary tragus are present, as "concha-type microtia." He describes the following two-stage procedure for the reconstruction of severe cup-ear deformities and the upper part of the auricle of mini-ears.

First operative stage. As with grade III dysplasias (see Fig. 5.**170**, p. 213), the position of the auricle is first marked with the aid of a template (Fig. 5.**135 a, c**) and then the incision is carried from the concha, across the transition from earlobe to rudimentary remnant (A), and onto the posterior

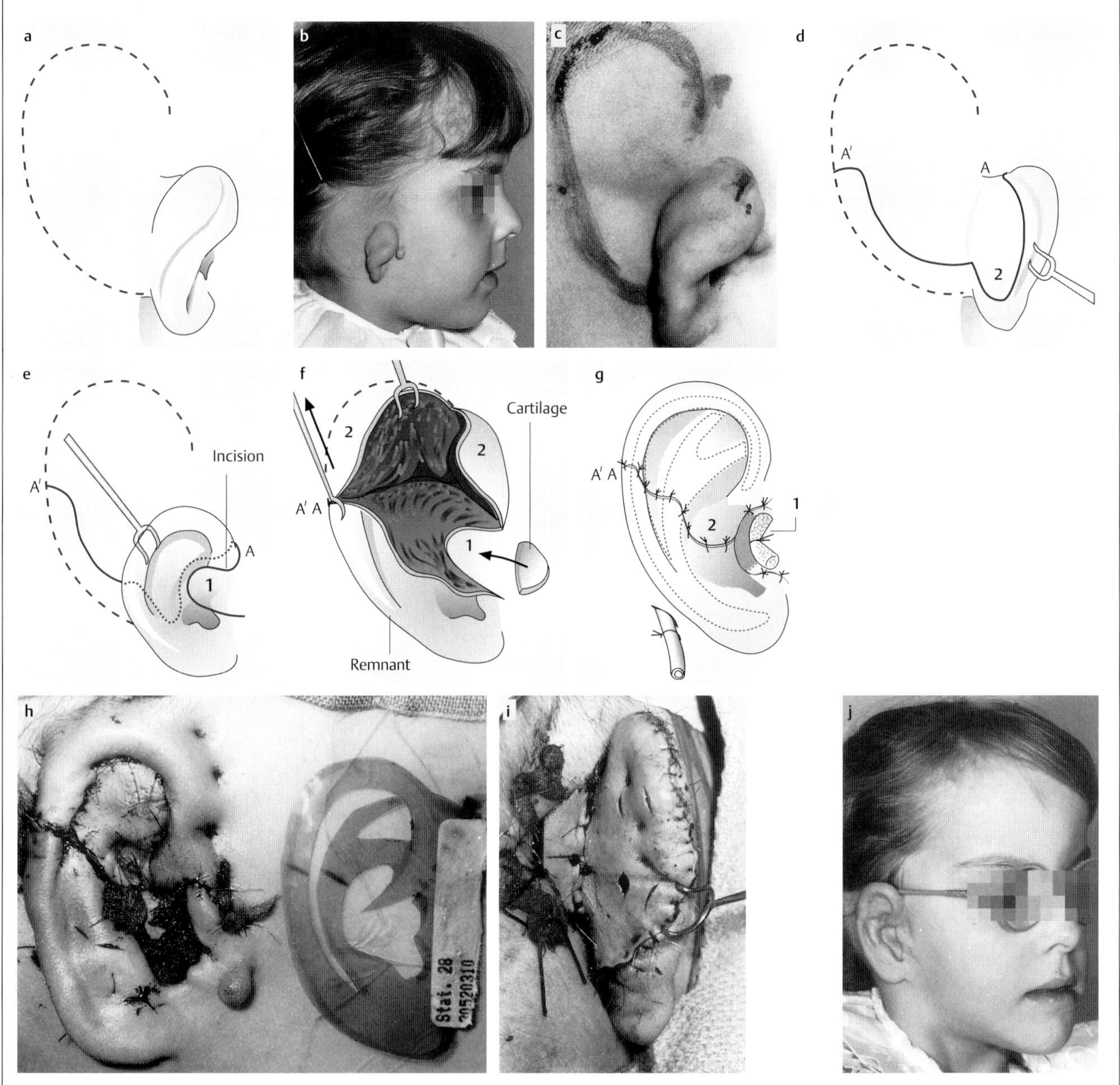

Fig. 5.132 Reconstruction of the dystopic type III cup-ear deformity as described by Weerda (1988 b).
First stage:
a–c Dystopic type III cup ear; the position of the normal auricle is marked according to a template of the normal ear (see **h**).
d Postauricular skin incision extending to the mastoid (see text).
e A flap (1) is raised for the tragus (constructed from rudimentary cartilage or rib). Incision through skin and cartilage at A and division of the cartilage (dotted line: incision on the postauricular surface; see **d**).
f Subcutaneous suture of the lower remnant with 5–0 braided polyglactic acid and cutaneous suture with 5–0 (6–0) monofilament suture material, bringing the remnant into a superior position (A'A). Dissection of a tunnel into the remnant and development of a pocket (2) in a superior and posterior direction, about 1 cm superior to the auricular contour (broken red line). Insertion of cartilage into the tragus and coverage with flap 1.
g, h Insertion of the cartilaginous support, skin suture using 6–0 monofilament material, formation of the auricular contours, vacuum drain (see Fig. 5.**135 k**).
Second stage:
i Elevation of the auricle after a minimum of 8 weeks and coverage with thick split skin or full-thickness skin (see section on grade III dysplasia, p. 215).
j Outcome (a similar method was systematized and published by Nagata 1993, 1994; see Fig. 5.**133**).

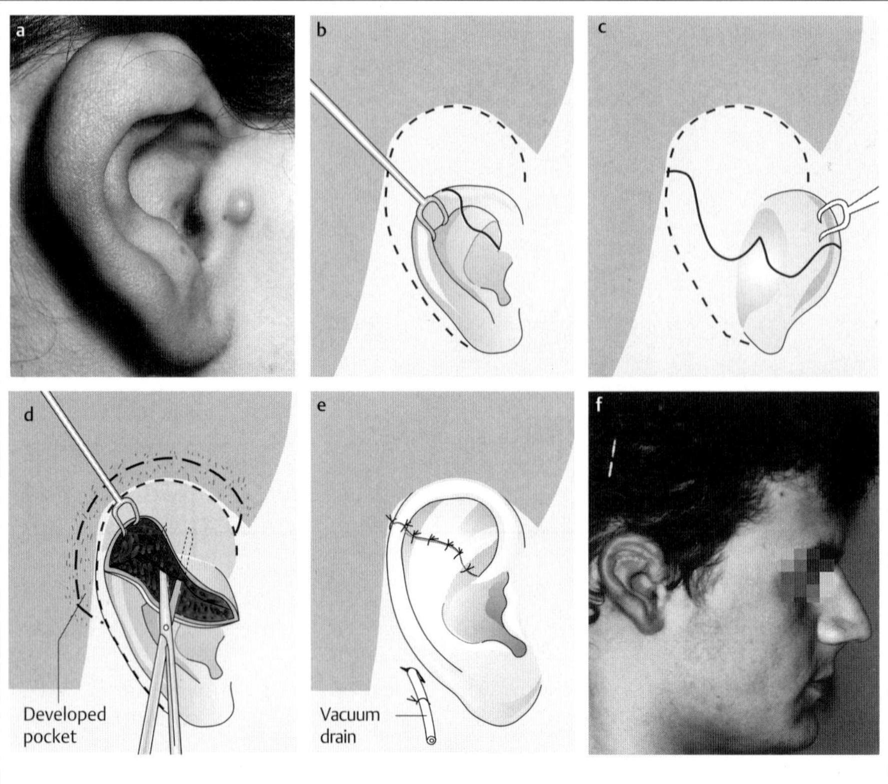

Fig. 5.**133** **Reconstruction of a mini-ear with deficits in the upper region (Weerda 1988 b; Nagata 1993, 1994 a–d; see also Fig. 5.132 and text).**

a, b Mini-ear, auricular height marked according to a template (broken red line), anterior incision in the upper part of the mini-ear extending into the concha.

c W-shaped posterior incision and division of the rudimentary cartilage.

d Development of the superior pocket after removal of the cartilage.

e Insertion of the cartilage support (see Fig. 5.**135 i, j**) followed by a subcutaneous suture using 5–0 braided polyglactic acid and a 6–0 monofilament cutaneous suture.

f Result after two stages (see Fig. 5.**135**; surgeon: R. Siegert).

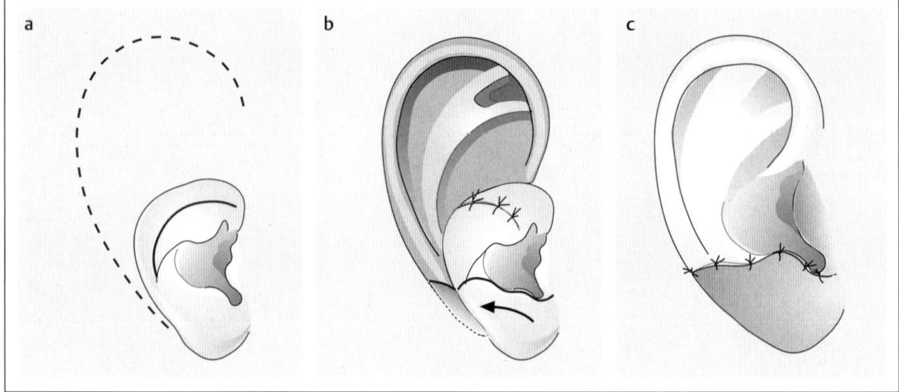

Fig. 5.**134** **Reconstruction of a mini-ear and severe type III cup-ear deformity using the technique described by Brent (1980, II; corresponding to a total reconstruction; see p. 207).**

First stage:

a Mini-ear or type III cup ear. Height: broken red line. Incision to remove the cartilage and undermining of the skin as far as, and including, the mastoid plane (see Fig. 5.**160 c**).

b The framework has been inserted and the incision closed.

Second stage:

Planning of the lobular transposition after a minimum of about 8–10 weeks.

c Tragus and concha have been designed from the upper part of the auricle, only the lower part has become the earlobe by exposing the lower part of the cartilage framework, transposing the new earlobe from the rudimentary auricle and insetting it with subcutaneous and cutaneous 6–0 monofilament suture material.

Third stage:

See text: elevation, see p. 209, Fig. 5.**162**.

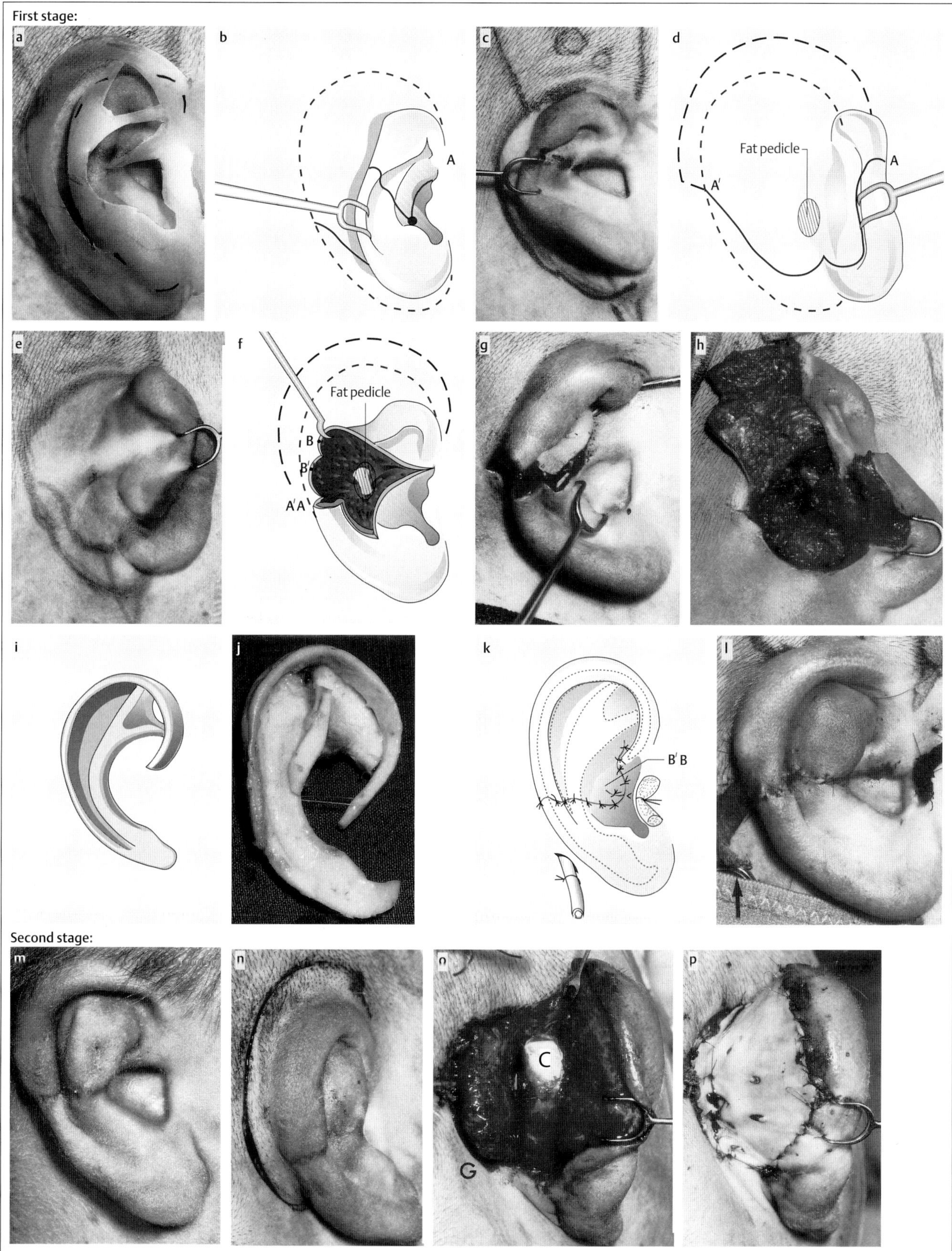

Fig. 5.**135 a–p**

Fig. 5.**135 q–s** ▷

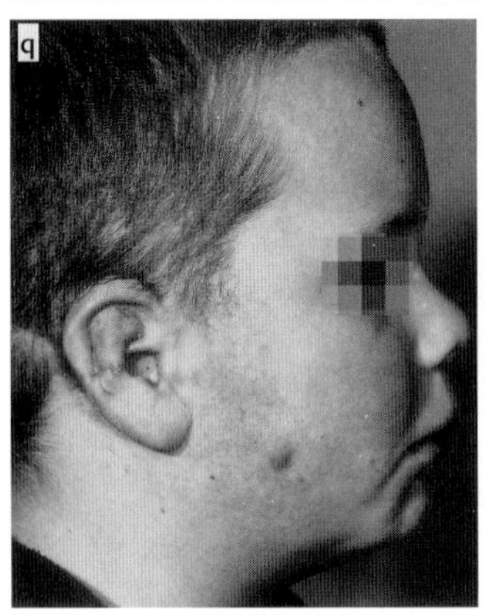

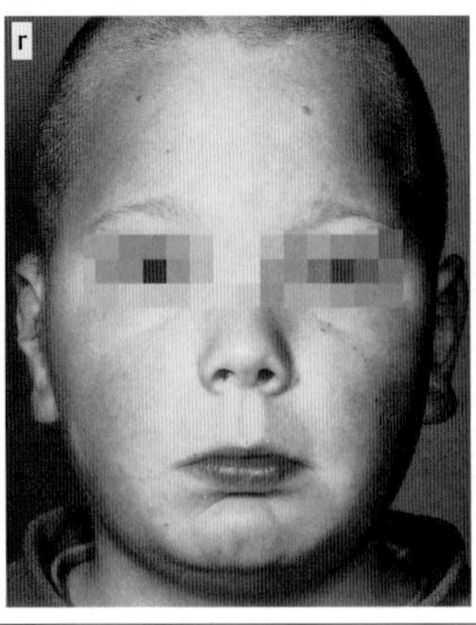

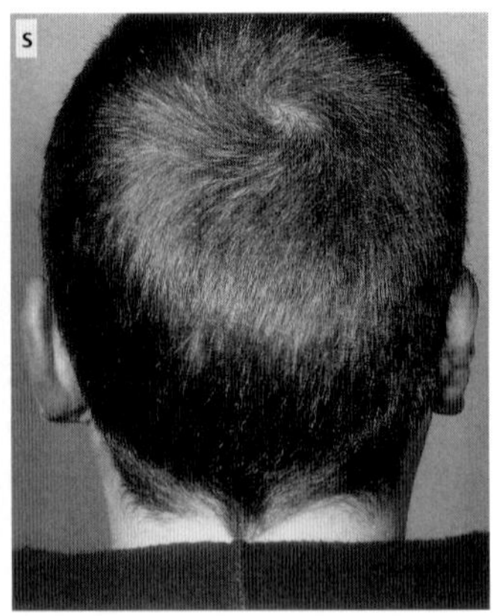

Fig. 5.**135** **Reconstruction of a severe type III cup-ear deformity and the upper auricle in a mini-ear (concha type microtia) as described by Nagata (1993, 1994a–d; see p. 209).**
Here, right mini-ear.
First stage:
a-c The normal position of the ear is marked (**b** broken red line) using a template of the contralateral ear (**a**; see pp. 202, 203); red line: anterior incision (**b**), axis about 20° (**c**).
d, e W-shaped incision, A to A′; broken black line: development of the pocket (see also **f**).
f–h Anterior (**g**) and posterior (**h**) incisions: removal of the upper rudimentary cartilage (preserve the specimen for use in tragal augmentation; see Fig. 5.**132 f**). The lower remnant is sutured to the mastoid (A to A′) using 5–0 braided polyglactic acid for the subcutaneous suture, and 5–0 monofilament material for the cutaneous one.
i, j Cartilage framework.
k, l Insertion of the cartilaginous framework; vacuum drain (arrow), and two-layer closure of the skin incision on the anterior surface (suture of BB′ after excision of a corresponding small skin-cartilage fragment; 6–0 monofilament suture material for the anterior surface).
Second stage (see p. 215: operative technique as described by Nagata 1994a–d):
m Appearance of the auricle approximately 12 weeks after the first stage.
n Elevation of a full-thickness skin flap, pedicled on the helix and above the hair follicles, for coverage of the helix (see pp. 214, 215; Fig. 5.**171 a**): good skin color match (see **n**, **o** and **p**).
o The auricle is exteriorized, leaving a layer of fibrous tissue on the framework. Insertion of a crescent-shaped cartilage spacer (C; see Fig. 5.**172 e**). Coverage of the cartilage with a musculofascial flap (G) (see p. 215).
p A thick split- or full-thickness skin graft is sutured and glued into place with fibrin adhesive.
q–s Result after the two-stage reconstruction.

surface. On the postauricular surface, the skin incision is continued in a W-shaped fashion. A pedicle of fat and fibrous tissue is preserved in the region of the sulcus (Fig. 5.**135 d–f**) in order to guarantee sufficient perfusion of the tissue. A pocket is then developed about 1 cm above the actual auricular contour (Fig. 5.**135 f, g**; broken black line). The superior part of the rudimentary auricular cartilage is excised, the inferior cartilage, including the inferior conchal region, is preserved (Fig. 5.**135 f–h**). A costal cartilage framework (Fig. 5.**135 i, j**; for its fabrication see pp. 206 and 211–212) is then drawn into the superior part, around the tissue pedicle, inserted into the previously dissected lobular segment, which has already been sutured to the posterior wound surface, and the incisions are then closed in two layers with fine 5–0 braided sutures and 6–0 monofilament sutures. One or two vacuum drainage systems are secured with sutures to give the auricle a good contour (Fig. 5.**135 k, l**).

Second operative stage. As with grade III dysplasia (see p. 215), the auricle is not elevated until after at least 8 weeks (Fig. 5.**135 m–p**).

Good results can be achieved with this method (Fig. 5.**135 q–s**).

Mini-ear (and Type III Cup-ear Deformity)

Special Forms of Reconstruction

Reconstruction/Expansion of the Middle Third of the Auricle — Since we usually reconstruct mini-ears using modifications of the Nagata technique (1994b; see Figs. 5.**132** and 5.**135**), as we do severe type III cup-ear deformities, reconstruction of the middle third of the auricle is occasionally required.

Weerda's U-Shaped Advancement Flap Method
(Fig. 5.**136**; Weerda 1981; see also section on reconstruction of defects of the middle third of the auricle, pp. 61, 62, 70 ff)

This technique is used only in the case of absent or mild dystopia (Tanzer 1977, p. 1706). The example shown here (Fig. 5.**136 d, i**) is taken from a very early reconstruction; we no longer do it like this (see below).

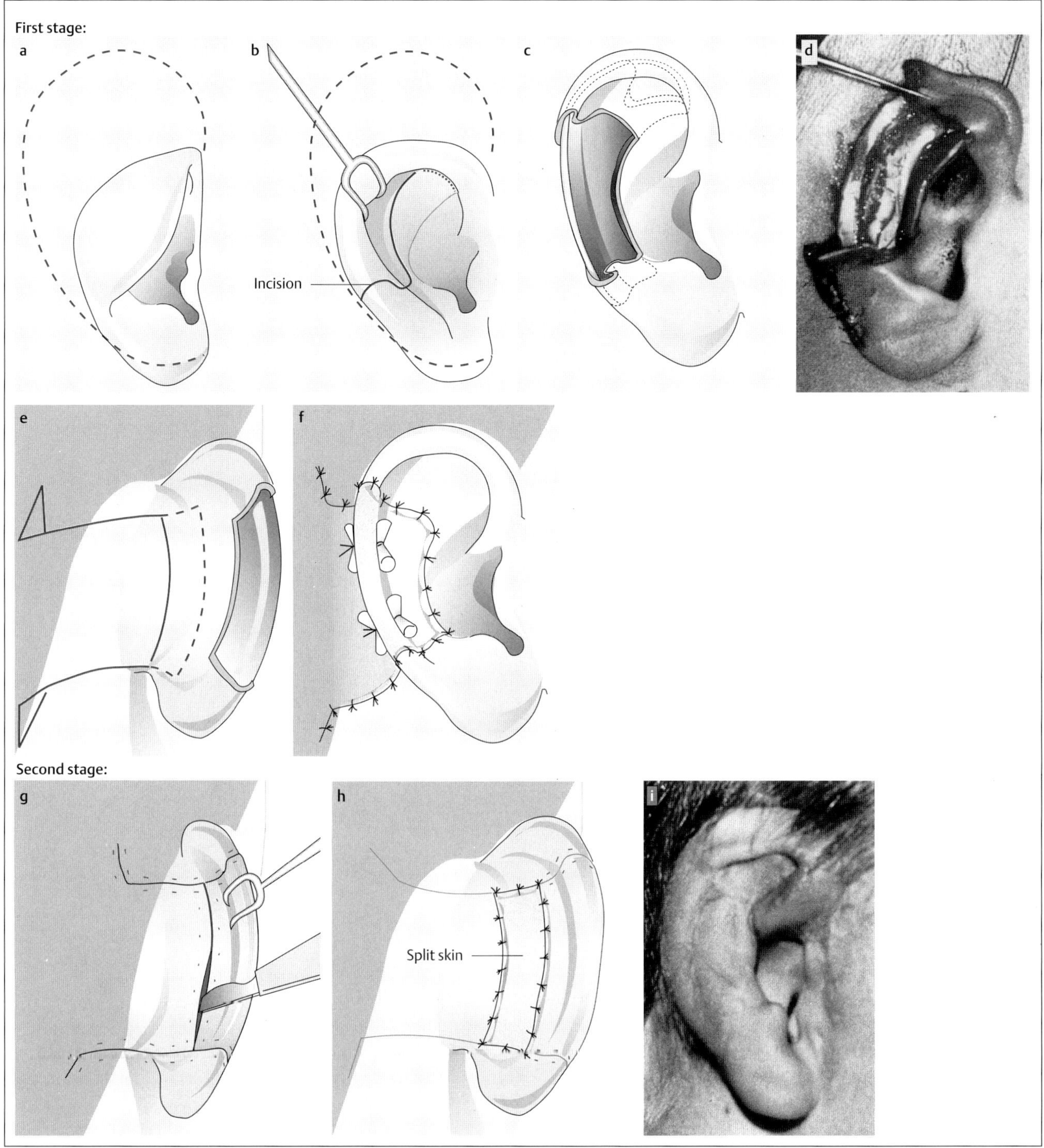

Fig. 5.**136** **Reconstruction of the middle third of the auricle in a mini-ear or severe cup-ear deformity using a U-shaped flap as described by Weerda (1981).**

First stage:

a Cup ear

b Mini-ear: Position of the normal auricle (using a template) is marked with a broken red line: Incision in the middle of the auricle, coursing upwards on reaching the concha (dotted red line: cartilage incision).

c, d Insertion of a delicate costal cartilage framework (2–3 mm smaller).

e, f Incision of a U-shaped advancement flap, with the option of extension over the sulcus (broken red line), inset and suture of the flap.

Second stage:

g, h If necessary, division of the flap (after 3–4 weeks) and coverage of the defect with thick split skin.

i, j Result after the two-stage reconstruction.

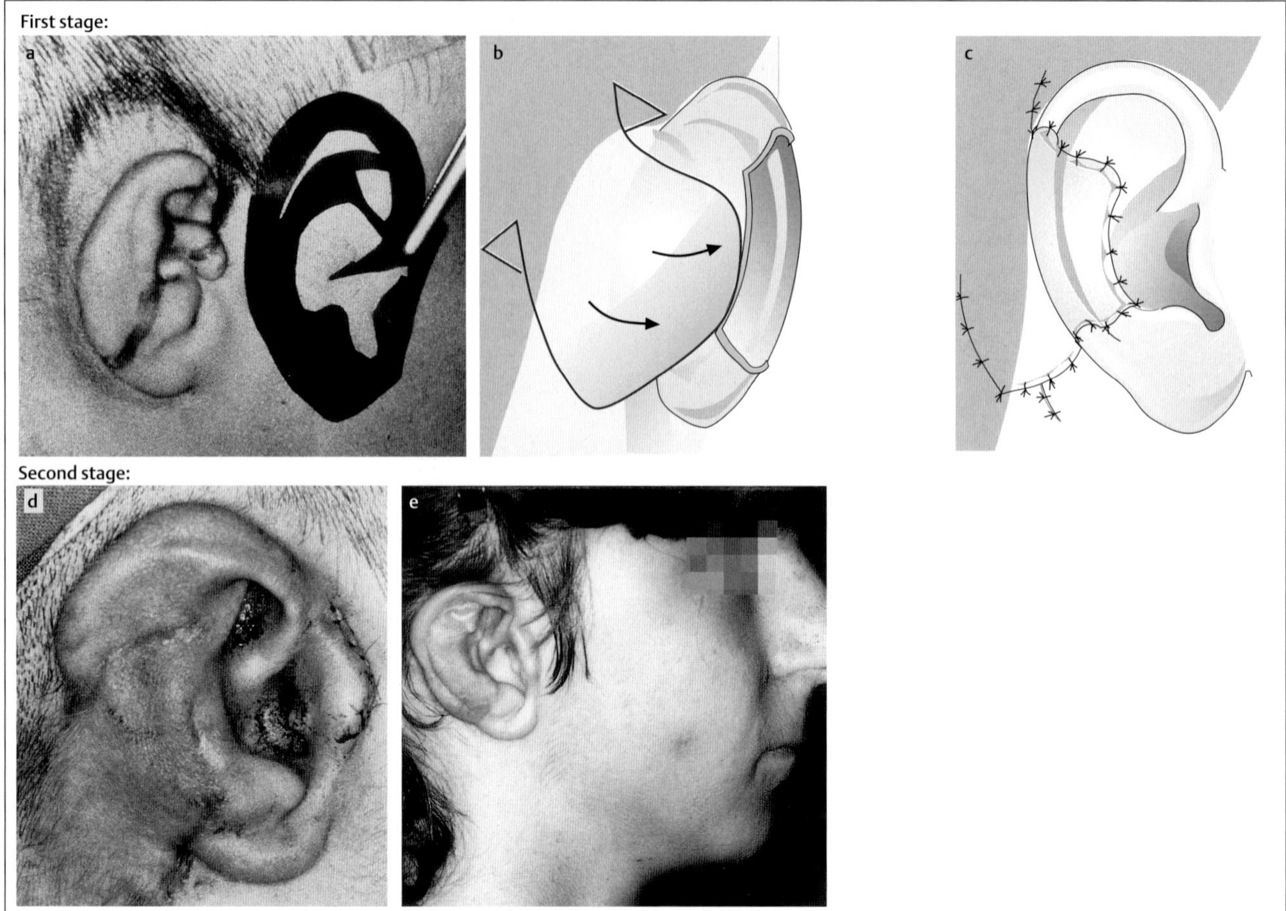

Fig. 5.**137** **Rotation flap to widen a mini-ear as described by Weerda (1982 d).**
First stage:
a Mini-ear; height of the ear marked from a template, inferior incision.
b The delicate framework has already been inserted (see Fig. 5.**136 c, d**) and the rotation flap has been marked out.
c, d The rotation flap has been sutured and has healed in.
Second stage:
e Division and final adjustments to the pedicle of the flap, coverage of the postauricular surface with thick split skin (see Fig. 5.**136**). Outcome after the second stage.

Expansion Using a Rotation Flap
(Fig. 5.**137**; Weerda 1982 d, 1984 c)

Instead of a U-shaped advancement flap, a rotation flap (Fig. 5.**137 b, c**) can also occasionally be used (Weerda 1982 d, 1984 c).

Expansion Using a Transposition–Rotation Flap
(Weerda 1982 c; see p. 73.)

Expansion Using a U-shaped Advancement Flap
(Fig. 5.**138**; Weerda 1999 b

This method uses a U-shaped advancement flap and VY-skin advancement on the postauricular surface.

First operative stage. In the presence of only a mild deficit in height (Fig. 5.**138 a**), the incision is extended inferiorly further into the concha and below the antitragus (red dotted line, Fig. 5.**138 b**), after marking the size of the auricle (red broken line) and after incising the helix anteriorly in the middle.

An inferiorly pedicled V-shaped flap is raised on the postauricular surface (Fig. 5.**138 c, d**). Then the costal cartilage framework is inserted (Fig. 5.**138 e**; Fig. 5.**136 c, d**) and covered with a U-shaped advancement flap (Fig. 5.**138 f, g**).

Second operative stage. The U-shaped flap is separated and inset after 3 weeks at the earliest (Fig. 5.**138 h, i**). At the same time the duplicated upper helix is narrowed and formed. The result is depicted in Figure 5.**138 j**.

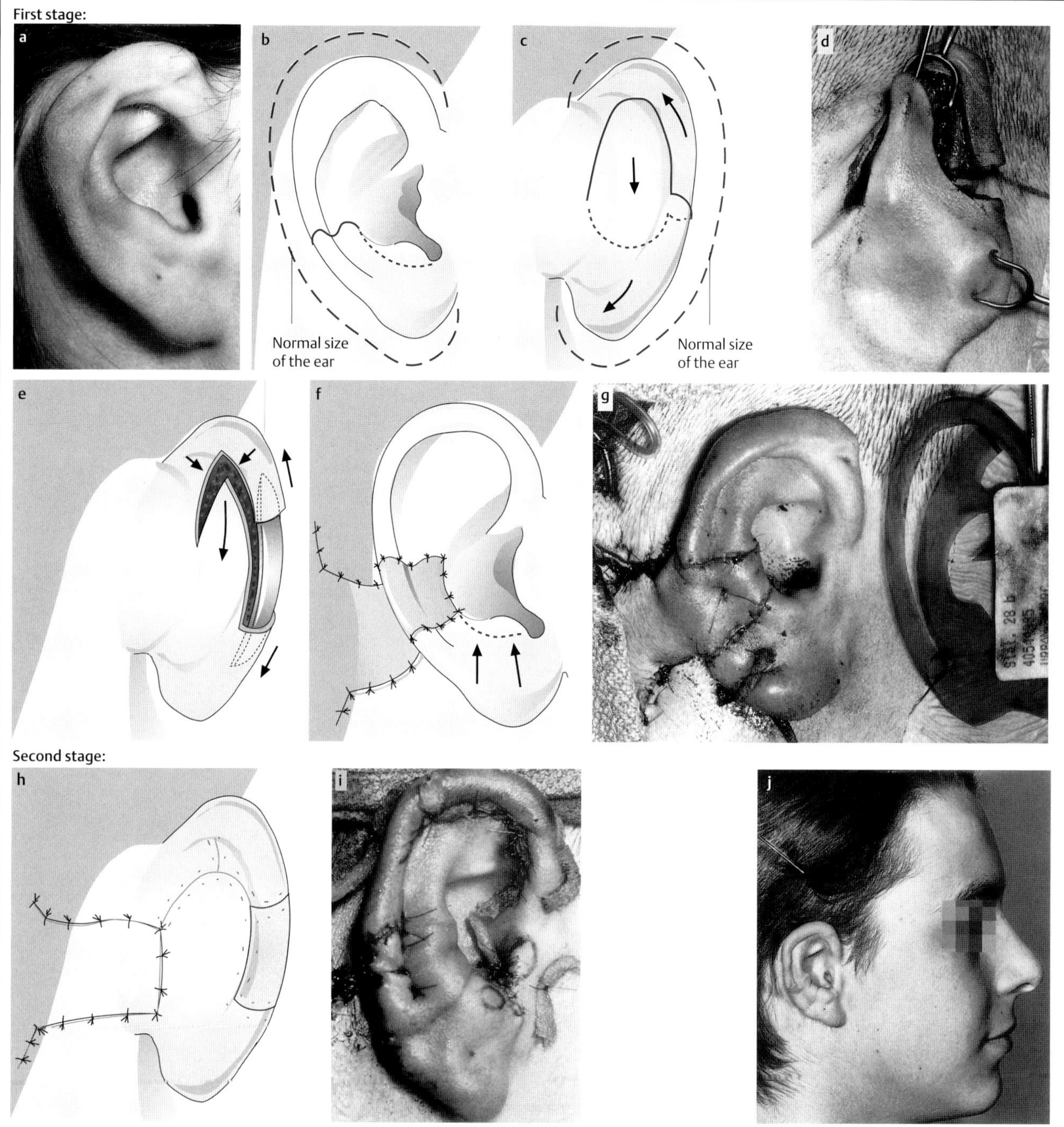

Fig. 5.**138** **Widening of the middle third of a mini-ear using a U-shaped advancement flap and posterior VY-advancement as described by Weerda (1999 b).**

First stage:

a Mini-ear with duplication of the superior helix (apparently similar to the malformation Beethoven had).

b The height of the normal ear has been marked out, incision in the middle of the ear, tunneling of the skin inferiorly, and incision only of the conchal cartilage down to, and below, the antitragus (dotted red line; see Fig. 5.**136 b**).

c, d Posterior incision of the VY-advancement flap (red line; the anterior incision shown as a dotted line).

e Insertion of a delicate framework, VY-advancement.

f, g The U-shaped advancement flap is inset and sutured, the auricle is enlarged according to the size of the template of the healthy ear (see also Fig. 5.**136**).

Second stage:

h, i Division of, and final adjustments to, the U-shaped flap (approximately 3–4 weeks later). The superior helix is made narrower.

j Outcome.

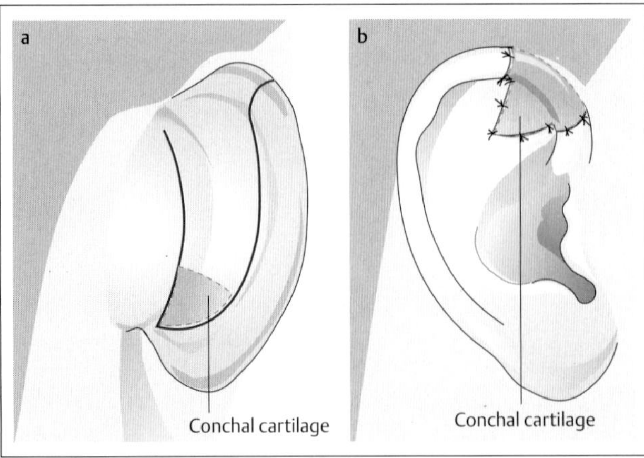

Fig. 5.**139** **Superiorly pedicled, chondrocutaneous postauricular transposition flap as described by Mavili et al. (1996).**
a Superior full-thickness incision and elevation of a transposition flap with cartilage harvested from the concha (fashioned from a template).
b The flap is inset into the defect (this technique is more suitable for type II cup-ear deformities; see Fig. 5.**131**).

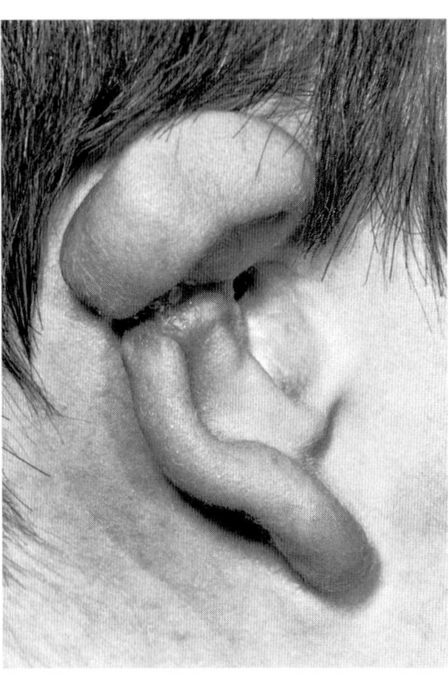

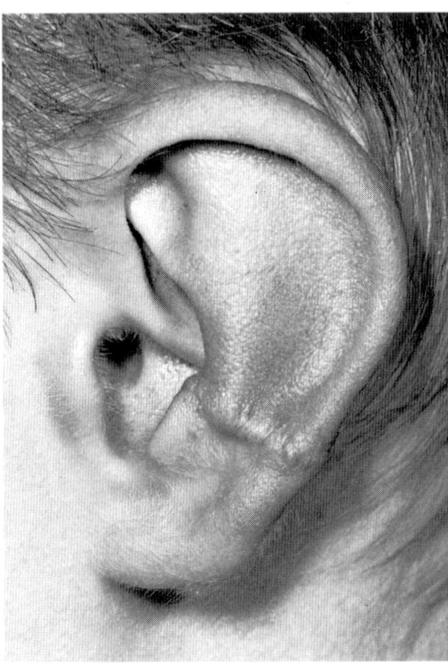

a b

Fig. 5.**140** **Widening of the auricle using a free full-thickness composite graft harvested from the contralateral ear as described by Quatela and Cheney (1995; see p. 57).**
a, b This child was referred to us after auricular reconstruction using this technique. Failure of the technique and loss of the composite graft. Deformation of the healthy left ear.

Use of Composite Grafts for Reconstruction

Mavili et al.'s Pedicled Composite Graft

(Fig. 5.**139**; Mavili et al 1996)

This graft is used for expansion of the auricle (Fig. 5.**139 a, b**).

Quatela and Cheney's Full-thickness Composite Graft

(Fig. 5.**140**; Quatela and Cheney 1995; see p. 57)

This full-thickness composite graft is harvested from the contralateral ear (Fig. 5.**140 a, b**).

Critique. All composite grafts are subject to a high risk of loss (Walter 1966, 1994 a; Fig. 5.**140 a**), with the additional risk of deforming the contralateral ear (Fig. 5.**140 b**), as with this child who was referred to us.

Park's Method

Park (1997) described a very elaborate one-stage method of reconstruction using postauricular skin and fascia flaps which are pedicled on the posterior auricular artery. He covered these fascia flaps with skin from the postauricular region of the contralateral ear (see p. 74, Fig. 5. **142**).

Reconstruction of the Lower Third of the Auricle

These techniques were also described earlier in the section on defects of the lower third of the auricle (see pp. 74 ff).

Gavello's Reconstruction

(Fig. 5.**141**; see p. 75)

Following the procedure described by Gavello (1907) for bilateral lower defects we were able to achieve as good a result (Fig. 5.**141 c, d**) using a large Gavello flap as we managed to obtain in the surgical management of defects.

For larger reconstructions of the lower auricular third, see section on surgical management of defects (pp. 75 ff).

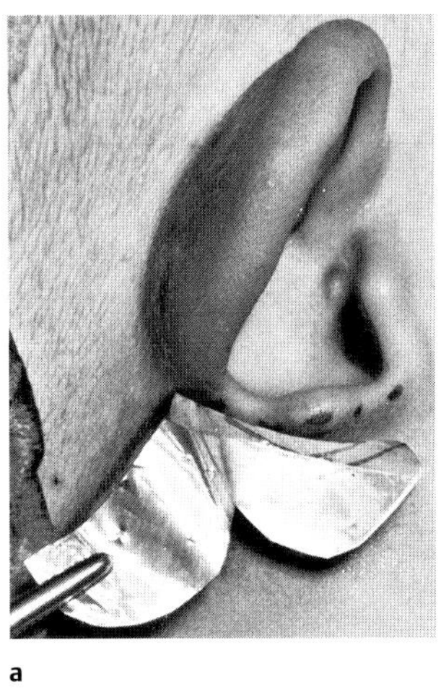

a

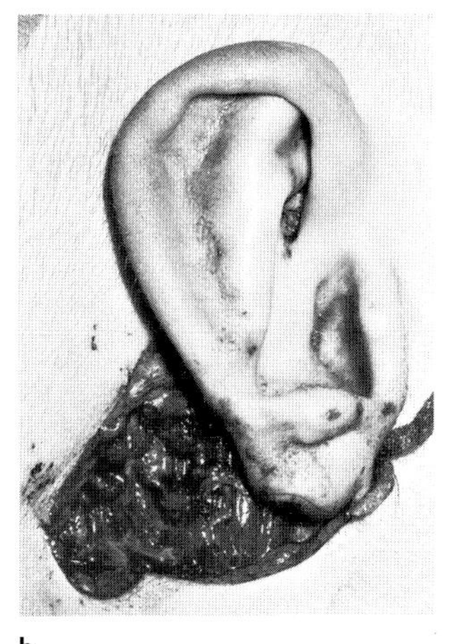

b

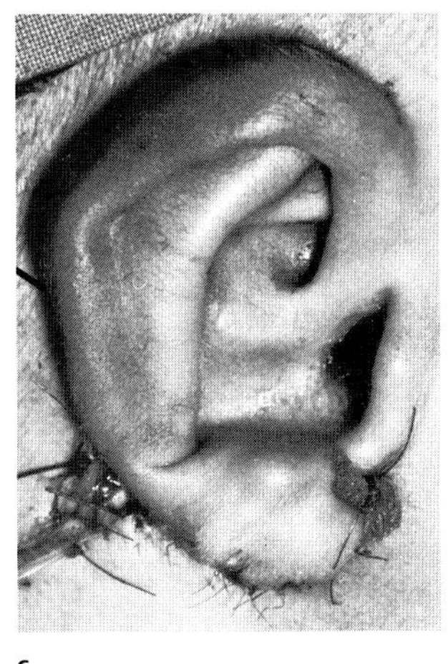

c

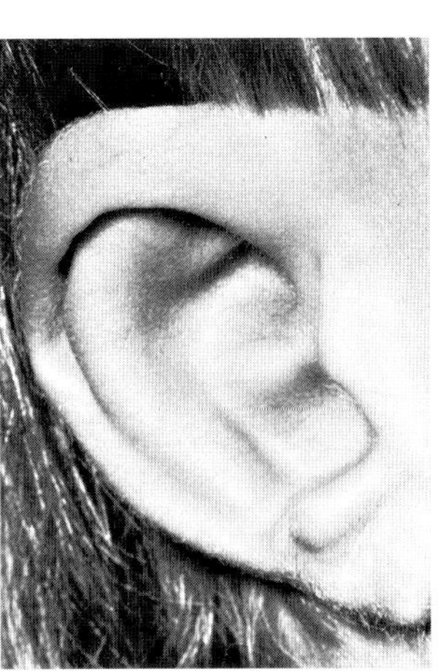

d

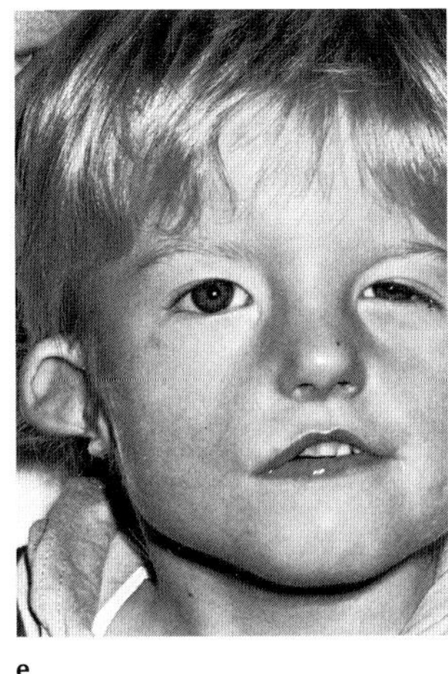

e

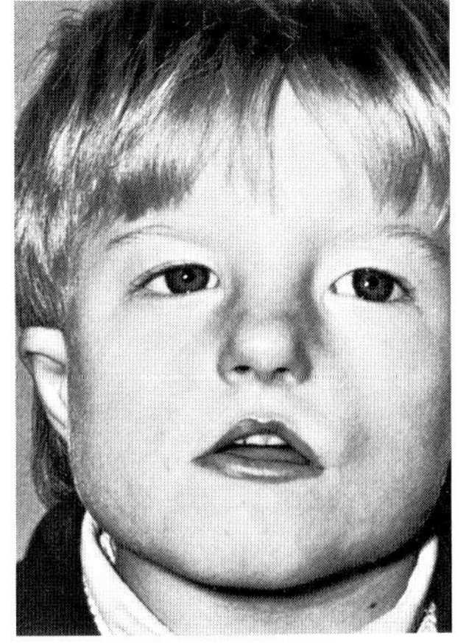

f

Fig. 5.**141** **Reconstruction of the lower auricle using the technique described by Gavello in 1903 (see also pp. 74–83).**
a A template is fashioned and Gavello's double flap is marked out (actually, this flap was described by Szymanowski in 1870). Then a cartilage strut is harvested from the contralateral concha using a template.
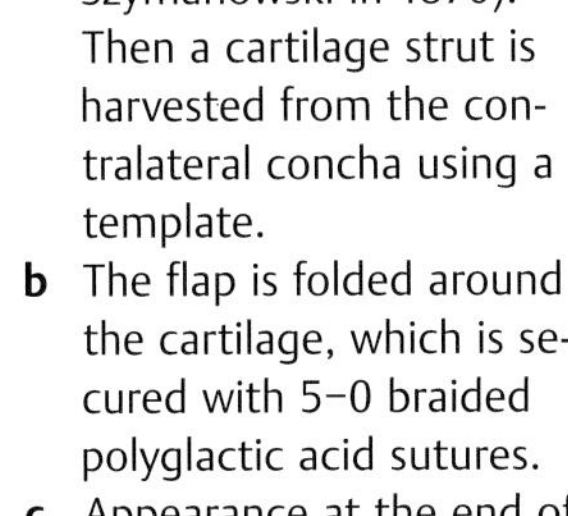
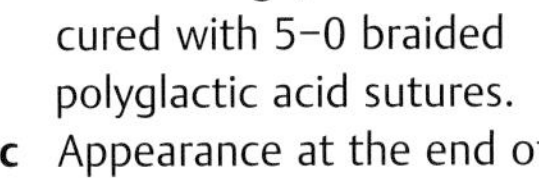
b The flap is folded around the cartilage, which is secured with 5–0 braided polyglactic acid sutures.
c Appearance at the end of the operation.
d Result.
e Bilateral mini-ear with a cup-ear form superiorly and absent earlobe.
f Appearance after bilateral reconstruction of the earlobe and expansion of the ear by antihelix reconstruction (according to Weerda 1979 a).

Mini-ears. Absent parts of the lower auricle of mini-ears are reconstructed with large Gavello flaps (see p. 75) or other flap techniques previously described in the section on defect surgery.

Auricular Reconstruction for Grade II Microtia with Dystopia of the Auricular Remnant and Presence of the Auditory Canal

P. Katzbach, S. Klaiber

In a small proportion of patients with grade II microtia, the auricular remnant is clearly displaced in comparison with its normal counterpart. This dystopia of the remnant is often combined with other malformations, such as hemifacial microsomia and facial nerve palsy. If the external auditory canal is also present, then classic auricular reconstruction will not achieve a cosmetically satisfactory result. In order to obtain the best symmetry possible, transposition of the auricular remnant and the external auditory canal is therefore advisable before auricular reconstruction, or else it is disregarded altogether (Brent 1980).

The few operative techniques described relating to this problem are based on transposition of the auricle or auricular remnant while preserving a cranial skin pedicle (Davis 1987, Hage 1967), using a fascia lata suspension sling around the cavum conchae (Kon 1996), and the cranial transposition of the auditory canal by placing drill holes in its bony wall (Lee 1999). These procedures either allow only minimal transposition, require a second intervention to divide the flap pedicle, or do not allow the combination with reconstruction of the auricle (Weerda 2004, see pp. 184, 185).

In 2002, Park published a new surgical technique for this problem (Fig. 5.**142**). He recommends transposing the remnant and the auditory canal while retaining the temporal fascia on the cranial part of the remnant. Perfusion of the remnant is via the fascia and the auditory canal. This enabled him to achieve transposition with a distance of as much as 3.5 cm without consecutive circulatory embarrassment, despite the circumferential incision of the skin (Fig. 5.**142 c**).

Patients and Methods

Between March 2003 and April 2004, three patients with a dystopic remnant (Fig. **5.143**) were treated in the ENT De-

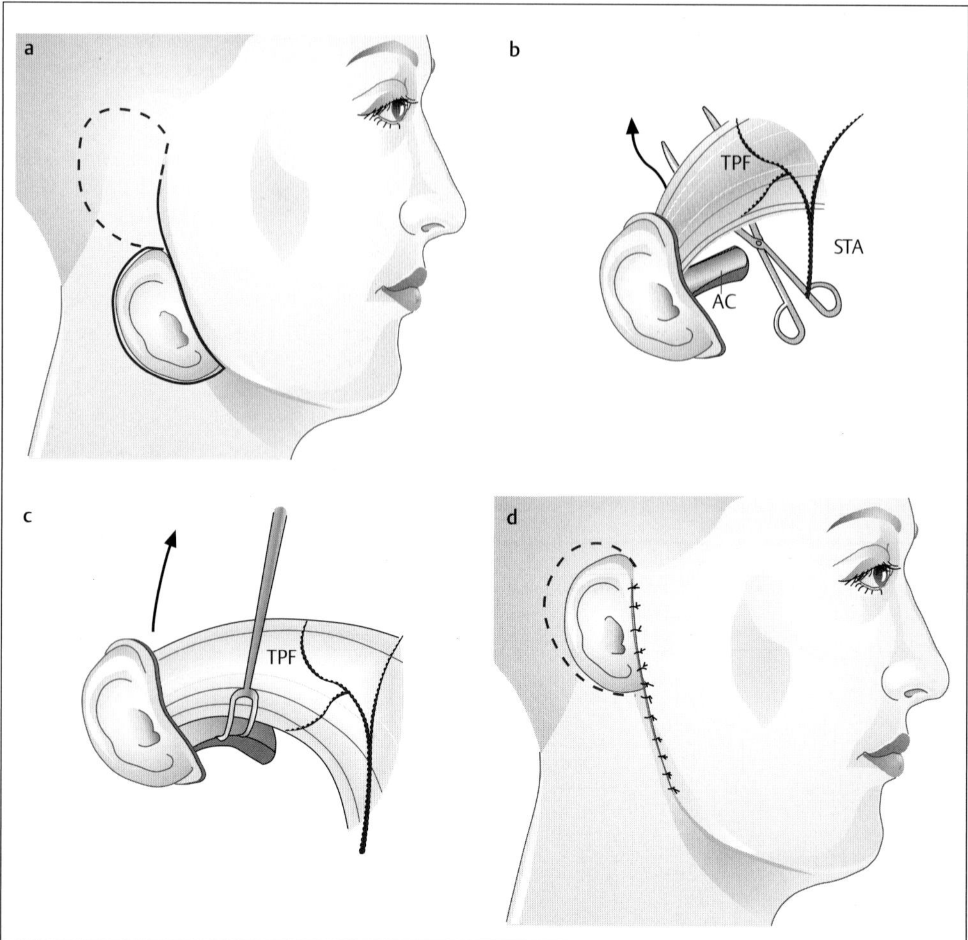

Fig. 5.**142** **YV-transposition of a dystopic auricular remnant in grade II microtia, as described by Park (2002, modified).**
a Identification of the superficial temporal artery using Doppler sonography (see p. 93, Fig. 4.**108 a**). Circumferential incision of the skin around the auricular remnant (see Fig. 5.**144 b**). Dissection of the surrounding skin with preservation of the vessels (dotted line = position of the auricle; see Fig. 5.**144 a**).
b Dissection of the auditory canal (AC), the temporoparietal fascia (TPF) and parts of the temporal muscle (arrow), while preserving the superficial temporal artery (STA). Fascia and muscle remained pedicled to the remnant.
c Transposition of remnant and auditory canal (arrow); sutures in layers.
d Position of the remnant after transposition and intended position of the auricle (dotted line; see Fig. 5.**144 c**).

partment of the University of Lübeck, Germany. All patients presented with unilateral grade II microtia, with obvious caudal dystopia, hemifacial microsomia, and incomplete facial nerve palsy.

We performed the transposition technique as described by Park (2002) in the first female patient: The relatively large remnant was completely incised circumferentially. The auditory canal was carefully dissected free under loupe magnification to avoid injury to the facial nerve. The temporal fascia was preserved at the superior end of the remnant. After excising suprameatal fibrous tissue, the cartilage was secured in its new position on the periosteum with the aid of non-absorbable sutures. The skin was closed primarily. This achieved a cranial transposition of 3.5 cm. Postoperative impairment of circulation prompted us to modify this method in the following patients by transposing parts of the temporal muscle along with the remnant.

Results

The first female patient developed subtotal necrosis of the transposed remnant during the postoperative phase. Only the auditory canal and parts of the cavum conchae were preserved. In order to avoid disturbances of circulation again in the following two cases, parts of the temporal muscles were also transposed together with the remnant (see p. 93, Fig. 4.**108**). No further complications were observed, despite transposition of a much as 4 cm (Fig. 5.**144 c**). There were no injuries to the facial nerve in any of the three cases. Auricular reconstruction with autologous costal cartilage was undertaken in each patient 3 months after transposition of the remnant (Figs. 5.**145**, 5.**146**).

Discussion

Park (2002) describes a surgical technique he used to transpose the auricular remnant on 18 patients. None of his patients experienced impairment of circulation during the postoperative phase, but the first patient on whom we performed a transposition using this technique suffered subtotal necrosis of the remnant. It should be pointed out that the transposed remnant in this case was very large and was moved a distance of 3.5 cm. In the following patients, we not only transposed temporal fascia together with the remnant,

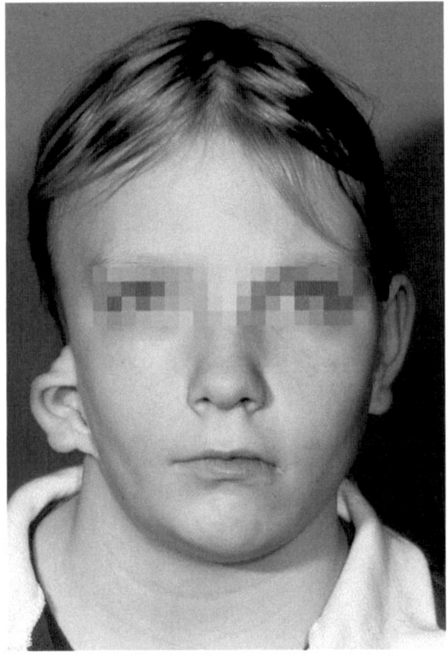

a

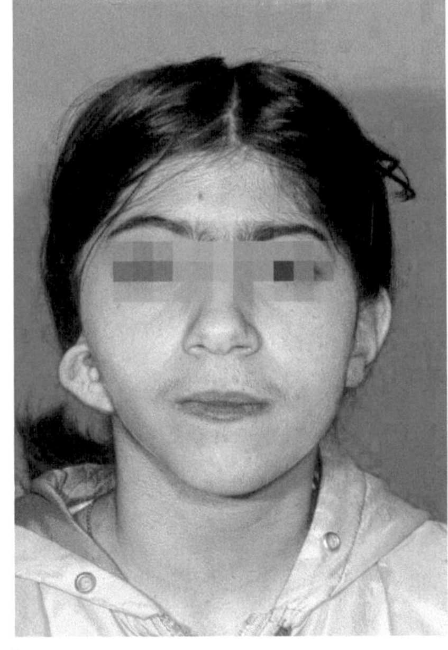

b

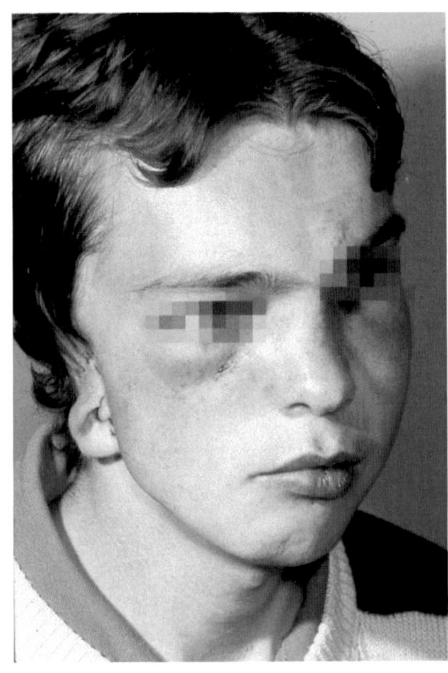

c

Fig. 5.**143**
a 13-year-old female patient.
b 16-year-old female patient.
c 17-year-old male patient with caudally dystopic remnant and the presence of an auditory canal, hemifacial microsomia, and incomplete right facial nerve palsy.

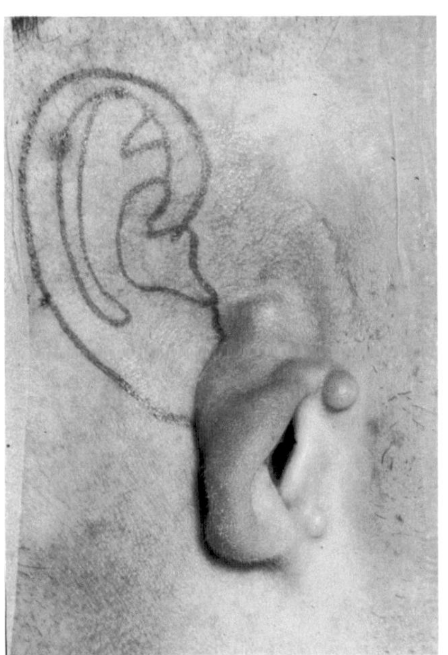

a

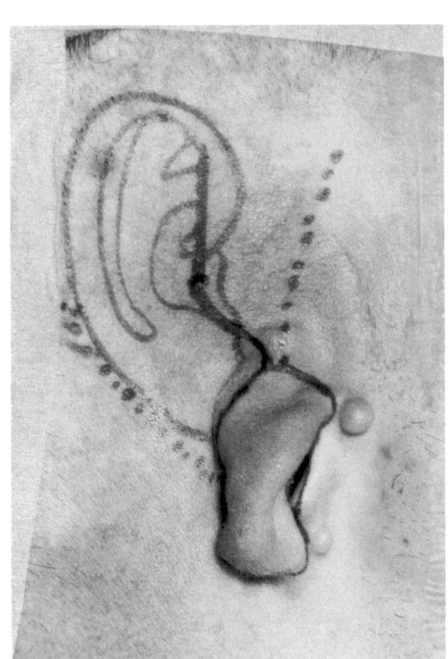

b

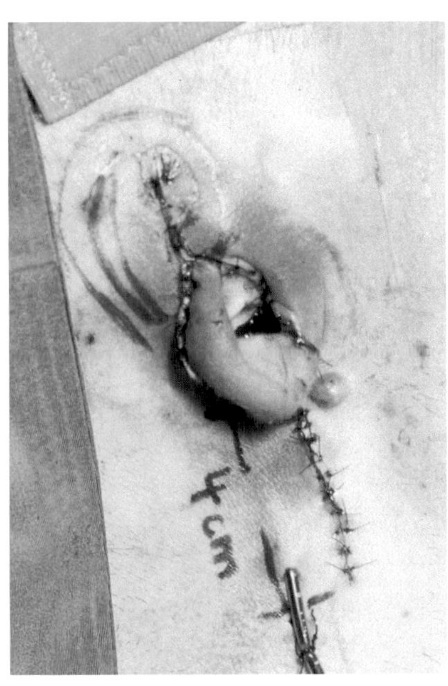

c

Fig. 5.**144** **Surgery for the patient in Figure** 5.**143 c**
a Desired position of the auricle.
b Course of the circumferential skin incision around the remnant and extended craniodorsally (continuous line), as well as the limits for mobilization of the temporal muscle (dotted line).
c Appearance on completion of the operation, with a transposed distance of 4 cm. Note also the pre- and postoperative position of the preauricular appendage relative to the remnant.

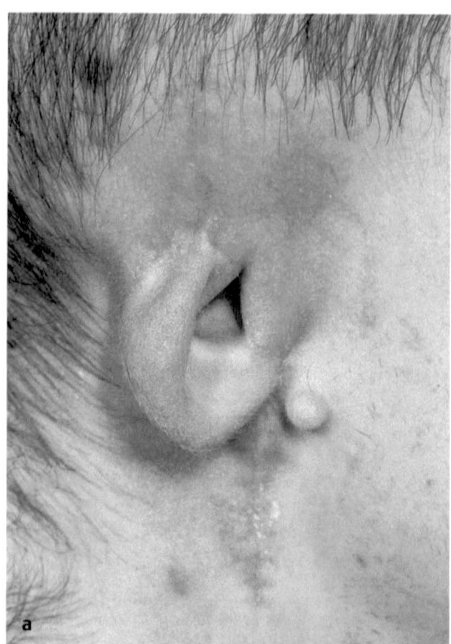

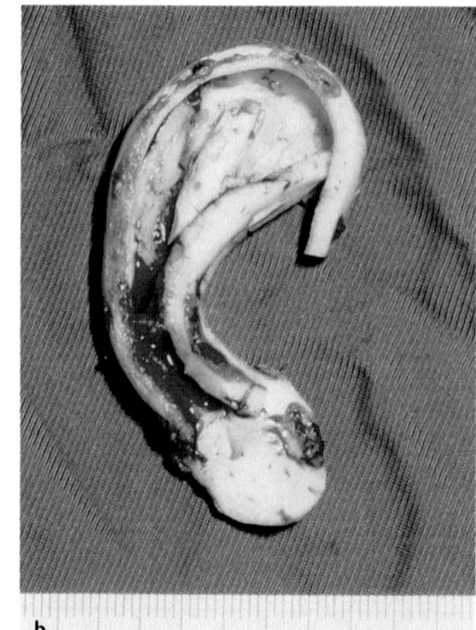

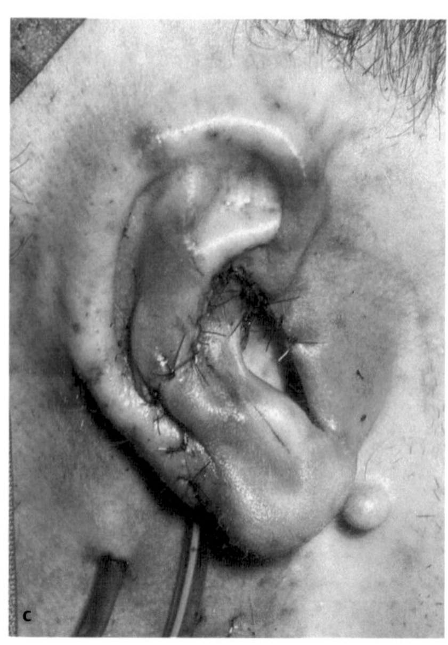

Fig. 5.**145**
a Appearance 3 months after transposition of the remnant in the patient shown in Fig. 5.**143 c**.
b Three-dimensional auricular framework fashioned from autologous costal cartilage (without the tragus).
c Inserted framework and appearance at the end of the first reconstructive stage (s. Fig. 5.**161 e, f**).

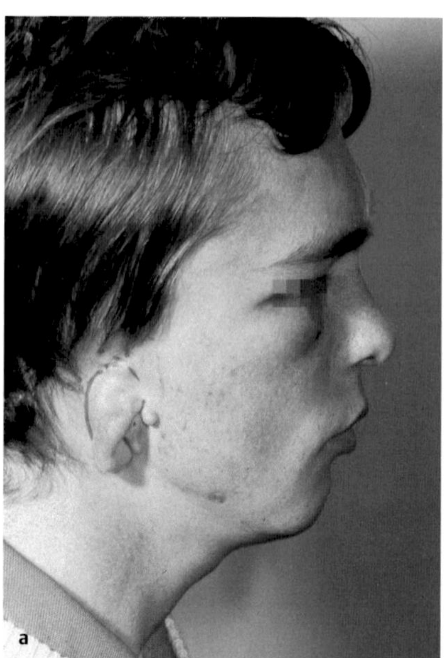

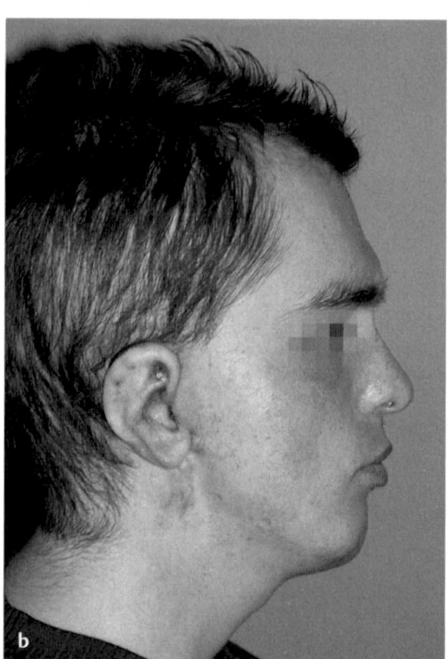

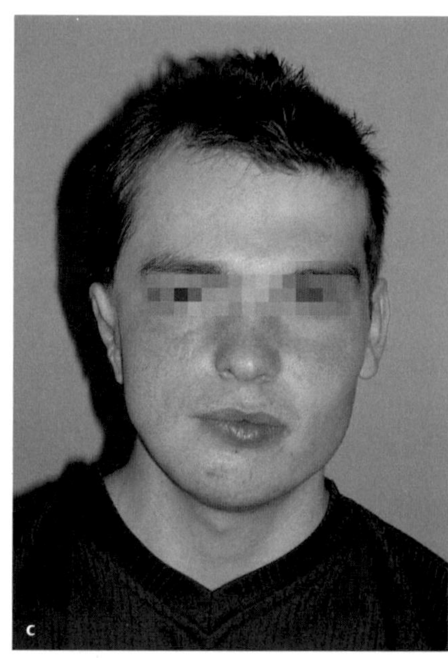

Fig. 5.**146**
a Preoperative findings.
b, c Postoperative appearance in the patient in Fig. 5.**143 c** after a total of four operations. Transposition of the remnant brought the reconstructed auricle to almost the same height as its counterpart.

but also a larger part of the temporal muscle. In our opinion, this reduced the risk to the perfusion of the fascia attached to the remnant. In addition, dissection had to proceed below the temporal muscle to expose the full circumference of the auditory canal down to its bony portion. It is probable that transposition merely on the temporal fascia and the auditory canal is sufficient for smaller remnants. However, we consider transposition together with parts of the temporal muscle to be safer for large remnants, with regard to impairment of circulation. It should be pointed out that this surgical technique is very atraumatic for the contiguous skin, so that after transposition of the remnant good preconditions are created for an esthetically pleasing result of the auricular reconstruction.

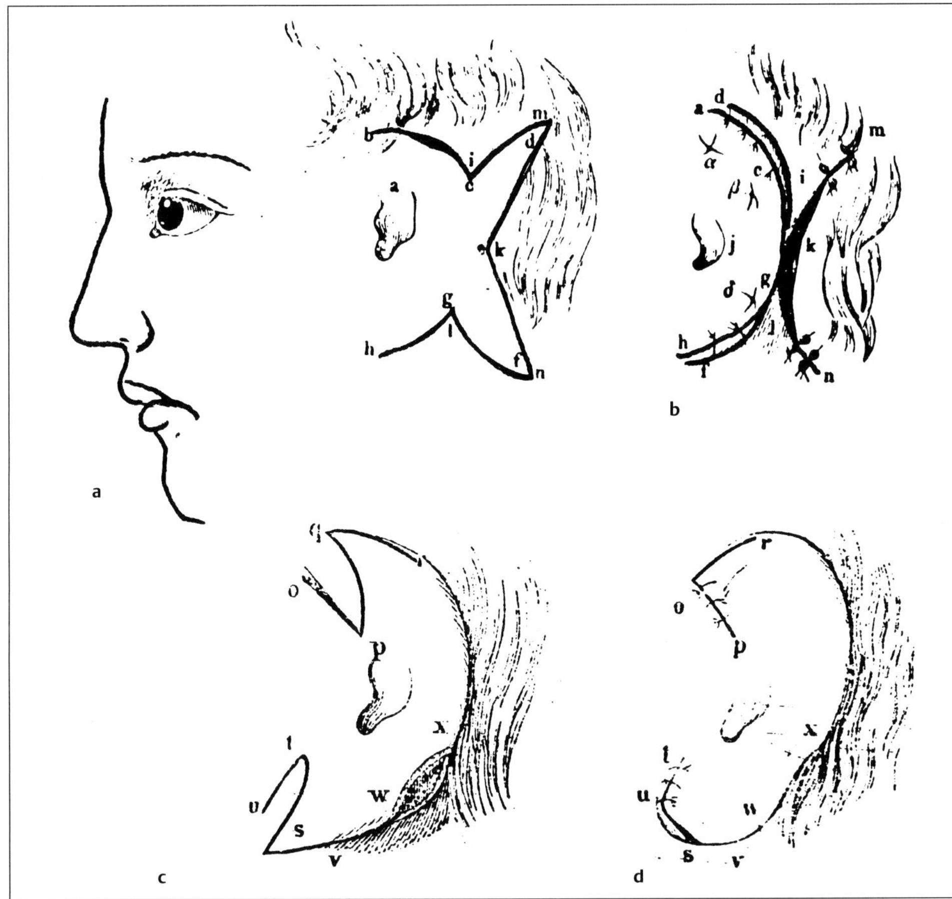

Fig. 5.**147** **Total reconstruction of the auricle as described by Szymanowski (1870).**
a Skin incision (the lower part corresponds to Gavello's double flap from 1907, see pp. 75–77).
b Folding of the auricle.
c, d Later corrections required to form the auricle.

5.4.3 Grade III Dysplasias (Microtias)

Synonyms: Grade III microtia and anotia (extreme, severe malformations of the auricle).

- **General definition.** No structures of a normal auricle are present.
- **Surgical definition.** Additional skin and cartilage (or allo plastic material) are required for total reconstruction.

Historical Review. Although in historical times repeated attempts were made to reconstruct parts of the auricle (see pp. 43 ff), total reconstruction of the auricle was thought to be impracticable right up to the late nineteenth century. Dieffenbach (1830) remarked that such an operation would only worsen the disfigurement; the result would be unshapely. Dieffenbach writes (1845 a): "I consider the replacement of the whole ear to be an entirely inappropriate experiment because it will be impossible to lend the ear its necessary form. Despite all attempts, the ear will remain an unshapely, disfigured lump." Similarly, Zeis (1838), Fritze and Reich (1845) and König (1885) did not consider total reconstruction of the auricle to be feasible. Sultan remarked in 1907: "The replacement of the missing ear with the aid of plastic surgery has been attempted, but any success has been less than satisfying, given the complexity of the auricular architecture." And Lexer wrote in 1921: "The replacement of a completely absent ear has been attempted for tumors, trauma and malformations, but so far no more than a fairly crude substitute of a construction has been created."

Beck (1923) also considered reconstruction of more than two-thirds of the auricle to be extraordinarily difficult, and Davis (1929) sarcastically remarks that although many attempts at total ear replacement have been made, the final result usually hardly resembles an auricle at all. Gillies (1937) even describes reconstruction with maternal auricular cartilage and reports on the disappointing results of his own reconstructive methods and of all those known to him.

Szymanowski reported on the first total auricular reconstruction in 1870 (Fig. 5.**147 a–d**). The illustration reproduced here shows that the main part of the skin material required for the posterior surface of the auricle lies in the hair-bearing part of the head, and also shows the lack of any form of support. Schanz (1890) was of the opinion that this lack of support must have resulted in a crude skin flap for the auricle, and that Szymanowski had probably never carried out such an operation. It should perhaps be pointed out that

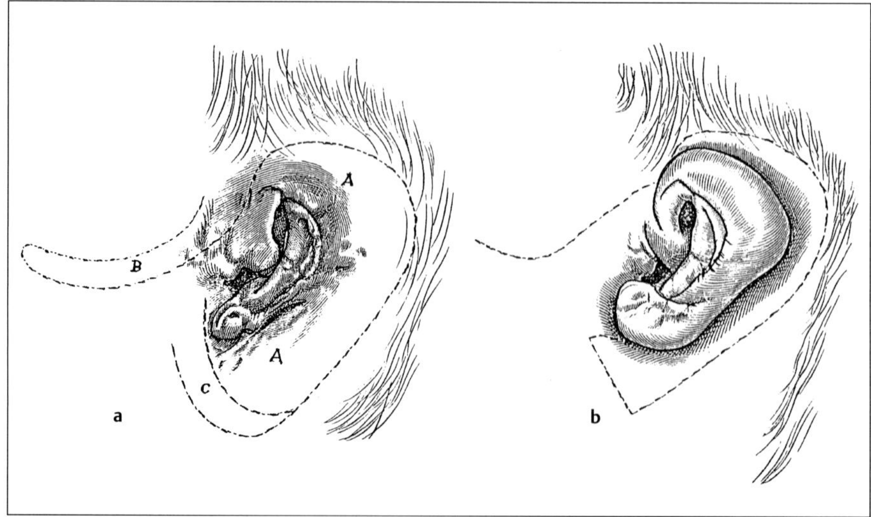

Fig. 5.**148** **Total reconstruction of the auricle as described by Schanz (1890).**
a Appearance after avulsion, reconstruction using the three skin flaps A, B, and C.
b Outcome.

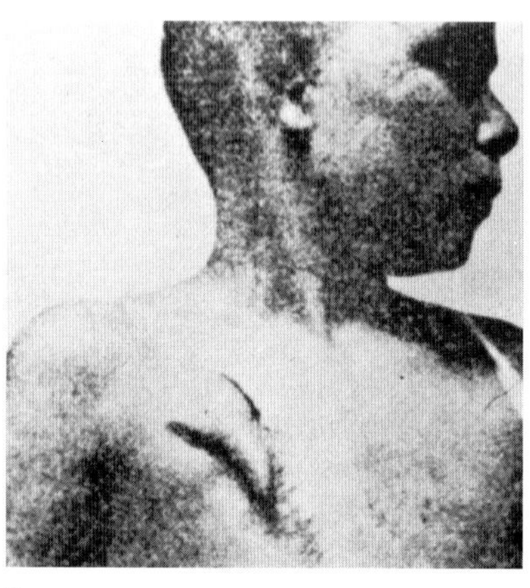
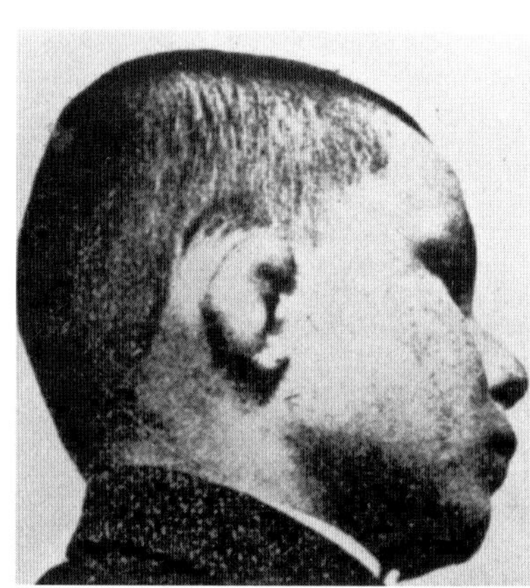

Fig. 5.**149 a, b** **Reconstruction as described by Schmieden (1908) using costal cartilage in a jump flap harvested from pectoral skin (a) which is transported via the arm to the ear (b), similar to the method described by Joseph (1931).**

the lower part of this reconstruction (Fig. 5.**147 a**) is still used today as the Gavello flap for the reconstruction of the lower auricular third (see Fig. 5.**141**).

Schanz (1890) describes a reconstruction after an almost complete avulsion where remnants of the helical crus were preserved and probably the antihelix was still available (Fig. 5.**148 a**) with some cartilage as well (Fig. 5.**148 b**).

Lexer (1910 b, 1921) modified the method described by Körte (1905) for a traumatic loss of the auricle, which Joseph also performed in 1931. Joseph explains that this method exploits the use of a triangular composite graft from the contralateral ear, similar to the transplantation described by König (1902) for the reconstruction of the nostril, provided the contralateral ear is sufficiently large.

Schmieden (1908) was the first to insert a supportive framework made of costal cartilage, although it was initially implanted into skin of the chest wall and then, via the upper arm, waltzed to the region of the ear. The outcome was a pathetic reconstructive result (Fig. 5.**149 a, b**; Schmieden 1908; Mündnich 1962 a). Joseph (1931) developed a method using an ivory framework which was implanted into the skin of the neck (Fig. 5.**150 a–d**).

Gillies (1920) was the first to take up Schmieden's (1908) suggestion again and developed a method of reconstruction which has become the model for later modern operative methods (Tanzer 1959). He implanted the carved cartilage framework into the mastoid region, directly after making an incision along the hairline, and then closed the wound. After healing, he elevated the cartilage framework and resurfaced it with an anteriorly pedicled cervical flap raised from the hairline.

Over the years, reconstructive methods have been recommended which, apart from the implantation of a framework fashioned from a wide variety of materials (Berghaus 1986; Toplak 1986; Goedecke 1995), employ the use of a range of techniques, including tube pedicle flaps from the neck or from the supraclavicular region (Pierce 1930; Padgett 1938; Kirkham 1940).

After implantation of a cartilaginous framework, a tube pedicle flap was raised in the supraclavicular region for reconstruction of the helix and waltzed as a jump flap to the region of the auricle (Pierce 1930, see p. 199). These flaps, especially when harvested from the region of the neck, result in scar formation and cosmetic impairment (Fig. 5.**151**; Mündnich 1962 a).

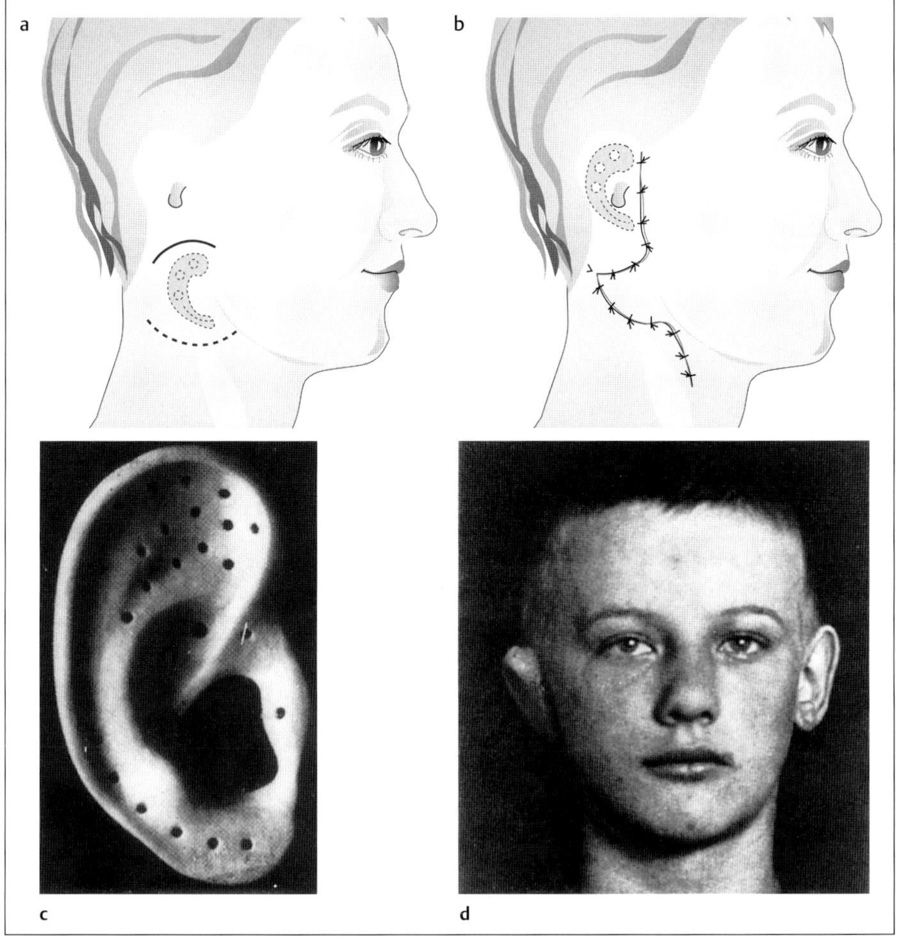

Fig. 5.**150 a–d** **Reconstruction with an ivory framework and a skin flap from the neck as described by Joseph (1931; a, b).** From Joseph J. Ohrdefekte (Otoneoplastik). In Joseph J. Nasenplastik und sonstige Gesichtsplastik. 3. Abteilung. Leipzig: C. Kabitzsch (1931: 717–736; **c, d**) [Ear defects (Otoneoplasty). In Joseph J. Rhinoplasty and other plastic surgery of the face].

An excellent overview of the various surgical methods, and in particular of the supportive frameworks used over the last 100 years, is to be found in the dissertation by Toplak (1986).

Esser (1921) and Esser and Aufricht (1922) published a technique which resembles our modern-day surgical methods even more than that of Gillies (1920). First, a framework carved from costal cartilage (Fig. 5.**152 a**) via a curvilinear incision was implanted (see p. 221, Fig. 5.**182**). After 2 months, or even later, the auricle was exteriorized, an impression was taken using a dental stent, and this impression then was enveloped by a split-thickness skin graft. This provided epithelialization of the postauricular surface and the mastoid region (Kirschner 1935). Brown et al. (1947) and Converse (1950, 1958) proceed in a similar fashion.

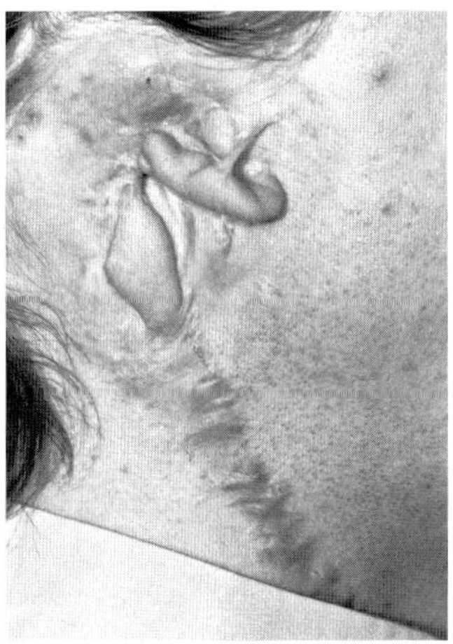

Fig. 5.**151** **A patient referred to us after several attempts at reconstruction using an alloplastic supportive framework and a pedicle tube flap from the neck.**

Summary. In the nineteenth century, plastic reconstruction of the auricle was regarded by plastic surgeons as impracticable (Zeis 1838 a; Dieffenbach 1845 a; Fritz and Reich 1845, amongst others). Although Szymanowski (1870) suggested a method of reconstruction, which was probably never performed (see Fig. 5.**147**), it was not until Victor von Schmieden (1908) first reported on an autologous supportive framework fashioned from costal cartilage that a rapid development of a large variety of methods for the total reconstruction of the ear was set in motion. Gillies (1920) and Esser (1921, Fig. 5.**152**) then went on to describe an operative technique of epithelializing the postauricular surface with split-thickness skin. They are regarded as the precursors of modern-day surgery.

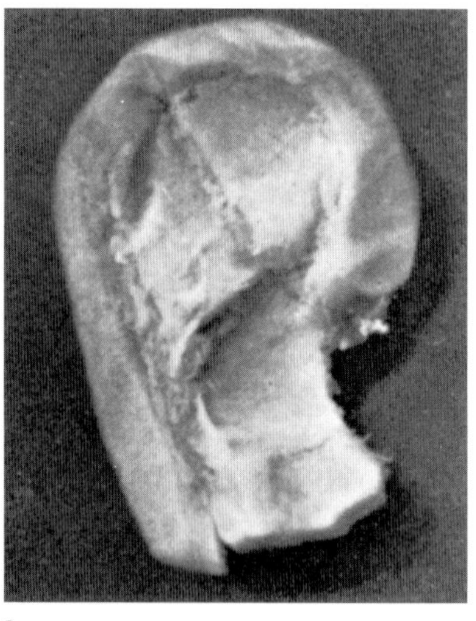

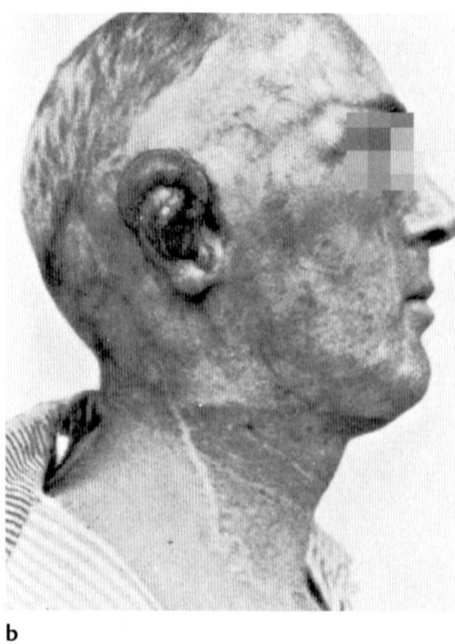

Fig. 5.**152** **Total auricular reconstruction as described by Esser (1921).**
a Carved costal cartilage framework.
b Result (scar on the neck); from: Kirschner M. Allgemeine and spezielle chirurgische Operationslehre. Vol. III/1. Berlin: Springer; 1935 [General and Special Manual of Surgical Operations].

Apart from the most frequently used autologous cartilage frameworks, alloplastic supportive materials, such as ivory (Joseph 1931) or hard rubber (Esser 1935), synthetic materials such as silicone (Cronin 1966, 1968; Edgerton 1969) or polyethylene (Edgerton 1969; Berghaus 1986) were also used. Furthermore, preserved cartilage, cartilage chips inserted into metal molds, maternal or paternal cartilage, bone, and other materials also found recommendation.

Toplak (1986) lists approximately 2500 cases of auricular reconstruction as reported in the literature, of which only about 165 date from before 1950. This shows that only after World War II was there an upsurge in total auricular reconstruction, with Burt Brent alone reporting 1200 total reconstructions of the ear in 1999. Our team has operated on about 1550 auricles and performed about 550 otoplasties, and over the last 30 years we have reconstructed about 630 grade III dysplasias out of about 950 malformations.

Supportive Frameworks

In his review, Toplak (1986) finds just over 2620 total reconstructions of the ear, of which approximately 1600, or about 60%, were performed using autologous cartilage, with the remaining 40% using various alloplastic materials or preserved cartilage, bone, or similar materials.

- **Costal cartilage** was used by Schmieden (1908), Gillies (1920), Esser (1921), Pierce (1930), and by all the famous ear surgeons such as Converse, Tanzer, Brent, Nagata, and Park, amongst others.
- **Auricular cartilage** was used by Körte (1905), Eitner (1914), Lexer (1919 b), Peer (1939, 1943) and many others. It was, however, used more frequently as a composite graft in the partial reconstruction of auricles (see section covering the surgical management of defects, p. 57).
- **Crushed (autogenous) cartilage** was used by Peer (1939), Young (1941, 1944 b), Nagel (1973, 1978) and others. Peer filled metal forms with crushed cartilage and allowed the framework to take shape in abdominal wall skin.
- **Allogenic cartilage.** Apart from maternal cartilage (Gillies 1937), allogenic cartilaginous materials were used, such as meniscal cartilage (Pitanguy 1958), or allogenic rib with various forms of preservation, as by O'Connor and Pierce (1938), Steffensen (1952), Pennisi et al. (1962), and by ourselves (Weerda 1982 d, 1984 a, Fig. 5.**153**).
- **Xenogenic cartilaginous implants.** Even Peer (1939; Mir and Mir 1952; Pitanguy 1981) worked extensively on the use of preserved cadaveric cartilage for the reconstruction of the external ear. Peer writes that cadaveric cartilage preserved in alcohol was used for a large number of operations. He concluded that fibrous transformation and partial absorption were observed in experimental studies of preserved cartilage implanted for up to 2 years, but for autogenous cartilage he witnessed no absorption even after 6 years.
- We also used cartilage conserved in thimerosal (Merthiolate) in 10 reconstructions between 1974 and 1976. This resulted in massive absorption in 7 patients (Fig. 5.**153**) and loss in 2 patients due to infection.
- **Metal, rubber, and other implants.** Especially in the early years of reconstructive auricular surgery, interesting and unusual materials were used. Thus Curtis (1920) recommends silver wire, Joseph (1931) and Eitner (1934) use ivory (see Fig. 5.**150 c**), Esser (1935) uses dental rubber, Greeley (1946) tried tantalum, and Bäckdahl et al. (1954) used, among other things, steel.
- **Silicone implants** play an important role and were used especially by Cronin (1966), Cronin et al. (1966, 1968, 1978), Brown et al. (1969), Lynch (1972), Fukuda (1974 a, 1988) and by the old master of ear surgery, Edgerton (1974). Thus, according to Toplak, the proportion of silicone implants in 1986 was 26% (679/2620). Toplak (1983) writes that, in a study, 116 of 426 implanted silicone frameworks (27%), had to be removed, with infection occurring in 46

(11 %). The infection rate was reduced when the implants were covered with the temporoparietal fascia.
- **Other artificial implants** which have been used include acrylate (Malbec and Beaux 1952; Zühlke 1960, 1964, Matthews 1961), X-ray film (Bäckdahl et al. 1954), and polyamide (nylon) (Boenninghaus 1952, Meyer 1955 b, Macomber 1960, Chmyrev 1967).
- **Teflon** has also been recommended for use as a supportive material (Meyer 1973).
- Berghaus (1986, 1988) recommends **porous polyethylene** together with temporoparietal fascia (fan flap).

Summary. Since König (1895) and Schmieden (1908) introduced cartilage transplantation to auricular reconstruction, reconstruction with autogenous costal cartilage has become the method of choice in reconstructive surgery of the external ear (see pp. 204–206).
- **Advantages** include good pliability, good supportive function, and the fact that its nutrition is that of bradytrophic tissues, subsequently resulting in low absorption and low complication rates.
- **Disadvantages** are the additional scar formation at the donor site (see pp. 204, 226), the deformation of the thorax, the time spent in fashioning the supportive frameworks and, above all, the rigidity of hyaline cartilage.

It is therefore the dream of every surgeon to implant prefabricated frameworks, but alloplastic frameworks or preserved cartilaginous frameworks have only shown good results in the short term, and reports on long-term results are few and far between.

The new methods of cultivating cartilaginous tissue are still in the development phase, yet the studies known to date show cartilage loss from absorption and low rigidity of the supportive framework (see p. 277).

Modern Surgery for Grade III Microtia

Unilateral Grade III Microtia

Converse (1958, 1963, 1967), Tanzer (1959) and his pupil Brent (1974, 1980, 1993, 1999 b) have distinguished themselves in the reconstruction of the auricle, particularly for cases of grade III dysplasia.

Until 1994, our group initially used the methods described by Tanzer and Brent and carried out versions of these reconstructive methods as modified by Nagata and presented in his publications (Nagata, 1993, 1994 a–d). When describing the reconstruction of grade III dysplasia in the sections of this chapter, we shall therefore present the two methods, which differ slightly, together with our own modifications.

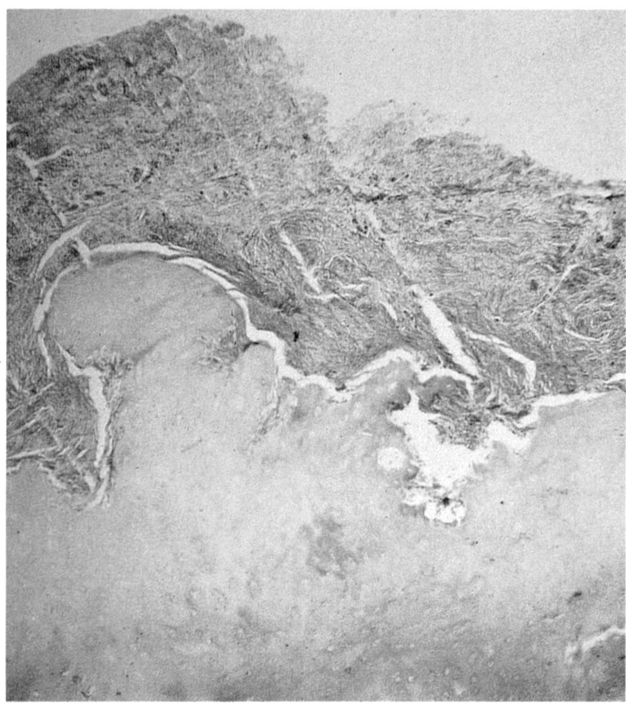

Fig. 5.**153** **Inflammatory absorption of Merthiolate cartilage (H&E stain).**

The following points should be observed:
- The size and position of the new auricle must correspond correctly to the contralateral ear.
- The contours must correspond to the contralateral ear.
- The degree of protrusion of both auricles must be equal.
- The height of both ears must be equal.
- Neither form nor size should change.
- Suitable material should be used.
- The skin color should match.

Age at Time of Surgery

Dupertuis and Musgrave (1959) recommend an age of 4 years, and Edgerton (1969) and Bauer (1984) recommend pre-school age, from 5 onwards. Bogdasarian and Baker (1983) as well as Brent (1980 I) suggest not starting before the sixth year of life. Brent (1999 a) believes that sufficient costal cartilage is available from the sixth year of life, but favors an age between 7 and 8 years.

Our eldest female patient requiring surgery for malformation was 56 years old; our eldest male patient (after amputation for a tumor) was 68 years old.

We used to prefer starting the reconstruction at 6 years of age, in accordance with Brent's recommendations, but we have found that at this age the cartilage is very soft and often insufficient, so we now prefer an age from 8 years onwards. Between 8–10 years of age children are more independent in their decision to have an ear operated, and this makes aftercare easier.

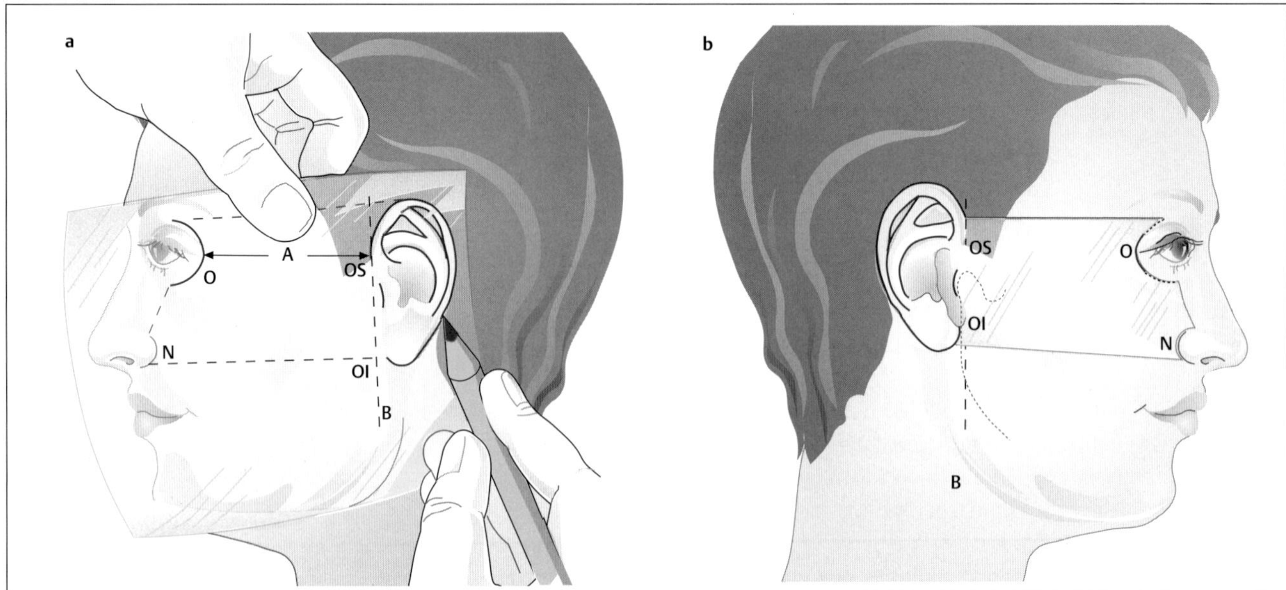

Fig. 5.**154** **Fashioning of template 1 from the intact (normal, here left) auricle (according to Weerda 1999 a).**
a The orbital margin (O), the nasal alar groove (N), the superior otobasion (OS), and the inferior otobasion (OI) are marked out. The distance A is measured from the orbital margin (O) to the line passing through OS and OI (= B; this line usually lies on the posterior margin of the ascending mandibular ramus). A transparent plastic foil (X-ray film) is superimposed on the face, the auricle, O and N are marked, and the template is excised.
b The template is superimposed on the side of the rudimentary auricle (here the right side) and the position of the new ear is marked out (see Fig. 5.**155 b, c**).

Preparation for Auricular Reconstruction and Information for Parents

The patients, or their parents, receive detailed information about the individual stages of the operation and informed consent is obtained (see surgery of the middle ear, pp. 245 and 255 ff; see Appendix 1, p. 301).

First stage. Costal cartilage is harvested, usually from the ipsilateral side, to fashion a framework for the reconstruction of the auricle, and the framework is implanted after planning the exact position of the ear (pp. 203 ff).

Second stage. Approximately 3–6 months later, the cartilage framework is elevated from its bed to resurface the postauricular surface with skin, which is harvested from the old wound in the region of the chest wall, from the buttock, or from the hair-bearing scalp. Remnants of costal cartilage are replanted into a pocket in the old chest wound after both the first and the second stage, because they may possibly be required later.

Third stage. Again, 3–6 months later, further fine tailoring of the auricular relief is carried out.

The length of stay in hospital can be very variable, lasting about 1 week or slightly longer for the first stage. The children can then go home, or stay with their parents in accommodation close to the hospital and return for further outpatient care. For the second stage, the hospital stay also lasts only a few days. A shorter stay, or even an outpatient procedure, can be considered for the remaining stages.

In-patient admission and photographic documentation. Admission is 1–2 days before the actual operation. The usual medical or pediatric pre-assessment examinations are conducted. The procedure, risks, and possible complications are once again extensively discussed with the parents, and, if this was not done during the first consultation, informed consent is obtained—signed by both parents, if possible. Standard photographs are then taken (p. 203, Fig. 5.**155 a, d**; see also p. 188, Fig. 5.**135 s**) after the hair has been generously trimmed in the proposed region of the operation: frontal view (Fig. 5.**155 a**), right and left lateral views of the head and a close-up view of the malformation (e. g., Fig. 5.**164 f**, close-up Fig. 5.**161**). Further views and other positions may also be included.

Construction of the Auricular Templates

In cases of unilateral grade III dysplasia (approximately 90 %) with practically normal configuration of the head, the healthy ear and the position of the healthy ear are measured and used as a guide for the position and size of the new auricle (see Fig. 5.**155** and Appendix 1, p. 301).

Template 1. Construction of template 1 is shown in Figure 5.**154 a, b**; see also Figure 5.**156**, Figures 4.**50**, 4.**51**, p. 64 and section on anatomy, p. 1.

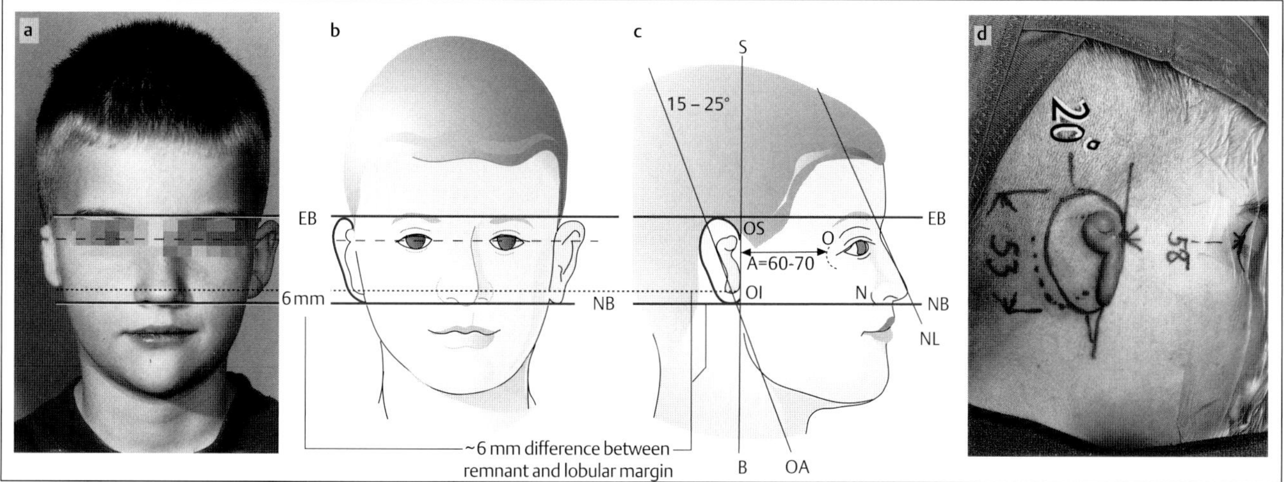

Fig. 5.**155** **Calculating the position of the auricle:** EB: eyebrow height; NB: base of the nose ≈ lobular margin (new ear); SB: base of the auricle, line through OS and OI (OS: otobasion superius ; OI: otobasion inferius); NL ≈OA: angle of the nasal line (NL) ≈ auricular axis (OA) = 15–25°; O = orbital margin; N = nasal alar groove; A = distance orbit–OS is about 60–70 mm (Fig. 5.**154**).

a, b Position of the auricle from the frontal perspective. The heights are determined by superimposing a transparent ruler.
c, d Calculating the position of the auricle from the lateral perspective.

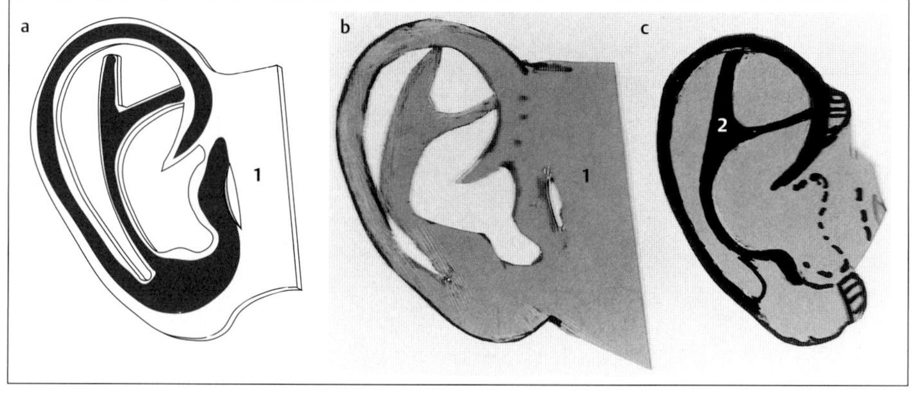

Fig. 5.**156** **Fashioning of framework template 2.**
a A framework template 2 is fashioned, based on template 1 (see Fig. 5.**154 a**). A transparent plastic foil (clear X-ray film) is superimposed on the main template 1 (normal auricular size), after which the framework template, approximately 2–3 mm smaller, is marked out using permanent ink and then cut out (template 2).
b Template 1.
c Template 2 (the light areas are then excised).

Determining the position of the new auricle. A series of points can be measured as additional controls, particularly in cases of highly varied or asymmetrical forms of malformation (Fig. 5.**155**):

- In most cases the upper auricular margin lies on the same level as the upper limit of the eyebrow arch (Fig. 5.**155 a–c**).
- The base of the auricle (SB = OS – OI) is located on a perpendicular formed by the posterior margin of the ascending mandibular ramus and the posterior border of the temporomandibular joint (Fig. 5.**155**).
- The auricular vestige is usually situated immediately behind this perpendicular (Fig. 5.**155 c**, **d**).
- The longitudinal axis of the auricle (OA) is inclined posteriorly at an angle of about 15–25° and is roughly parallel to the nasal bridge (Fig. 5.**155 c**, **d**; NL = OA, approximately).
- The lobular margin of the normal auricle is situated about 5–6 mm below the rudimentary auricle and on a level with the base of the nose (Fig. 5.**155 a–c**, NB).
- The helical attachment lies on a level with the lateral canthus, the distance (A) between orbital arch and the otobasion superius (OS) amounts to about 60–70 mm in this case (Fig. 5.**155 c**, **d**).

Converse (1958, 1963), Tanzer (1959, 1974 a, c), and Brent (1974, 1980, 1987 b) have described determining the position of the new auricle in a similar way. The position of the new auricle should also be checked from an anterior view by holding a straight edge at the level of the eyebrows and at the level of the base of the nose while the patient holds the template in the correct position (Fig. 5.**155 b**).

Template 2 (Fig. 5.156 a–c). Converse (1963), Tanzer (1974 a), and Brent (1980) recommend first constructing for the framework a template which is about 2–3 mm smaller in size. Reducing the size of the template, and thus constructing a smaller framework, is necessary because the final size of the

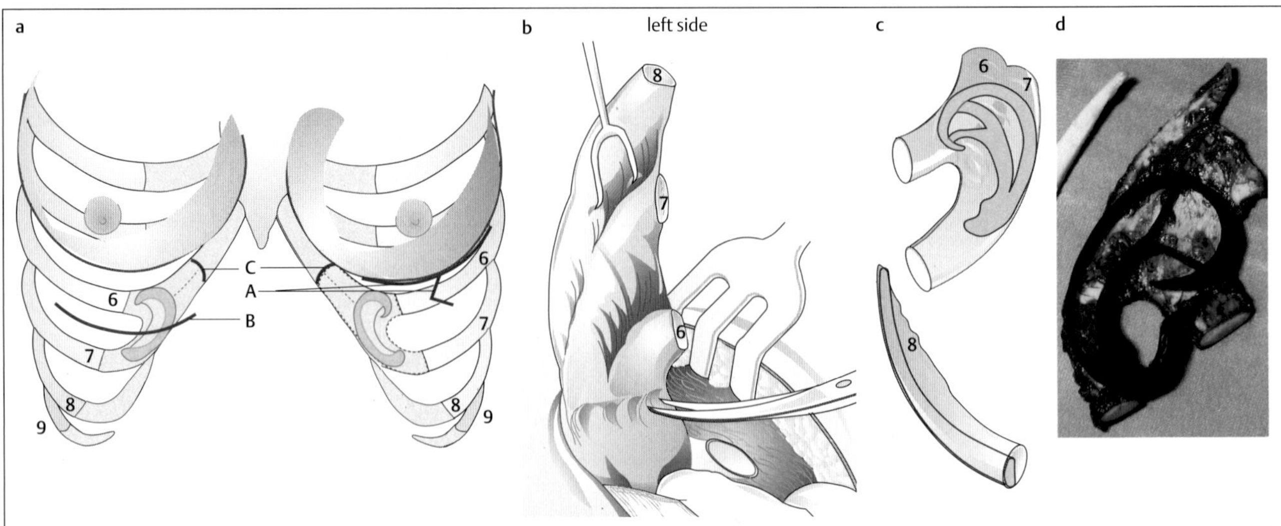

Fig. 5.**157** **Harvesting of costal cartilage (we take this from the same side as the ear to be reconstructed).**
a The incision in women lies in the submammary fold (A), alternatively a small additional Z-shaped incision. In men the incision is placed between the 7th and 8th ribs (B); C: incision of the cartilage.
b Full-thickness incision down to the 6th, 7th, and 8th ribs. Division at the osseous transition and careful dissection close to the rib or between cartilage and perichondrium (risk of injury to the pleura; the use of an electric knife is also an option).
c, d Harvesting of the 6th, 7th and 8th (or 7th and 8th) ribs for auricular reconstruction. Cartilaginous remnants or the 9th rib are preserved in the subcutaneous pocket of the chest for use as a spacer for the second stage. The costal block is then reversed to carve the framework, and the main framework is marked out after superimposing the template (**d**).

auricle also includes the enveloping skin. The length of the ear axis should also be 4–5 mm shorter.

A film is placed over the previously prepared template 1 to mark and cut out the smaller template (Fig. 5.**156 a**).

For the methods of reconstruction described by Tanzer (1974 a) and Brent (1980), marking out the tragus is not necessarily required for the construction of template 2, but is useful later for tragal reconstruction.

Harvesting Costal Cartilage

The advantages and disadvantages of the costal cartilage framework have already been discussed (see p. 201). Which donor site is the more favorable for the reconstruction is a matter of debate. Many authors favor the contralateral side (Tanzer 1974 a; Manach et al. 1987; Aguilar 1996); on the other hand, Conway (1948), Converse (1958, 1963), Cloutier (1968), Senechal and Pech (1970), Furnas (1991), Eavey (1995), and Weerda (1982 IV, 1999 a, 2001, 2004) have all reported the ipsilateral side. Frameworks fashioned from costal cartilage of the contralateral side have a somewhat more favorable shape. Harvesting from the same side as the auricle to be reconstructed is, however, preferred by some of surgeons for convenience of positioning, and being able to place the anesthetist and his equipment on the contralateral side.

We no longer use the **open-type** or **cantilever frameworks** (Brent 1974, 1977) because pressure from the scar may cause them to lose their form. They incorporate larger "windows," especially in the scapha, and experience has shown that such large gaps in the structure render it unstable, resulting in warping of the helix from the effects of scar formation.

Expansile frameworks. From the 1990s onward, Brent preferred "closed" or expansile frameworks, with at most small gaps in the triangular fossa. This construction was more robust and stable against the effects of scar formation. For reconstruction of the auricle a **basic framework** is carved from the 6th and 7th ribs (Fig. 5.**157 a**); the **helix** is usually obtained from the 8th rib (Fig. 5.**157 c**). Depending on the size of the framework, the 8th rib should ideally be 8–10 cm long. If sufficient length cannot be obtained or if the 8th rib is broken, as is often the case in adult patients with areas of calcification within the costal cartilage, then the helix will have to be assembled from individual parts (see Figs. 5.**158**, 5.**159**).

Harvesting is usually performed under general anesthesia, so smaller amounts of cartilage can also be taken from the 4th, 5th, or 6th ribs, close to the sternum.

Approach. If possible, we incise along the inframammary fold in women (Fig. 5.**157 a**, A), and in men parallel to the donor region over the 7th rib (Fig. 5.**157 a**, B). The 7th rib is the last one still attached to the sternum (Rauber-Kopsch 1955); the 8th rib is slightly shorter and thus often connected to the 7th rib by synchondrosis.

For the auricular reconstruction, we harvest the 6th and 7th ribs ***en bloc*** to provide the cartilaginous base (Fig. 5.**157 b–d**, Fig. 5.**158**). The 8th rib is usually taken for the helix (Fig. 5.**157 c**).

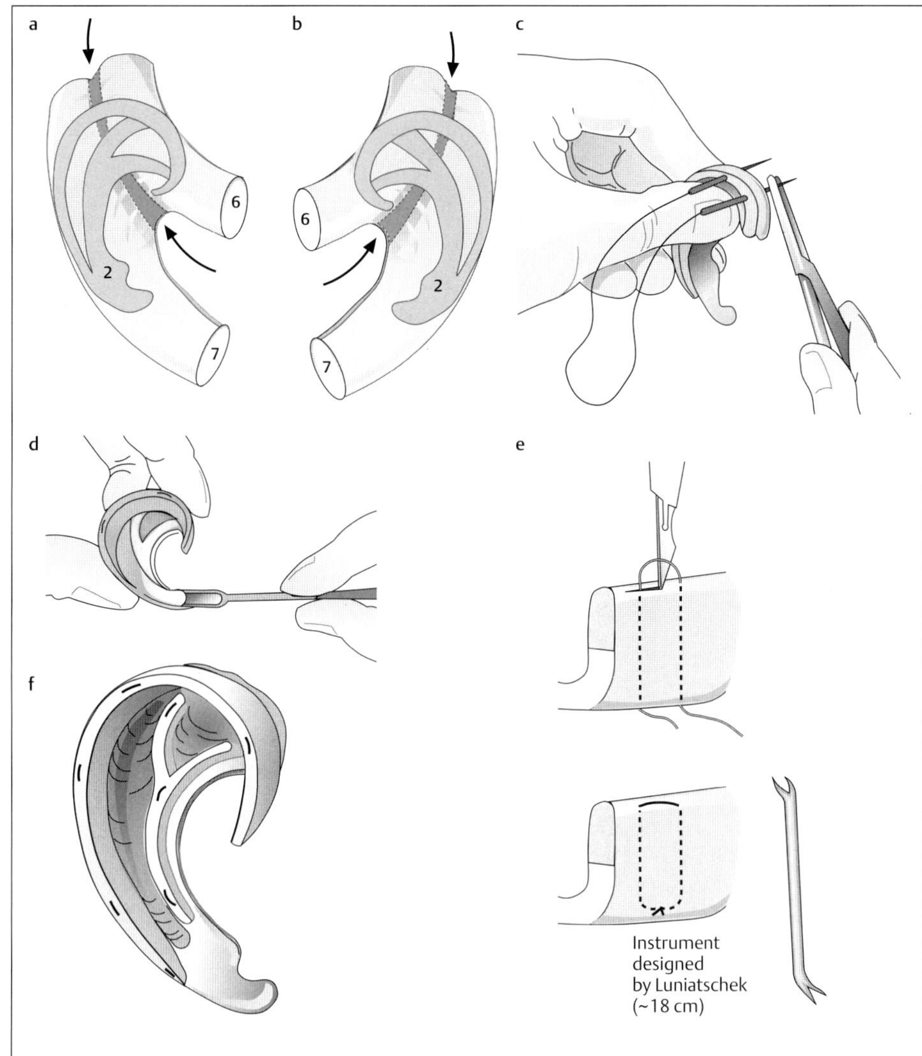

Fig. 5.**158** **Fashioning of a framework as described by Brent (1987 a; modification from Weerda and Siegert 1999 b; the same framework is also suitable for total reconstruction of the auricle).**

- **a** Right ear: harvesting from the right side and reversal of the block (parietal side superior).
- **b** Left ear: harvesting from the left side (see above; proceed in a corresponding fashion when harvesting rib from the contralateral side).
- **c** After carving the helical framework (see Fig. 5.**159**), it is sutured into place with 4–0 braided polyglactic acid (Brent) or 5–0 steel wire (Converse 1963; Nagata 1994 a–d; Weerda 1999 a), double-armed (5–0 steel wire with 2 ST-4 plus needles, sharp; 19.1 mm; see Appendix 2, p. 305).
- **d** Deepening of the scapha.
- **e** The steel wire is buried using a size 11 blade and the bifurcated instrument designed by Luniatschek.
- **f** Finished framework. (For practice, frameworks may be carved from porcine or bovine cartilage, or even from potato, bars of soap, or plaster-of-Paris blocks.)

Operative approach. The operation is performed under general anesthesia and we generally infiltrate the incision area with a local anesthetic plus epinephrine, diluted 1 : 200 000. The skin is incised parallel to, or above, the 7th rib, and the fascia and muscle layers divided down to the rib. The 6th, 7th, and 8th ribs are dissected, the 9th if necessary. The wound is held open with a self-retracting clamp or by the assistant. When removing whole cartilaginous ribs, the muscles of the posterior surface are divided superficially with an electric knife, parallel to the rib and close to the cartilage. Template 2 (see Fig. 5.**156**) is placed over the 6th and 7th ribs (Fig. 5.**157 d**). While holding away the parietal pleura, the ribs are divided at the bony region. When, on occasion, the antihelix needs expansion (see Fig. 5.**158**) and a cartilaginous spacer is required for the second stage (see Fig. 5.**171 b**), parts of the cartilaginous 6th and 7th ribs are also removed towards the sternum (Fig. 5.**157 a, c**). The 6th and 7th ribs, together with the 8th rib, are then removed ***en bloc***, taking care to protect the pleura (Fig. 5.**157 b**). Where there is insufficient cartilage, the 9th rib is also removed (Fig. 5.**157 a**, 9).

Pleura check, pleura defect. The integrity of the pleura is checked by passing Ringer's solution into the defect in the chest wall and observing whether bubbles appear when the lung is expanded. If there is a defect in the pleura, it is repaired with fibrin glue using a pedicled or free piece of fascia. We like to insert a collagen fleece, soaked with blood, into the larger defects. Siegert (2001, personal communication) places small pieces of spare cartilage into nets made of resorbable braided sutures, sewn into the form of ribs, to fill out the defects. He was able to observe contiguous **costal neoformation**, particularly in children, thus avoiding deformities of the chest. Analgesics can also be infiltrated into the wound for pain control. The incision is closed in layers after inserting a vacuum drain into the defect. Skin closure is accomplished with intracuticular 4–0 monofilament suture material to avoid hyperplastic scar formation. These mea-

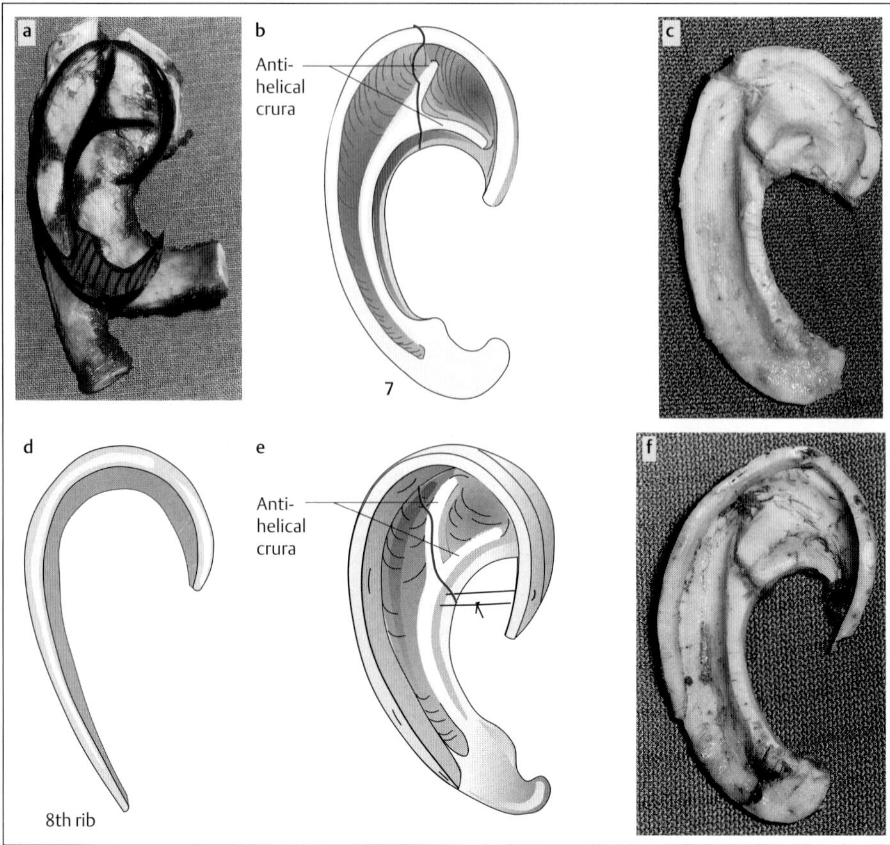

Fig. 5.**159** **Fashioning of a framework as described by Weerda (1999 a; Tanzer 1974 a–d; Nagata 1994 a–d; from Weerda 1999 a, 2001).**
a–c Main framework harvested from the 6th and 7th ribs of the ipsilateral side (**a**), deepening of the scapha and fossa (arrow: synchondrosis between the 6th and 7th ribs).
d The helix is carved from the 8th costal cartilage (approximately 8–10 cm long).
e, f The helical rim is sutured onto the main cartilage with wire sutures (see Fig. 5.**158**; double armed 5–0 steel wire, straight needle, or ST-4 plus needles (sharp) (see Appendix 2; helical depth about 6–8 mm down to the scapha, in the fossa and supero-inferiorly). The wire sutures are buried (see Fig. 5.**158**). The curve of the helical root can be improved with the aid of a 4–0 braided polyglactic acid suture (see Fig. 5.**168 b, c**)
For practice suggestions, see Fig. 5.**158**.

sures obviate fears of any further complications, even after injury to the parietal pleura. Postoperative pain control is achieved in children using patient-controlled analgesia (Lindig et al. 1997).

Brent's Method of Reconstruction of the Auricle for Grade III Dysplasia

Fabrication of a Cartilage Framework

(Brent 1980, 1987 b, 1993, 1999 a; Fig. 5.**158**)

Positioning and draping (see p. 129). The face should be covered with a transparent foil.

Although Brent preferred an open-type framework until about 1980, in his more recent work he recommends only the use of an expansile framework (see Fig. 5.159).

After harvesting costal cartilage (see p. 204), a cartilaginous framework is fabricated as described by Brent (1987 b, 1993, 1994). After removing the 6th and 7th costal cartilages from the ipsilateral side (Fig. 5.**158**) and the 8th rib for the helix, the body of the framework is fashioned from template 2 (see p. 203, see also p. 212 for measurements), making it approximately 2–3 mm smaller than the intended auricle (template 1, see Fig. 5.**156**).

Brent first sutures the previously carved helix (approximately 2–2.5 mm wide, 5–7 mm high, and as near to 9–10 cm in length as possible, Fig. 5.**158 c**, **f**) onto the basic framework (Fig. 5.**158 c**) using double-armed braided sutures or 5–0 wire. Only then does he deepen the scapha (Fig. 5.**158 d**).

As previously suggested by Converse (1963), wire should be buried in the cartilage when used (Fig. 5.**158 e, f**). For this purpose, small incisions are placed in the cartilage over the helix (Fig. 5.**158 e**) using a size 11 knife and the wire drawn in. Similarly, an incision is made in the posterior surface of the framework before twisting the wire and the knot is buried in the cartilage using a special bifurcated instrument designed by Luniatscheck.

Our modification. Following the suggestions made by Tanzer (1974 b) and Nagata (1994 a–d), we first carve the base and deepen the scapha and triangular fossa (Fig. 5.**159 a–f**) before affixing the helix (see Fig. 5.**159**). The antihelix may also be expanded if required (see framework as described by Nagata 1994 a, p. 212).

Important. Only a relatively short antihelical crura should be carved (Fig. 5.**159 b**, **e**); the scapha in this region needs the same width and depth as behind the superior crus (indentation of the skin).

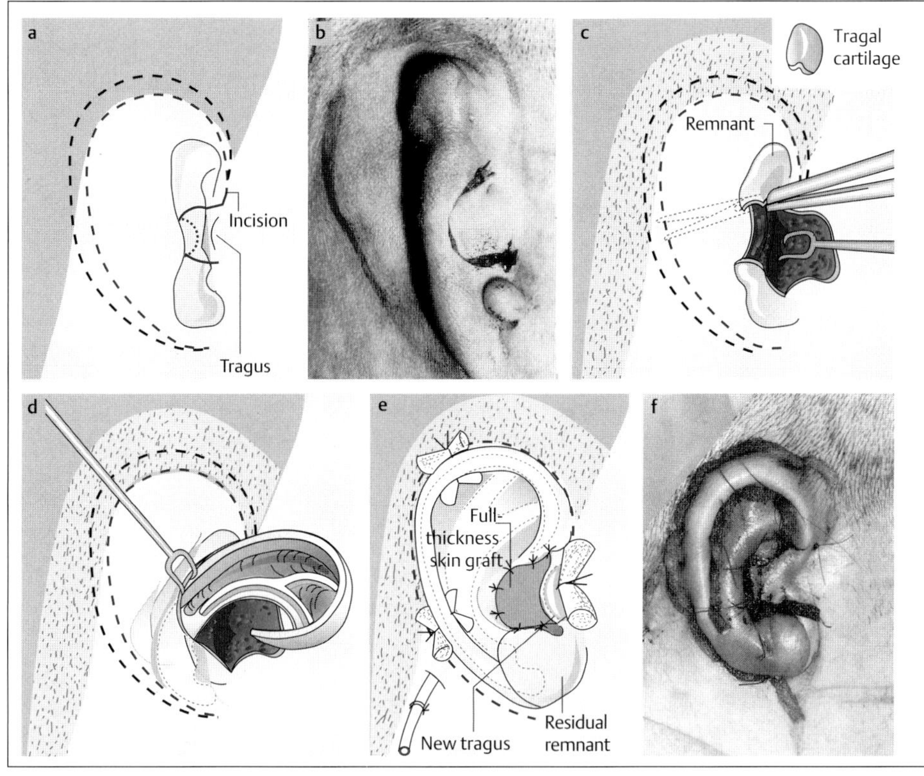

Fig. 5.**160** **First stage of reconstruction of grade III dysplasia (microtia) as described by Brent (1987 a, 1992), modified according to Weerda and Siegert (1994 b; see also Fig. 5.177, p. 219).**
Insertion of the cartilaginous framework.

a, b Position of the auricle (broken red line), superior and inferior incision anterior to the remnant and extending into the remnant in the region of the tragus (flap to be draped over the tragus).
c Removal of the rudimentary cartilage, a part of which is fashioned as a cartilaginous strut (tragal cartilage), and tunneling of the skin as far as the broken black line.
d Insertion of the cartilaginous framework, secured by mattress sutures tied over cotton bolsters (**e**).
e Placement of 1–2 vacuum drains; the shape of the auricle is formed using mattress sutures tied over cotton bolsters. If there is insufficient skin in the concha, a full-thickness skin graft harvested from the contralateral auricular sulcus is sutured to the tragal skin (tragal cartilage formed from remnant cartilage).
f Here the shape of the earlobe has already been sufficiently formed, rendering any transposition of the remnant unnecessary. Brent (1992) rejects mattress sutures because of the risk of necrosis (in which case a vacuum drain over 6–7 days is essential).

Reconstruction Procedure

Surgery for grade III dysplasia as described by Brent (1987, 1993 modified).

First stage. Insertion of the costal cartilage framework (Fig. 5.**160 a–f**). A dressing is carefully applied without pressure, and the vacuum drain is removed after about 7 days. After about 12 days the entire dressing is taken down. The child must refrain from sports for approximately 3 weeks. The child should also sleep on the contralateral side and use a soft pillow to guarantee a good contour to the helix (for dressings, see p. 223).

Second stage. If necessary, the auricular vestige is transposed to create the earlobe (Fig. 5.**161 a–f**).

Brent (1987 b) reports that he prefers transposing the earlobe after 8 weeks at a second stage, when, as he states, the exact positioning of the earlobe is possible (see Fig. 5.**160 e**, Fig. 5.**161 c**, **d**). In addition, the concha is excavated during the same session and, if necessary (if this was not done at the first stage), the resulting defect is covered with a full-thickness graft taken from the sulcus of the contralateral auricular region (Fig. 5.**161 c**, **e**).

Third stage. The posterior surface is dissected free and epithelialized with thick split-thickness skin (Fig. 5.**162 a–g**).

At this stage, and occasionally together with the lobular transposition at the second stage, the skin behind the framework is incised in the region of the upper helix, particularly in cases with small, hair-bearing areas (Fig. 5.**162 a**; better: Nagata's method 1994 a–d, see p. 215) and a thick split-skin graft applied (see Fig. 5.**162 b–e**).

Next, a sponge tie-over dressing (see p. 216, Fig. 5.**172 f**) with the sutures left long is applied under mild pressure and left until the free graft has taken. Brent (1999) reported on 1200 auricular reconstructions using autogenous costal cartilage. After attending our symposium in Lübeck in 1997 (Weerda and Siegert 1998 e) he followed our suggestions and made slight alterations to his method of reconstruction. During the first stage he attached the tragus to the framework along the lines of Nagata's suggestions (Nagata

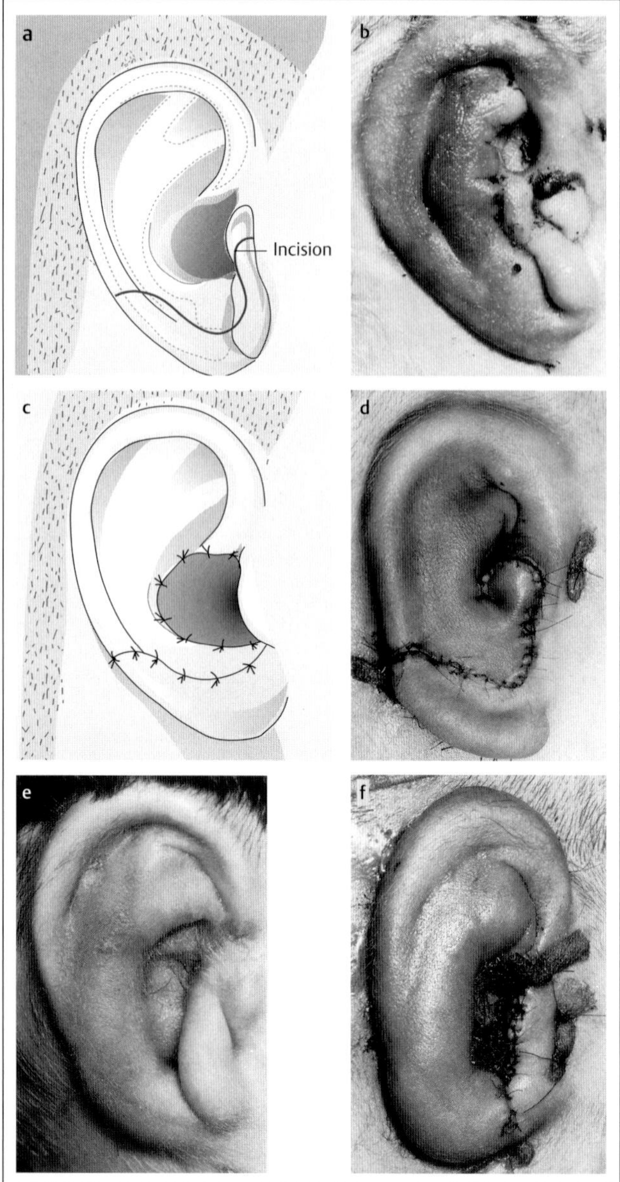

Fig. 5.**161** **Second stage of reconstruction for grade III dysplasia (microtia), as described by Brent (1987 a, 1992), modified.**

Transposition of the remnant to form the earlobe.

a, b Incision of the remnant and exposure of the inferior cartilaginous framework at the corresponding site (if the shape of the tragus was not formed during the first stage, it can be done now; see Fig. 5.**160**).

c, d Transposition of the earlobe and suture (using a template of the ear). At this stage the postauricular surface can be epithelialized, especially if there is no tragus to be formed (see also Nagata's technique).

e, f Transposition of the remnant is not necessary in the case of this ear; it is used instead to form the tragus (see Fig. 5.**160**).

1994 a–d) and, to augment ear projection, incorporated into his operative procedure a crescent-shaped piece of cartilage (Nagata 1994 a) and, following our suggestions, a musculofascial flap (Weerda 1998 a; see Fig. 5.**172**; following the description of Nagata's method 1994 a–d).

Fourth stage. Construction of the tragus as described by Brent (1987 b, 1992, Fig. 5.**163**; our modification in Fig. 5.**160** and Fig. 5.**161**).

The fourth stage is undertaken some months later. A new tragus is created from the contralateral auricle (Fig. 5.**163 a**). Since a small defect usually remains below the new tragus in the region of the concha, it is covered with a small full-thickness skin graft taken from the postauricular region of the contralateral ear (Fig. 5.**163 b**; see also p. 219, Figs. 5.**177**, 5.**178**).

Brent's technique is currently used by many authors (Boudard and Portmann 1987; Aguilar and Jahrsdoerfer 1988; Aguilar 1996; Simmen 2001 personal communication).

Deepening of the scapha and concha. The scapha may be deepened during the same session (Fig. 5.**164 a–f**; see also p. 205), if necessary combined with augmentation of ear projection (Fig. 5.**165 a, b**; see Fig. 5.**177**, p. 219).

If the second stage of Brent's method is performed using neither Nagata's technique (see p. 212) nor our modified Nagata technique (see p. 215), projection of the auricle is augmented during the third stage, if necessary combined with a reduction of the contralateral auricle (see Figs. 5.**165**, 5.**166**), by dissecting a tunnel from an incision in the sulcus and inserting a piece of cartilage approximately 35–40 mm long and 8 mm high (see Fig. 5.**164 e** and Fig. 5.**165**; result shown in Fig. 5.**164 f**).

Adjustments to the contralateral ear. Occasionally the malformed auricle cannot be recreated to the same size as the contralateral ear, in which case we suggest reducing the normal ear, usually with the modified Gersuny technique (1903; see p. 155; see Figs. 5.**74**, 5.**75**).

An additional otoplasty can also be performed (measurements of the reconstructed and contralateral ears taken before the operation; see p. 120).

Reconstruction in the presence of previously damaged skin. If the skin has been previously damaged, expansion may be used to gain a sufficient amount of skin (see p. 231). Otherwise, the use of temporoparietal fascia is possible, provided the temporal vessels are intact (see pp. 74, 93). If the auditory canal is well positioned, the auricle can also be reconstructed with the available skin of the external ear as described by Brent (Fig. 5.**167 a–c**).

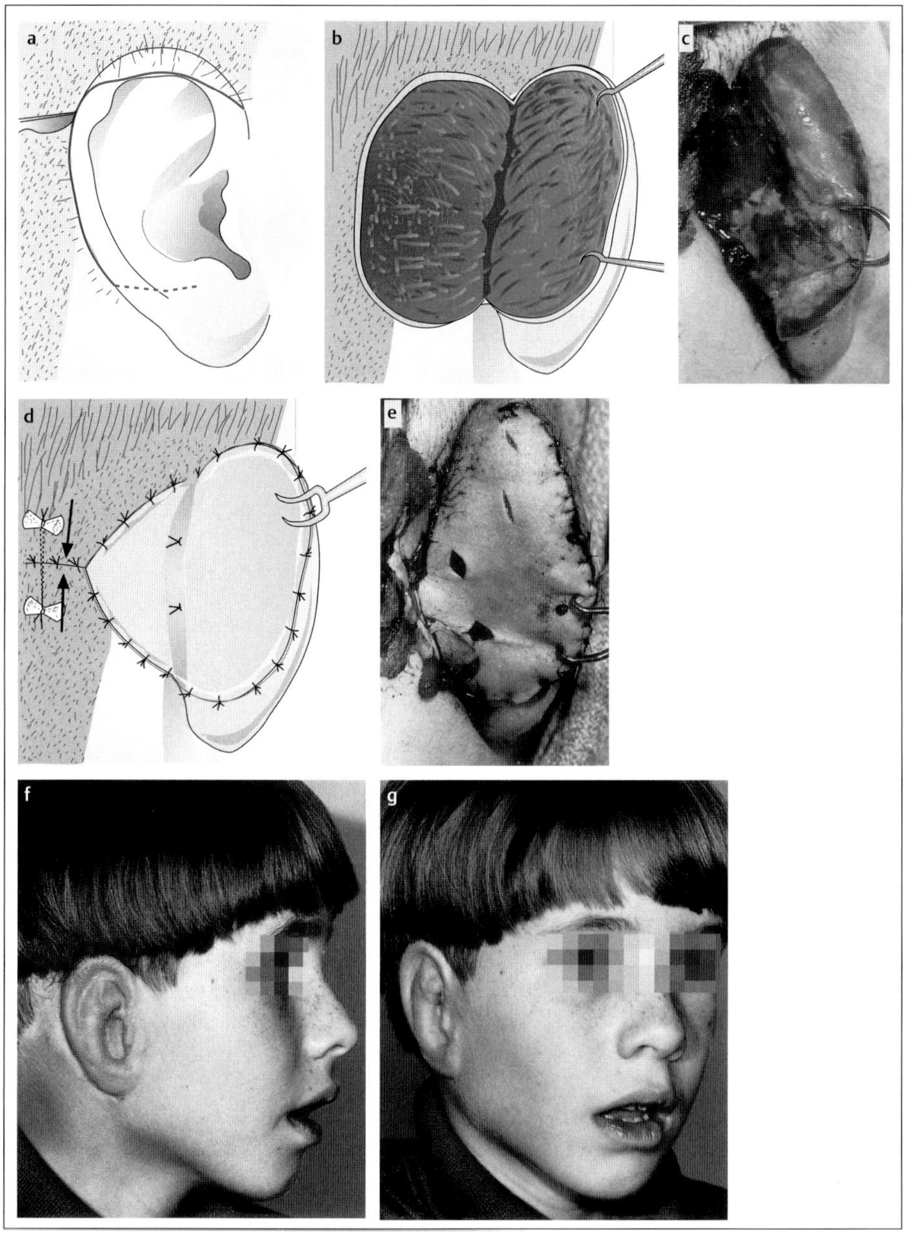

Fig. 5.**162** **Third stage of the reconstruction as described by Brent (1987 a, 1992 b, 1998 a).** Epilation and epithelialization of the postauricular surface (see also pp. 220, 221, 275 ff).

a Incision (red line).

b, c Careful dissection of the hair-bearing skin from the anterior and posterior auricular surface (we prefer Nagata's technique, see p. 215). A nutrient layer of fibrous tissue is left on the cartilage.

d, e The size of the wound on the mastoid is reduced and resurfaced with thick split skin (from the chest wall or buttock), glued with fibrin adhesive, and sutured using 5–0 monofilament material. Individual sutures are inserted in the sulcus for fixation (S).

f, g Result (dressing see p. 223).

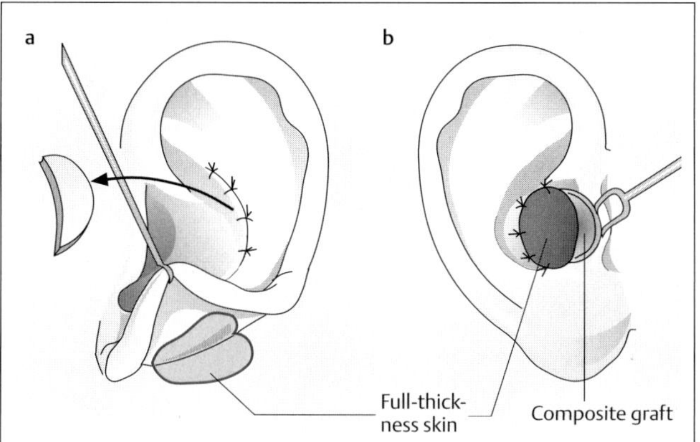

Fig. 5.**163** **Reconstruction of the tragus using a composite graft from the contralateral side as described by Brent (1987 a, 1992 b, 1998 a).**

a A two-layer composite graft is harvested from the concha of the contralateral side according to a template. The wound is closed.

b Incision in the concha of the reconstructed ear. Insertion of the composite graft and suture. Coverage of the residual defect in the concha with skin from the contralateral postauricular region (see **a**).

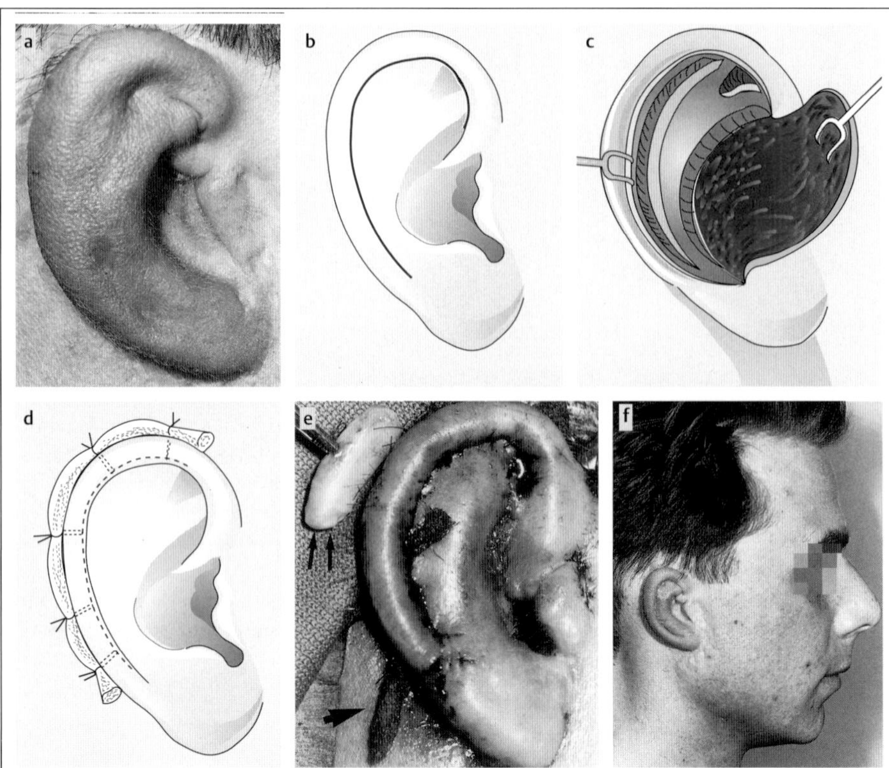

Fig. 5.164 **Deepening of the scapha (also of the concha, if required) in cases of flat contours or hyperplastic scarring (see also p. 72, Fig. 4.66 g).**
a Flattened scapha.
b Incision in the scapha (red line), near to the antihelix (see also Fig. 5.**174**).
c The skin is dissected around the helix and over the antihelix. Scapha, fossa and concha are deepened. If required, epilation by removing hair follicles from the helix.
d, e Suture of the incision in the scapha using 6–0 polydioxanone, or a similar material. The suture line is brought into the scapha using 5–0 polydioxanone (FS 2 needle) and knotted over cotton bolsters (broad arrow). Ear projection is augmented with the aid of cartilage (two arrows, see Fig. 5.**165**). If necessary, 1–2 mattress sutures to form the shape of the concha (long straight needle, 5–0 or 4–0 monofilament suture material).
f Result (see Fig. 5.**174**, p. 218).

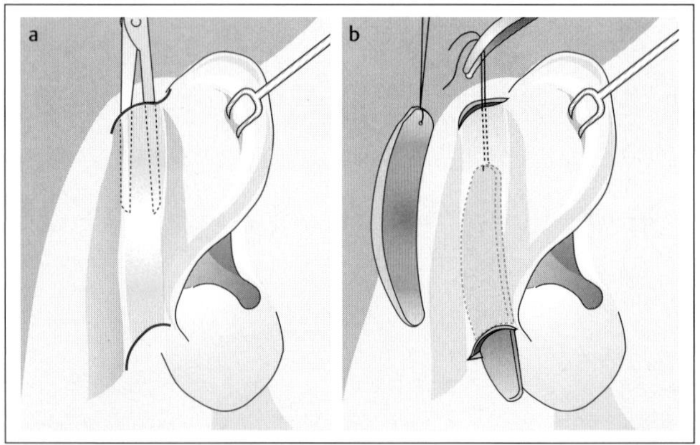

Fig. 5.165 **Augmentation of auricular projection.**
a Superior and inferior incision in the sulcus and creation of a skin tunnel.
b A slightly curved cartilaginous graft, previously deposited in a chest-wall pocket, approximately 35–45 × 8 × 8 mm, is inserted into the tunnel using stay sutures and a clamp (if required, additional insertion of cartilaginous chips; see Fig. 5.**164 e**; two small arrows).

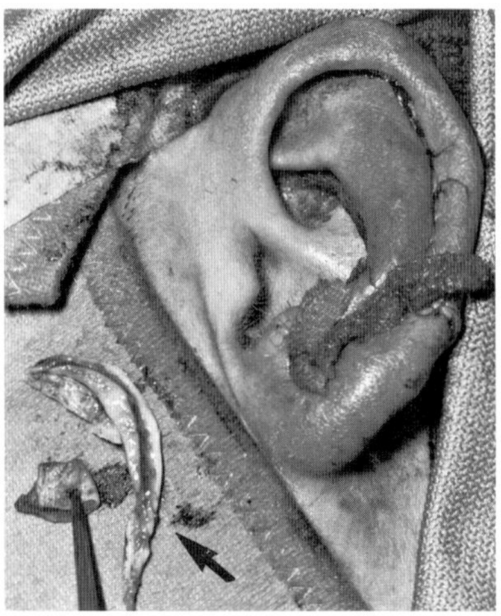
a

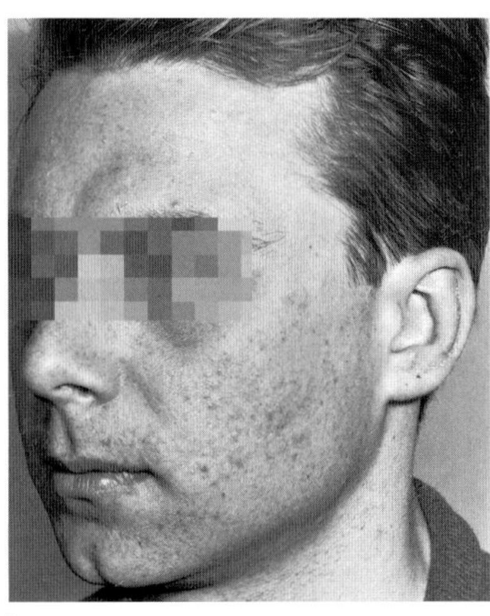
b

Fig. 5.166 **Reduction of the contralateral ear as described by Gersuny (1903; see pp. 54–56).**
a The contralateral ear is reduced according to a template of the reconstructed ear (see pp. 208, 209) using our modified Gersuny technique and set back if necessary; arrow: excised scapha and helix.
b Result (same patient as in Fig. 5.**164**).

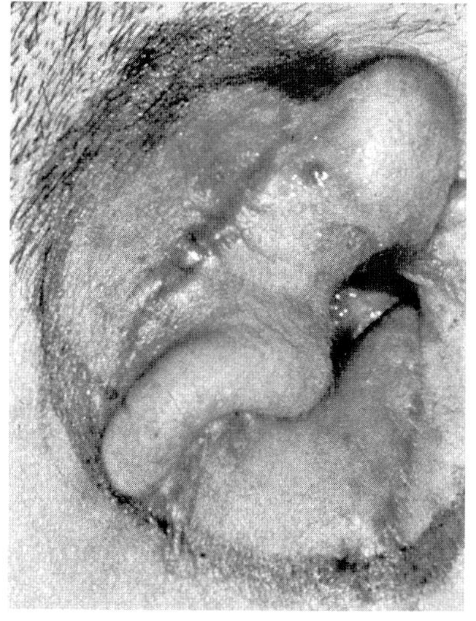
a

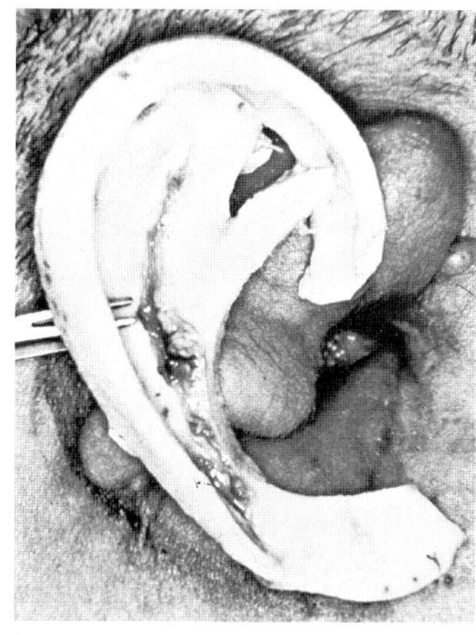
b

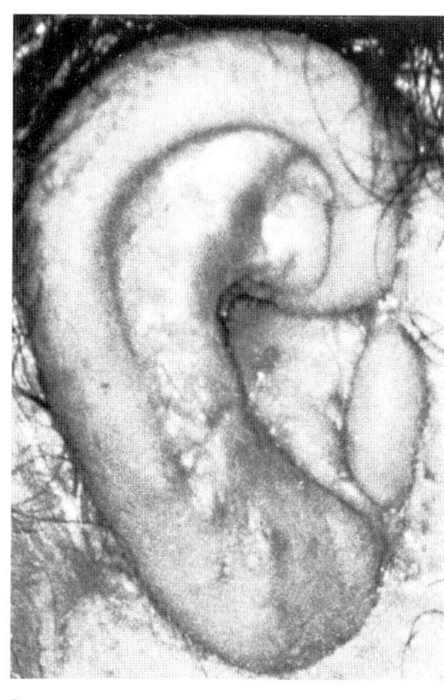
c

Fig. 5.**167** **Reconstruction in a case of previously damaged skin, transposed remnant and auditory canal created elsewhere using microsurgical technique, before auricular reconstruction.**
a Position of the transposed remnant and position of the planned auricle, with scars anterior and posterior to the remnant.
b Position of the framework. Prolonged use of an expander before insertion of the framework (p. 207).
c Result after three reconstructive stages.

Nagata's Reconstructive Techniques: First Stage

Reconstruction for Grade III Dysplasia (Microtias)
(Nagata 1993, 1994 a–d)

First stage. Framework (Fig. 5.**168 a–g** and Fig. 5.**169 a–c**).

Nagata adopted the operative technique developed by Tanzer (1959) and his school (see p. 207) and systematized and elaborated both the auricular framework and the individual operative stages (see Fig. 5.**168**). The basic framework is carved from the 6th and 7th ribs, as previously described for the reconstruction of the auricle after total loss and for grade II dysplasia (see pp. 89, 187, see Fig. 5.**168 a**). Any absent parts of the basic framework, especially the upper helical dome, are supplemented (pink). The helix (Fig. 5.**168 a**) is carved from the 8th rib, emphasizing the helical crus, and the helix of the basic framework is expanded (Fig. 5.**168 b**). Antihelix and tragus (Fig. 5.**168 a–d**) are constructed in the same manner. The individual parts are then assembled to form a three-dimensional framework (see Fig. 5.**158**, p. 205) using fine, double-armed 5–0 wire with an ST-4-plus needle (see Appendix 2), which is buried in the cartilage (see Fig. 5.**158 e**, **f**).

Figure 5.**168 c** demonstrates the posterior surface of the framework, with the helical crus and the tragus held in position by 4–0 braided sutures. Figure 5.**168 f** shows the profile of the helix, and Figure 5.**168 g** shows how the base is affixed to the individual parts. Average measurements (widths and depths) are shown in Figure 5.**169 a–c**.

Reconstruction for Grade III Dysplasias: Incisions for Lobule Type Microtia and Small Concha Type Microtia
(Nagata 1993, 1994 a–d)

First stage. Insertion of the cartilaginous framework and transposition of the lobule (Fig. 5.**170 a–j**).

The rudimentary cartilage is preserved, as we like to use it to reconstruct the tragus. In the region of the intertragic notch, a small amount of skin is excised (Fig. 5.**170 a**). The tragal element has not yet been attached to the framework (see Fig. 5.**168 b**, **c**), which, with its lobular part first (Fig. 5.**170 g**), is now rotated around the fat pedicle into the pocket where the cartilaginous earlobe part is now held in its new position within the cutaneous earlobe, the latter having been formed from the rudiment (Fig. 5.**170 f**) and already sutured in its new position with 5–0 braided sutures and 5–0 or 6–0 monofilament sutures. **Only now do we affix the new tragal framework to the main framework, unlike Nagata** (1994 a–d), because this facilitates insertion of the framework into the pocket (see Fig. 5.**168 a**, **b**, T; Weerda and Siegert 1998 h). It is also important to insert one or two vacuum drainage systems (Fig. 5.**170 h**, **j**).

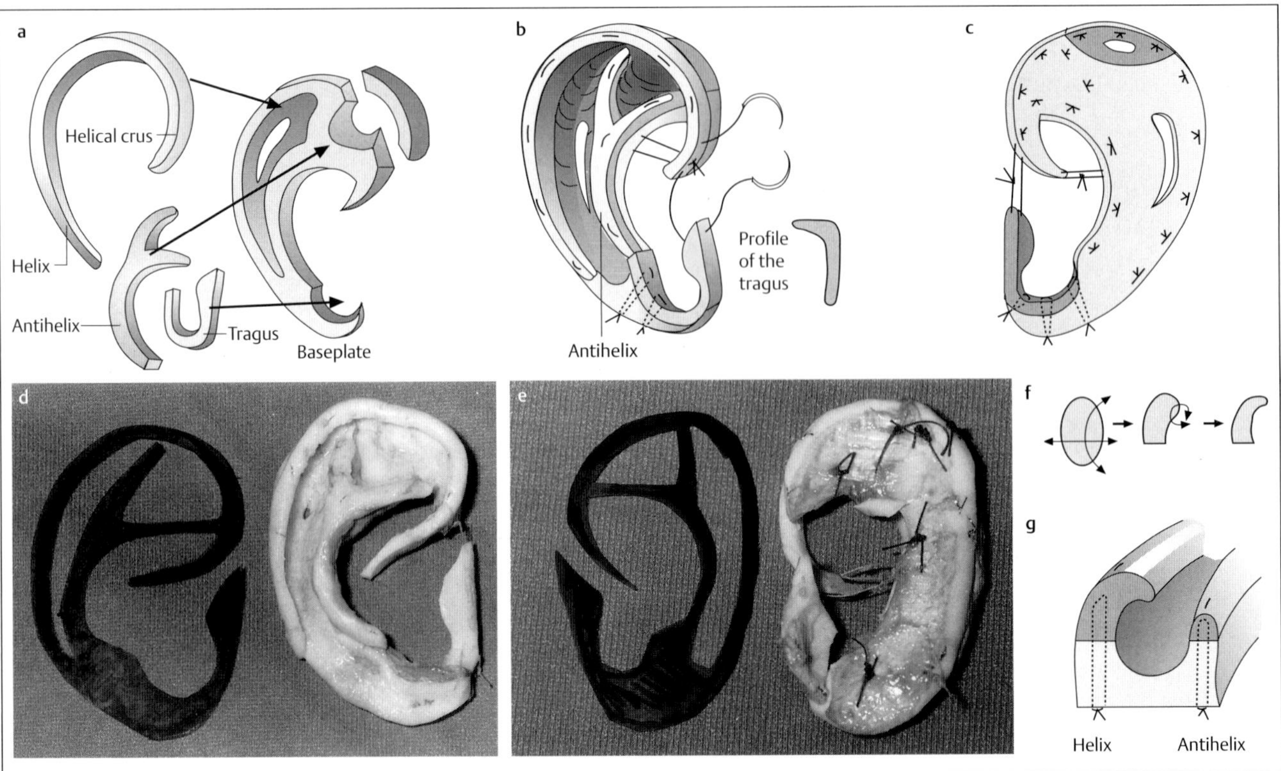

Fig. 5.**168** **Three-dimensional framework as fashioned by Nagata (1993, 1994 a–d; see also Fig. 5.158).**

a Baseplate fashioned from the 6th and 7th ribs (Nagata prefers to use the contralateral side, we prefer the ipsilateral; see pp. 202–206), the perichondrium of the postauricular surface remains largely intact (see **e**). Parts for supplementation (pink) derived from cartilaginous remains. We construct helix and helical crus from the 8th rib; antihelix and crura, as well as the tragus are taken from corresponding remains of the 7th or 8th rib.

b–e The individual parts are affixed with wire sutures (see Fig. 5.**158**; armed with two straight needles; see Appendix 2); **b**, **d**: anterior view; **c**, **e**: posterior view.

f Forming the shape of the helix from the 8th rib (cross-section).

g Helix and antihelix are sutured on: the wire sutures are buried in the cartilage (see Fig. 5.**158 e, f**).

For practice suggestions, see Fig. 5.**158**, p. 205.

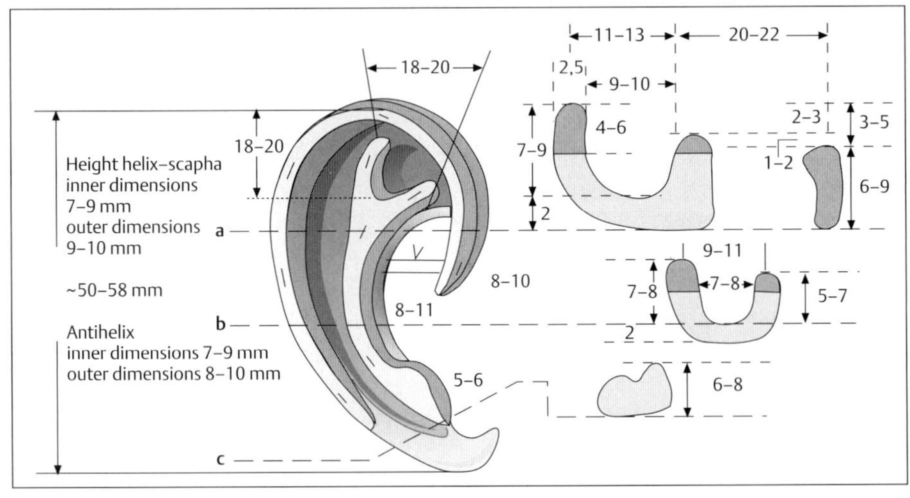

Fig. 5.**169** **Average dimensions of the framework in mm with three cross-sections; pink: cartilage superimposed onto helix and antihelix. All measurement are mm.**

a Upper.

b Middle.

c Lower.

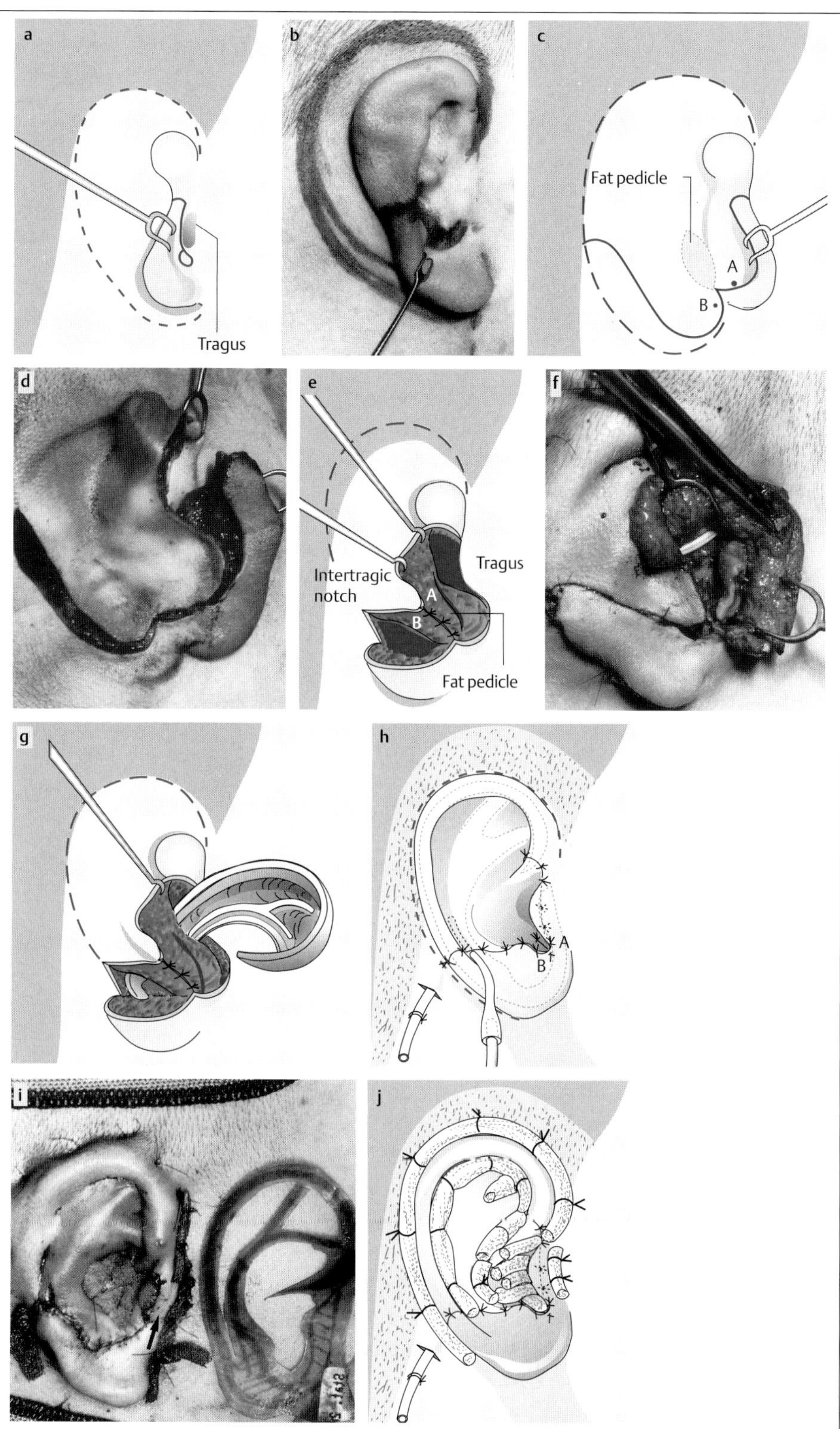

Fig. 5.**170** **First stage of the reconstruction of grade III (microtia) dysplasias (lobule type and small concha type microtia) as described by Nagata (1993, 1994 a–d).**
Insertion of the cartilaginous framework and transposition of the remnant to the earlobe.

a, b Incision of the anterior aspect of the remnant, skin excision for the intertragic notch. Some cartilaginous remnant remains in the region of the tragus. Position of the auricle, see pp. 202 ff.

c, d Incision on the postauricular surface and on the mastoid. A fat pedicle remains intact in order to ensure improved nutrition of the flap. A is sutured to B.

e, f Removal of the rudimentary cartilage. Suture of A to B and to the notch.

g The cartilaginous framework is drawn in (see Fig. 5.**160**) around the fat pedicle. Only now do we suture the tragal cartilage to the main framework (s. Fig. 5.**163 b**). The tragal cartilage is draped with anterior skin (see **f**, double skin hook).

h Suture using 6–0 monofilament material (polydioxanone, polypropylene; see Appendix 2, p. 305) after insertion of 1–2 vacuum drains, well-formed tragus (arrow, **i**).

i, j Only a few mattress sutures tied over cotton bolsters. Brent (1992) rejects these due to the risk of necrosis.

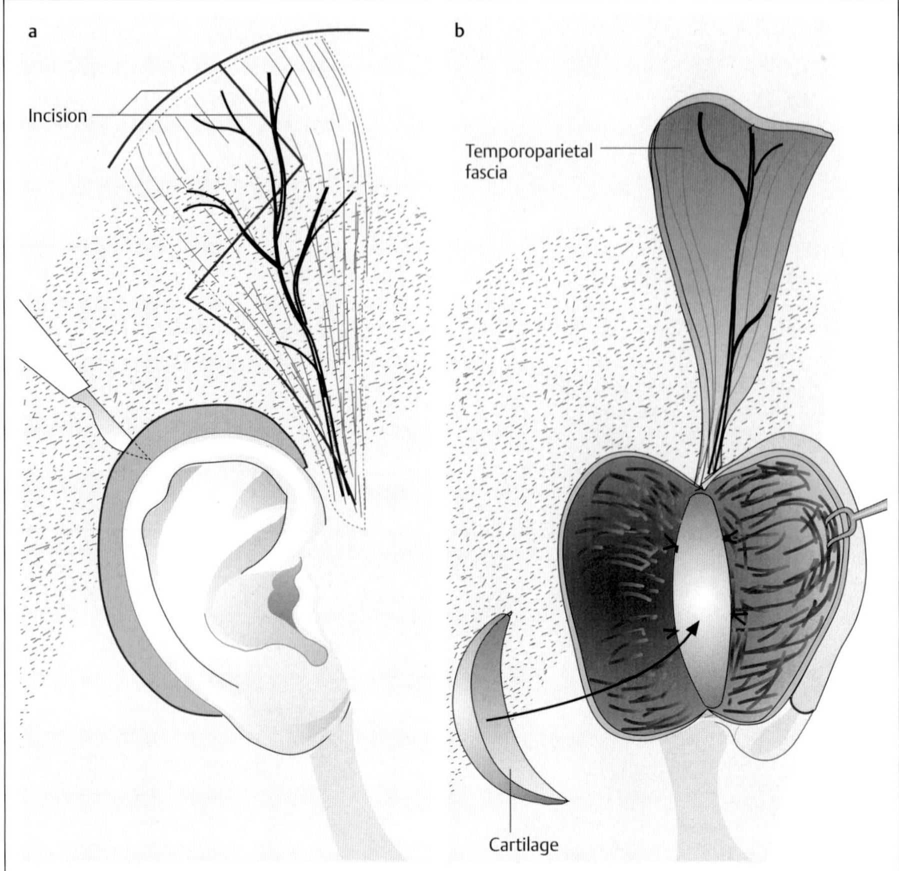

Fig. 5.**171** **Second stage of the reconstruction of grades II and III dysplasias, as described by Nagata (1993, 1994 a–d).** Exteriorization and epithelialization of the posterior surface. Insertion of the cartilage, resurfacing with temporoparietal fascia and epithelialization with skin (for a description of the individual steps in our modified form see Fig. 5.**172**).
a Generous shaving of an approximately 10 cm wide margin. Zigzag incision (see pp. 74, 93) and dissection of the fascia along its pedicle. Thin dissection of full-thickness skin 1 cm above the framework (red line) and dissection of the framework, leaving a sufficient layer of fibrous tissue on the framework.
b Elevation of the auricle, suturing of a crescent-shaped strip of cartilage 35–40 × 10 × 8–10 mm, coverage with the fascia, reduction of the mastoid wound (see Fig. 5.**172 g**, **h**) and suturing of split-thickness skin graft (see Fig. 5.**172 j–l**).

Unlike Brent (1980, 1993, 1999 a), Nagata forms the shape of the auricle with the aid of additional mattress sutures (without pressure) (Fig. 5.**170 j**). Next, the dressing with a fenestrated sponge and gauze is applied, also without pressure (see p. 223).

First Stage for Grade II Dysplasia (Concha Type Microtia, Severe Cup-ear Deformity, Mini-ear)
(Nagata 1993, 1994 a–d; see pp. 187, 188, 193 ff)

Nagata's Reconstructive Techniques: Second Stage

Second Stage of the Operations for Grades II and III Dysplasia – (Nagata 1993, 1994 a–d; Figs. 5.**171 b**, 5.**172 e**)

Dissection and epithelialization of the posterior surface. Nagata waits 6 months before the second operative stage and has reported a few innovations for the reconstruction of the postauricular surface which differ from the method of the Tanzer–Brent group:

- Insertion of a crescent-shaped piece of cartilage approximately 10 mm high as a spacer (Fig. 5.**171 b**, Fig. 5.**172 e, f C**).
- Coverage of the cartilage with a vascular-pedicled temporoparietal fascia.
- A full-thickness graft attached to the helix and dissected with a scalpel to achieve a good texture and color match, also in the region of the superior and posterior helix (Figs. 5.**171 a**, 5.**172 a–d**).

The skin is incised about 1 cm above the framework (Fig. 5.**171 a**, red line). A zigzag incision is made for the dissection of the temporoparietal fascia (Fig. 5.**171 a**; see also Figs. 4.**108**, 4.**109**; pp. 93, 94). The temporoparietal fascia is raised, a crescent-shaped piece of cartilage, which had been stored in the old chest wound during the first stage, is carved to 8–10 × 35–40 × 8–10 mm and inserted using wire sutures (see also Fig. 5.**172 e**). The cartilage is then covered with a previously prepared vascular-pedicled temporoparietal fascia (Fig. 5.**171 b**; see also pp. 74, 93).

The defect on the mastoid is reduced by mobilizing the surrounding skin and forming one or two Burow's triangles (see Fig. 5.**172 h**, Fig. 5.**162 d**) and covered by thick split- or full-thickness skin harvested from the chest wall, the groin or buttock (see Fig. 5.**172 j–l**). We always glue the free grafts into place with fibrin adhesive. The postoperative edema initially obscures the contours of the auricle.

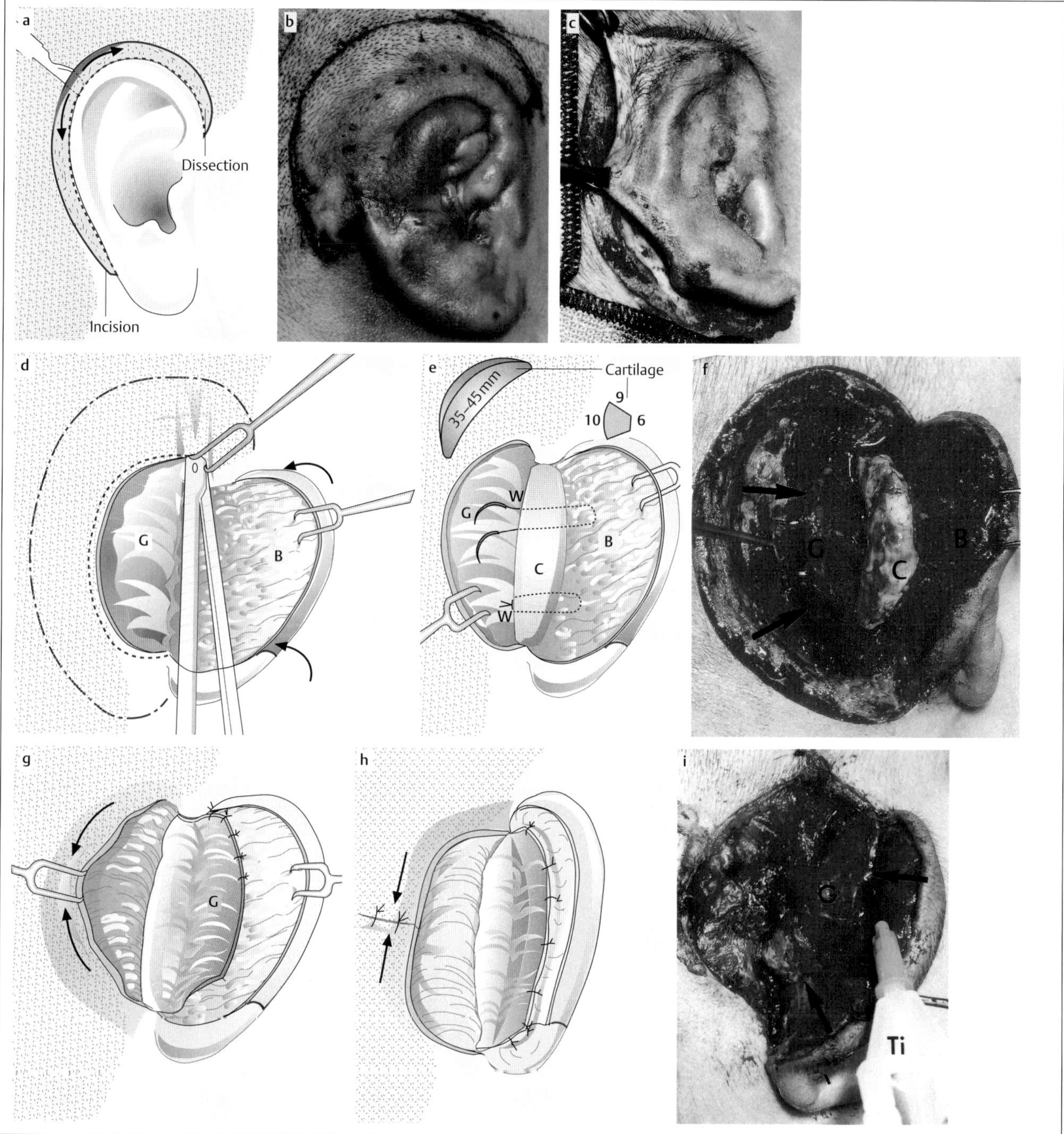

Fig. 5.**172** **Second stage of the reconstruction of grade III (microtia) dysplasias as described by Nagata (1994 a–d), in the modified form described by Weerda (1996 b, 1999 a) and Weerda and Siegert (1997 b).**

a–c Marking and incision approximately 1 cm above and behind the framework. Using a size 15 blade, dissection of a full-thickness skin flap above the hair follicles until almost reaching the framework (the framework must not be exposed), the hairs are removed (**b, c;** see Fig. 5.**171 a**, **b**).

d The posterior surface is dissected off, **leaving behind a covering layer of fibrous tissue** (**B**) over the framework. The galea–fascia–muscle flap (**G**) is then incised **large enough** over the mastoid and elevated. The area surrounding the defect is mobilized.

e, f A crescent-shaped segment of cartilage (**C**), approximately 35–40 × 9–12 mm, is inserted as a spacer and sutured. It is adapted to the antihelix with 5–0 wire sutures (W) (in **f**: G = galea–fascia–muscle flap, two arrows).

g–i Coverage of the cartilage with the galea–fascia–muscle flap (G) which is sutured and glued with fibrin adhesive (**Ti**) into place. The size of the wound surface over the mastoid plane is reduced and the Burow's triangle sutured (**h**).

Fig. 5.**172 j–r** ▷

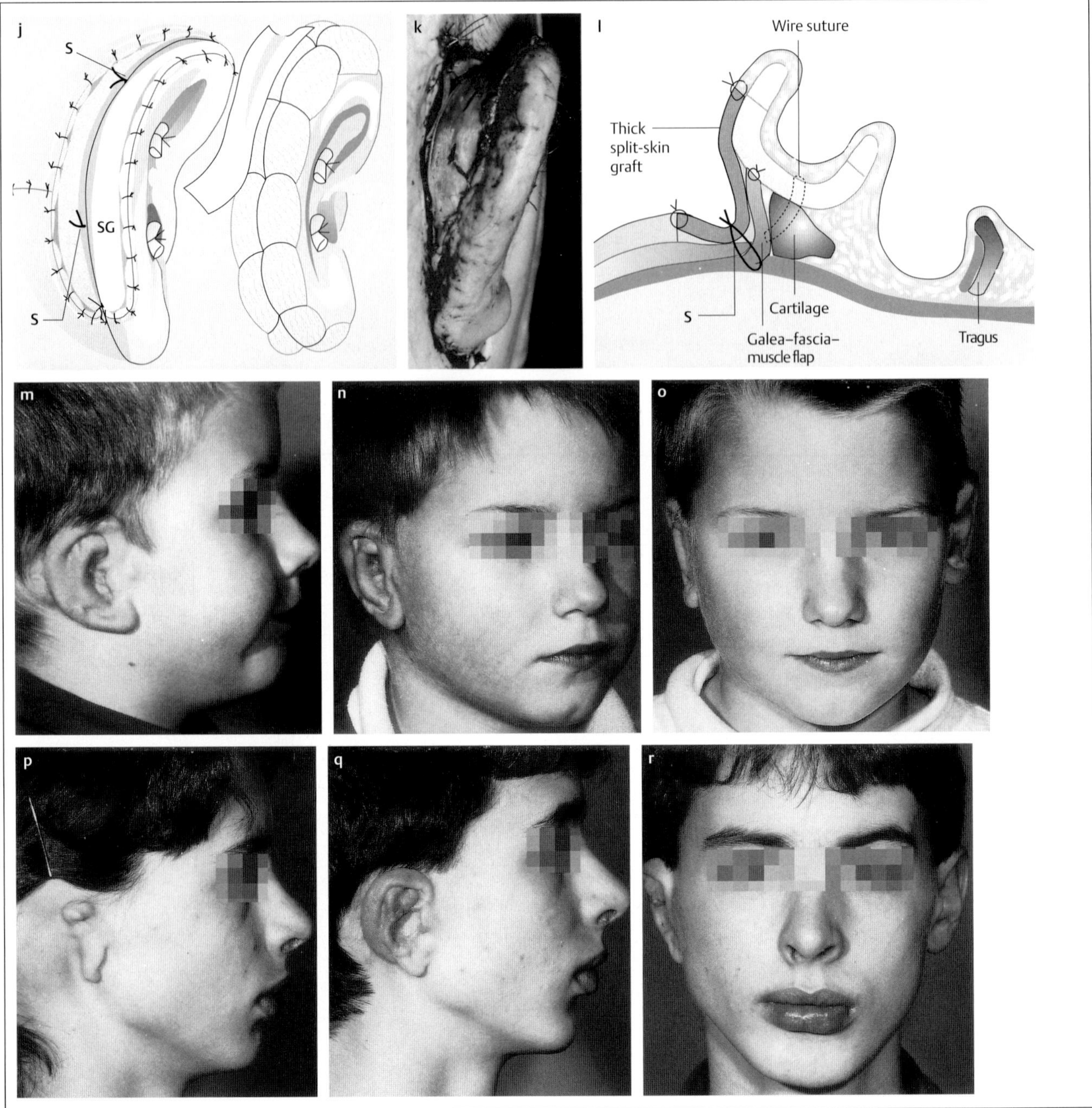

Fig. 5.**172** **j–r**

j, k 1–2 thick split-thickness or full-thickness skin grafts (SG) are glued and sutured into the defects, stay suture (S) in the sulcus, mild compression bandage with ointment-soaked packs, secured by adhesive plaster (see Fig. 5.**185** **a–d**; p. 223).

l Demonstration of the individual stages in cross-section. S = sulcus suture

m–o Result; patient 1 (Figs. **5.170**, 5.**172** **a–i**).

p Preoperative appearance of patient 2.

q, r Result.

We have developed a special fenestrated sponge dressing for this operation (see Fig. 5.**185**). The ear is kept bandaged for 6 days to allow the thick split- or full-thickness skin to heal.

Over the past years, we have not lost a single free skin graft because the graft was glued down under mild pressure.

Weerda and Siegert's Modifications of the Second Stage of Reconstructions of Grade II and III Dysplasias

(Weerda 1996 b, 1997 a, 1998 b, 1999 a, b, 2001; Weerda and Siegert 1997, 1998 h, 1998 f, 1999 b; Fig. 5.**172**).

With only minor differences, we perform this operation using the technique described by Nagata (see p. 186). As previously explained when describing the costal cartilage

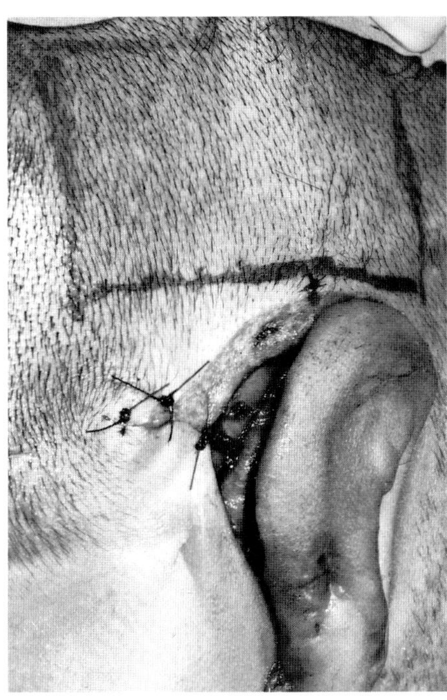

a

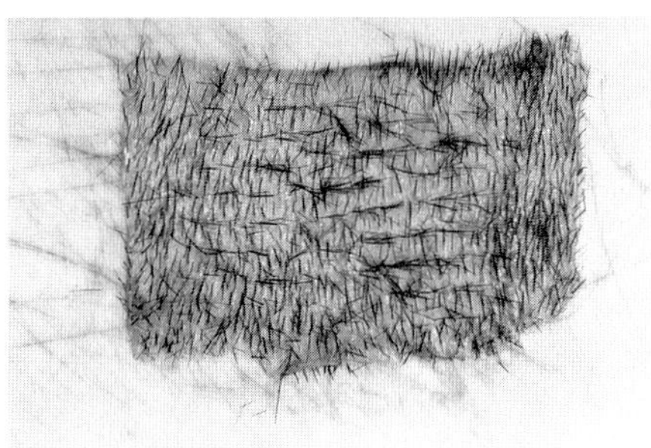

b

Fig. 5.173 **Harvesting of a split-skin graft (approximately 0.3 mm) with a dermatome above the hair follicles.**
a The skin required for harvesting.
b The split-skin graft after harvesting and before de-epilation.

framework derived from Nagata (see Fig. 5.**168**), our auricular framework is initially carved without the tragus. The helix is 2–3 mm higher than the antihelix, particularly in the upper auricular region (see Figs. 5.**168**, 5.**169**).

Second stage. Dissection and epithelialization of the posterior surface (Fig. 5.**172 a–r**).

After total loss of the auricle, and for grade II or III dysplasias, we have modified the second stage according to Nagata's suggestions (Nagata 1993, 1994 a–d; Weerda 1996 b, 1999 a, 2001; see Figs. 5.**135**, 5.**172**).

After at least 8 weeks an incision is made 1 cm above the framework using a size 15 blade (Fig. 5.**172 a**), and a full-thickness skin flap is dissected superficial to the hair follicles towards the framework (Fig. 5.**172 a–c**), leaving enough fibrous tissue on the aspect facing the framework. Then the postauricular surface is dissected free, ensuring that enough fibrous tissue remains on the framework (Fig. 5.**172 d**; see also Fig. 5.**162**). The previously dissected full-thickness skin graft is draped around the helix, rendering the entire helix optimally epithelialized in both color and texture. The mastoid skin is then undermined with the scalpel and, instead of a temporoparietal fascial flap, a fascia–galea–muscle flap is raised (Fig. 5.**172 d**, G; dotted red line).

A template is fashioned from the defect in the postauricular surface and in the mastoid using the aluminum foil of a suture pack, and a full-thickness skin graft is dissected to the corresponding size from the skin of the old chest wound (to be harvested before opening the wound and removing the cartilage). This skin can also be taken as a split- or full-thickness skin graft from the groin, the buttock region, or the hair-bearing scalp (Fig. 5.**173 a, b**). It is sutured and glued onto the defect (Fig. 5.**172 k, l**).

After attending our symposium in Lübeck in 1997, Brent (1999) subsequently modified his reconstructive technique. Results are shown in Figs. 5.**172 m–o, q, r**.

Fine-tailoring After Operations for Dysplasias

Occasionally we find that the contours of the scapha are not readily apparent (Fig. 5.**174**; see also Fig. 5.**164 a**), or there is a lack of depth to the concha (Fig. 5.**175**), a poorly defined tragus, or distortions from scar formation.

Deepening of the scapha and the triangular fossa, and epilation of the helix. An incision is made in the scapha, directed somewhat more towards the antihelix (Fig. 5.**174 a**). If necessary, the skin is dissected as far as the upper concha and the scapha is deepened (Peer and Walker 1957; Fig. 5.**174 b**). In addition, refinements may also be made to the antihelical framework, the triangular fossa excavated, and the concha slightly enlarged (Fig. 5.**174 c, d**). When hair is present on the helix, it is dissected off the framework and the hair follicles are removed with fine pointed scissors (Fig. 5.**174 c, d**).

The incision is closed with 6–0 monofilament sutures. Placing the incision close to the antihelix now allows the skin to reach down into the base of the scapha. By removing the scar tissue and lowering the antihelix and the crura, the

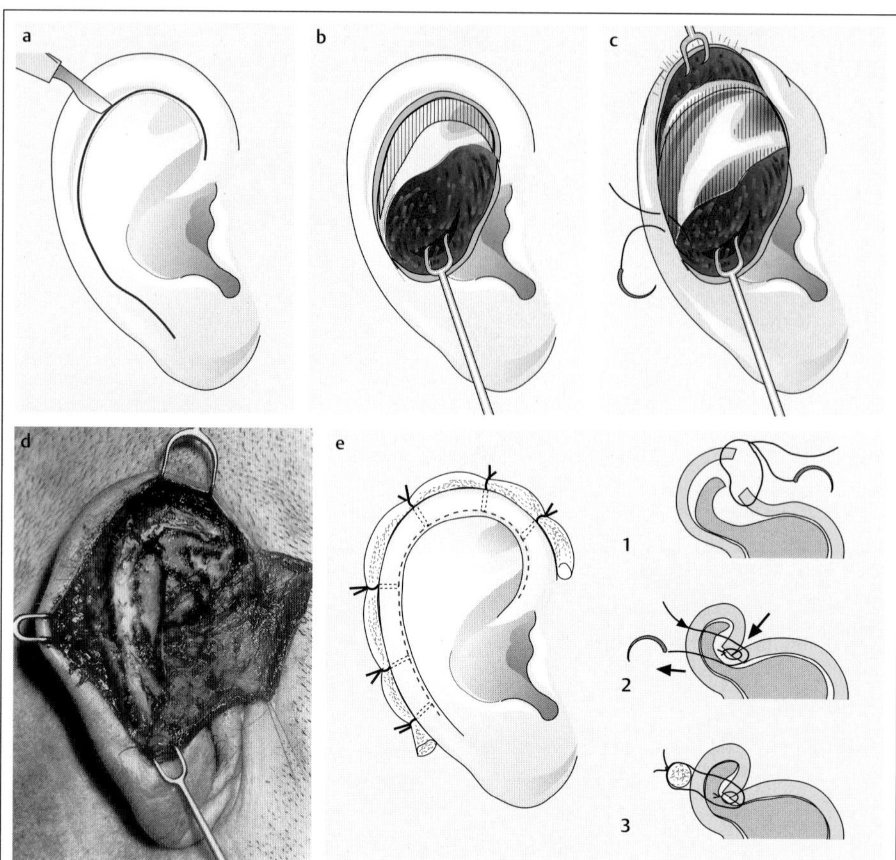

Fig. 5.**174** **Corrective surgery for grade III dysplasia. Deepening of the scapha and fossa and epilation (see Fig. 5.164).**
- **a** Incision in the scapha, near the antihelix, dissection of the skin.
- **b** Deepening of the scapha and scar excision.
- **c, d** If required, deepening of the triangular fossa and widening of the concha. Lowering of the antihelix. Dissection around the superior helix and (**d**) removal of the hair follicles (sharp/sharp fine scissors; see Fig. 5.**180**).
- **e** The skin incision is sutured with 6–0 (1) polydioxanone mattress sutures, knotted over a long cotton bolster soaked in petroleum jelly (2,3), and also, if necessary, glued with fibrin adhesive. Result: see p. 210, Fig. 5.**164 e–f**.

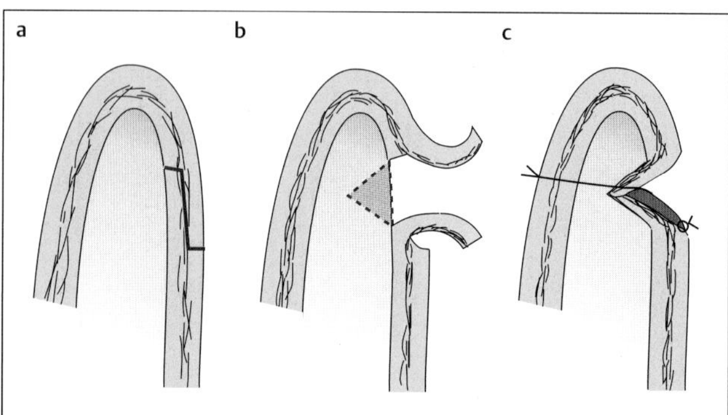

Fig. 5.**175** **Contouring of the helical margin as described by Bethmann for total reconstruction of the auricle (from Mündnich 1962 a) (an arduous technique, not recommended).**
- **a** Stepped incision of the skin.
- **b** Skin and subcutaneous tissue are dissected in the form of two flaps, the pedicles of which lie opposite one another. The hatched area is excised from the cartilage in the form of a triangular strip, creating a groove.
- **c** The cartilage of this groove is covered with the two flaps. A strip of split-thickness skin is placed over the de-epithelialized flap. The result is secured by a full-thickness suture and interrupted sutures.

skin of the antihelix also suffices to lend a good form to the scapha. The skin incision is closed (Fig. 5.**174 e**, 1). Mattress sutures (5–0 monofilament sutures, P3 or PS-3 needle), knotted behind the helix over long, thin bolsters soaked in a mixture of petroleum jelly and povidone-iodine, draw the skin into the scapha (Fig. 5.**174 e**, 2, 3).

Bethmann and Zoltan (1968) suggested incising the skin in the region of the scapha in a stepwise manner (Fig. 5.**175 a–c**).

Tanzer (1974 a) suggests making only 3–4 incisions in the scapha, 7–8 mm in length, instead of a long incision, and deepening the scapha via these.

Converse (1958) suggests a different procedure (Fig. 5.**176 a, b**), but here the excision should not reach down as far as the cartilage.

Deepening of the scapha and improving the contour of the tragus (Fig. 5.**172 a–e**). Should deepening of the scapha prove unnecessary, any fine-tailoring of the auricle can also be performed during stage 3 (Kirkham 1940; Peer and Walker 1957; Brent 1974, 1980l, 1987 b; Bogdasarian and Baker 1983; Davis 1987).

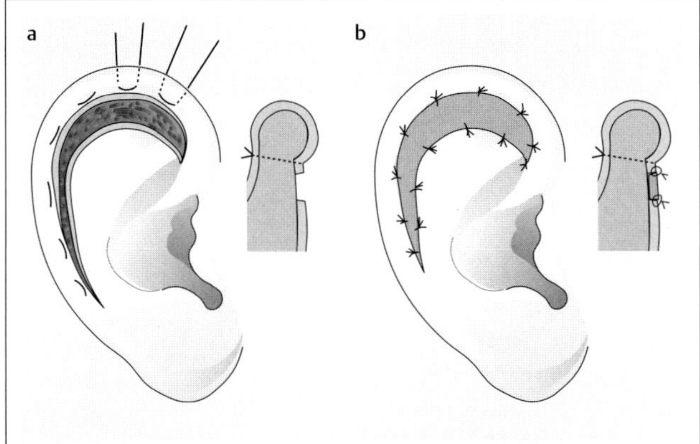

Fig. 5.**176** **Additional contouring of the helix as described by Converse (1958; from Mündnich 1962 a) (a difficult technique, not recommended).**

a Skin incision; advancement of the peripheral wound margin towards the auricular margin; the resulting fold over the helix is secured with transfixion sutures.

b The resulting crescent-shaped defect is resurfaced by a split-thickness skin graft (Fig. 5.**173**)

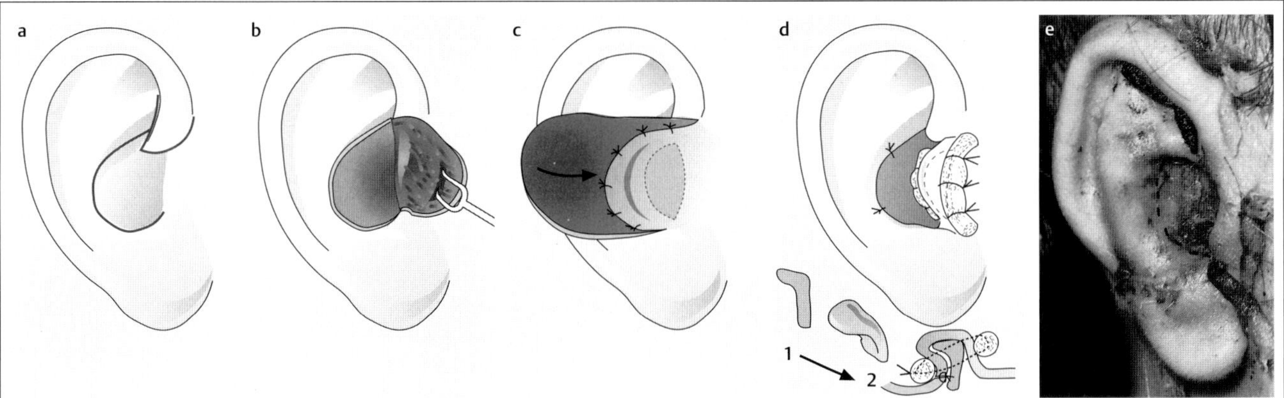

Fig. 5.**177** **Deepening of the concha and formation of the helical crus and the tragus as described by Tanzer (1974 a), modified (see also Fig. 5.160, p. 207), coverage of the concha with a full-thickness skin graft.**

a Incision around the helical crus and in the transition from concha to antihelix.

b Elevation of the skin anteriorly by dissection. The concha is deepened down to the mastoid and anteriorly. If necessary, antihelical cartilage is excised.

c A full-thickness skin graft, fashioned from a template and harvested from the sulcus of the contralateral ear, is sutured to the tragal skin.

d A L-shaped segment of cartilage is inserted as a tragal strut, the full-thickness skin graft is glued into place with fibrin adhesive and the shape of the tragus is formed using mattress sutures tied over cotton bolsters; 1 and 2: schematic illustration.

e 7th postoperative day.

Because we usually fix the skin onto the concha using fibrin glue, suturing is often unnecessary (Fig. 5.**177 d**).

Forming the shape of the helical crus, concha, antitragus, and intertragic notch. Figure 5.**178 a**, **b** demonstrates Weerda's method.

Davis's (1987) method of forming the helical crus is shown in Figure 5.**174 a**, **b**.

In the absence of the helical crus, or if it is poorly defined, transposition of tissue from the preauricular region in the form of a Z-plasty (see Fig. 4.**20** p. 51 and Fig. 5.**178 a**, 1) can create a helical crus.

Corrective Measures for a Low Hairline—Epilation (see pp. 275 ff)

Hairs present only in the region of the superior helix. When hairs are present in the helical area, we place an incision in the region of the scapha as a final step on completion of all

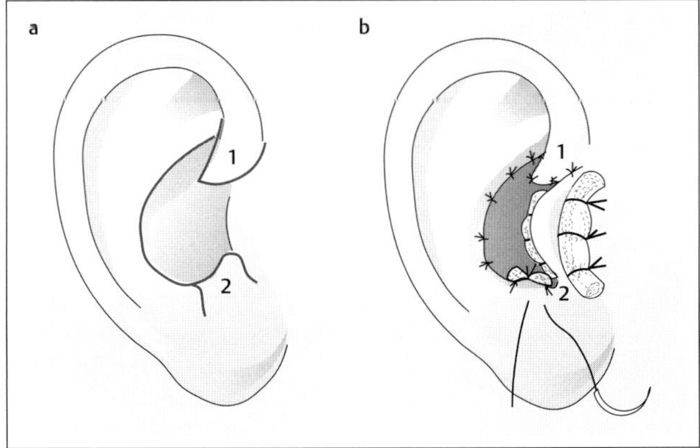

Fig. 5.**178** **Formation of the helical crus and intertragic notch and deepening of the concha (see also Fig. 5.177).**

a Pattern of the incisions for formation of the helical crus (1) and intertragic notch (2).

b After elevation of the skin flaps, scar tissue and, if necessary, cartilage (including the antihelix) are excised. A mattress suture is also used to form the notch (2).

Epithelialization of the concha: see Fig. 5.**177**.

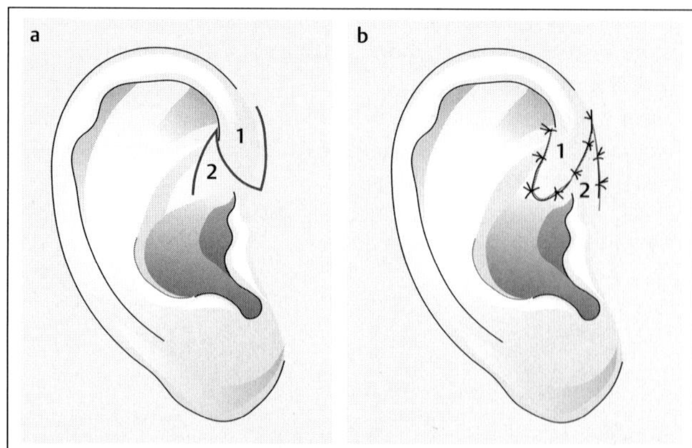

Fig. 5.**179** **Formation of the helical crus (helical root) using a Z-plasty as described by Davis (1987).**
a Z-shaped incision (1, 2).
b Z-plasty and suture, if necessary, the crus can be underlaid with some fibrous tissue or cartilage (1; see also Fig. 5.**178**).

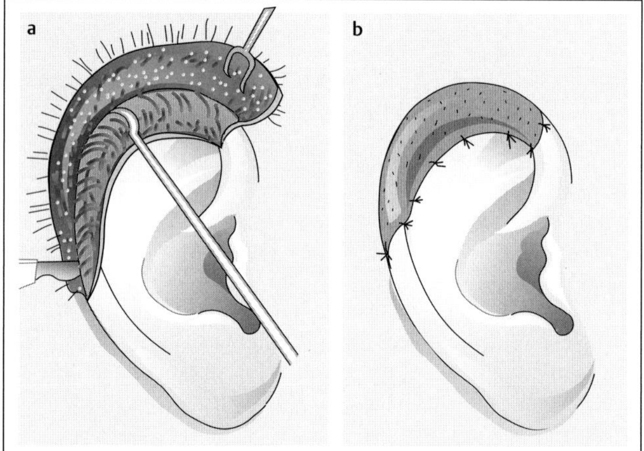

Fig. 5.**180** **Epilation performed from the scaphal surface (second stage of the operation).**
a The hair-bearing skin is dissected off in the second stage of the reconstruction (Brent 1987 a), leaving a layer of fibrous tissue on the framework, removal of hair follicles.
b Resurfacing with full-thickness skin from the sulcus region of the contralateral ear.

the operations (see Fig. 5.**174**; see also Fig. 5.**162**, p. 209) and dissect the helix, removing the hair follicles with pointed scissors.

Preoperative laser epilation. This is recommended particularly for dark-haired patients with a low hairline (Goldberg et al. 1997; Lask et al. 1997; Nanni and Alster 1997; Gault et al. 1998; Brent 1999 a; Landthaler and Hohenleutner 1999; Liew et al. 1999).

Postoperative laser epilation. About 6 months after completion of treatment, laser epilation is performed over several sessions (see p. 275). Admittedly, long-term results are still lacking, so no conclusive results can be provided here.

Depilatory cream achieves only short-term removal of hair.

Epilation during the second or third stage as described by Brent is shown in Figure 5.**180 a, b**).

Electroepilation. This is the only sure method of epilation (Goldberg et al. 1997; Löffler et al. 1996, 1998 a, b).

We followed up 14 patients in a study involving a total of 27 patients. Based on the results of an experimental histological examination, we found that during a single treatment session with electroepilation using a fine epilation needle, about 40% of the hair follicles in the region of the papilla are targeted, making several electroepilation sessions necessary (Fig. 5.**181 a–c**; Löffler et al. 1998 a, b).

If, in the region of the ear to be reconstructed, more than one third of the skin bears hairs (Brent 1999 a), then we have so far covered the framework with a temporoparietal flap, broadly based in the sulcus, and resurfaced the fascial flap with skin from the sulcus and the retroauricular region of the contralateral ear (see p. 93).

Approach in the hair-bearing scalp. In the presence of strong hair growth, an attempt may also be made, after marking the position of the auricle, to place the incision about 15 mm above the ear (Fig. 5.**182 a, b**) and, after dissecting out a pocket, to achieve epilation by removing the hair follicles with sharp scissors. The results are satisfactory (Fig. 5.**182 c**).

Scalp roll and free graft. In earlier work methods were reported in which a scalp flap was raised as a tube, while the skin needed for the reconstruction was placed over the fascia in the form of a full-thickness skin graft (Lettermann and Harding 1956; Kazanjian and Converse 1959 a; Converse 1963; Brown et al. 1969; Brent 1980 II). These methods must be considered unadvisable; the fan flap (see pp. 74, 93) is better.

Corrective Measures for a High Hairline

(Fig. 5.**183**)

In very rare cases too high a hairline, of either congenital or iatrogenic origin, may necessitate later revision surgery to lower it. Since it is most commonly a case of hairless regions secondary to defect coverage with a free graft, attempts can be made to remove this cosmetic defect by scar revision and lowering of the hairline, at the earliest 3 months after completion of the reconstruction.

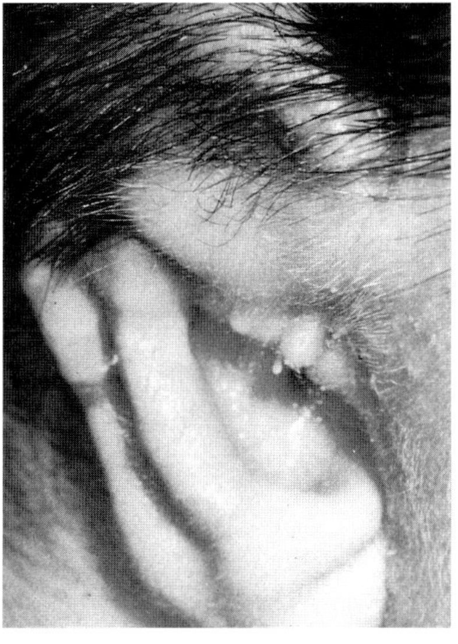
a

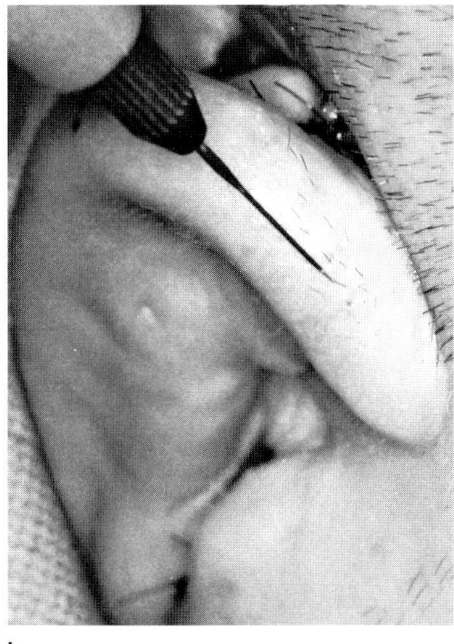
b

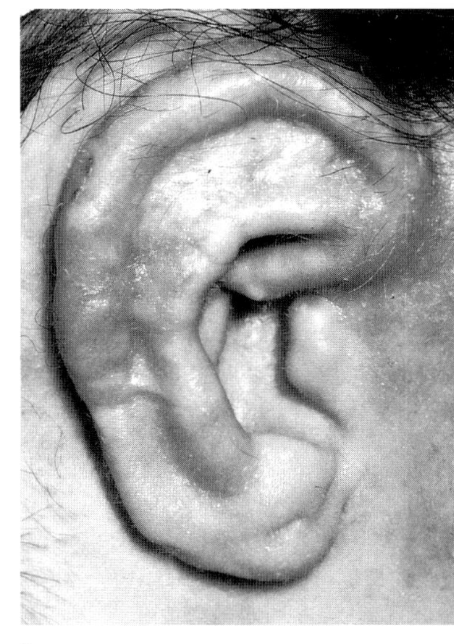
c

Fig. 5.**181** **Electroepilation.**
a Strong hair growth.
b Appearance after three sessions.
c Result after four sessions (surgeons: R. Siegert, A. Löffler).

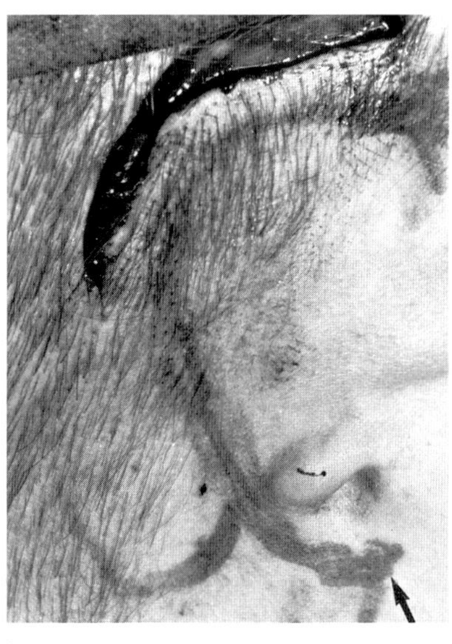
a

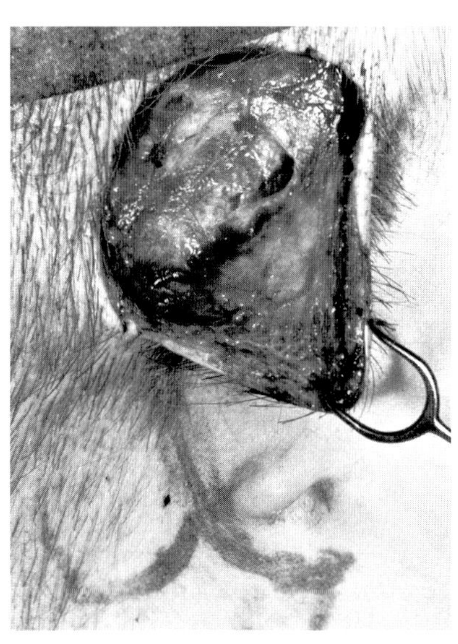
b

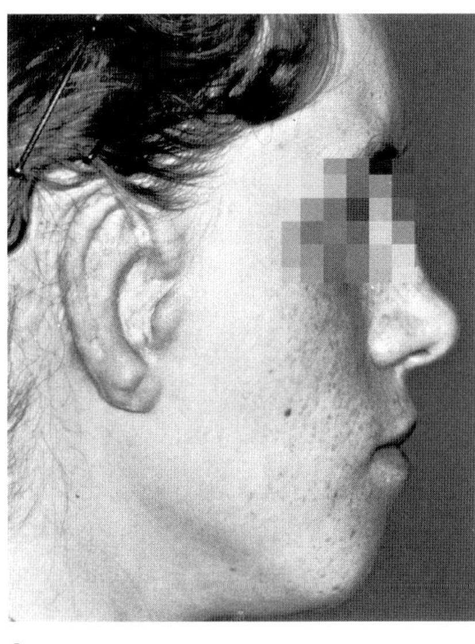
c

Fig. 5.**182** **Epilation via an approach originating from an incision in the hair-bearing scalp in a case of anotia and low hairline.**
a Position of the auricle (arrow) and the mastoid. Incision approximately 15–20 mm above the contour of the ear.
b Epilation by separation of the follicles with sharp/sharp curved scissors after developing a pocket.
c Result.

Tanzer's Procedure for Lowering the Hairline
(Fig. 5.**183**; Tanzer 1963 c)

Tanzer excises a crescent-shaped strip along the hairline and above the ear (Fig. 5.**183 a**), mobilizes the scalp, excises a posterior Burow's triangle, and thus manages to lower the hairline (Fig. 5.**183 b**).

Peer's Procedure for Lowering the Hairline
(Fig. 5.**184 a, b**; Peer and Walker 1955)

After excising the scar, a Z-shaped incision is placed in the scalp (Fig. 5.**184 a**) and the hairline is lowered with the aid of a Z-plasty (Fig. 5.**184 b**).

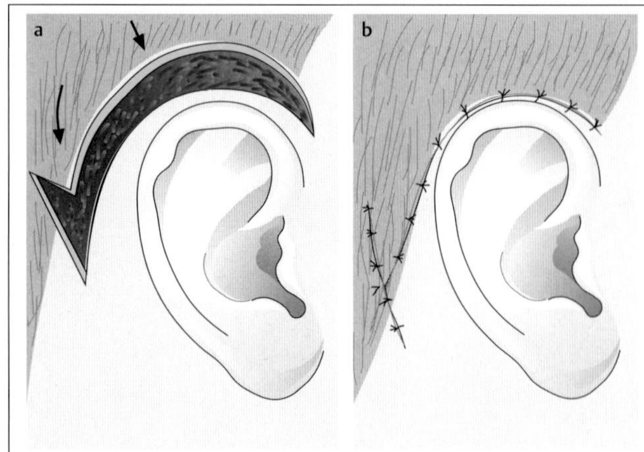

Fig. 5.**183** **Lowering of the hairline (following auricular reconstruction), as described by Tanzer (1963 a).**
a Scar excision and removal of a large Burow's triangle after scalp mobilization.
b Lowering and closure of the wounds.

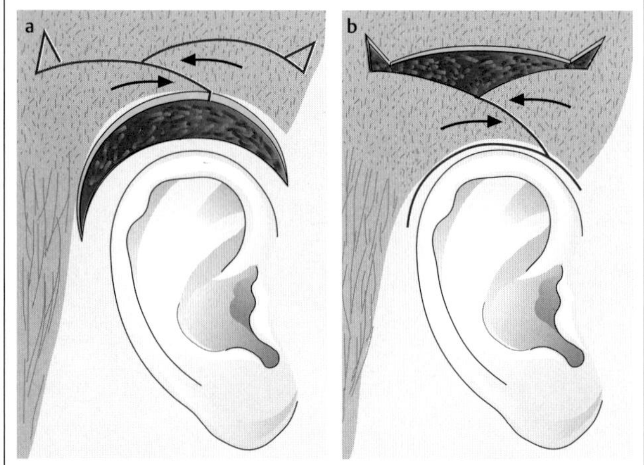

Fig. 5.**184** **Lowering of the hairline as described by Peer and Walke (1955).**
a Scar excision and Z-shaped flap incision with Burow's triangles.
b Z-plasty and closure.

Siegert and Firmin's Procedure for Lowering the Hairline after Skin Expansion

(Siegert and Weerda 1994 a, b; Firmin 1995)

A further option is the insertion of an expander (Firmin 1995; see also p. 231). After several weeks of expansion the hairless skin is excised after resurfacing.

Critique. We used expanders quite frequently in the early 1990s (Siegert et al. 1998 b). The high complication rate encountered with long-term expansion over a period of 8 weeks (see Fig. 5.**188**) and the fibrous capsule that forms around the expander, thickening the otherwise supple skin required for the reconstruction, have prompted us to use an expander (35 ml) only on rare occasions (Nordström et al. 1988).

Dressing the Ear

(Fig. 5.**185**)

We use ointment dressings soaked in a mixture of povidone–iodine and petroleum jelly for all of our dressings, supplemented with additional steroid ointments for otoplasty and after individual operative stages. The auricle is covered with a fenestrated sponge dressing developed especially for this purpose, to avoid pressure on the external ear. We also apply additional cotton-wool cushioning. Then a circular dressing is put on, secured with a tubular dressing (see also p. 131).

At the **second operative stage** (coverage of the posterior region with a free graft), the whole cavity behind the ear is sealed off with the ointment dressing described above (Fig. 5.**185 a, b**) and the auricle is bandaged under mild compression for 1 week (Fig. 5.**185 c, d**). Fibrin adhesive is used to glue the thick split- or full-thickness graft over the postauricular surface, so partial or total loss of the split-thickness grafts has become very rare. With problem cases and for secondary interventions, we administer perioperative antibiotics, extended over at least 5 days.

A fenestrated sponge and a circular bandage covered by a tubular bandage, particularly at night, secure the entire dressing (Fig. 5.**185 e–h**).

Removal of Sutures

This is done 6–8 days after surgery, preferably on the 8th day. The same applies for the chest wound, because of the intracutaneous suture used there. We then recommend the short-term use of adhesive tape for 3–4 days to secure the wound.

Discharge

After the first stage: children are discharged on the 7th or 8th day, following removal of the vacuum drain, and may stay for a few more days in the hotel with their parents if they do not live in the vicinity.

After the second stage: discharge back to the hotel is on the 3rd or 4th day; removal of the adhesive plaster dressing (soak the adhesive plaster beforehand in rubbing alcohol or something similar) and free-graft check with removal of sutures on the 6th to 7th day; wound check on the 8th day; and then discharge home.

All the other, less demanding, operative stages are performed on an outpatient basis, or the patient may be admitted to hospital for 2–3 days.

See p. 131 for the dressing for otoplasty.

Complications

Brent (1997, personal communication, 1998 b, 1999 a) no longer places mattress sutures to coapt the skin of the auricle onto the framework during the first stage, and states that since then he has had no problems in the form of skin necrosis. Nagata (1993, 1994 a–d), on the other hand, uses

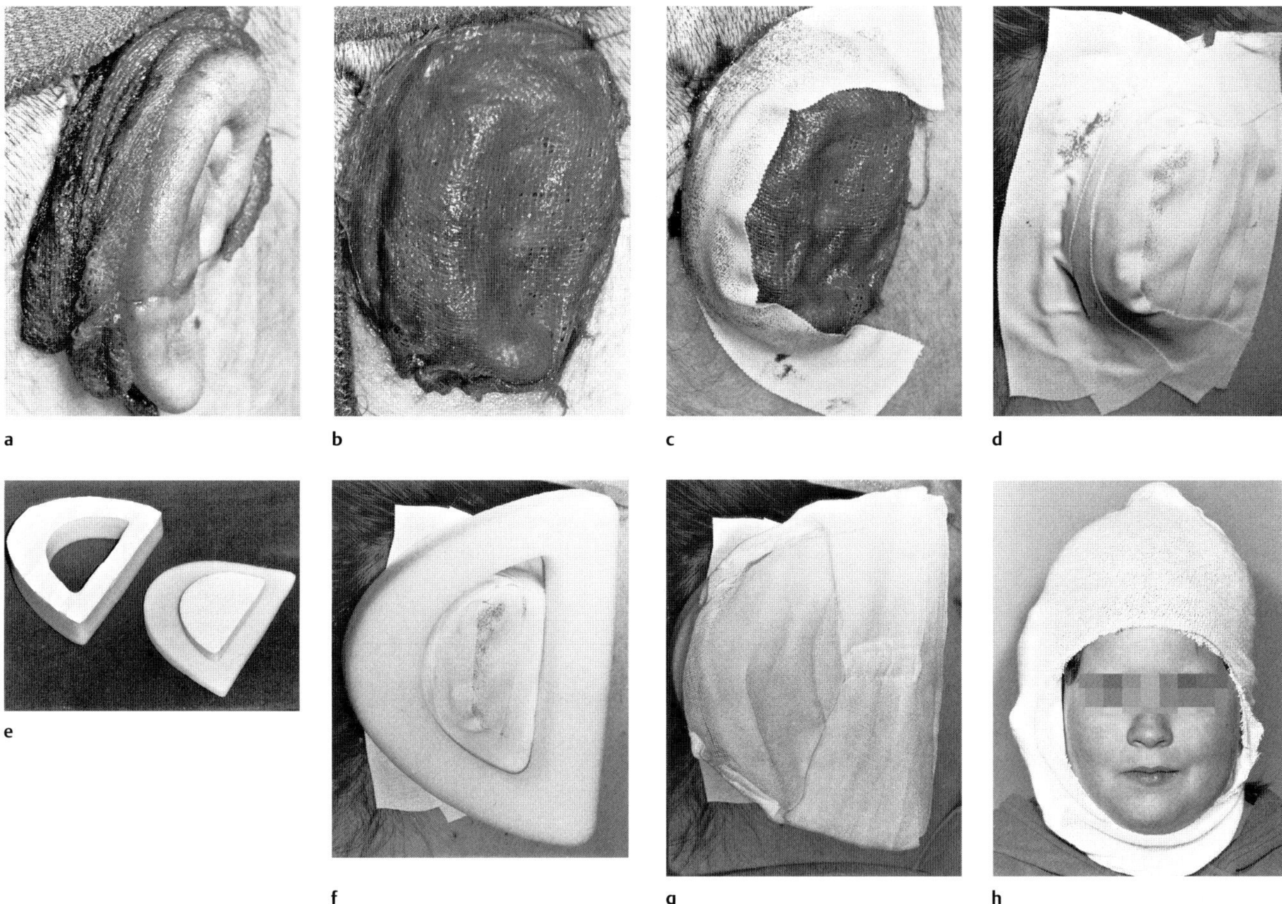

Fig. 5.185 **Dressing for the second and third stages of surgery for dysplasia using a thick split- or a full-thickness skin graft (harvested from the chest wall or buttock: 0.35–0.40 mm).**
a Padding out of the posterior graft (see Fig. 5.**172 j–l**, p. 216).
b Coverage of the auricle with ointment-soaked gauze swabs (mixture of povidone–iodine and petroleum jelly ointment).
c The skin is prepped with rubbing alcohol and the first strips of adhesive plaster (2 cm) are applied to provide mild compression on the posterior (**a**) padding and skin.
d Application of the adhesive-plaster dressing.
e, f Fenestrated sponge dressing which is also used without the adhesive-plaster dressing for the first stage, as for all other operations.
g Cotton-wool cushion.
h Circular dressing secured with a tubular bandage.

many mattress sutures tied over long, soft cotton bolsters (see Fig. 5.**170 j**, p. 213), and also does not report any skin necrosis as a complication.

We make very sparing use of mattress sutures, knotted without pressure over thin cotton bolsters to mold the form of the auricle (see Fig. 5.**160 e**, p. 207). Yet even without placing mattress sutures, and leaving a wide pedicle of fatty tissue when using Nagata's technique for total reconstruction of the auricle, we still occasionally see dark discoloration and venous congestion of the superior skin flap (Fig. 5.**189 a, b**), in addition to marginal necroses. **Brent's technique is the safer option** (p. 224).

As a rule, for this technique we administer a steroid bolus of approximately 250 mg in adults and 150–200 mg in children, and in addition we also apply a steroid-containing ointment or cream to the skin over the first 3 days. Furthermore, the **operative site is also checked 1 hour after the operation**. If the auricle demonstrates a livid discoloration, it is stroked out in the direction of the flap pedicle and, if necessary, mattress sutures are removed. Causes for the livid discoloration are (1) the administration of epinephrine before the operation, which causes vascular constriction (2) edema, and (3) strangulation of the venous limb in the presence of an intact arterial inflow. This results in increasing autostrangulation and reduced venous return. In the presence of any livid discoloration, the ear is stroked every 1–2 hours until the flap edema has subsided, which is usually around the second—at latest the third—postoperative day. The blood is stroked out of the flap in the direction of the pedicle, using a steroid-containing ointment and a cotton bud.

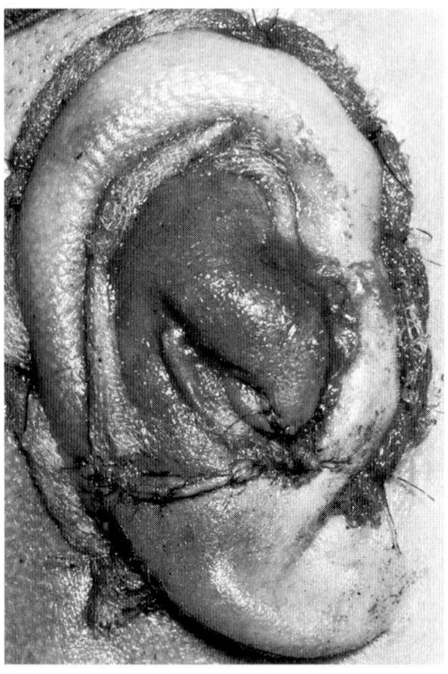

a

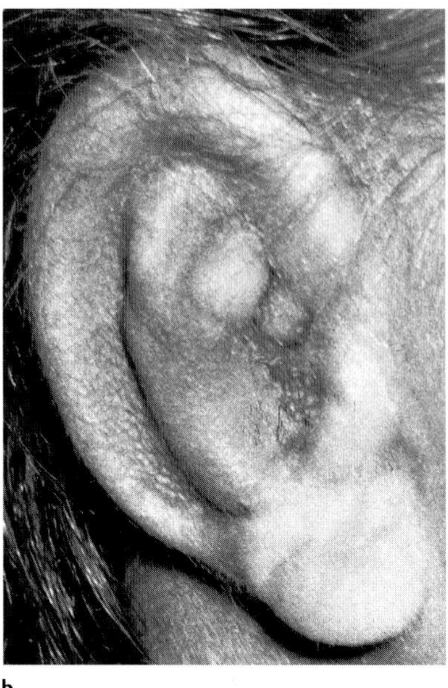

b

Fig. 5.**186** **Disturbances of circulation.**
a Livid discoloration of the remnant following Nagata's technique with subsequent necrosis.
b Result after excision of the necrosis.

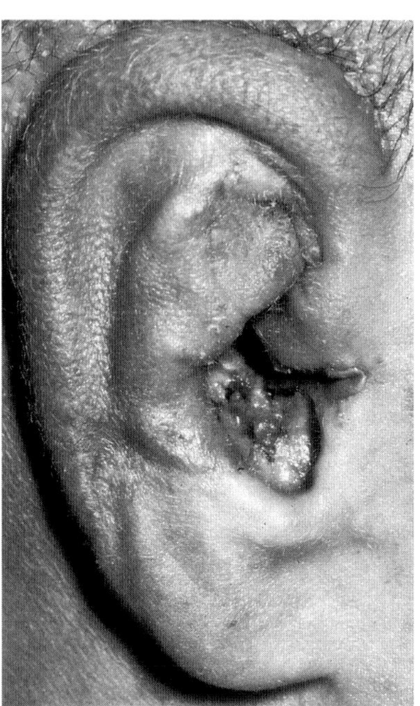

Fig. 5.**187** **Mild necrosis of the full-thickness skin graft in the concha (usually heals by secondary intention, as in this case).**

Furnas (1990) has looked into the complications of auricular reconstruction in great detail. He lists the following categories of errors and complications:

Errors in Planning or Technique

- Malpositioning of the auricle
- Poorly designed cartilage framework
- Inexperience and poor technique
- Wrong material, e. g., silicone rubber or polyethylene instead of cartilage
- Wrong size
- Wrong free graft in a conspicuous area
- Hair on the auricle

Errors in Harvesting the Costal Cartilage

- Pneumothorax
- Hypertrophic scarring
- Deformity of the chest

Errors in Managing Skin Coverage

- Ischemia and skin necrosis (Figs. 5.**186**–5.**189**)
- Problems of circulation due to lack of skin
- Problems of circulation due to excessive height of the helix or antihelix (reduction in the height of the cartilage, see Fig. 5.**189 a**)

Errors of Expander Implantation

Furnas suggests the use of expander implantation especially for post-traumatic auricular defects and scars (see p. 231).

- Expander leakage
- Skin necrosis due to accelerated filling and exaggerated tension (Fig. 5.**188**)
- Infection, extrusion

Hematoma and Seroma

It is imperative:

- To obtain meticulous perioperative hemostasis (Brent 1980 I, 1999 a)
- To avoid the use of epinephrine
- To use bipolar coagulation under good visualization
- To have good drainage and constant vacuum within the drainage bottles, especially when changing them

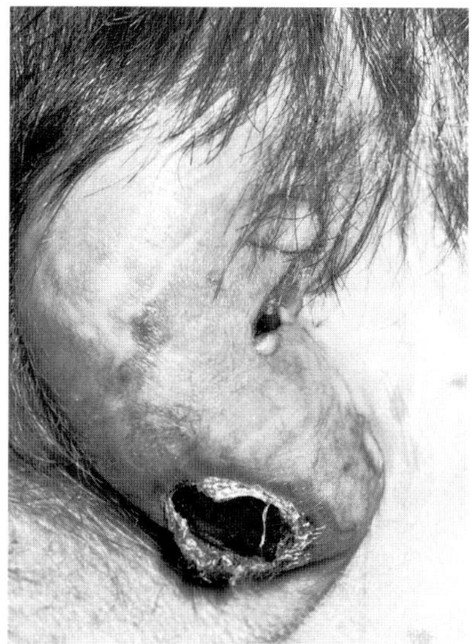

Fig. 5.**188** **Pressure necrosis after insertion of an expander in the presence of scars secondary to previous surgery** (Treatment: removal of the expander, excision of the necrosis, and closure of the defect).

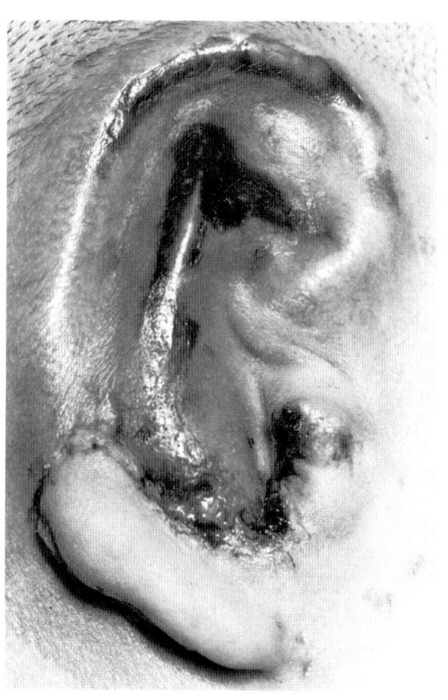

a

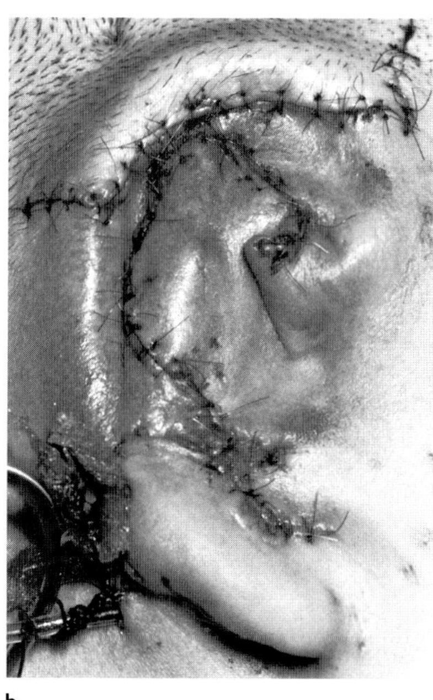

b

Fig. 5.**189** **Necrosis with defect of the superior helix and superior antihelical crus: reconstruction by skin transposition.**

a Necrosis of the superior helix and antihelix.

b Excision of the necrosis and cartilage, mobilization of the scalp, removal of hair follicles, and U-shaped advancement. Similarly, skin is mobilized anteriorly, followed by closure (additional lowering of the cartilages).

Necrosis of Skin Coverage and Ischemia of Transposed Earlobe -

- We have already described the protection of the ear by using appropriate dressing techniques (Tanzer 1963; see Figs. 5.**185**).
- **Mattress sutures** should be used only sparingly, if at all (Brent 1997, personal communication), and without great pressure. They should be removed immediately if the tissue is at risk.
- Furnas (1990) suggests only the use of ointment dressings for small skin defects, while larger skin losses are covered by local flaps (see p. 227 and Chapter 4).
- In addition, fan flaps (Brent 1980 II), postauricular artery flaps, and hair-bearing flaps are recommended for temporary coverage (see Chapter 4).
- For extreme cases, Furnas recommends removing the framework and banking it in the chest wall until the skin has recovered. He also recommends hyperbaric oxygen treatment.

Cartilage Absorption and Necrosis

Exposure of the cartilage and rare infections result in absorption and cartilage necrosis (Fig. 5.**189 a**, **b**; see also Fig. 4.**39**, p. 59). The skin pocket must therefore be large enough to avoid pressure on the cartilage (see Fig. 4.**40 a**, p. 59).

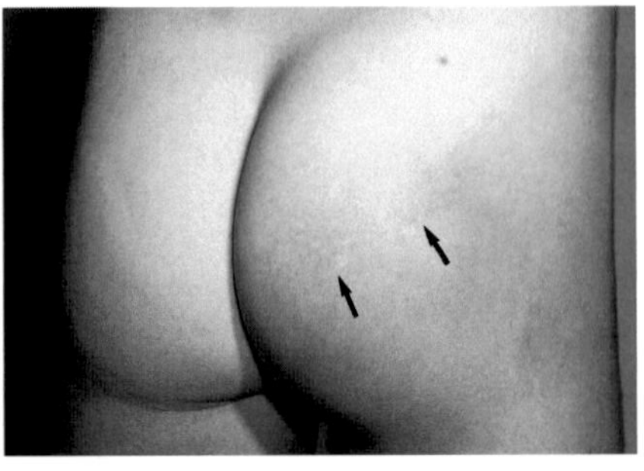

a

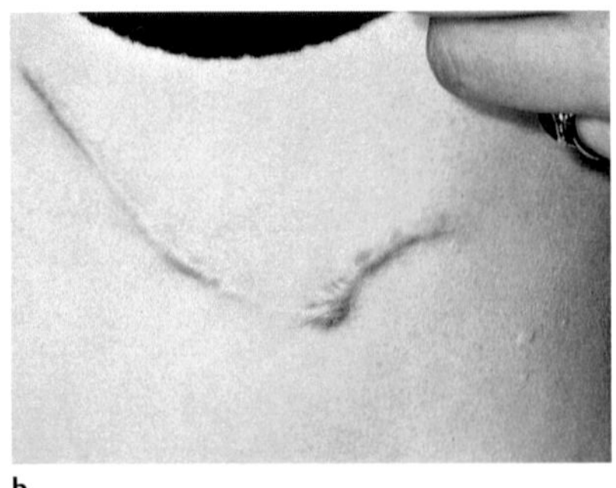

b

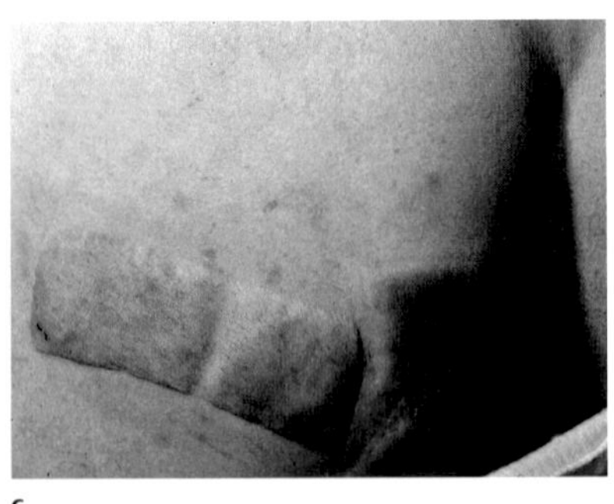

c

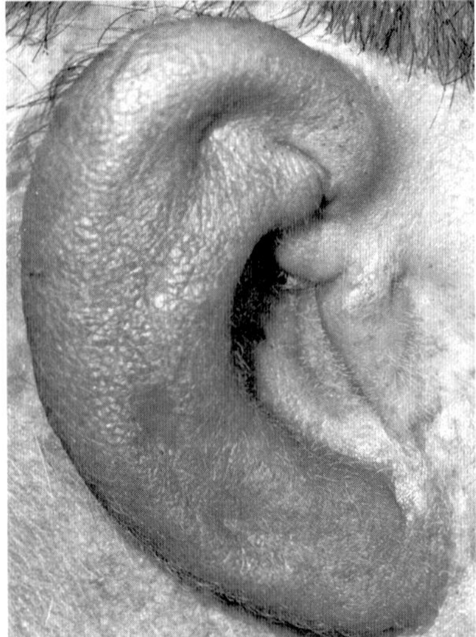

d

Fig. 5.**190** **Hypertrophic scarring after surgery for dysplasia.**
a Normal wound healing after harvesting skin from the buttock.
b, c Hypertrophic scarring over the chest wall and buttock (steroid infiltration may be used, or scar revision).
d Loss of contour of the reconstructed auricle secondary to hypertrophic scarring, especially in the scapha and concha (for improvement of contour see Figs. 5.**164**, p. 210, 5.**174**, see p. 218).

Small defects can be allowed to heal by secondary intention. The cartilage is covered with ointment to protect it from drying out. Larger defects are resurfaced with local flaps (see Figs. 5.**191**–5.**193**; see also Chapter 4). Like Bogdasarian and Baker (1983), Fukuda (1988, 1990), and Boudard et al. (1989), we recommend allowing healing by secondary intention for smaller defects and unexposed cartilage. Fukuda (1988, 1990) reports that he experienced necrosis in 20% of the skin covering the cartilage and in 10% there was necrosis or partial necrosis of the free grafts (see Fig. 5.**187**). Much less often, he saw cartilage absorption, dislocation of the helical cartilage, wire suture exposure, and hypertrophic scar formation.

Partial necroses of the cartilage are repaired with spare cartilage from the skin pocket in the chest wall, the helix dislocation is corrected surgically, and the helix is expanded and sutured to the corresponding point on the framework (5–0 wire or 4–0 braided sutures). Wire sutures are removed.

Further revision operations correspond to the methods previously described for the reconstruction of defects (see Chapter 4).

Infections

Infections are rarely reported in the literature when perioperative prophylaxis is initiated. We personally have experienced, at most, small foci of infection where local necrosis has developed; we have never encountered losses secondary to infection. A broad-spectrum antibiotic is administered should an infection occur. The antibiotic therapy may require adjustment after identification of the pathogen. More important is careful changing of dressings without pressure, ointment packs and, if necessary, the incision and drainage of an abscess.

A perichondritis of the residual framework occasionally occurs.

Suture Fistulas

Mechanical erosion of sutures, especially wire sutures, is occasionally observed and requires cutting and removal of the suture.

Hypertrophic Scarring and Keloids

(Fig. 5.**190**)

In a long-term postoperative observation, Yanai et al. (1985) followed up 166 patients for 1 year after reconstruction of the auricle and witnessed cases ranging from slight fibrosis to moderate fibrosis with loss of contour, as well as extreme changes with keloid formation. Their findings in the region of the scar on the anterior chest were similar, leading them to postulate a predisposition for hypertrophic scar formation here.

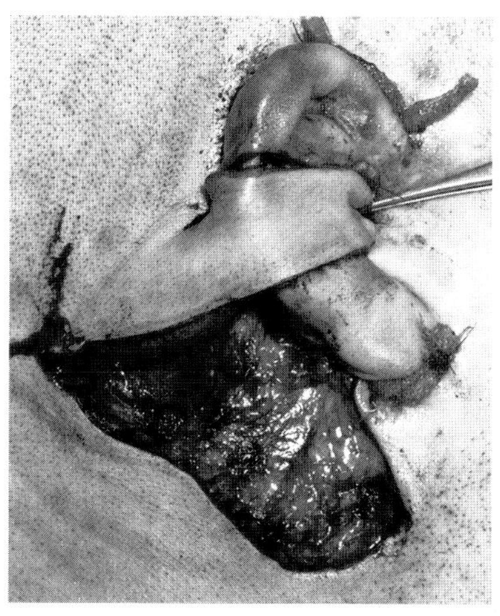

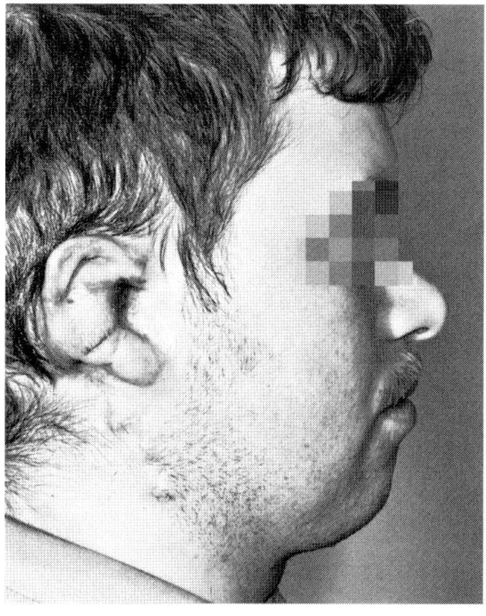

a b

Fig. 5.**191** **Necrosis and defect of the middle third of the auricle after total ear reconstruction: coverage with a transposition flap.**
a Elevation and transposition of the flap.
b The flap has been divided and inset. Further smaller corrections are necessary, such as formation of the scapha (see Figs. 5.**164**, 5.**174**) and of the concha (see Figs. 5.**177**, 5.**178**).

On reviewing the chest donor site, Thomson et al. (1995) found a number of hypertrophic scars, even to the extent of keloid formation (for treatment see p. 145). Scar revision requires the usual corrective measures, such as excision, Z-plasty, W-plasty, or staggering of the scar using the broken-line technique (Weerda 1999 a, 2001).

Loss of Contour

We have previously given a detailed account of the molding of the auricular form after loss of contour of the scapha (see p. 210), the concha (see p. 218), the helical crus, and the intertragic notch.

Thoracic Deformities

These can occur especially after the very generous removal of cartilage undertaken when using Nagata's technique (1994 a–d).

Siegert (2001, personal communication) fills cartilage remains into a net rather than a sock (Fig. 6.**29**, p. 256) made of resorbable braided sutures, shaped like a rib, and hopes to eliminate chest wall deformity by cartilage neoformation, especially in young patients.

Local flaps are used in the attempt to repair defects. The techniques are described in Chapter 4.

Defects After the First Operative Stage

Posterior helix and antihelix, defect of the anterior region of the auricle. With Brent's technique (1980, 1999 a), defects after the first operative stage can occasionally be resurfaced by a pedicled flap raised from the residual vestige in the concha or from accessory auricles (see Fig. 5.**189**). In the region of the transposed earlobe, in the anterior region, as well as in the region of the helical crus and the superior helix, we like to use a superiorly or inferiorly based preauricular flap, even after the second or third operative stage (see Fig. 5.**192**).

Defects of the posterior helical and antihelical regions. The necrosis can be excised; in some cases cartilage requires excision and replacement, while the defect can be closed by anterior advancement of skin after mobilization of the hair-bearing scalp (see Fig. 5.**189**). On occasion, a larger, superiorly based transposition flap will be necessary (Fig. 5.**191 a, b**; see Figs. 4.**20**, 4.**22**, 4.**38**, 4.**39**, 4.**44**).

Occasionally, a **fat/fibrous-tissue flap** can also be used, which will then require coverage with a free skin graft. This flap is dissected out below the hair follicles. The temporoparietal fascia and the galea should be left untouched, as they will be required for the second stage.

Defects After the Second Operative Stage

Defects of the posterior helical and antihelical regions. Here an attempt is made to cover the defect with a fascial flap or a flap from the superoposterior region of the neck (see Fig. 5.**191**) or another type of flap (Figs. 5.**192 a**, **b**, 5.**193 a**, **b**). If necessary, a flap from the hair-bearing scalp will have to be used. First, an attempt is made to resect the hair follicles. Hair is left untouched and de-epilated later only when necessary, or the skin is removed together with the hair follicles, leaving a fibrous layer over the cartilage, and the defect is resurfaced with a free graft from the contralateral postauricular region.

Malposition

An auricle set too high is rarely a problem; we have yet to encounter it in our entire reconstructive experience. More common, however, is an auricle lying too low, because of a low hairline. Here the auricle will require dissection far enough anteriorly until sufficient mobility is achieved to allow its fixation in a higher position, perhaps even held in place with a strip of fascia.

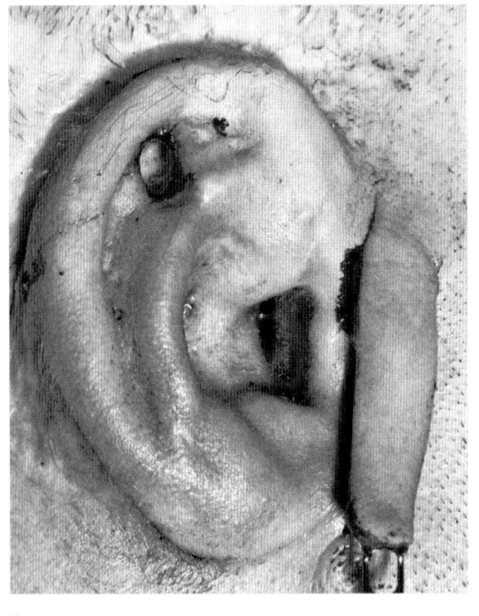
a

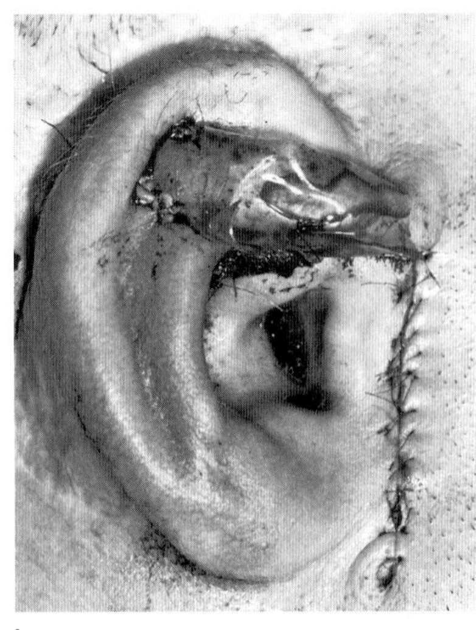
b

Fig. 5.**192** **Necrosis in the superior scapha: coverage with a preauricular flap.**
a Necrosis; the flap has been elevated.
b The flap has been inset, the wound closed. The ear is protected from partial digestion by a thin silicone film (see p. 59, Fig. 4.**39**).

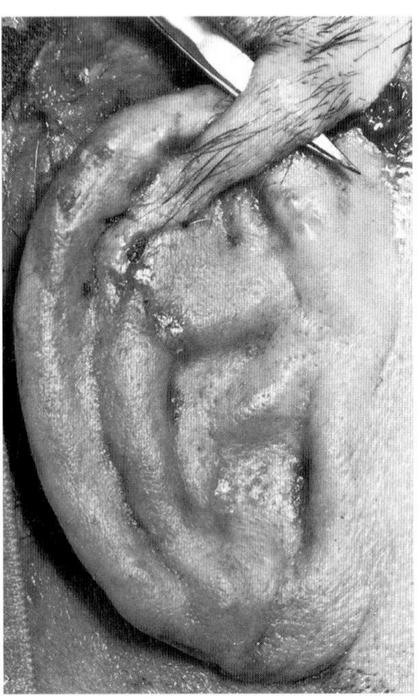
a

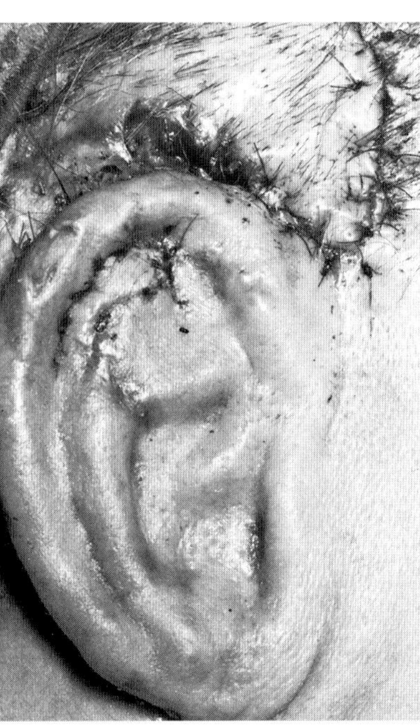
b

Fig. 5.**193** **Coverage of a scaphal defect with a preauricular flap (second stage).**
a, b Division and inset.

Auricular Reconstruction and Microsomia

Nowadays attempts are increasingly being made to harmonize the dysplastic face by distraction therapy and augmentation plasty (see p. 271).

For the auricular relationships on the healthy side to be transferred to the malformed side, the patient in Figure 5.**194** would have to undergo auricular reconstruction within the hair-bearing occipital region. We therefore try to place the auricle as far posteriorly as possible, recognizing of course that here the hairless skin is the limiting factor (Fig. 5.**194**). In addition, it is also possible to reconstruct the ear slightly smaller than the healthy auricle, possibly setting back and reducing the prominent ear of the healthy side (see Fig. 5.**166**, p. 210).

Auricular Reconstruction and Otoplasty

In our cases of unilateral grade III dysplasia, we have frequently encountered a prominent ear on the healthy side. The auricle will then require setting back at the final stage of the reconstruction to achieve a harmonious final result (see pp. 137 ff).

Bilateral Dysplasia

In cases of grade III dysplasia on the one side and less severe dysplasia on the other, reconstruction begins with the less

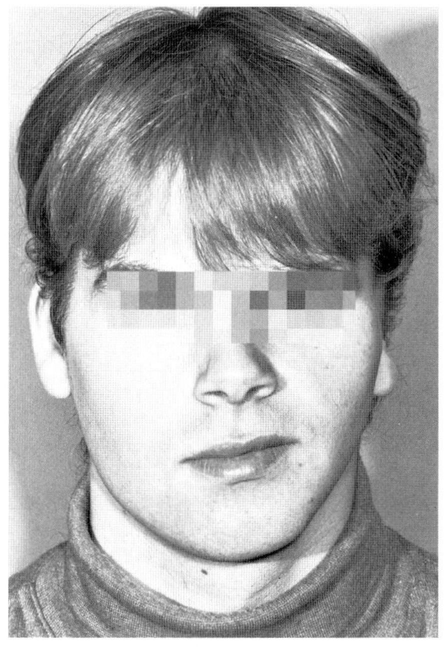

a

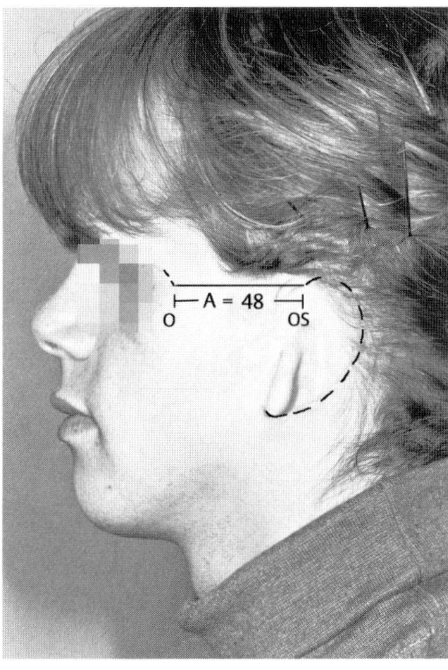

b

Fig. 5.**194** **Position of the auricle in a case of microsomia.**
a Microsomia.
b The distance A between orbita (O) and otobasion superius (OS) is 67 mm on the right and 48 mm on the left.

severe side. At the first stage, the auricles can be reconstructed in succession, with an interval of 3–4 days. From the second stage onwards, we then try to reconstruct both ears simultaneously.

We try to supply children with bilateral congenital atresia of the auditory canal with a bone conduction hearing aid during the first weeks of life (see p. 260). We are able to provide patients with bilateral bone-anchored hearing aids from the third year of life (Oppermann et al. 1996). Middle-ear reconstruction is commenced at the second stage at the earliest (see pp. 245, 255; Weerda 1985c, Weerda et al. 1985).

Anotia

If there is no auricular vestige or rudimentary remnant (Fig. 5.**195**) that can be utilized to reconstruct the earlobe, the lobular part of the cartilage framework is fashioned slightly larger and the auricle is then reconstructed as for cases of loss of the auricle (see pp. 90 ff).

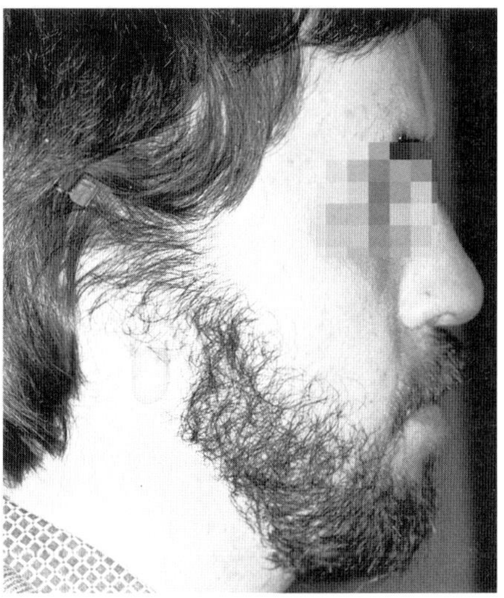

Fig. 5.**195** **Anotia.**
Apart from congenital atresia of the auditory canal, a low hairline is also frequently encountered. An auricular appendage or a fistula-like pit is seen behind the temporomandibular joint (see p. 221, Fig. 5.**181**).

5.4.4 Classification of Stenosis of the Auditory Canal and Atresia (Figs. 5.196–5.198)

The skin around the auricular region should remain untouched, as it will be required for the reconstruction.

Stenosis of the auditory canal can occur in association with a malformation of the auricle (see Embryology, p. 106). An axial CT will provide information on the extent of the stenosis (see p. 230; Mehra et al. 1988; Weerda 1985 a, b). Many classifications for stenosis and forms of atresia have been reported; they commonly include malformations of the auricle, the auditory canal, and the middle ear (Cremers et al. 1984). We have modified the various classifications for stenosis to permit reference to the auditory canal alone (Fig. 5.**196 a–c**). Malformations of the auricle, auditory canal, and middle ear should be classified separately (Weerda 1994 e).

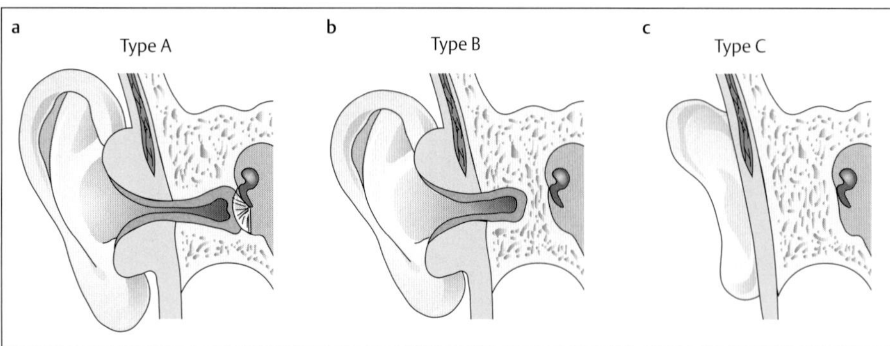

Fig. 5.**196** **Classification of malformations of the auditory canal in the presence of auricular malformations (from Weerda 1994 e).**
a Type A: stenosis of the auditory canal with severe stenosis of the auditory canal with an intact skin envelope.
b Type B: bony atresia plate near the middle ear.
c Type C: complete bony atresia of the auditory canal.

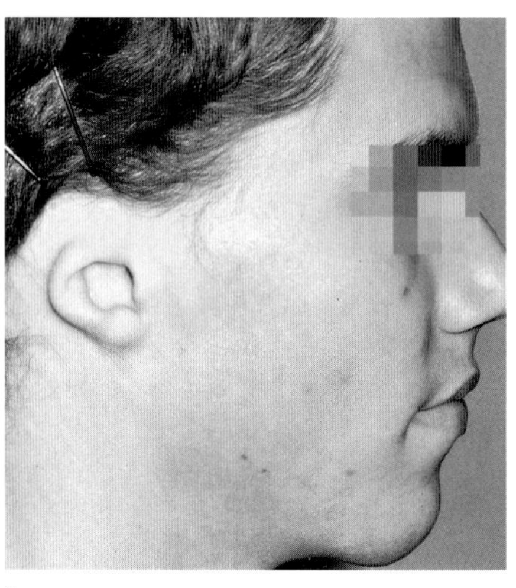
a

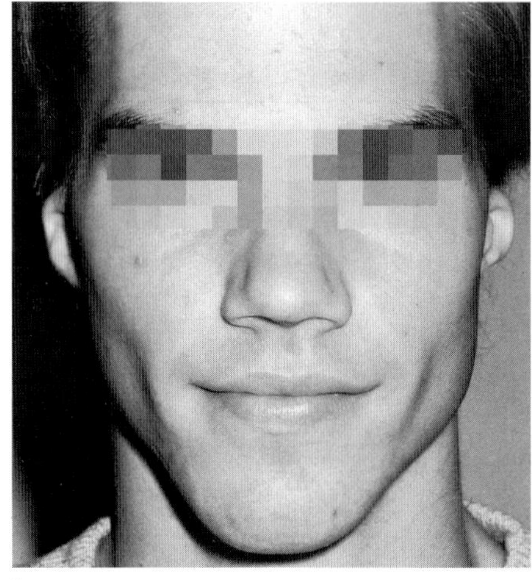
b

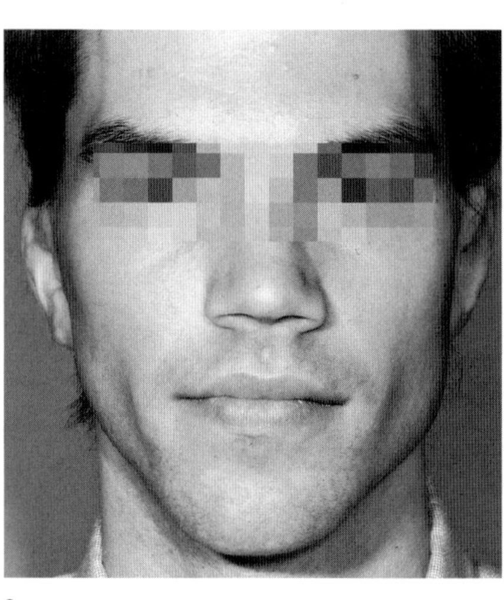
c

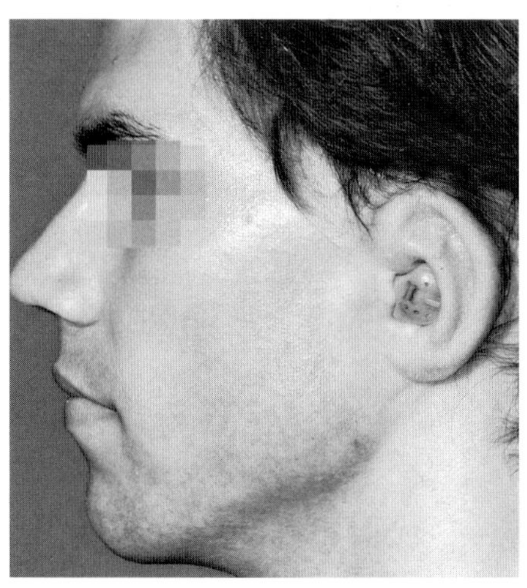
d

Fig. 5.**197** **Surgery for bilateral type B stenosis of the auditory canal with subsequent provision of two hearing aids (see also pp. 260).**
a, b Bilateral grade III dysplasia (microtia) with type B stenosis of the auditory canal.
c Appearance after bilateral auricular reconstruction and reconstruction of the auditory canal.
d Additional provision of two in-ear hearing aids.

Malformations of the Auditory Canal

- Type A: stenosis (Fig. 5.**196 a**)
- Type B: partially preformed auditory canal with an atretic bony plate in its medial segment (Fig. 5.**196 b**, see Fig. 5.**197 a–d** for surgery)
- Type C: complete atresia of the auditory canal (Fig. 5.**196 c**). Additional provision of a hearing aid is commonly required (Fig. 5.**198 a, b**).

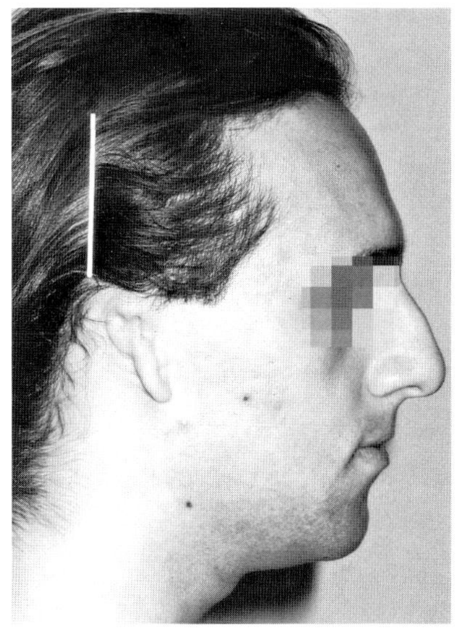

a

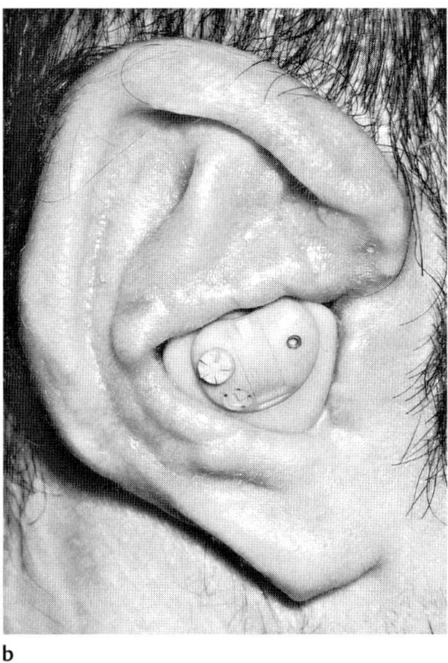

b

Fig. 5.198 **Surgery for type C atresia of the auditory canal with subsequent provision with a hearing aid.**

a Grade III dysplasia (microtia) and congenital atresia of the auditory canal.

b Appearance after auricular reconstruction, reconstruction of the auditory canal and the middle ear as well as provision of an in-ear hearing aid (surgeon: R. Siegert; see p. 255).

5.4.5 Skin Expansion in Preparation for Auricular Construction or Reconstruction

R. Siegert

Introduction

The principle of skin expansion can be witnessed in the natural world in pregnant women, in the development of the female breast during puberty, or in the subcutaneous growth of tumors. Since primeval times, various African tribes have used special forms of skin expansion to stretch lips, earlobes, or, with the aid of rings, the skin of the neck (Burnett 1945; Caputo 1983).

The first use of the principle of expansion dates back to Neumann who employed it in 1957 to treat a 52-year-old patient who had suffered a traumatic partial loss of the auricle (Neumann 1957). He implanted a balloon beneath the scalp and filled it with air several times a week via an externally placed port. The amount of inflated air depended on the clinical assessment of the skin, whereby "an attempt was made to avoid blanching and at the same time to keep the tissues under tension." Expansion was over a period of 2 months.

Neumann's innovative technique remained relatively unknown for many years and was only later rediscovered by Radovan in 1976 when he used it for breast reconstruction (Radovan 1980).

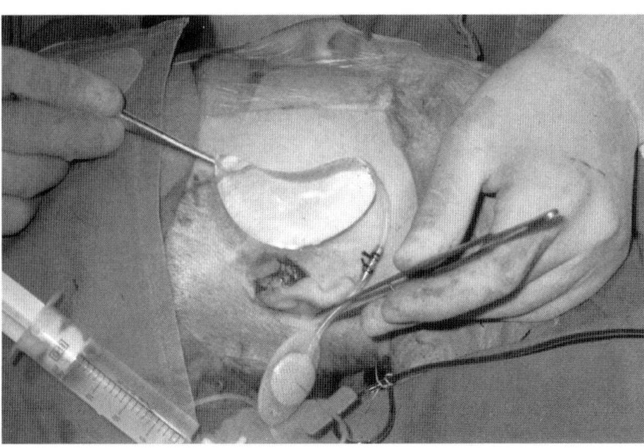

Fig. 5.199 **Expansion treatment: incision anterior to the auricular rudiment; development of a pocket: trial filling of the expander before implantation (35 mL expander with port below).**

Basic Principles

Expanders. Balloons with a silicone shell, ports, and cannulae are required for skin expansion (see Fig. 5.199).

The balloons and ports together are referred to as the "expander." The ports are either integrated into the balloon or connected to it via a tube (see Fig. 5.199).

Expanded tissue. The expansion results in specific biological reactions which can be used to prepare for auricular (re-)construction and defect coverage.

The **epidermis** and **dermis** undergo hardly any morphological changes, although an increase in the mitosis rate of the epidermis as early as the first day and increased collagen

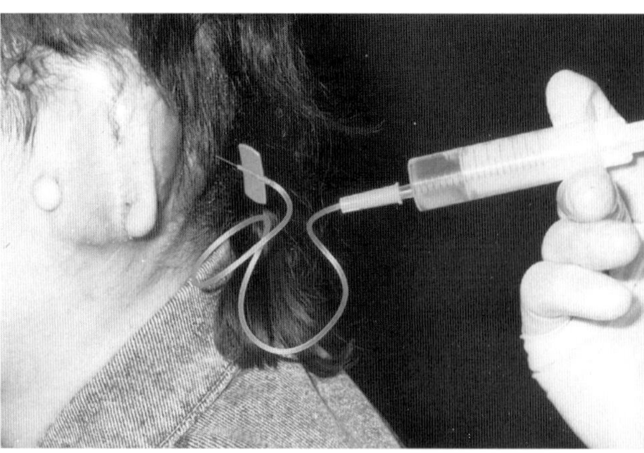

Fig. 5.**200** **Expansion treatment: inflation of expander 2 weeks after implantation; filling with sterile physiological saline solution via the port with a thin cannula.**

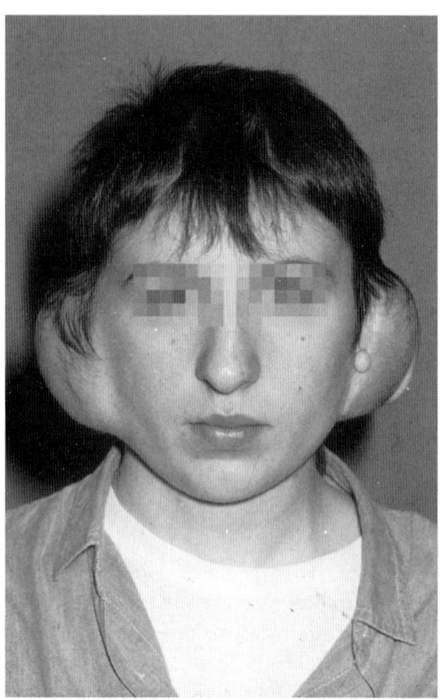

Fig. 5.**201** **Expansion treatment: appearance after 2 months of repeated expander infiltration.**

synthesis can be detected about 2 weeks after commencing expansion. During expansion the **subcutaneous fatty tissue** is initially compressed, only to be slowly and partially absorbed afterwards. The **capsule** is of great clinical importance, and develops in the immediate vicinity of the silicone foreign body in the course of a few weeks. It is a fibrous, reversible structure comprising histiocytes, fibrocytes, macrophages, and myofibroblasts, as well as newly formed collagen fibers which degenerate over a period of months after explantation of the expander.

Immediately after filling the expander, skin perfusion initially decreases relative to the volume applied and the subsequent rise in pressure, followed by a compensatory increase in perfusion. This initial increase in **microcirculation** is the result of functional reactions. Morphological changes, accompanied by increases in the relative volumes of the vessels in the dermis, may be observed after about 2 weeks.

Surgically useful skin. The linear expandability of unscarred skin amounts to about 15–20% in the region of the ear. Since the elastic properties of skin only begin to normalize about 2 weeks after expansion with the remodeling of the dermal fibrous system, refilling the balloon after only a short interval is of little use. Genuine surgically useful skin is only obtainable with expansion sessions carried out over several weeks to several months.

Clinical Use

Expander size. For most cases, a kidney-shaped expander with a nominal volume of 35–50 ml is advisable for auricular reconstruction (see Fig. 5.**199**).

Incision and mobilization. The incision is placed anterior to the auricular remnant (Fig. 5.**199**, see also p. 207, Fig. 5.**160 a**).

The size of the subcutaneous pocket required for implantation is determined by the surface area of the expander base.

Port. The port (see Figs. 5.**199**, 5.**200**) is implanted beneath the scalp near the expander. The incision is then closed. Care should be taken not to damage the balloon with needle or forceps.

Expansion. The expander should be pre-filled with about 5 ml of sterile physiological saline or Ringer's solution at the time of implantation. The immediate filling reduces the dead space of the expander pocket and so reduces the risk of hematoma formation. Needless to say, a vacuum drain should also be inserted.

Further fillings depend on the individual objective and the expansion protocol employed (Fig. 5.**200** and see Fig. 5.**201**).

Objective and Expansion Protocols

Depending on the duration, there are three different types of skin expansion with entirely different biological effects:

- **Intraoperative expansion** over a period of about 2 hours results in subcutaneous mobilization.
- **Short-term expansion** over a period of 1–2 weeks results in the increase of flap circulation.
- **Long-term expansion** over a period of about 2 months; this results in genuine skin growth, in addition to the frequently undesired formation of a capsule.

Long-term expansion. Depending on the surface area of skin needed for the reconstruction, this type of expansion requires several weeks to months (Fig. 5.**201**). After a postoperative healing phase of 2 weeks, the expander is inflated at intervals of 1–2 weeks, similar to the short-term form of expansion. Because of the sluggishness of the dermal fibrous tissue, a more frequent filling is biologically not recommendable.

Explantation and treatment of the expanded skin. A capsule forms after long-term expansion and contributes not only to the stability of the skin, but also to its thickness. Initially expanded skin also conforms more poorly to the convolutions and relief of the cartilage framework. The capsule should therefore be removed very carefully, taking care to protect the dermal vascular network.

Complications and Their Prevention

Apart from **pain**, which should not be regarded as a complication in its narrower sense, **skin necrosis** with extrusion of the expander and subsequent **infection** are the most serious, and by no means infrequent, complications (see Fig. 5.**188**, p. 225). They are reported in the literature as occurring in as may as **one third** of cases (Siegert and Weerda 1994 a, b; Siegert et al. 1995 a). Their main causes are embarrassment to circulation and excessive thinning of the skin.

Skin thinning can result from pressure and the actual weight of the expander and lead to perforation over the implant and necrosis, especially with skin flaps which have already been dissected very thinly during implantation (see p. 225, Fig. 5.**188**).

Conclusion

Depending on the type of expansion protocol used, tissue expansion provides the option of preparing for (re-)construction of the auricle by either gentle subcutaneous mobilization, increase in the blood circulation of the skin, or by genuine skin growth (see Fig. 5.**201**). The latter is admittedly very time-consuming, but creates skin for coverage of the framework which, given its color and texture that are specific to its location, is superior to any skin flap or graft. **This therapeutic option should be considered only for difficult cases with scarring in the region of the ear.**

6 Diagnostics and Auxiliary Therapy

6.1 Radiological Examination of Malformations of the Petrous Temporal Bone

S. Gottschalk and D. Petersen

6.1.1 Introduction

During the preoperative diagnostic work-up of malformations of the external ear, much emphasis is placed on the radiological assessment of the petrous temporal bone, in addition to standard audiological examinations (Bockenheimer, Weerda et al. 1984). The planning and prognosis of any surgical reconstruction demand a precise anatomical definition of the associated middle ear and inner ear malformation.

Since its introduction in the 1980s, computed tomography (CT) has largely replaced traditional radiography and tomography in the diagnostic examination of the petrous bone. The demonstration of the bony structures of the middle ear and the skull base is the domain of high-resolution CT (HRCT) (Alexander et al. 1998). Assessment of the inner ear is also undertaken primarily with the aid of CT, supplemented by magnetic resonance imaging (MRI) for the examination of membranous structures (Swartz 1996). CT sections allow easy identification of the course of the facial nerve along its tympanic and mastoid segments, while evaluation of its intracranial portion and assessment of the vestibulocochlear nerve are done with the aid of MRI. The bony demarcations of the vessels of the skull base reflect the course of the vessels in great detail on plain CT sections, and both CT angiography and MR angiography are also used as noninvasive methods (Rodgers et al. 1993).

Table 6.**1** CT score according to Jahrsdoerfer (0–10 points)

Finding	Score
Normal external auditory canal	1
Middle ear space, pneumatized	1
Mastoid well pneumatized	1
Malleus–incus complex present	1
Incus–stapes connection	1
Stapes present	2
Oval window open	1
Round window normal	1
Course of the facial nerve normal to a large extent (this means that the present course of the facial nerve makes any damage to the nerve during surgery improbable)	1

6.1.2 High-Resolution CT (HRCT)

The **scan volume** should extend from the jugular foramen to the superior margin of the petrous pyramid. The traditional slice orientation to display the petrous bone is the **axial plane**, parallel to the German horizontal plane or to the orbitomeatal line. This plane is easy to position, displays the petrous bone in comparison with the contralateral side, and provides good anatomical information in the standard plane. However, it is not possible to image all the anatomical structures adequately in one plane. The most important supplementary images which should also be available are **coronary sections** perpendicular to the orbitomeatal plane and extending from the tragus to the convexity of the posterior semicircular canal (Yeakley and Jahrsdoerfer 1996). For reasons of radiation protection, the primary orientation can also be selected so as to avoid including the lens of the eye within the scan volume. Modern image-processing techniques allow the reconstruction of secondary sections along any desired plane, primarily using isotropic voxels without any loss of quality. Additional three-dimensional surface reconstructions and virtual images can be reconstructed from high-resolution image data sets (Seemann et al. 1999; Himi et al. 2000).

6.1.3 CT Scores for Assessing Malformations of the Petrous Bone

Jahrsdoerfer et al. (1992) developed a CT score comprising a maximum of 10 points for the prognostic assessment of the surgical reconstruction of the middle ear in patients with congenital aural atresia (Table 6.1). The score takes into account the appearance of the external auditory canal, pneumatization of the mastoid, pneumatization of the tympanic cavity, presence or absence of the stapes, the incus–stapes connection, the incus–malleus complex, the patency of the round and oval windows, and any variations in the course of the facial nerve (see Table 6.1). The authors consider a score of **8 points for unilateral** atresia and more than **5 points for bilateral** atresia to be an **indication for surgery.**

Based on their experience with a large population of their own patients with malformations of the middle ear, Siegert, Weerda et al. (1996 b) sought to refine the preoperative assessment of prognosis. They introduced a CT score with a maximum of 28 points (Table 6.2). Their score differs from that of Jahrsdoerfer in that the stapes is assessed as normal, dysplastic, or absent. Oval and round windows are allocated a higher score. The size of the tympanic cavity is subject to a more differentiated grading system, given that it represents the spatial prerequisite for a tympanoplasty. Pneumatization of the mastoid and pneumatization of the tympanum are regarded as proof of the functioning of the Eustachian tube. The multitude of variations in the course of the facial nerve and additional aberrant vessels are included in the assessment, since they can increase the degree of difficulty of the operation. Siegert and Weerda consider score of **20 points or more for unilateral** malformation and **15 points or more for bilateral** malformation to be an **indication for surgery** (Table 6.2).

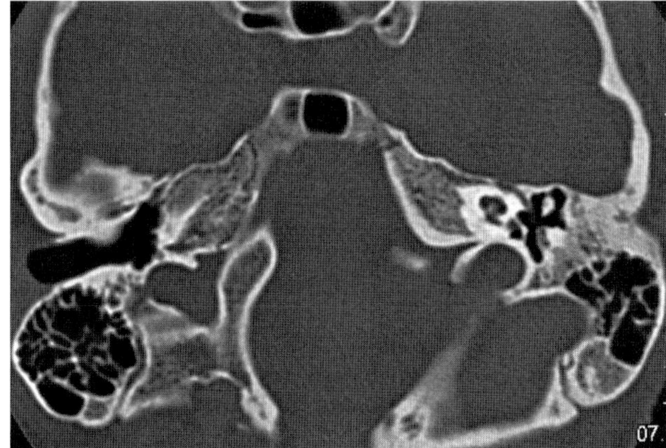

Fig. 6.**1** **CT of external auditory canal and tympanic cavity.** Left grade III microtia; axial CT section.
Left: Atretic bony plate (0 points according to the Jahrsdoerfer score and to the Siegert and Weerda score). Reduced size of tympanic cavity (no loss of points according to the Jahrsdoerfer score as width is more than 3 mm; 1 point deducted according to the Siegert and Weerda score). Dysplasia of the ossicles (see discussion and text for Figs. 6.**7**–6.**9**). The mastoid is bilaterally pneumatized (no loss of points according to both the Jahrsdoerfer score and the Siegert and Weerda score).
Right: Normal findings.

Table 6.**2** CT score according to Siegert and Weerda (0–28 points)

Finding	Score
External auditory canal: normal/atresia of soft tissue/ bony atresia	2/1/0
Tympanum size: large/moderate/sclerosed	2/1/0
Tympanum pneumatization: marked/moderate/ absent	2/1/0
Mastoid pneumatization: marked/moderate/ absent	2/1/0
Incus–malleus complex: normal/dysplastic/absent	2/1/0
Stapes: normal/dysplastic/absent	4/2/0
Oval window: open/closed	4/0
Round window: open/closed	4/0
Facial nerve: normal/slightly displaced/extremely displaced course	4/2/0
Vessels: normal/slightly displaced/extremely displaced course	2/1/0

6.1.4 Radiological Analysis—Normal and Pathological Anatomy

All the important anatomical structures of the petrous bone are assessed primarily with reference to the CT scores; certain indications will require supplementary imaging.

External Auditory Canal

The **external auditory canal** may be absent, shortened, stenotic, or end blind in cases of microtia. Instead of a normal auditory canal, there is a fibrous or bony atretic plate (see Fig. 5.**196**, Figs. 6.**1**–6.**3**). Adjacent structures of the skull base, such as the glenoid fossa of the temporomandibular joint, are often dysplastic and displaced.

Mastoid Process

The **mastoid** is often small and may also appear deformed, together with the bony skull base. The degree of pneumatization is noted. In addition, it should also be documented whether the cells are pneumatized or clouded at the time of investigation (Figs. 6.**4**, 6.**5**, cf. Figs. 6.**1**–6.**3**).

Tympanic Cavity

The **auditory (eustachian) tube** has a bony portion in its dorsal third, which can be well defined on the axial CT image to be lateral to the exit of the internal carotid artery through the foramen lacerum. A functioning tube should appear pneumatized on the CT images. A foreshortened tube which is widened in its bony portion is often found in cases with a diminished hypoplastic cavity. The functioning of the tube determines the pneumatization of the tympanic cavity.

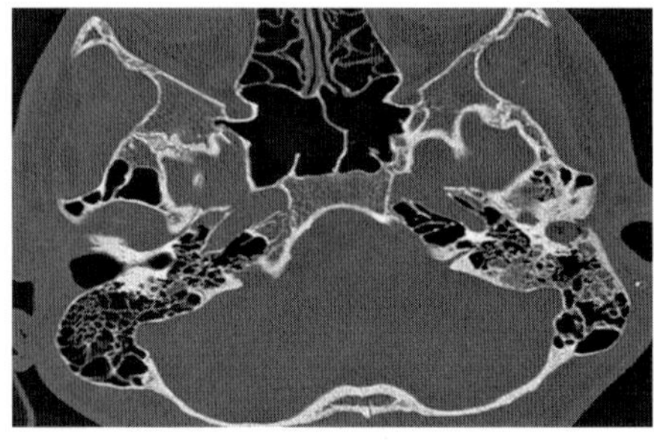

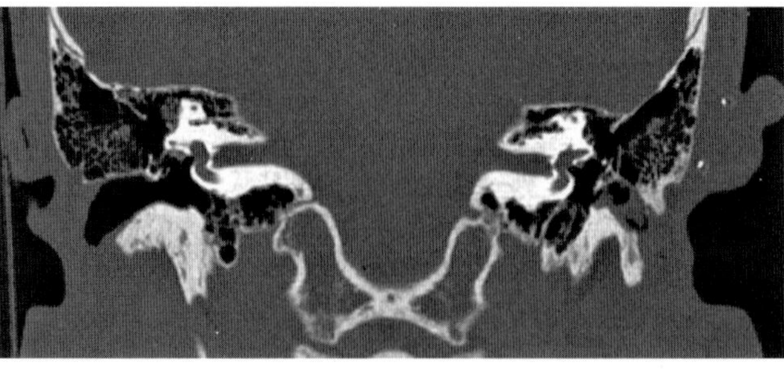

a b

Fig. 6.2 **CT of external auditory canal and tympanic cavity.** Left grade II microtia.
a Axial image.
b Coronary image.
The right external ear and middle ear are normal. The left ear shows fibrous atresia (no loss of points according to the Jahrsdoerfer score, 1 point deducted according to the Siegert and Weerda score). The external auditory canal on the left is normal in form and shows mild bony stenosis at the level of its entrance. There is narrowing along its course to varying degrees due to fibrous tissue. The tympanic cavity is pneumatized and normal in width. The mastoid demonstrates extensive pneumatization, and on the left individual cells are clouded (no point reduction according to the Jahrsdoerfer score or to the Siegert and Weerda score for tympanum and mastoid).

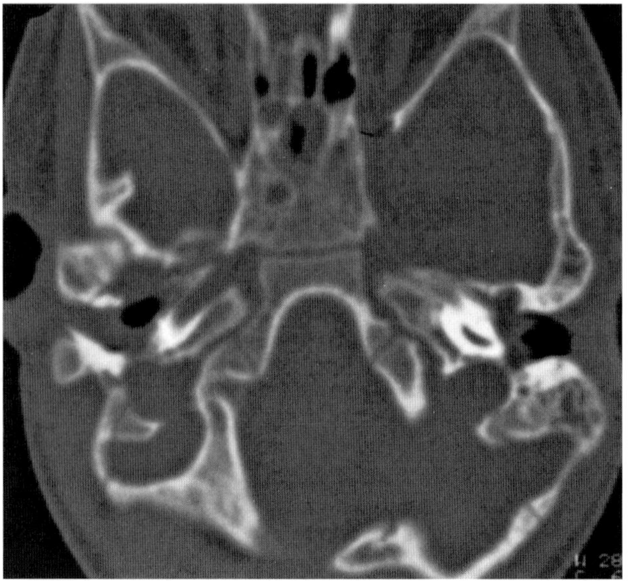

Fig. 6.3 **CT of external auditory canal and tympanic cavity.** Bilateral grade III microtia.
There is bilateral fibrous atresia of the external auditory canal. Complete cloudiness of the tympanic cavity on the left, with partial pneumatization of the external auditory canal with cloudiness of the hypotympanum on the right. The mastoid is hypoplastic and not pneumatized on the right, cells are developed on the left but are cloudy (according to the Jahrsdoerfer score, deduction of 2 points for the left side and no loss of points for the right; according to the Siegert and Weerda score, deduction of 4 points for the left side and 2 points for the right).

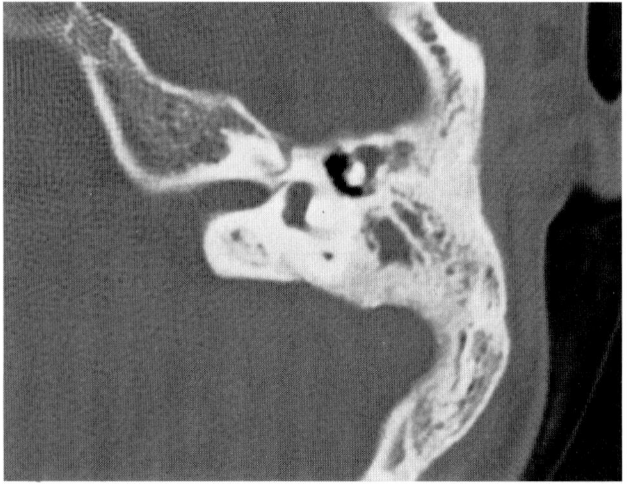

Fig. 6.4 **CT of external auditory canal and tympanic cavity.** Left grade III microtia.
Atretic bony plate. Slightly reduced size of the tympanic cavity with partial cloudiness at the level of the epitympanum (cloudiness presumably caused by fluid) as well as cloudiness of the antrum. Reduced pneumatization of the mastoid.

The tympanic cavity is contiguous with the atretic plate medially and can be virtually normal, reduced in size, or completely obliterated (Fig. 6.6; see Figs. 6.1–6.5). The maximum width of the tympanic cavity at the level of the promontory in a healthy individual is 7–10 mm on the axial CT slice. Yeakley and Jahrsdoerfer (1996) regard a width of at least 3 mm as a prerequisite for surgical reconstruction.

Occasionally the roof of the tympanic cavity appears collapsed caudally. This finding is usually identifiable with any degree of certainty only on coronary slices. Careful note should be made of the complete pneumatization of an embryonically preformed tympanic cavity (cf. Figs. 6.3–6.6). The tympanic membrane can be preformed in the presence of auditory canal stenosis, and a cholesteatoma may be present. Cole and Jahrsdoerfer (1990) discovered cholesteatomas in 91 % of their series of patients with an extreme stenosis of the auditory canal. In such cases a partially clouded tympanic cavity appears on CT, typically in the mesotympanum, with some cases also demonstrating destruction of the auditory ossicles. If the tympanic cavity appears completely clouded in the presence of atresia of the auditory canal, then CT imaging does not always allow unequivocal differentiation between a temporary blockage by fluid and mesenchymal tissue. For these cases Yeakley and Jahrsdoerfer recommend a follow-up CT after 6 months (cf. Fig. 6.5).

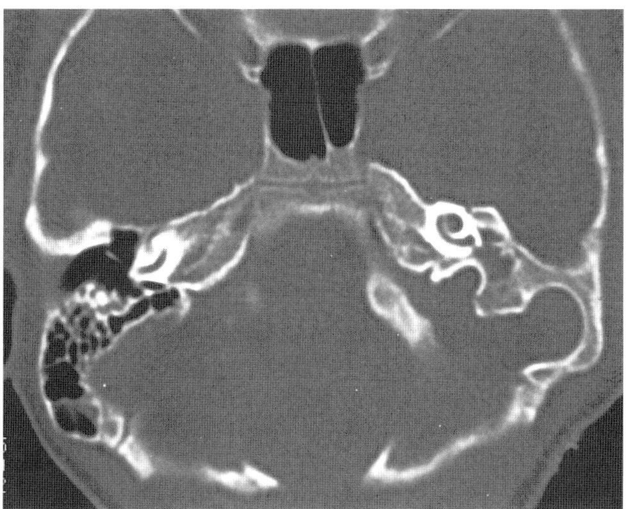

Fig. 6.5 **CT of external auditory canal and tympanic cavity.** Left grade III microtia.
Hypoplastic and completely clouded tympanic cavity. No distinction possible between mesenchymal tissue and fluid. The examination should be repeated at a later date. Lateralization and ventralization of the sigmoid sinus. Slight protrusion and slightly high position of the jugular bulb (see discussion on vessels).

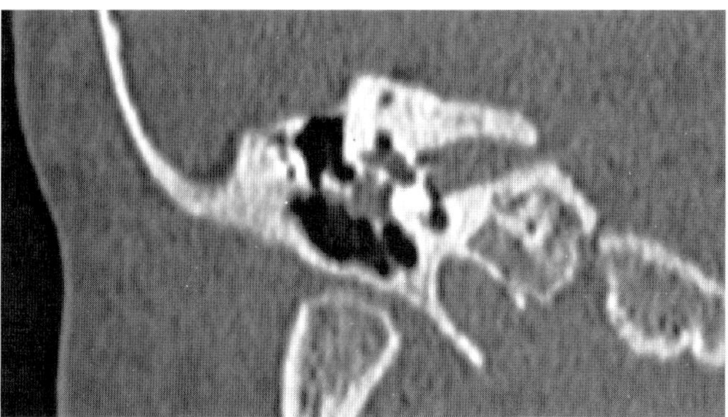

Fig. 6.6 **CT of external auditory canal and tympanic cavity.** Cholesteatoma with destruction of the incudostapedial joint.

Auditory Ossicles

Incus–Malleus

The incus–malleus complex is readily assessable on both the coronary and the axial slice orientations (Fig. 6.7 a–c). The joint surface is particularly well demonstrated on the axial slice. In their patient population with middle ear malformations, Siegert et al. (1996 b) used CT to identify a dysplastic incus–malleus complex in 69 % of patients, and this auditory ossicle was completely absent in 27 % of the patients. The hammer handle (manubrium mallei) was almost always absent.

In particular, dysplasias such as the absence of the long process of the incus or short fusions of the joint are frequently recognizable on high-quality CT images. There is often a fixation of the dysplastic complex to the atretic plate (Fig. 6.8).

The incus–malleus complex is occasionally found far laterally in a deformed tympanic cavity, with no connection to the stapes (Fig. 6.9).

In addition to primary sectional views, secondary three-dimensional reconstructions, for example in the form of virtual endoscopy, are also helpful when analyzing the ossicles (Himi et al. 2000).

Incus–Stapes

The **incudostapedial joint** is usually identifiable on a coronary slice, although fixation in this joint is not distinguishable from a functioning joint (Fig. 6.10, cf. Fig. 6.7 c). Its very small size does not always allow depiction of the **stapes** in its entirety, which is only possible using the most modern CT scanners with slice thicknesses of as little as 0.5 mm (Fig. 6.11). Individual types of stapedial dysplasia, such as the absence of a limb (crus) or a thickened footplate, are detectable, but do not allow any final conclusions regarding stapedial function. During surgery, a mobile stapes is identified in only about 70 % of patients with malformations of the middle ear (Weerda et al. 1985), and fixation of the

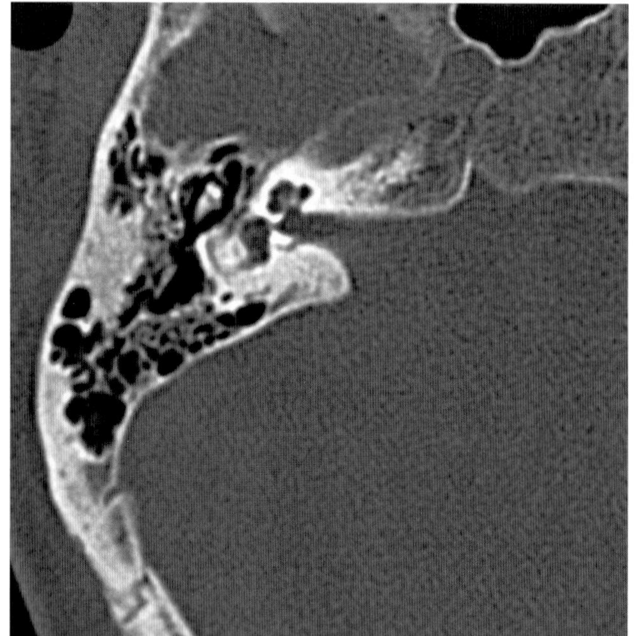

a

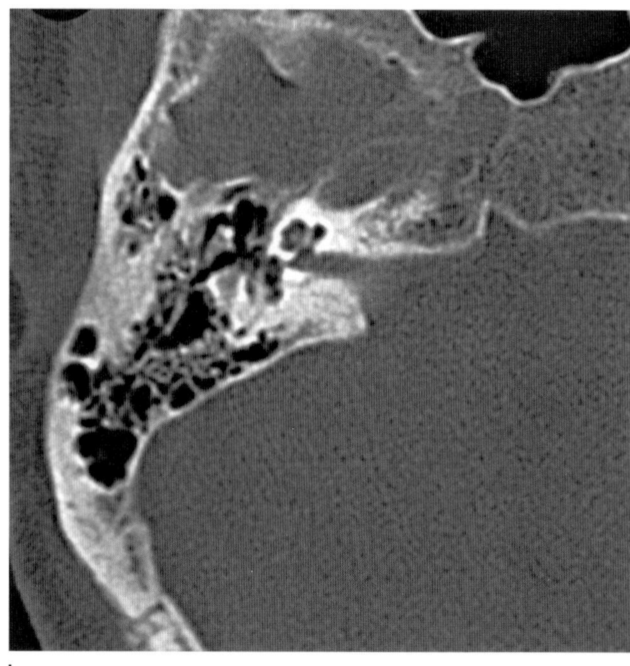

b

c

Fig. 6.7 **CT of the ossicles.**
Physiological demonstration of the ossicles on the axial CT view. Contiguous slices with 1 mm slice thickness.
a Incus–malleus complex at the level of the joint surface. The auditory ossicles resemble an ice-cream cone. The incus represents the cone, the head of the hammer forms the ice-cream.
b Incus–malleus complex with the transition to the long limb of the incus.
c Incudo-stapedial joint on the axial CT view. The crura of the stapes course outside the level of the section and are therefore not visible (the malleus is seen ventrally as a dot, the incus is dorsal, while the tensor tympani muscle is seen to course in a ventral transverse direction).

stapes footplate is not primarily recognizable by radiology. Hypoplastic forms of the stapes with its structure still preserved may be partially below the resolving power of CT, or cannot be imaged with enough richness in contrast because of their low bone density. It is not possible here to show good enough quality reproductions of original CT images depicting a dysplastic stapes. Yeakley and Jahrsdoerfer (1996) state that aplasia may be assumed with all probability if CT assessment using a primary slice thickness of 1.5 mm fails to identify any stapedial suprastructure. However, if the tympanic cavity is not pneumatized, then identification of a more or less normally developed stapes can become impossible using CT scanning. The limitations of CT assessment of the stapes are particularly disappointing from a diagnostic standpoint, given its central role for potential surgery. It may be possible to obtain detailed assessment of the stapes using transtubal fiberoptic videoendoscopy, which provides information superior to that of CT imaging (Karhuketo et al. 2001).

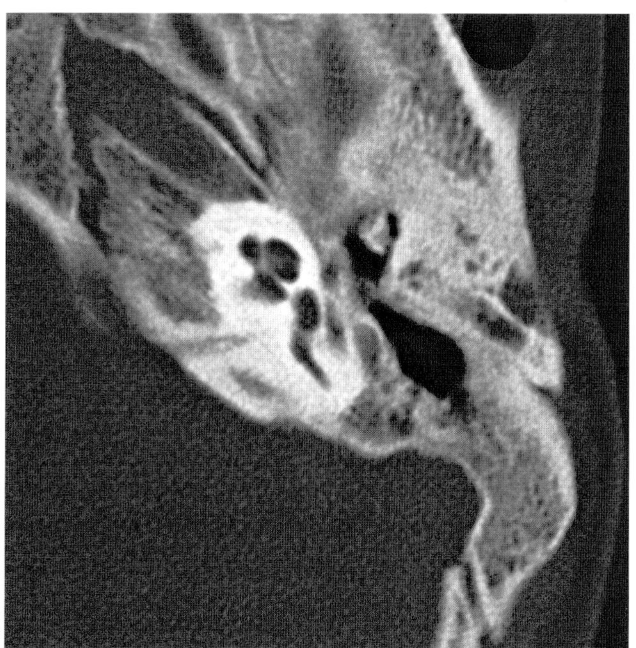

Fig. 6.8 **CT of the ossicles.**
Short fusion of malleus and incus with fixation of the dysplastic complex to the atretic plate. Deduction of 1 point for severe deformity according to the Jahrsdoerfer score (there would have been no point loss for mild dysplasia). Loss of 1 point on the left, irrespective of the degree of dysplasia, on using the Siegert and Weerda score. Tympanic cavity and antrum are pneumatized; the tympanic cavity is smaller than normal. The mastoid is not pneumatized.

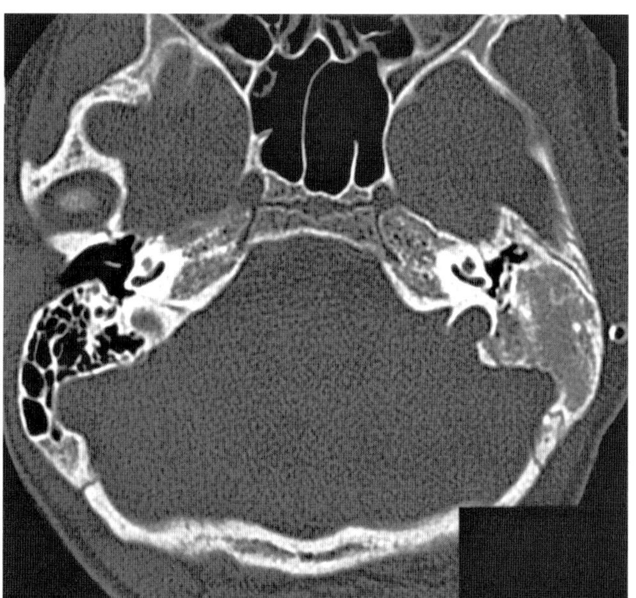

Fig. 6.9 **CT of the ossicles.**
Severe dysplasia of the ossicles in the form of a dissociation of the incus–malleus complex from the stapes. Incus and malleus are severely dysplastic and displaced far laterally in a deformed tympanic cavity. There is no bony connection with the stapes. Loss of one point on both the Jahrsdoerfer and the Siegert and Weerda scores. The tympanic cavity does not reach a width greater than 3 mm at the level of the promontory. An operation would not be appropriate in Jahrsdoerfer's view (narrow tympanum).

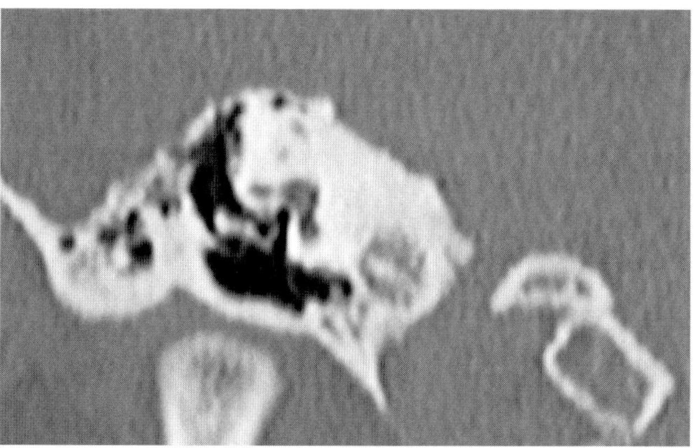

Fig. 6.10 **CT of the ossicles.**
Incudostapedial joint: coronal view showing a physiological appearance.

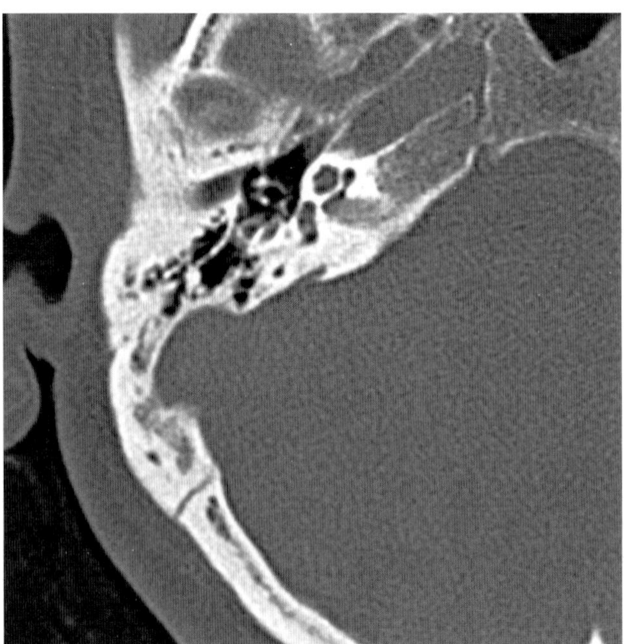

Fig. 6.**11** **CT of the ossicles.**
Normal stirrup with demonstration of the crura stapedis. The slice orientation in the axial plane is slightly angulated (approximately 15°) towards the coronary plane. The tensor tympani muscle with its insertion on the incus is also displayed ventral to the stapes. The dorsal spot represents the incus (at the level of its articulation with the stapes).

Labyrinthine Windows

Normally, both **round and oval windows** are sufficiently assessable on CT imaging at a slice thickness of 1 mm. The oval window has a maximum diameter of about 2 mm (Fig. 6.**12 a**). Congenital absence of the oval window can be diagnosed using CT imaging (Zeifer et al. 2000). Stenosis of the oval window with a diameter down to about 1 mm can be identified by combined axial and coronary slices, and is treated in the Jahrsdoerfer score as being absent (Yeakley and Jahrsdoerfer 1996; Fig. 6.**12 c**). Variations in the round window are less frequent. Adequate patency of at least 1 mm is identifiable dorsal to the promontory on axial CT images at fine slice thicknesses.

Facial Nerve

Numerous variations in the course of the facial nerve have been described for congenital aural atresia (Jahrsdoerfer 1995; Schwager and Helms 1995). The labyrinthine segment of the facial nerve is easily recognizable on the axial CT slice by its convex course. The facial nerve takes a more acute bend in a dorsal direction at its "external knee" (second genu) after giving off the greater petrosal nerve (Fig. 6.**13**). In this segment, the nerve is covered by bone to a varying extent. It is readily seen on the coronary projection that the facial nerve courses physiologically above the oval window in its tympanic segment (Fig. 6.**14**). Problematic displacements of the facial nerve caudally, accompanied by narrowing of the oval window recess, can be demonstrated by CT scanning of optimal quality on the coronary image.

After leaving the tympanic cavity, the facial nerve normally proceeds slightly laterally and dorsally, before coursing relatively perpendicularly in the mastoid segment and proceeding slightly laterally to emerge from the skull base through the stylomastoid foramen (Figs. 6.**15**, 6.**16**). Should identification prove difficult on the axial image, sagittal or coronary reconstructions may be of help. A common variation in the mastoid segment, particularly in patients with a bony atretic plate, is a slight displacement of the facial nerve in a ventral direction to the edge of a possible surgical approach, which is identifiable on CT (Jahrsdoerfer and Lambert 1998, Benton and Bellet 2000; Fig. 6.**17**). Wide lateral displacement in the tympanic segment is only rarely observed (Fig. 6.**18**).

Vessels

Apart from documenting the variations of the facial nerve, it is important to identify aberrations of the major vessels of the skull base.

The normal course of the **internal carotid artery** is recognizable by the position of the carotid canal and the foramen lacerum. Agenesis of the carotid artery is a rarity. Important vascular anomalies include a persistent stapedial artery and the so-called **aberrant internal carotid artery**. These arterial variations influence the operative risk and result in a loss of 2 points on the Siegert and Weerda score (see Table 6.**2**).

The **persistent stapedial artery** branches off the internal carotid artery to enter the anterocaudal segment of the tympanic cavity. It courses along the promontory and enters the posterior segment of the tympanic facial canal. The artery is recognizable on CT as a soft-tissue density within the tympanic cavity, with enlargement of the bony margin of the facial canal. The middle meningeal artery arises from the maxillary artery and normally enters the skull base through the foramen spinosum. If the stapedial artery is persistent, then the middle meningeal artery also emerges from it and the foramen spinosum is absent. Failure to identify the foramen spinosum on CT is thus important additional evidence of a persistent stapedial artery (Silbergleit et al. 2000; Benton and Belett 2000).

In the presence of segmental hypoplasia of the internal carotid artery in an extracranial segment, the **inferior tympanic artery**, which arises from the ascending pharyngeal artery, can assume the arterial blood supply as far as the anastomosis with the normally formed intracranial part of

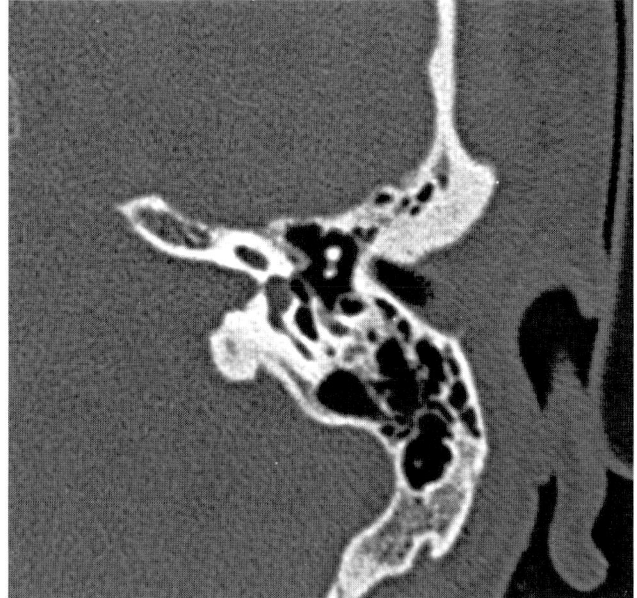

a

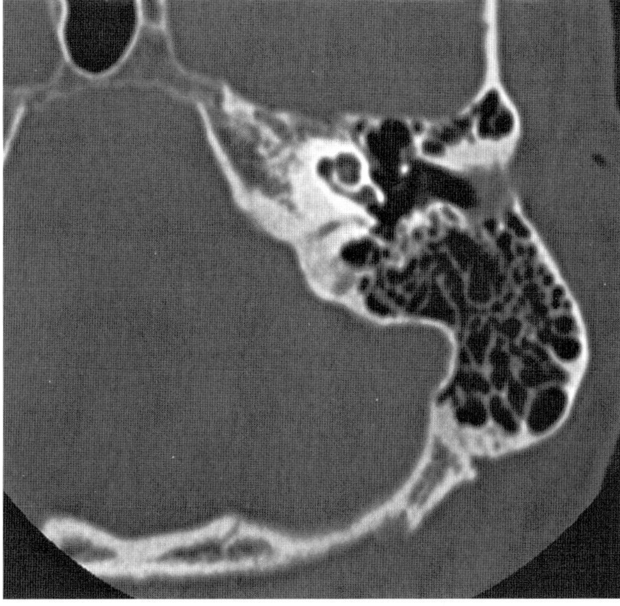

b

c

Fig. 6.**12** **CT of the labyrinthine windows, axial view.**
a Normal oval window.
b Normal round window.
c Axial CT image at the level of the vestibulum.
Bilateral grade III microtia. There is bony atresia on the right and fibrous atresia on the left. There is normal delineation of the oval window on the left. The oval window is absent on the right. Reduction of 1 point according to the Jahrsdoerfer score and 4 points according to the Siegert and Weerda score. The tympanic cavity is almost completely sclerosed on the right (see discussion on tympanic cavity).

the internal carotid artery (Lasjaunias and Berenstein 1987). This inferior tympanic artery is consequently enlarged and is also referred to as the **aberrant internal carotid artery**. It enters the lower part of the tympanic cavity, recognizable on native CT images as a roundish soft-tissue structure, and runs in the tympanic cavity in a ventral and medial direction to the foramen lacerum (for image examples see Caldas et al. 1998). On analysis of the CT images, the altered bony margins of the vessels already strongly support the diagnosis which can be finally established using MR angiography. Catheter angiography is usually no longer necessary.

Relevant anomalies of the major **venous vessels** primarily involve the jugular bulb (Atilla et al. 1995), less frequently the sigmoid sinus. The **sigmoid sinus** is occasionally displaced ventrally, secondary to deformations of the skull base which are also associated with meatal atresia. The **jugular bulb** normally lies caudal and dorsal to the hypotympanum, and even physiologically demonstrates a wide range of variations, with a continuous transition to pathological variations. Caldemeyer et al. (1997) differentiate between a protruding ventral bulb and a high bulb, with the possibility of combinations. Where the bulb merely protrudes ventrally, it appears as a soft-tissue structure in the hypotympanum. When in a high position, it bulges into the dorsal wall of hypo- and mesotympanum. Analysis of the CT images should not only describe localization of the bulb, but careful

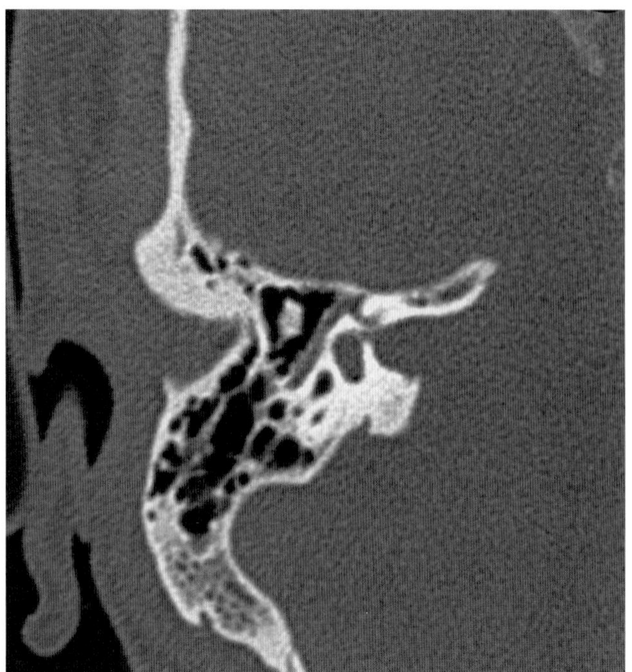

Fig. 6.**13** **CT of the facial nerve segments, axial view.** Labyrinthine segment of the facial nerve as far as the external knee and tympanic segment of the facial nerve, demonstrating a physiological course. The bony lamella within the tympanic segment is intact.

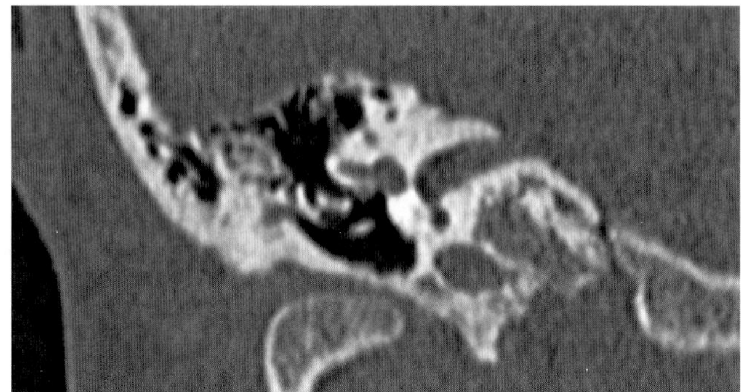

Fig. 6.**14** **CT of the facial nerve segments, coronal view.** The facial nerve shows a physiological course immediately above the oval window.

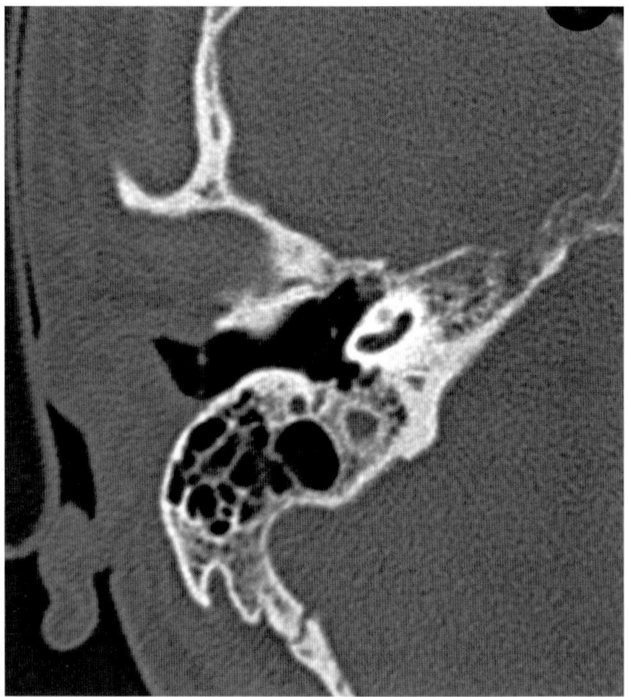

Fig. 6.**15** **CT of the facial nerve segments.** Physiological course of the facial nerve in the mastoid segment. Here the nerve initially continues to take a strictly vertical course.

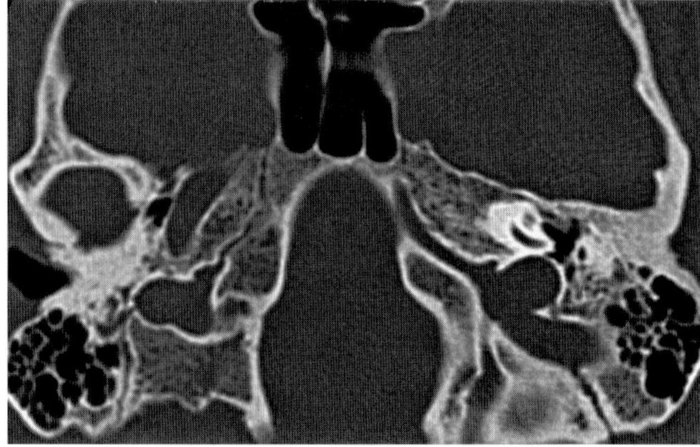

Fig. 6.**16** **CT of the facial nerve segments.** Right-sided physiological course of the facial nerve. The nerve then exits the mastoid segment in a slightly lateral direction and leaves the skull base via the stylomastoid foramen. Left-sided ventral displacement of the facial nerve in the mastoid segment in the presence of bony congenital aural atresia with a tympanic cavity severely reduced in size. Any potential surgical approach would endanger the nerve.

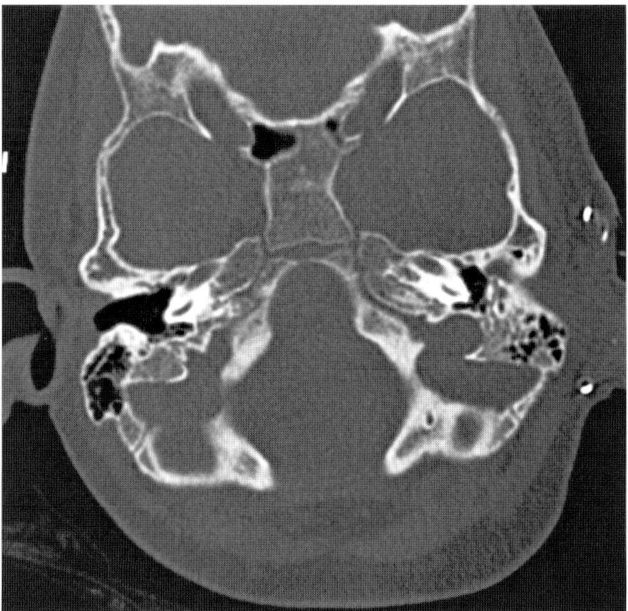

Fig. 6.**17** **CT of the facial nerve segments.**
Right normal middle ear with physiological course of the facial nerve. Bony atresia on the left. Ventral displacement of the facial nerve in the mastoid segment with superior displacement of the exit point of the facial nerve at the level of the dysplastic glenoid fossa of the temporomandibular joint.

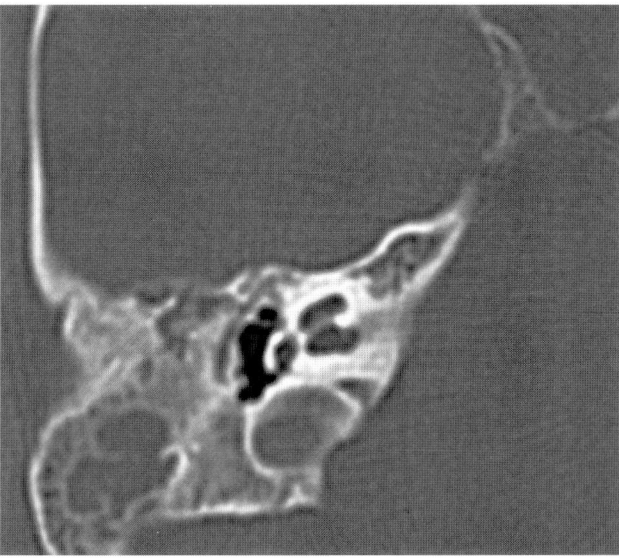

Fig. 6.**18** **CT of the facial nerve segments.**
Left-sided bony atretic plate. Displacement of the facial nerve to the lateral margin of the tympanic cavity. Loss of 1 point according to the Jahrsdoerfer score, with a deduction of four points according to the Siegert and Weerda score. Necrolysis within the mastoid and high location of the jugular bulb are also recognizable.

examination should also investigate to what extent its bony wall is attenuated (Figs. 6.**19**, 6.**20**).

In comparison with arterial anomalies, the diagnosis of venous anomalies is usually easy to establish on CT. If the jugular foramen is ill-defined or displays signs of destruction, thus indicating the presence of a tumor, then MRI examination together with MR angiography should be performed initially. Catheter angiography is required only when a glomus tumor or any other highly vascularized lesion is suspected (Rodgers et al. 1993; Atilla et al. 1995).

Inner Ear

The presence of an audiologically relevant malformation of the inner ear together with a malformation of the middle ear represents a contraindication for surgical reconstruction of the middle ear (Yeakley and Jahrsdoerfer 1996). Careful examination of the cochlea, each semicircular canal, the aqueduct of the vestibule, and the inner auditory canals will in most cases allow a diagnosis with CT (Benton and Bellet 2000). Two and a half turns of the cochlea must be identifiable. **Mondini's malformation** is characterized by one and a half turns, and a mere rudimentary cavity is distinctive of **Michel's deformity**. The semicircular canals can be absent individually or completely. Bony expansion of the vestibular aqueduct is commonly associated with other cochlear malformations.

Although anomalies and calcified obliterations of the inner ear are recognizable on CT, membranous causes of a sensorineural hearing loss find no correlation on CT (Lowe and Vezina 1997). When assessed together with CT, high-resolution fluid-sensitive MRI sequences, such as 3DFT-CISS, can demonstrate optimally the anatomy of the inner auditory canal and the inner ear (Figs. 6.**21**, 6.**22**). For example, the diagnosis of an occlusion in the cochlea or the semicircular canals can be established, while a labyrinthitis is sometimes detectable by pathological contrast uptake in the semicircular canals (Casselman et al. 1993; Mack et al. 1997).

HRCT, however, is always the method of first choice in the radiological analysis of malformations of the inner ear as well as for examinations of the middle ear. Unlike with secondary acquired disorders, CT allows a diagnosis or makes the exclusion of inner ear disorders possible in the majority of cases of congenital lesions.

Since embryological development does not usually produce combined malformations of the middle and inner ear, MRI is not routinely used for the diagnostics of congenital aural atresia, but rather employed as a supplement for specific questions.

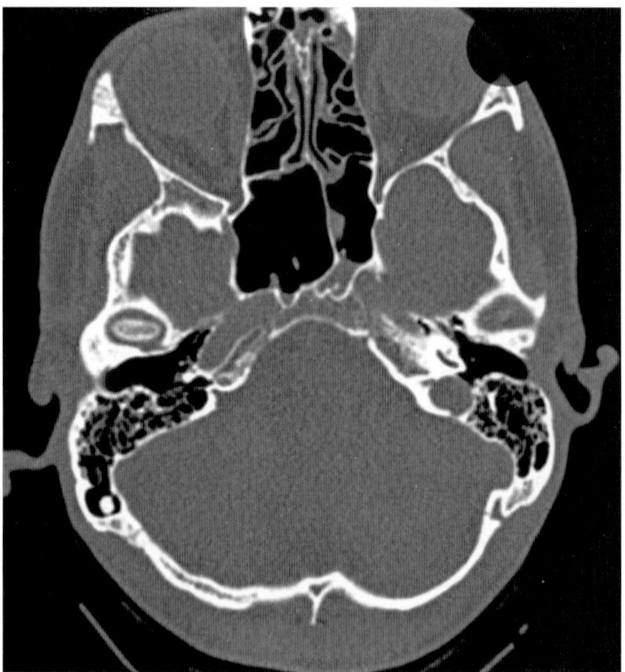

Fig. 6.**19** **Vessels.**
Patient without any malformations. The jugular bulb lies in a physiological position below the hypotympanum. In a normal case, therefore, the jugular bulb would not be visible at the level of the hypotympanum on an axial CT image (right side). On the left side, there is a high location of the jugular bulb. The dorsal bony delineation against the tympanic cavity is partially missing.

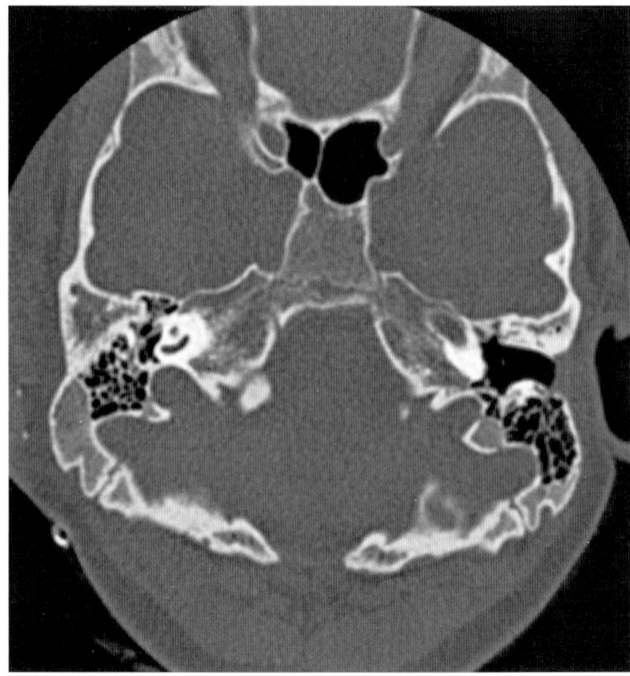

Fig. 6.**20** **Vessels.**
Patient with bony atresia on the right. The bulb demonstrates a high position with a slight protrusion in a ventral direction. The bony delineation against the dysplastic tympanic cavity is retained. The finding has no effect on the Jahresdoerfer score, but has 1 point deducted on the Siegert and Weerda score. Mild high location of the bulb on the healthy left side.

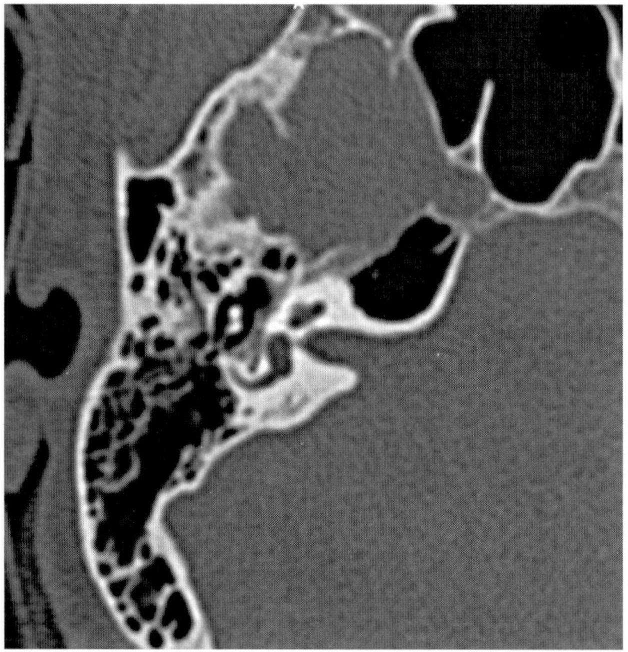

Fig. 6.**21** **Inner ear.**
Axial CT image of a normal finding demonstrating the inner auditory canal, parts of the cochlea, the vestibulum, and the posterior semicircular canal.

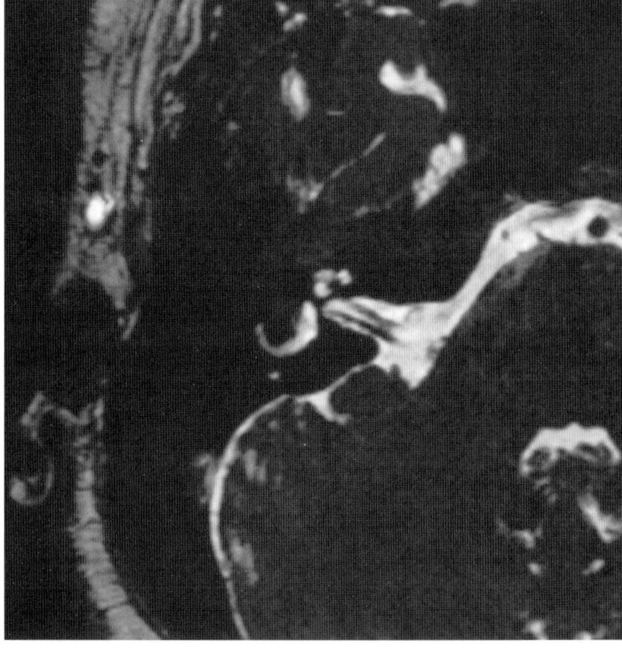

Fig. 6.**22** **Inner ear.**
MR image (fluid-sensitive CISS image of the same patient using an exactly corresponding slice). Good presentation of the facial nerve and the vestibular nerve (superior part) in the inner auditory canal and the lymphatic fluid of the cochlea, the vestibulum, and the semicircular canals.

Summary

- HRCT is the procedure of choice for the anatomical demonstration of the petrous bone.
- The calculated CT score is essential for the indication and prognosis of any surgical reconstruction of middle-ear dysplasias.
- MRI is capable of solving problems of differential diagnosis in cases of a concomitant disorder of the inner ear or the major vessels.

6.2 Treatment of the Malformed Middle Ear—Techniques and Results

R. Jahrsdoerfer and J.H.N. Kim

6.2.1 Introduction

Congenital ear malformations can be broadly classified into two main categories, major malformations and minor malformations. **Major malformations** are those in which there is atresia or stenosis of the external ear canal, often seen along with a corresponding malformation of the external ear. **Minor malformations** are those in which the problem is largely confined to the middle ear. There is a patent external ear canal, and a tympanic membrane is present (see pp. 229–231).

In the senior author's experience of 3000 patients evaluated and 1400 patients operated, most of the patients had aural atresia and were referred for surgical consideration as an initial event. Fewer patients with minor malformations were seen because these patients were often first operated elsewhere and only referred to us after a diagnosis of a congenital middle ear malformation was suspected or confirmed.

The surgical repair of congenital aural atresia should be done by an experienced otologist. Even in expert hands there is significant risk of facial nerve injury and the hearing being made worse. Advances in otologic and imaging studies, and microsurgical instrumentation and techniques, allow otologists to restore hearing in selected patients with aural atresia.

6.2.2 Incidence

Congenital aural atresia occurs in approximately 1 in 10000 births. Unilateral atresia is 7 times more common than bilateral atresia. The ear malformation may be inherited in 20% of cases, and in 10% of cases is part of a syndrome, such as Treacher Collins, Goldenhar, or hemifacial microsomia (see p. 272). Most cases of aural atresia are the result of a spontaneous genetic mutation. Any family with a child who has a congenital ear malformation should seek genetic counseling, especially if they wish to have further children.

Approximately 0.05% of cases are associated with a history of teratogen exposure. The use of vitamin A derivatives and fertility drugs taken during an unsuspected pregnancy are incriminating medications for ear malformations. Although it is not unusual to find complete atresia associated with a well-formed auricle, the reverse—a normal ear canal and tympanic membrane in the presence of congenital microtia—is rare. However, this can be seen in thalidomide patients.

6.2.3 Clinical Evaluation

When a neonate is found to have a malformed auricle, a thorough physical examination of the craniofacial structures should be undertaken. An assessment of the hearing is mandatory. A combined anomaly of microtia and aural atresia is usually obvious, but patients with a normal or only slightly malformed auricle may have their atresia go undiagnosed for many years. It is important to note the appearance of the external ear since it has been found to correlate well with the development of the middle ear (Kountakis et al. 1995). A patient with unilateral atresia should have the contralateral ear examined under a microscope, particularly if a conductive hearing loss is present or suspected. An abnormal shape or size of the malleus and tympanic membrane may suggest the presence of a congenital middle ear malformation. Preauricular skin tags or fistulae as well as a facial nerve weakness or paralysis are often associated with an abnormal development of the ear. It is not uncommon to have a weakness or absence of the mandibular branch of the facial nerve.

It is also important to inquire about associated congenital problems involving the heart, kidney, or cervical spine. Patients with congenital craniofacial malformations such as hemifacial microsomia and Treacher Collins syndrome may present a challenge for airway management during surgery. A consultation with a pediatric anesthesiologist is clearly indicated. Cervical spine and skull base abnormalities such as vertebral fusion and platybasia with occipitalization of the atlas are associated with Goldenhar and Klippel–Feil syndrome. During endotrachal intubation, extreme caution must be exercised in these patients when manipulating the neck in order to prevent cervical subluxation.

Hearing Assessment (see p. 260)

The most important initial evaluation in patients with microtia and atresia is hearing assessment. In bilateral atresia there will be a 45–60 db conductive hearing loss in each ear. In unilateral atresia it is important to document hearing in the normal-appearing contralateral ear. In children 3 years of age and over, routine behavioral audiologic testing can usually be done. **Auditory brainstem response** (ABR) testing may be necessary in children less than 2 years of age. Patients with bilateral atresia present a masking dilemma. It is important to determine ear-specific thresholds and sensorineural cochlear function in order to avoid operating on an only hearing ear, or on an ear with little or no potential for hearing improvement. Otoacoustic emission testing can be of use in unilateral atresia if the contralateral ear appears normal.

Generally, the **sensorineural acuity level** (SAL) can be used to resolve the masking dilemma in determining cochlear status in each ear. The SAL measures air conduction thresholds in the presence of fixed-level bone conduction masking noise (Dirks 1994). The masked and unmasked air conduction thresholds are compared, with the difference between the two compared to that of normal-hearing listeners. A conductive loss produces a significant threshold shift similar to that seen in normal-hearing subjects, while sensorineural loss produces no or small threshold shifts. The side with the better reserve is then operated upon to achieve the best postoperative hearing result.

In younger patients or children who are difficult to test, simultaneous multichannel recording of the ABR in both air and bone conduction modes is the procedure of choice. Analysis of ABR wave I from the mastoid electrodes placed ipsilateral and contralateral to the stimulus allows evaluation of sensorineural function for each ear (Jahrsdoerfer et al. 1985). If there is any doubt concerning hearing, a bone conduction hearing aid should be placed as early as possible.

Once a child with unilateral or bilateral atresia has been determined to have one normal hearing ear, or has been aided for hearing loss, they are allowed to mature until 5 years of age. At that time, a plastic surgeon and an otologic surgeon who are both familiar with auricular reconstruction and atresia surgery should be consulted. A repeat audiologic evaluation should be obtained as well as high-resolution CT (HRCT) performed in the 30° axial and 105° coronal planes. MRI is not the modality of choice here since it does not image bone. HRCT will image bony structures within the temporal bone including the ossicles, cochlear, atretic plate, and fallopian canal. The appearance on CT will primarily determine the patient's suitability for atresia surgery.

The resolution of new spiral CT scanners with improved software allows imaging to be done in the axial plane only, with reformatting to coronal images. These images are almost as good as true coronal images. This method also avoids undesirable radiation to the eye (see p. 234).

Grading System to Predict Surgical Outcome: Jahrsdoerfer Score (see Table 6.1)

A grading scheme based on high-resolution CT (HRCT) was developed in an effort to select those patients who would have the best chance of success (Jahrsdoerfer et al. 1992). This scheme was based primarily on the preoperative CT scan, and points were assigned according to the degree of development of vital temporal bone structures. The presence of a well-defined stapes rated two points, and all other parameters were assigned one point each (p. 234, Table 6.1). The appearance of the unoperated external ear was factored in because, as mentioned earlier, this was found to correlate well with the development of the middle ear. The significance of the grading system is that it allows prediction of the surgical outcome. For example, a grade of 7/10 translates to a 70% chance of restoring hearing to normal or near normal levels (15–30 dB) postoperatively.

There are two absolute criteria which the patient must meet in order to qualify for surgery:

- Good cochlear function
- No imaging evidence of a malformed inner ear (CT confirmation is required)

Surgery is also deferred if the mastoid and middle ear have failed to aerate. In this case, the CT scan is repeated in 1 year. If the mastoid fails to aerate, it usually indicates chronic or absent Eustachian tube function. On rare occasion, the Eustachian tube may not connect with the middle ear. The result will be a persistence of primitive mesenchymal tissue in the middle ear and mastoid. The reason this ear is not amenable to corrective surgery is that the best possible postoperative hearing result is 35 db, which would still require amplification.

Only 50% of all patients seen and evaluated qualify for surgery. In patients who have a craniofacial syndrome, the percentage is even less. In Treacher Collins syndrome, only 25% of patients qualify, and in hemifacial microsomia, only 15%.

The grading system is based on a best possible score of 10. The presence of a stapes is the single most important factor for successful surgery. Most patients selected for surgery are graded 7 or 8. A grade of 5 or below disqualifies the patient as the risk of the operation outweighs the potential benefits.

6.2.4 Minor Malformations

Minor malformations are those in which the problem is limited to the middle ear. The auricle and external ear canal are normal in appearance, or almost so, and the tympanic membrane can be identified. Minor malformations typically involve the stapes/oval window/facial nerve axis. Embryologically, the stapes develops slightly later than the facial nerve. In the early part of week 7 of gestation, Reichert's cartilage (precursor of the stapes) first appears, but by this time the horizontal portion of the facial nerve has already been established. If extrinsic forces have occurred, i. e., shifting of the hyoid arch, the nerve may be displaced anteriorly before the stapes has developed. This would explain those rare middle ear anomalies where a bare facial nerve is located anterior and inferior to an intact stapes and oval window. A more common scenario results from a time-related migration of the facial nerve anteriorly while the stapes is forming. The nerve may then be interposed between the stapes blastema and the labyrinth, preventing formation of the footplate and oval window. Additionally, one or both stapes crura may fail to develop, or the crura may be small and the rudimentary stapes free-hanging.

It is not necessary for the facial nerve to assume a final position over the area of the oval window to prevent normal stapes development. It is sufficient for the facial nerve to have migrated anteriorly over the area of the stapes blastema to disrupt normal development of this ossicle. The many reported cases of bare and anteriorly and inferiorly displaced facial nerves in concert with an absent oval window and a primitive stapes attached to an incus strongly support this contention. It is the authors' opinion that the development of the facial nerve influences the development of the stapes, rather than the reverse.

Surgical Techniques

When an absent oval window is found at surgery, the choices available to the surgeon are to terminate the operation or to attempt hearing restoration by creating a vestibulotomy. If the latter approach is chosen, there should be a defined oval window area which can be targeted for drilling, and mature ossicular development to enable placement of a prosthesis. A well-formed long arm of the incus helps. If the incus long arm and malleus handle are poorly developed, a **total ossicular replacement prosthesis** (TORP) may be selected.

Once a vestibulotomy is drilled, the opening should be covered with temporalis fascia or other appropriate soft tissue seal. On occasion, the long arm of the incus will be vertical to the new oval window and the use of a wire loop prosthesis is not feasible. Only a bucket prosthesis can accommodate the tip of a vertical incus. The distance between the new oval window and the ossicle may vary greatly. A wide assortment of prosthesis lengths should be available. Even then, the surgeon may find it necessary to modify or construct a prosthesis in the operating room.

A bare facial nerve will not infrequently be found to overlie the area where the new oval window should be drilled. In malformations limited to the middle ear, it is not possible to transpose the facial nerve as it is in atresia surgery. There simply is not room enough in which to work. A decision must be made to drill above or below the bare facial nerve. Again, a well-defined oval window area helps in this decision. Lacking this, drilling may begin superior to the nerve using a saucerizing technique. If the vestibule is not encountered at a depth of 2 mm, the procedure is terminated as there is a heightened risk of sensorineural hearing loss from surgical violation of the membranous labyrinth. If there is insufficient room to saucerize, a cylindrical opening may be drilled.

If a bare facial nerve obscures the oval window superiorly, a promontorial window may be drilled according to Plester (Plester and Katzke 1983). The promontorial bone should be saucerized down to an intact endosteal membrane. Disruption of the endosteal membrane carries a greater chance of nerve loss from cochlear injury. A prosthesis can be inserted between the endosteal membrane and the malleus handle, or the tympanic membrane if the handle is unfavorable.

The older otologic literature stated that an opening made through the bony capsule of the labyrinth would endure because the bone was endochondral and had poor powers of regeneration. This is a myth. Over the past few years, we have operated two patients in whom an opening drilled through the bony capsule was closed by new bone growth. This was confirmed upon reoperation when the initial good hearing result faded.

The most important aspect in exploring the middle ear of a patient with a conductive hearing loss is an awareness that one may be dealing with a congenital malformation. This awareness must include the possibility of finding a bare and displaced facial nerve. Failure to recognize this possibility places the patient at a huge risk of facial nerve injury. There are reported cases wherein the stapes was found to descend for a short distance into the soft tissue of a bare facial nerve (Welling et al. 1992). If this anomaly goes unrecognized, the surgeon may elect to dissect the "soft tissue" to better define the stapes crura and oval window. The resulting facial nerve paralysis alerts the surgeon too late to the distorted middle ear anatomy.

A bare and displaced facial nerve may also be camouflaged by an enveloping layer of adipose tissue or concealed by a choristoma. Any abnormal soft tissue encountered during middle ear exploration should give the surgeon pause.

Congenital primary incus fixation is rare. Fixation of the malleus in the epitympanum is not. There are two surgical methods to correct malleus head fixation:

- Excision of the malleus head and incus, and placement of an incus strut from the malleus handle to the stapes
- Drilling away the bony attachment in the epitympanum and interposing silicone rubber sheeting as a barrier to bony refixation

Ossicular fixation may also be attributable to a "malleus bar." This is a term coined by Nomura (Nomura et al. 1988) to describe a bar of bone running from the malleus neck to the posterior bony annulus. This bony bar is about 1 mm in thickness and firmly fixes the malleus in place, producing a conductive hearing loss. The chorda tympani nerve frequently runs in a bony groove in the bar, and must be considered when drilling away the bar. Freeing the ossicular chain from the malleus bar will usually correct the conductive hearing loss, but not always. If the chain remains fixed, additional sites of fixation must be searched for. It is our preference that any suspected congenital middle ear malformation be approached through a postauricular incision. The ossicular anomaly, commonly the stapes/oval window/facial nerve complex, is often concealed by overhanging bone. As much as 3–4 mm of bony overhang may need to be drilled away to access the area of concern.

Vascular Anomalies of the Middle Ear

Vascular malformations (see pp. 240–244), particularly an anomalous internal carotid artery and a high, uncovered jugular bulb, should be diagnosed preoperatively. HRCT will show the course of the internal carotid artery through the middle ear, and this can be confirmed by MRI and/or MR angiography. An aberrant internal carotid artery may also be diagnosed preoperatively by examination under the operating microscope. A suspicious pink mass in the middle ear may be seen to blanch upon gentle pressure on the common carotid artery in the neck, and the bruit heard on auscultation may temporarily disappear. A persistent stapedial artery is usually an incidental finding at middle ear surgery and will infrequently be seen on preoperative imaging.

A high, uncovered jugular bulb may be diagnosed on HRCT or MR venography. The problem with these jugular bulbs is their vulnerability to penetration from a surgical instrument when a tympanomeatal flap is raised. As a high, uncovered jugular bulb presses against the undersurface of the tympanic membrane, the bare bulb is easily punctured. When an unsuspected vascular anomaly is encountered in the middle ear, it is best to work around it. We do not endorse attempts to displace, bury, or cover the vascular structure, as any manipulation risks severe hemorrhage. The patient, or parents if the patient is a child, must be made aware of the vascular problem so that any subsequent surgery can be avoided, or the surgeon forewarned of the potential problem.

6.2.5 Major Malformations—Congenital Aural Atresia

Timing of the Operation

Microtia repair should precede atresia repair. This allows the plastic surgeon to construct an external ear using an autologous rib graft placed in a virgin surgical field. Performing atresia repair first can compromise the blood supply in that area and incite soft tissue scarring. **There is no rationale for making a hole in the side of the head independent of external ear reconstruction.** Exceptions to this are the presence of cholesteatoma, or a patient who has no interest in the cosmetic appearance of the external ear.

Although atresia surgery can take place any time after the second stage of microtia repair (transposition of the earlobe), we prefer the plastic surgeon to finish the auricular reconstruction before carrying out surgery for hearing (see pp. 255 ff).

As auricular reconstruction entails the harvesting of autologous rib cartilage which is then sculpted into an ear framework, the rib cage must have achieved optimal growth. Harvesting of rib usually takes place at age 6–7 years if the atresia is unilateral. If bilateral, the time table can be advanced to allow atresia repair to be completed in one ear before the child starts school.

Cholesteatoma and Aural Stenosis

One of every seven patients with a major ear malformation will have stenosis of the external ear canal. Usually these patients require the same operation as those with complete atresia. Patients with canal stenosis have a predisposition to cholesteatoma formation, particularly those patients who have an hourglass configuration of the external ear canal (s. pp. 229–231). These ears are incapable of self-cleaning because of a narrow isthmus. An earlier publication from our series reported a 90 % incidence of cholesteatoma in patients older than 12 years of age in whom a canal diameter less than 2 mm was found (Cole and Jahrsdoerfer 1990). More recently we have encountered patients younger than 12 years who had signs of destructive cholesteatoma. Patients with canal stenosis should be carefully followed and may need to undergo a canalplasty at 6–12 years of age if the cholesteatoma shows signs of infection or early bone modeling.

Surgical Treatment

Positioning of the Patient

The patient is placed in a slightly reversed Trendelenburg position with the ear to be operated facing up. The hair is shaved for a short distance above the ear (less than 2.5 cm). The postauricular sulcus and soft tissue medial to the cartilage implant are infiltrated with lidocaine 1 % with epinephrine 1 : 50 000. Facial nerve monitoring is used routinely and the needle electrodes are positioned. Facial nerve monitoring is particularly helpful when the nerve is significantly displaced, rerouted, or previously injured. The anesthetist is instructed not to use paralytic agents other than those necessary for induction, and then only short-acting drugs. Nitrous oxide is avoided except for induction as needed.

Before the patient is brought to the operating suite, the parents are informed that the operation will take 4–5 hours and they will not receive periodic progress reports during this time. Rather, the surgeon will meet with them after the operation. Most cases of atresia repair are completed in 3–3 $^{1}/_{2}$ hours.

Before scrubbing up we routinely review the CT scan in the surgical suite. Particular attention is paid to the slope of the tegmen, the depth of the middle ear from the lateral surface of the mastoid, and the course of the facial nerve (see pp. 234 ff).

Surgical Approach

A postauricular approach is used routinely. If the plastic surgeon has completed all stages of reconstruction there will be an adequate postauricular sulcus and usually good projection of the external ear off the side of the head. An incision is made in the postauricular crease (see p. 256, Fig. 6.**30**). If the plastic surgeon has not yet elevated the ear off the head, the postauricular incision is made 1 cm posterior to the cartilage implant. If the incision is made close to the implant, the skin will contract anteriorly over the cartilage and may adversely affect future efforts of the plastic surgeon to elevate the ear.

Temporalis fascia is harvested for later use as a tympanic membrane graft. Soft-tissue dissection is carried anteriorly and the posterior lip of the glenoid fossa identified. A crescent incision is made just posterior to the glenoid fossa, preserving an anterior rim of periosteum for later use in anchoring a tragal-based pedicle flap. A second incision is made through the periosteum paralleling the temporal line. A periosteal elevator is used to lift the periosteum off the lateral surface of the mastoid bone. It is important to insert a word of caution here: On rare occasions, the facial nerve may exit the temporal bone on the lateral surface of the mastoid and be directly beneath the periosteum. In this location it is vulnerable to injury when the periosteum is elevated.

A tympanic bone remnant is searched for. A tympanic bone is found in approximately 10% of patients. It is unwise to dissect deep in the glenoid fossa in search of a tympanic bone remnant, as this may jeopardize the facial nerve. Remember that in 25–30% of atresia patients the facial nerve makes a sharp turn anteriorly at the second genu to cross the middle ear and exit the temporal bone into the glenoid fossa. Indiscriminate dissection within the fossa may stretch the facial nerve, or worse yet, avulse it.

If a tympanic bone remnant is found on the surface of the lateral mastoid, drilling should begin in that area, as the middle ear is usually located directly medial. If a tympanic bone remnant is absent, drilling should begin over the cribriform area. As drilling proceeds medially, the degree of pneumatization of the temporal bone is assessed. A highly pneumatized temporal bone may lack well-defined atretic bone and cause the surgeon to go astray. A densely sclerotic temporal bone indicates a lack of development rather than infection or chronic ear disease. Moreover, an underdeveloped temporal bone will have increased vascular structures—veins and sinuses—which may contribute to nuisance bleeding during drilling.

Beginning at the cribriform area, a direct approach by drilling is taken to the middle ear. Surgical entry into the mastoid should be avoided. Although a mastoid approach may soothe the anxiety of an insecure surgeon, it does the patient no favors. It produces a large, unsightly cavity which is hard to skin graft and is more susceptible to infection.

Drilling is continued medially, staying high and anterior. The tegmen may be the first landmark encountered and can be tracked medial to the epitympanum. However, it is best to follow the dense atretic bone to the atretic plate. The atretic bone is found anteriorly.

We define the atretic plate as that layer of atretic bone contiguous to the middle ear. This differs from the definition employed by neuroradiologists, who include the entire width of the atretic bone from the middle ear to the lateral skull. This definition serves no useful purpose for the otologic surgeon. Under the neuroradiology definition the width of the atretic plate may fluctuate widely, depending on the coronal CT cut through the temporal bone.

The atretic plate is normally found at a depth of approximately 1.5 mm. If the atretic plate has not been identified at a depth of 2.0 mm, we will backtrack in our search for the middle ear. In extensively pneumatized temporal bones, it is possible to overshoot the middle ear and drill into the petrous apex.

Once the atretic plate has been identified (Fig. 6.**23 a**), it is thinned to eggshell thickness with a diamond burr and the bony fragments carefully picked away. Usually the first sign of the middle ear occurs when the epitympanum is entered. Further exposure of this area will reveal a fused incus–malleus complex which looks similar to the derrière of a newborn infant (Fig. 6.**23 b**). We have named this appearance the **"buttock sign"** (Jahrdoerfer et al. 1991). Gentle palpation of the fused incus–malleus will yield important information about the mobility of the ossicular chain. An absence of movement will indicate bony fixation of the ossicular chain at the junction of the malleus neck and the atretic plate. The chain may be fixed in other locations as well. A moderate degree of movement will indicate an intact (but malformed) ossicular chain that is fixed to the atretic plate by periosteum (Fig. 6.**23 c**). A "floppy" incus–malleus complex, where there is excessive movement, probably indicates a lack of connection to the stapes (Fig. 6.**24**). Remember that in aural atresia the handle of the malleus is almost always absent and the malleus neck is fixed to the atretic plate by either bone or periosteum.

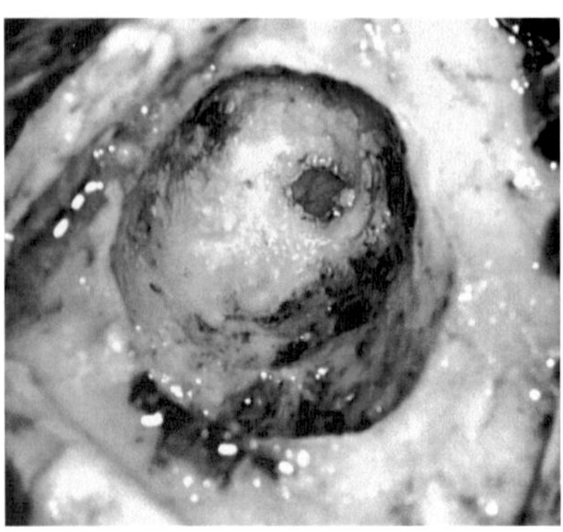

a

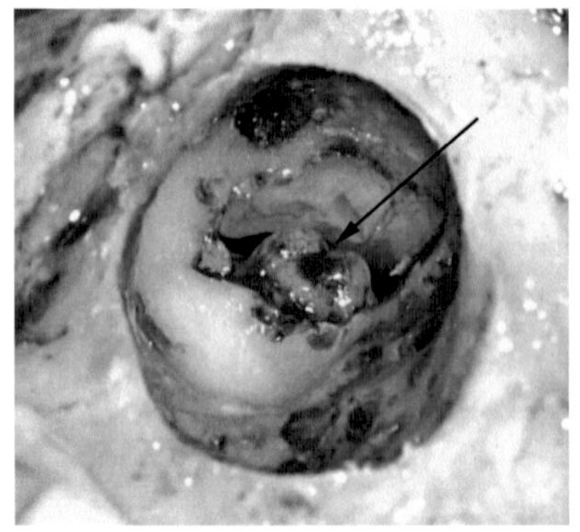

b

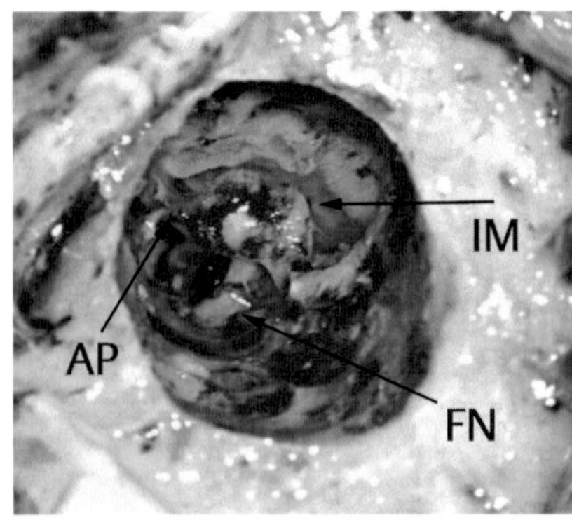

c

Fig. 6.**23** a–c **Surgical approach for congenital aural atresia.**
a Atretic plate with early opening into the middle ear.
b Epitympanum has been opened. The finding demonstrates a fused incus–malleus complex (the "buttock sign," arrow).
c The remnants of the atretic plate have been drilled away. View of the middle ear. Note the fused incus–malleus complex (IM), the facial nerve (FN), vertical long arm of the incus, and the connection of the atretic plate (AP) to the neck of the malleus.

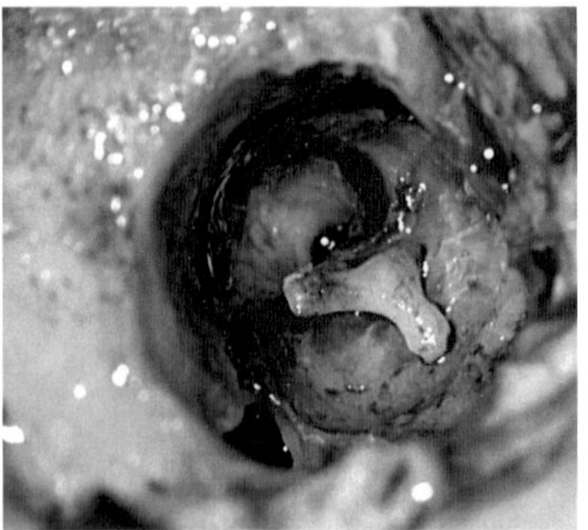

Fig. 6.**24** **Primitive development of the incus–malleus complex; feels "floppy" on palpation; no connection with the stapes.**

As the remainder of the atretic plate is drilled away, the contents of the middle ear are revealed (Fig. 6.**25**). A chorda tympani nerve is found in less than 50% of cases, and when present will be running in the bony atretic plate far inferior. In this location it cannot be spared without compromising the success of the operation. Occasionally, the chorda tympani nerve will be found in a more favorable position and can be saved. In these cases there may be a partial malleus handle and early formation of a fibrous tympanic membrane.

Once the atretic plate has been removed, bone peripheral to the ossicular mass is drilled away to center the ossicles in the approximate middle of the new tympanic membrane. Great care must be exercised at this junction to prevent the drill from brushing the ossicles and possibly incurring a sensorineural hearing loss.

It should be appreciated that the absence of a malleus handle makes reconstruction with a homograft tympanic membrane unfeasible. Moreover, the cone-shaped configuration and size of a homograft tympanic membrane would fit poorly in the atretic middle ear. Temporalis fascia is the tissue of choice for the new tympanic membrane.

Before the tympanic membrane is constructed, a split-thickness skin graft is harvested from the ipsilateral arm. The skin graft is taken at the time that it is needed and not at the inception of the operation. We routinely use a Zimmer air dermatome with the 2 inch (5 cm) template. The circulating nurse extracts the arm from beneath the drapes and places it on an arm board with the elbow bent and the medial upper arm exposed. The arm is prepped with a sterilizing solution and draped with sterile towels. The area of the skin graft is liberally swabbed with mineral oil to facilitate lubrication. The dermatome is set at a thickness of 0.006 inches (0.152 mm). The anesthesiologist is alerted that the patient needs a deep level of anesthesia to prevent involuntary movement of the upper arm from pain.

A split-thickness graft measuring approximately 5 × 7 cm is harvested, rinsed in lactated Ringer's solution, and placed on a dermacarrier. The graft is trimmed and shaped to conform to the new ear canal. Usually one side of the graft is thinner than the other, and this side is chosen to be used at the level of the tympanic membrane. The thicker side is used at the meatus. Four notches are cut in the thin side to form five skin tabs. While the surgeon is preparing the skin graft, the surgical assistant dresses the arm with a scarlet red dressing, a nonadherent dressing, and a gauze wrap.

Before positioning the fascia graft and the skin graft, the area of the new meatus is liberally injected with lidocaine 1% with epinephrine 1 : 50 000. At this point in the operation the surgeon can tell if the new ear canal will align with the new meatus. If alignment is poor, the external ear needs to be transposed (Fig. 6.**26**). We have found that in approximately 50% of cases the auricle must be repositioned, al-

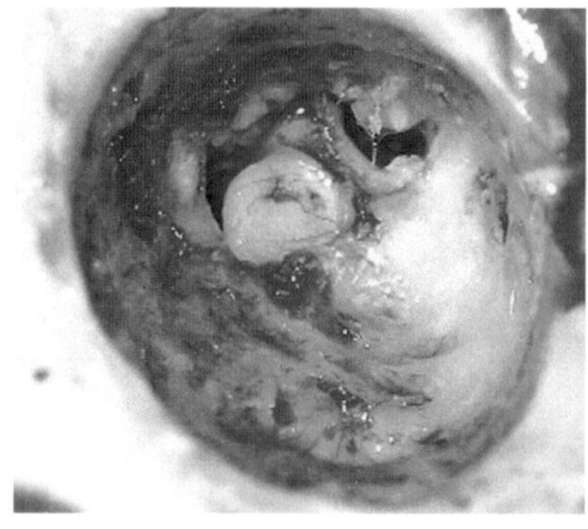
a

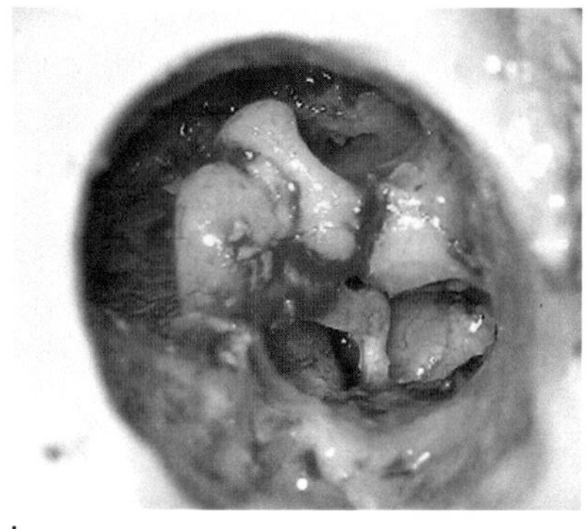
b

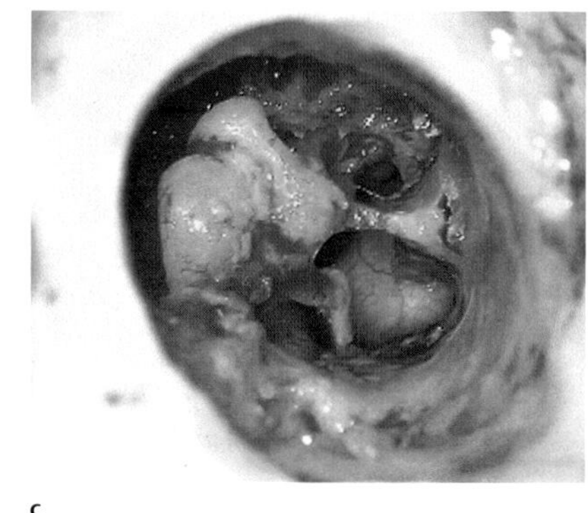
c

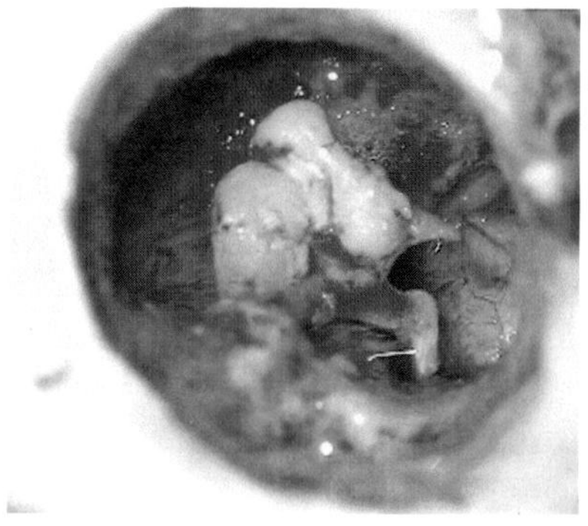
d

Fig. 6.25 a–d **Right congenital aural atresia.**
Series showing the gradual removal of the atretic plate down to a bony bridge and, finally, its completed removal and mobilization of the ossicular chain.

most always in a superior and posterior direction, occasionally in a superior only direction. Injecting lidocaine with epinephrine at this point in the operation ensures there is good hemostasis by the time the meatoplasty is done and the external ear needs to be relocated.

The temporalis fascia graft which had been allowed to dry is now hydrated and placed in the new ear canal to cover the ossicles. This serves as a lateral graft. The edges of the fascia are reflected onto the bony canal wall for a short distance, about 2–3 mm. The split-thickness skin graft is placed in the new ear canal to line the bare bone. The graft is inserted in a manner so the vertical slit faces anteriorly. This prevents skin edges from migrating into mastoid air cells posteriorly. The skin tabs are systematically placed over the fascia graft starting anteriorly and proceeding in a clockwise direction (Fig. 6.26). The skin tabs provide a second epithelial layer to the tympanic membrane.

A silicone rubber button approximately 1 mm thick is cut and placed over the new tympanic membrane. This step is absolutely key to the success of the operation. It creates a sulcus anteriorly and inferiorly and prevents lateralization of the drum and blunting of the medial ear canal. PVA sponge ear wicks are inserted and hydrated with an ear drop preparation. Upon expansion the PVA sponge stabilizes the skin graft in the new bony ear canal. The lateral edges of the skin graft are folded over the wicks and attention is turned to the new meatus.

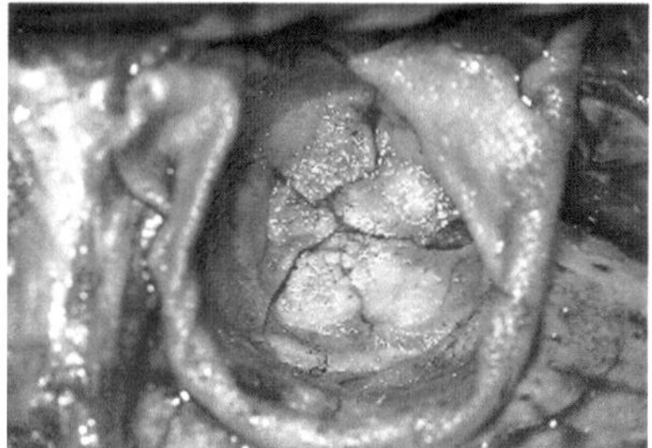

Fig. 6.26 **Order of the skin tabs. Note the clockwise ordering of the five skin tabs to cover the fascial tympanic membrane.**

If the external ear needs to be repositioned, the preauricular soft tissue and skin are undermined by blunt dissection. It is important that the plane of dissection be lateral to the parotid gland to avoid a postoperative salivary fistula. Repositioning is possible because the external ear is not yet tethered by an ear canal. With this maneuver the external ear can be mobilized up to 3 cm.

A U-shaped pedical flap hinged at the tragus is outlined. The skin is elevated off the underlying conchal cartilage, if present, or off conchal soft tissue if cartilage is absent. With the skin flap held anteriorly, a scalpel is used to excise a core of soft tissue which is discarded. This opens the new meatus to the new ear canal. Minor adjustments are made to the position of the external ear to facilitate alignment. The pedicle flap is swung down into the new ear canal and sutured to a cuff of periosteum at the level of the mastoid cortex. This periosteum had been previously preserved to accommodate attachment of the pedicle flap. The pedicle flap provides excellent skin coverage for the anterior ear canal in its lateral soft tissue part. It is also instrumental in decreasing the incidence of postoperative meatal stenosis.

The external ear is sutured in its final position with absorbable 4–0 sutures. Deeper nonabsorbable sutures may be necessary if there is tension on the ear. If the external ear requires transposition of 1 cm or more, a crescent of postauricular skin is excised to accommodate retroplacement of the auricle. Addition PVA sponge wicks are inserted in the lateral ear canal and hydrated. The postauricular incision is closed with a running subcuticular absorbable suture, a mastoid dressing is placed, and the patient is returned to the postanesthesia care unit.

All canal packing and the silicone rubber button are removed 1 week postoperatively. At the 4 week postoperative visit, the desquamated crusty layer of the skin graft is removed and a postoperative audiogram is obtained. As the skin of the split-thickness skin graft does not have memory and is not self-cleaning as in a normal ear canal, the ear canal should be cleaned every 6–12 months indefinitely.

Anesthesia Gases and Middle Ear Pressure

Unless required in the induction phase of anesthesia, nitrous oxide is not used. The reason for this is the release of nitrous oxide into the middle ear space by mucosal capillaries. This is a well-known problem in middle ear surgery, and can cause ballooning of a tympanic membrane graft due to increased middle ear pressure. This is also true of oxygen. If the partial pressure of expired oxygen is 30% or greater, more oxygen will be released into the middle ear. This may be of little consequence in routine tympanoplasty, but when a tympanic membrane needs to be totally reconstructed, the graft will balloon. In atresia the new tympanic membrane is a lateral graft over fused ossicles and ballooning may lift the graft off the ossicles where it is lateralized, it and may not reattach. To circumvent this potential problem, the anesthesiologist is asked to lower the expiratory partial pressure of oxygen to 25% or less before proceeding with fascia graft placement. Ideally, the best possible situation is to have a patient spontaneously breathing on room air.

Alternative Methods of Ossicular Chain Reconstruction

In 25% of cases the ossicular chain will need to be reconstructed. This is mandatory when one finds a disconnected ossicular chain, a fixed chain which requires disconnection, a fibrous incudostapedial joint, or absence of the incus–malleus complex. The preoperative CT scan will alert the surgeon to these conditions.

In 4% of patients, the stapes will be fixed. This condition cannot be diagnosed from the preoperative CT scan. A fixed stapes is one of only a few intraoperative findings that obliges a surgeon to stage the operation. The reason for this is that a stapedectomy requires an oval window seal with soft tissue. This then creates an unstable membrane at each end of the prosthesis—the oval window seal and the new tympanic membrane. As the new ear canal is packed with expandable packing, excess pressure on the prosthesis may result in medial displacement of the TORP into the vestibule, labyrinthine irritation, and a dizzy patient.

Another reason to stage the atresia operation occurs when the middle ear is found far anterior, medial to the temporomandibular joint. In this anatomic variation, one can drill down to the middle ear but, because the anterior bony wall is missing, there is no way to maintain a canal lumen. Soft tissue anteriorly will prolapse into the ear canal and obliterate the opening. When this problem is encountered, a bone graft composed of mastoid cortex shavings, bone paté collected while drilling, and hydroxyapatite is inserted between the mastoid and the temporomandibular joint. A meatal opening is not created and the ear is simply returned to its preoperative position. A second-stage operation 6 months later allows the surgeon to create a bony external ear canal by drilling through the bone graft. We use this technique infrequently, in perhaps 1–2% of cases. Others, however, use it routinely. Professor Vicente Diamante in Argentina has developed a technique whereby a bone plug is harvested from the mastoid tip and inserted between the mastoid and temporomandibular joint as a first-stage procedure.

The choices available to the surgeon to reconstruct the ossicular chain involve **partial** and **total ossicular replacement prostheses** (PORP and TORP). If there is a well-defined head to the stapes, a PORP may be used. The shaft of the PORP can be further modified by notching the distal end to accommodate the arch of the stapes when the head and neck are absent. In the majority of cases the arch of the stapes will be bent either toward the facial nerve or toward the promontory. This tilt of the stapes allows access to the footplate. A TORP is selected that has an hydroxylapatite flange and a shaft of either hydroxylapatite or Teflon depending on the proximity of other tissues. For example, a bony facial nerve canal contiguous to a hydroxylapatite shaft encourages bony bridging and subsequent fixation of the prosthesis. To avoid this, the shaft is positioned through the obturator foramen of the stapes and onto its footplate (Fig. 6.**27 a**). The prosthesis is stabilized with pledgets of Gelfoam. The new tympanic membrane is a lateral graft onto the flange of the prosthesis, or onto a cartilage wafer interposed between the drum and prosthesis (Fig. 6.**27 b**).

Hearing results with TORPs and PORPs are not as predictable as a lateral graft over the malformed but intact ossicular chain. However, on occasion the use of a middle

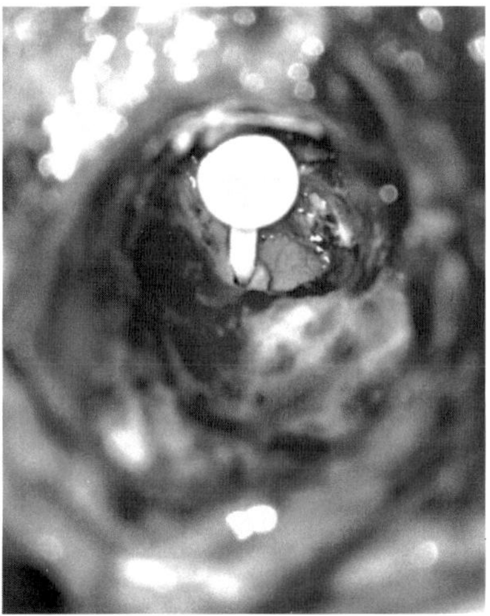

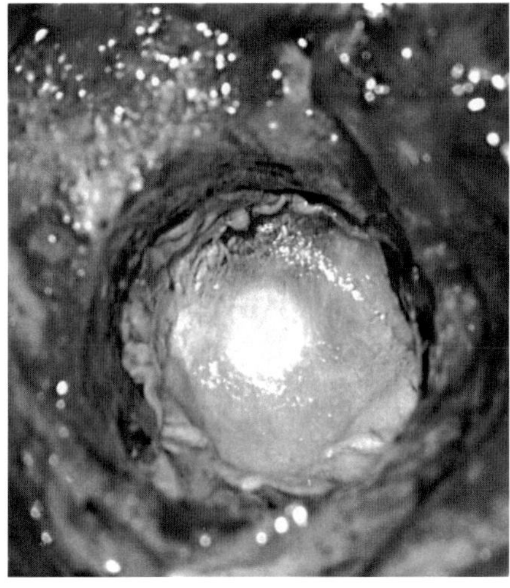

Fig. 6.**27** **Total auricular prosthesis (TORP).**
a Positioning of the shaft through the obturator foramen of the stapes and onto the footplate of the stapes.
b New tympanic membrane replacement using the temporal fascia over the flange of the prosthesis (the author would use additional cartilage on the prosthesis; s. Fig. 6.**31**, p. 257).

ear prosthesis will produce a truly outstanding hearing improvement.

Titanium implants, long used in Germany, are only now obtaining some measure of popularity in the United States. One obvious advantage of these implants is a slotted flange that enables the surgeon to better visualize the distal end of the shaft.

Facial Nerve Injury

Fear of facial nerve injury is the single most important concern that parents and patients have about atresia surgery. It is also the greatest deterrent to otologic surgeons who may contemplate performing this operation. For the inexperienced surgeon, the risk of facial nerve injury is the single most compelling reason to avoid these cases (Jahrsdoerfer and Lambert 1990).

In congenital aural atresia, the facial nerve is displaced in 25–30% of cases. The displacement occurs at the second genu where there is a sharp bend anteriorly with the nerve crossing the middle ear at the level of the round window to exit into the glenoid fossa.

What is not generally recognized is that although the nerve makes a sharp bend anteriorly, it pursues a medial-to-lateral course through the middle ear. Thus, after the facial nerve makes an acute turn and tracks anteriorly, it ascends. This has great clinical significance. The nerve at the level of the round window may be as much as 4 mm lateral to its position at the oval window. As the nerve is encased in atretic bone and is now lateral to the middle ear space, it is largely concealed. In this location it is vulnerable to injury from the drill before the middle ear is reached (Fig. 6.**28 b**). Thus, the anterior approach to the middle ear by drilling directly through atretic bone poses a substantial risk to the facial nerve in the hands of the novice surgeon.

The greatest risk to the facial nerve is seen in those patients who have low-set ears and are not otherwise candidates for atresia surgery. However, cholesteatoma may be present in a patient with a stenotic ear canal requiring surgery despite a poor grading score. Patients who are not otherwise surgical candidates, but need the operation, may have facial nerves that pursue an abnormal course through the temporal bone to exit into the lateral face. As the facial nerve now is in soft tissue, it is impossible to track on routine imaging. Our one case of facial nerve transection occurred during the postauricular skin incision when the nerve was severed at the superior helix. We advocate that facial nerve monitoring be routine in every case.

Transposition of the Facial Nerve

In 1995, we published an account of six patients who underwent atresia surgery with the intent of transposing the facial nerve to better access the oval window and stapes (Jahrsdoerfer 1995). This series was updated in 1998 with the inclusion of six additional nerve transpositions. Nerve transposition is restricted to those patients with bilateral atresia in whom the preoperative CT scan has indicated the presence of a stapes, albeit covered by an overhanging facial nerve. In the atresia operation there is sufficient room to remove the bony facial canal and displace the nerve from its bony groove. The facial nerve then assumes a position inferior to the stapes and oval window, and allows access to the foot plate for placement of a prosthesis. We have now performed 20 cases of facial nerve transposition. In these cases, the senior author has discovered an anatomic defect in the floor of the bony fallopian canal just lateral to the oval window. This is a dehiscence in the bone and a persistent membrane which, when incised, reveals the underlining stapes and oval window. This has been opportunistically named

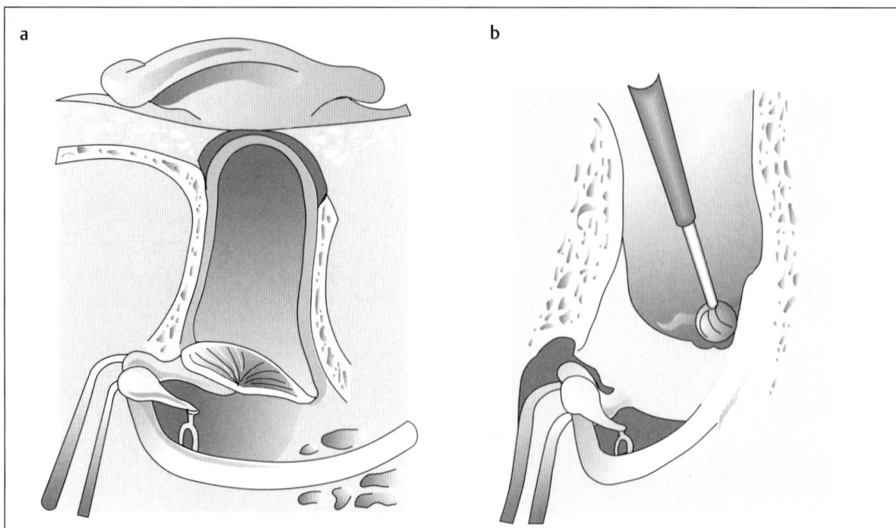

Fig. 6.**28 a, b** **Ascending facial nerve in a case of congenital aural atresia (b) as compared with a normal finding (a).**

"Bob's window." (Please refer to the otologic literature describing "Bill's bar" and "Mike's dot" after Bill House and Mike Glasscock.)

Results

It should never be forgotten that this operation is done to improve hearing. One does not make a hole in the side of the head for cosmetic reasons. If there is little chance of improving hearing, surgery should be avoided.

The grading scheme has helped us considerably in our choice of surgical candidates (see Tables 6.1, 6.2, pp. 234, 235). It not only allows us to avoid impossible cases (those with little chance of hearing success) but also allows for a prediction of outcome. Most patients who undergo surgery will grade 7–8/10. This translates to a 70–80% chance of achieving normal, or near normal, hearing through surgery. By that is meant a postoperative speech reception threshold (SRT) of 15–30 db.

There is no significant difference in hearing results between unilateral and bilateral cases. Patients with bilateral atresia who achieve normal hearing through surgery exhibit a dramatic response to unaided sound for the first time. In patients with unilateral atresia, the response is less dramatic, but significant. Binaural auditory processing enables one to localize sounds in space and to detect sounds in background noise. Successful atresia surgery will immediately allow the patient to hear better in the presence of other noise (Wilmington et al. 1994). Tests for sound localization show some improvement and appear to gradually improve over months following surgery.

Do the hearing results endure, and is the atresia operation worthwhile? Lambert studied this a few years ago and concluded that while long-term hearing results show some degradation, 53% of patients maintained an SRT of 25 dB or less, and in 64% of cases an SRT of 30 dB was sustained (Weerda et al. 1985, Lambert 1998). The senior author's experience is similar to that of Lambert. However, much of this is dependent on the patient conforming to a protocol for the periodic cleaning of the ears and the willingness to seek early treatment in the face of potential postoperative complications. Ten to fifteen percent of operations now entail revision atresia surgery because of meatal stenosis, late stenosis from new bone growth, graft lateralization, or refixation of the ossicular chain.

Risks and Complications

The two greatest risks to the patient in atresia repair are facial nerve injury and hearing being made worse. Facial nerve injury has been addressed previously. In our experience in 1400 operations, 12 patients have incurred a facial nerve injury. Eight of these 12 patients were ours; 4 had their surgery elsewhere. One of these 4 patients sustained a permanent facial nerve paralysis from microtia repair.

In only 1 of our 8 patients was the facial nerve transected. However, this patient has normal function of the upper one-third of his face, with good eyelid closure. All others, except one, had a temporary weakness of the facial nerve which subsequently progressed to normal facial function. The lone exception is a teenage boy in whom the facial nerve was damaged while elevating the periosteum over the lateral mastoid. Of clinical interest in this series of 12 facial nerve injuries is that 6 occurred within the temporal bone and 6 were extratemporal. Again, for the experienced surgeon, the facial nerve is at greatest risk when it prematurely exits the temporal bone on its lateral surface.

Hearing Loss. A high-frequency sensorineural hearing loss occurs in 15% of surgical cases. The loss usually occurs in the 6–8 kHz range, and does not significantly affect the SRT or the speech discrimination score. The transfer of acoustic energy from drilling on or near the atretic plate may account for this type of hearing loss. Extra care must be taken when drilling near the ossicles to prevent their being brushed by the burr.

Meatal Stenosis. Postoperative meatal stenosis may occur in fully one-half of patients in whom the microtia is grade III and there is no conchal cartilage. If conchal cartilage is present, adding some stiffness and support to the new meatus, the problem is much less. The use of a tragal-based anterior pedicle flap has significantly ameliorated this problem.

The size of the new meatus is generous, about 1.5–2 times normal size, in anticipation of postoperative scarring. Moreover, if meatal stenosis is apparent early (1 month) 0.5 mL of triamcinolone 40 mg/mL is injected. This may need to be repeated 2–3 times. Triamcinolone is a depot steroid used to soften the scar and prevent additional scarring. Approximately 10% of patients with postoperative meatal stenosis will require revision surgery.

Siegert and Weerda recently published a two-step external ear construction in patients with atresia in concert with microtia surgery (Siegert and Weerda 2001). In their series, 33/36 patients showed little or no evidence of postoperative meatal stenosis. Only 14/36 patients were candidates for tympanoplasty to improve hearing, although all 36 had a new ear canal drilled. They state that a new ear canal is made for esthetic reasons and to allow the placement of an air conduction hearing aid.

Canal Stenosis. Bony canal stenosis is one of the long-term complications associated with atresia surgery. Canal stenosis resembles occlusive exostosis and develops from new bone growth in the ear canal. This osteoneogenesis can trap epithelial debris and can cause a deterioration in hearing from encroachment on the tympanic membrane. This process develops 3–10 years after initial atresia repair. Revision surgery may be required, and has a very good chance of restoring hearing to previous levels.

6.3 Surgery of the Middle Ear for Grade III Microtia in the Presence of Congenital Aural Atresia

R. Siegert

6.3.1 Introduction

Tympanoplasty of malformed ears associated with congenital aural atresia is regarded as one of the most difficult operations in the region of the middle ear, often with uncertain results (Weerda et al. 1985; Hildmann et al. 1992). Although some highly specialized surgeons have reported their own acceptable results (Jahrsdoerfer 1978, 1980; Weerda et al. 1985; Schuknecht 1989), the outcome in patients not operated at these specialized centers is rather more sobering. In such cases, the preoperative sound conduction block of around 60 dB was on average only reduced to about 50 dB.

One of the most common complications is recurrent stenosis of the newly formed auditory canal (Weerda et al. 1985). According to Jahrsdoerfer (1978, 1980), Helms (1987) and others, drilling is directed into the mastoid and through the atretic plate, to be covered with a split-skin graft and packs to be inserted (see above; Figs. 6.**23**–6.**28**).

In order to avoid complications, efforts have been made to create a very wide new auditory canal and maintain its patency by using various obturators. Apart from the risk that recurrent stenosis will still develop despite obturators—and sometimes one even has the impression that recurrent stenosis is even encouraged by the irritation caused by the obturators—this technique results in aesthetically unsatisfactory, funnel-shaped auditory canals, which allow a combined reconstruction of the outer ear only with difficulty.

Whereas we essentially rely on those techniques that have established themselves over the decades for the reconstruction of the sound-conducting apparatus, we have developed special techniques for the combination of auricular reconstruction and tympanoplasty in the presence of atresia, in which the auditory canal is created in several stages and which, in combination with the reconstruction of the external ear, do not require any additional procedures. This procedure will now be presented.

6.3.2 Middle Ear Surgery Combined with Reconstruction of the Auricle: Method

Reconstruction of the sound apparatus is in three stages, as with reconstruction of the auricle (see pp. 201 ff).

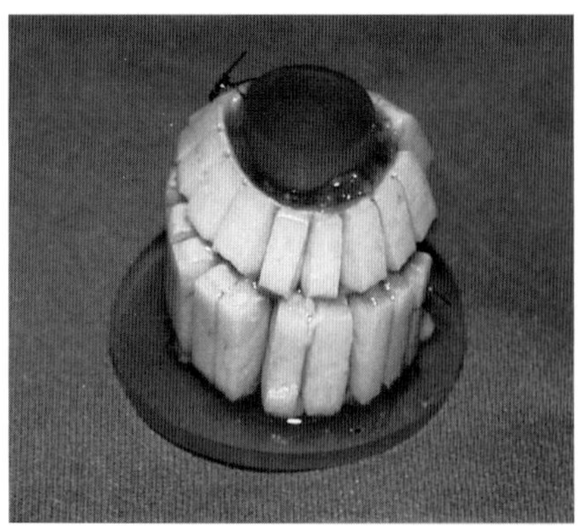

a

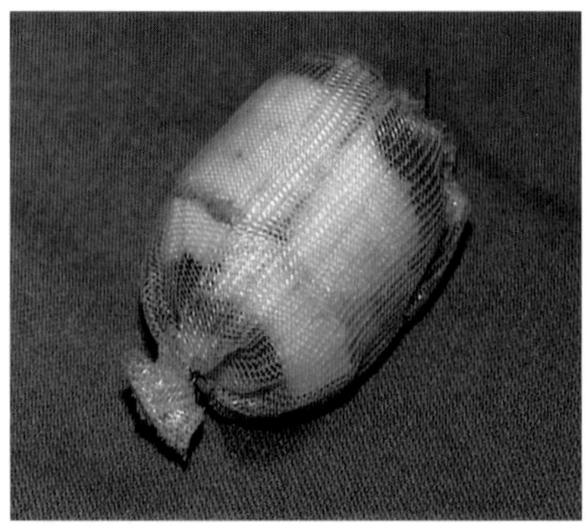

b

Fig. 6.**29 a, b** **Silicone rubber cylinder invested by small pieces of cartilage (a) and wrapped in an absorbable mesh (b).**

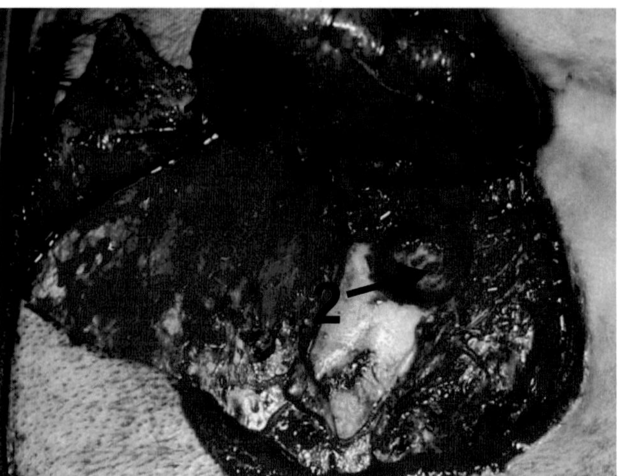

Fig. 6.**30** **Cartilage framework (1) mobilized from a dorsal direction and elevated, exposure of the mastoid plane and creation of the auditory canal (2).**

Preoperative Preparation

As with any form of surgery for atresia, a preoperative HRCT scan of the temporal bone should be obtained (see p. 234). The anatomical structures are assessed using a points system (see Tables 6.**1**, 6.**2**; pp. 234, 235), in order to calculate the chances of a successful tympanoplasty and to provide orientation for the second stage of the operation. This system uses Table 6.**2** to assess those individual anatomical structures which are essential for the atresia operation by assigning points between 1 and 4. The individual scores are added together and can reach a maximum value of 28 in a healthy individual. At present, we offer surgery for the middle ear at scores of 20 and above (Siegert et al. 1996 b; see p. 235).

Surgery

First Operative Stage

- Construction of the cartilage framework for the auricle
- Formation of the auditory canal

For the first operative stage, autologous costal cartilage is harvested, from which the cartilaginous framework for the auricle is created (see p. 204) and, if a suitable remnant is available, its lower part is transposed to form the earlobe (for details see pp. 213 ff; Aguilar and Jahrsdoerfer 1988; Brent 1992; Nagata 1994 a; Weerda and Siegert 1999 b).

At this stage, the future auditory canal is also prepared using more costal cartilage. For this purpose a special silicone rubber cylinder with a diameter of 11 mm is used (Fig. 6.**29 a**). This is "invested" by small pieces of cartilage, ensuring that the perichondrium comes to lie on the inside (Fig. 6.**29 a**). Once the pieces of cartilage have been tightly packed and attached together with absorbable sutures, this preformed new auditory canal is wrapped in an absorbable polydioxanone mesh (Fig. 6.**29 b**) and stored in a subcutaneous chest pocket until the second operative stage, which is performed about 6 months later.

Second Operative Stage

- Elevation of the auricular framework
- Formation of the retroauricular fold
- Creation of the external auditory canal
- Tympanoplasty, including construction of the tympanic membrane

About 6 months after the first stage, the cartilaginous framework is elevated from a dorsal approach and the retroauricular fold is formed (for details see pp. 214 ff; Nagata 1994 d; Weerda and Siegert 1999 b).

The periosteum, which has been left on the mastoid plane, is now incised in the shape of an "H" and the bone is exposed. The mastoid is opened between the temporal line, the glenoid fossa, and the mastoid process (see p. 250, Fig. 6.**23 a–c**) and an auditory canal is created with a diameter of about 20 mm (Fig. 6.**30**). A CT of the temporal bone, obtained preoperatively using the thin-slice technique, is used for orientation. The entire operation of the middle ear is performed under **intraoperative nerve monitoring** to avoid injury to the facial nerve, which is often displaced in these malformations (pp. 240 ff).

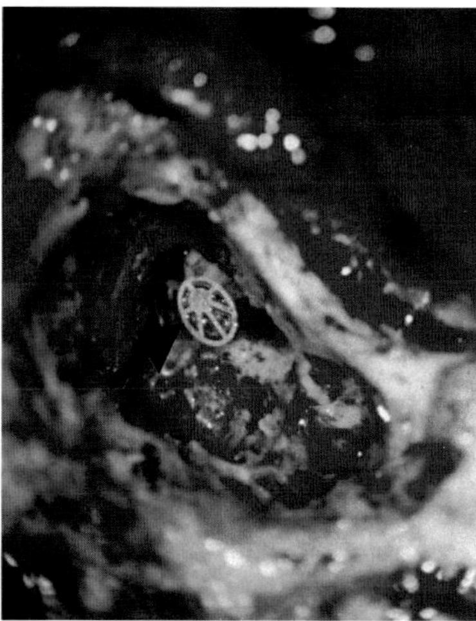

Fig. 6.**31** **Titanium prosthesis (arrow) in situ on the stapes.**

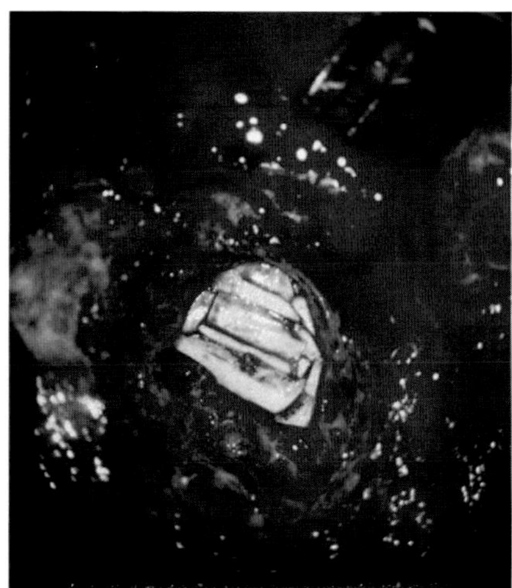

Fig. 6.**32** **Tympanic membrane reconstructed from thin slices of cartilage.**

First, the mastoid is drilled down to the atretic plate. Then the skull base is exposed, beginning posteriorly, and the antrum identified. After more of the atretic plate is carefully drilled away with a diamond burr, the malformed incus–malleus complex is exposed (see p. 251 and Fig. 6.**28**, p. 254). It is advisable here to remove the final fine bony lamellae with a House curette to avoid contact of the rotating tools with the ossicular chain. It is not uncommon to find fine bony bridges between the atretic plate and the auditory ossicles, which can wrongly create the impression of perceptive deafness in the preoperative audiogram. After further drilling away of the atretic plate, the chorda tympani is encountered, which courses through the atretic plate and must therefore be sacrificed.

It is important to identify the facial nerve canal early and with certainty (see p. 254). The facial nerve can also run through the atretic plate, which will render the tympanoplasty considerably more difficult or even impossible. Congenital aural atresia shows a great variety of course variations of the facial nerve which are not always amenable to diagnostics, even with the best of radiological techniques (see pp. 240 ff). Displacement of the stapes is a common observation. Only when a free view of the mobile stapedial suprastructures is possible can the sound conduction apparatus be reliably reconstructed. For this purpose we use extralong titanium prostheses (8–10 mm). A bell basket is used to position them onto the head of the stapes (Fig. 6.**31**). Since structures such as a hammer handle or residual tympanic membrane, under which the prosthesis plate can be anchored, are absent, the prosthesis with its shaft and supporting surface are initially suspended in "free space." To prevent it from tipping over, it is stabilized either with a few drops of blood in the oval window recess or with an absorbable sponge.

Reconstruction of the tympanic membrane now follows, employing the well-known palisade technique and using very thin slices of cartilage which are laid onto the plate of the prosthesis and laterally supported by the bone (Fig. 6.**32**). Here it is important to maintain drainage of the antrum open.

Meanwhile, the silicone rubber cylinder with its surrounding pieces of cartilage, which has been stored in a subcutaneous pocket since the first stage and from which a stable cartilaginous cylinder has meanwhile developed, is harvested (Fig. 6.**33**). After removal of the silicone rubber cylinder, a stable preformed auditory canal appears which is very soft on its inner surface. Its length is now adapted to the proportions within the temporal bone and the cylinder is positioned onto the new tympanic membrane (Fig. 6.**34**). The transitions between the medial end of the new auditory canal and the new tympanic membrane are sealed off with small cartilage chips and fibrous tissue. Another press-fit silicone rubber cylinder is now placed into the new auditory canal as a spacer (Fig. 6.**34**, 2).

The gap between the lateral end of the new auditory canal and the bone, i. e., the former mastoid plane, is reconstructed with further pieces of cartilage and bone chippings (see Fig. 6.**34**). The periosteum is then replaced and sutured.

This concludes this stage of the so-called atresia operation and the second stage to reconstruct the auricle is continued as described on p. 215. For this purpose, a supportive cartilage (Fig. 6.**35**, 3; Danter et al. 1997) is placed beneath the base plate of the auricular framework and secured in this new elevated position. The supportive cartilage and the reconstructed mastoid plane are covered by the previously dissected and pedicled superficial temporal fascia (Fig. 6.**35**, 4) and a full-thickness skin graft (Fig. 6.**36**; Ginsbach et al. 1979; see also pp. 214, 215).

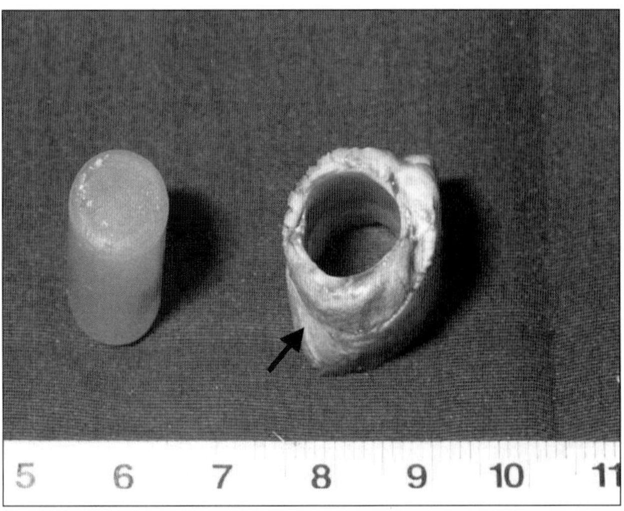

Fig. 6.**33** **New auditory canal (arrow) from Figure 6.29 6 months after preformation around the silicone rubber cylinder.**

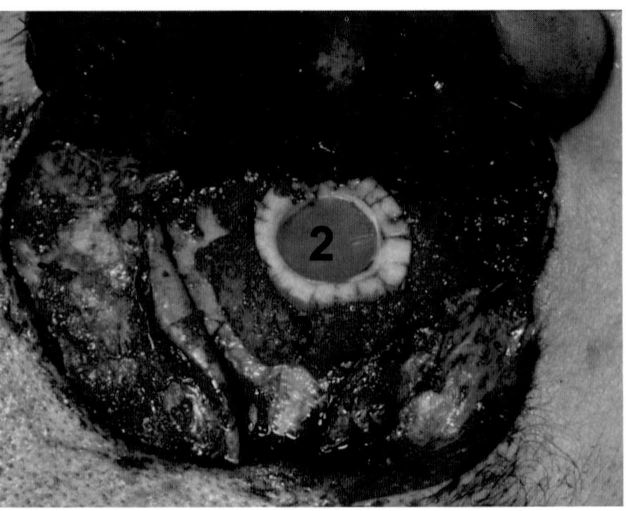

Fig. 6.**34** **New auditory canal (1) in situ with silicone rubber cylinder (2) and bone pati (3).**

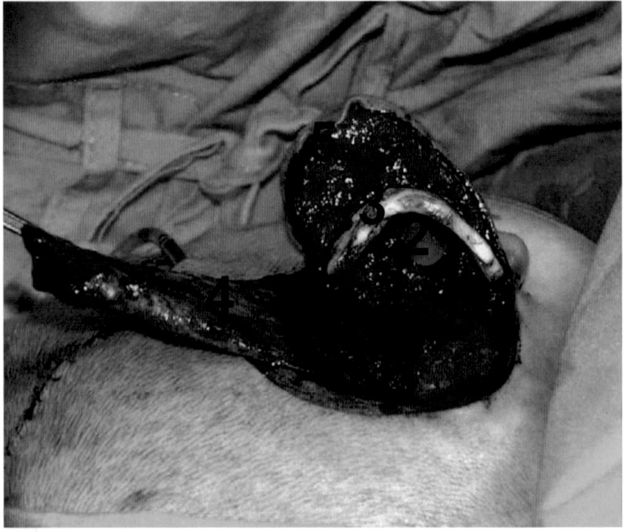

Fig. 6.**35** **Continuation (from Fig. 6.34) of the second stage of auricular reconstruction after reconstruction of the middle ear and creation of the auditory canal.** 1: New auditory canal with silicone rubber cylinder; 2: silicone rubber spacer in the auditory canal; 3: cartilage strut beneath the conchal base; 4: superficial temporal fascia pedicled on the temporal vessels; 5: dorsal view of the reconstructed auricle, covered by connective tissue.

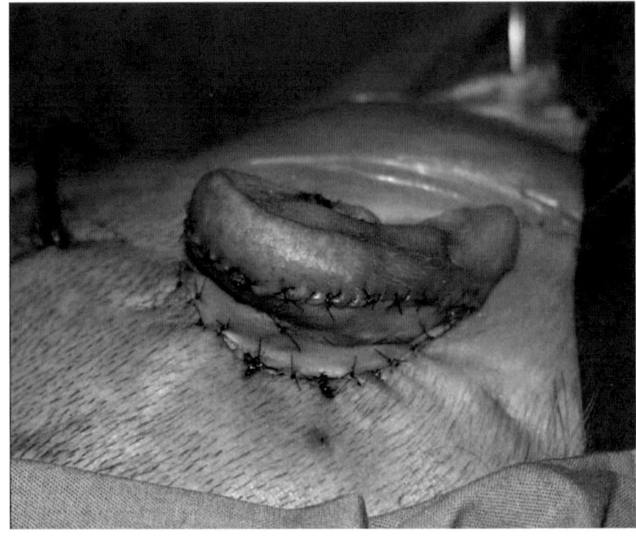

Fig. 6.**36** **Retroauricular fold covered with a full-thickness skin graft (continued from Fig. 6.34, see pp. 213 ff).**

Third Operative Stage

- Excavation of the cavum conchae
- Opening and epithelialization of the auditory canal

The contour of the auricle is formed at this third operative stage, 6 months at the earliest after the second stage. For this purpose, the skin over the cavum conchae is incised and raised as a thin flap and fibrous tissue is removed to excavate the cavum conchae. The silicone rubber cylinder in the new auditory canal is exposed (Fig. 6.**37**) and removed from its bed. A firm smooth auditory canal now appears, bounded in the depths by the new tympanic membrane (Fig. 6.**37**). The canal is then lined with a full-thickness skin graft. For this purpose, the graft is cut to size so that it envelopes a silicone rubber tube with a diameter of 10 mm in the shape of a goblet (Fig. 6.**38**), with the epithelial surface facing towards the

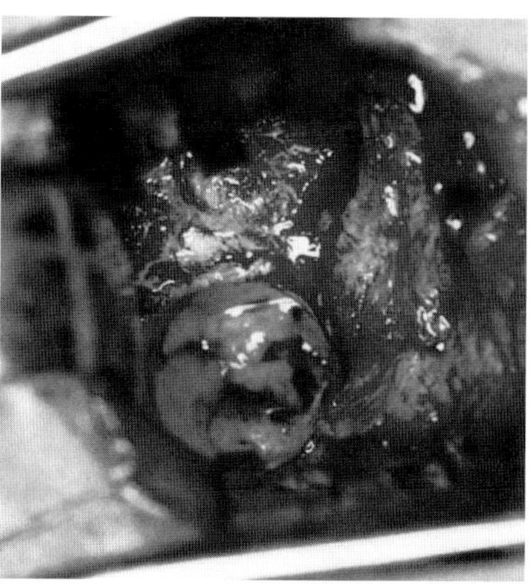

Fig. 6.37 **Operative site from Figs. 6.34–6.36 after removal of the silicone rubber cylinder. A firm, smooth new auditory canal is apparent, bounded below by the new tympanic membrane.**

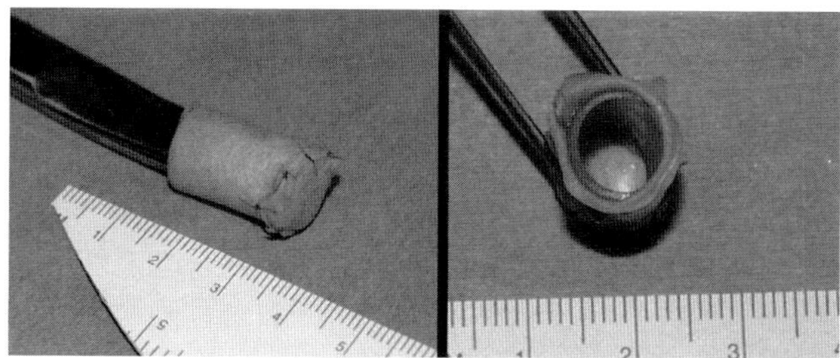

Fig. 6.38 **Silicone rubber tube with full-thickness skin graft.**

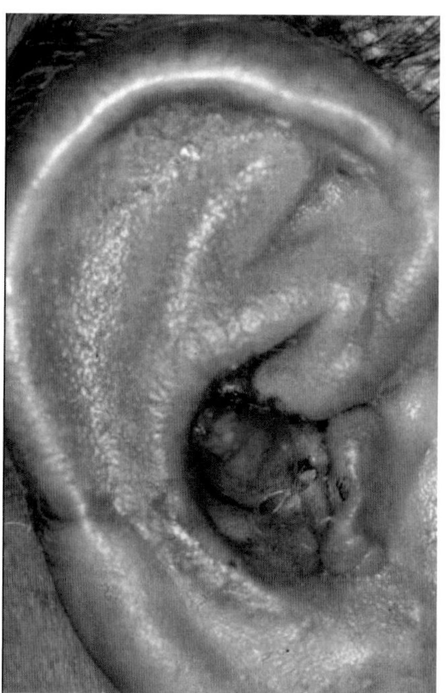

a

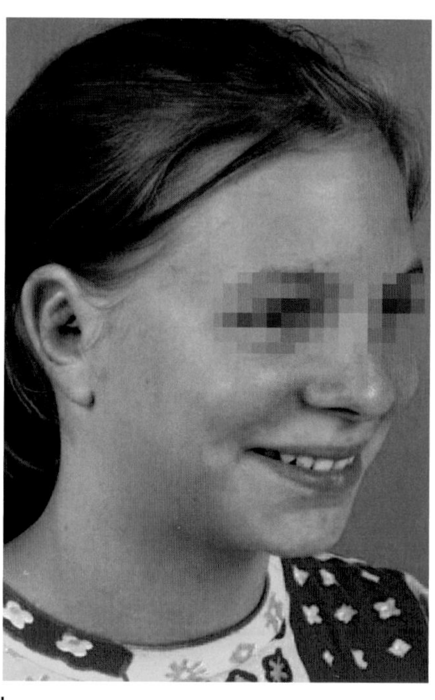

b

Fig. 6.39 **Results.**
a Appearance after 2 weeks after lining the new auditory canal with a full-thickness skin graft.
b Appearance after reconstruction of the auricle in combination with a multistaged, so-called "atresia" operation with reconstruction of the middle ear.

silicone rubber cylinder. Some fibrin adhesive is inserted into the new auditory canal and the 10 mm-thick silicone rubber cylinder, together with the split-skin graft, is pressed into place. The split-skin graft is thus well-positioned and well-fitted in the newly formed auditory canal. The cavum conchae skin flap is then replaced and secured in the excavated concha (Moore et al. 1984; Weerda and Siegert 1999 b, 2001).

Postoperative Care

The silicone rubber tube remains in situ for 1–2 weeks. During this time the graft heals sufficiently stably. After removing the tube (Fig. 6.39), the still-fresh wound area is covered with a moisturizing ointment and cared for as after a "classic" tympanoplasty. We have never witnessed a clinically relevant recurrent stenosis after using this staged technique.

6.4 Provision of Hearing Aids for Congenital Aural Atresia

H. Sommer and R. Schoenweiler

In almost all cases of congenital microtia with atresia of the auditory canal and middle ear, the inner ear is usually intact. This is typically associated with a so-called conduction block. A pantonal air-conduction hearing threshold of about 60 dB is the result (Figs. 6.**40**, 6.**41**).

In exceptional cases, additional inner-ear deafness is present, for example in cases of thalidomide embryopathy, where in some patients a combined form of deafness is found.

A hearing aid should be fitted as early as possible, i. e., during the first weeks of life. Various options are available for providing a patient with a hearing aid which will now be presented.

6.4.1 Bone-Conduction Hearing Aids (Fig. 6.42)

Principle

Sound is picked up is via a microphone. The cochlea is stimulated directly via bone conduction, i. e., sound travels within the bone, under the direction of an oscillator which is in contact with the skull bone. Various types of devices are available.

Bone-Conduction Receiver, Bone-Conduction Spectacles

Figure 6.**42 a** shows a bone-conduction receiver with clip, Figure 6.**42 b** a bone-conduction receiver integrated in a headband, and Figure 6.**42 c** bone-conduction spectacles.

Advantages. Simple fitting without surgery, no interference with any later reconstruction of the outer ear, provision can be initiated very quickly.

Disadvantages. Skin macerations at the pressure points; problems at contact points due to moisture, e. g., from sweat; instability during physical activity; e. g., during sport, stigmatizing optical appearance.

Bone-Anchored Hearing Aid (BAHA)

(see Fig. 6.48 **b**; p. 266).

Advantages. Good acoustic properties, good stability during physical activities.

Disadvantages. An operation is required with the disadvantage of early and late complications, which cannot always be ruled out (skin necrosis, inflammatory reactions, screw loosening), emotional impairment from the implanted foreign body on the head.

Audient Bone Conductor

Advantages. Implant not visible from the outside.

Disadvantages. An operation is required, moderate acoustic properties.

Air-Conduction Hearing Aids

Advantages. Comparatively good acoustic properties, minimal stigmatization ("normal hearing aid"), highly comfortable to wear.

Disadvantages. Required is the presence of a cavum conchae, auditory canal, and an auricle (which can be surgically constructed if necessary; see Fig. 5.**197**, p. 230; Fig. 5.**198**, p. 231 and Fig. 6.**39**, p. 259).

6.4.2 Strategies for Provision of Hearing Aids

Unilateral Atresia of the Auditory Canal: Early Provision of a Hearing Aid

If only unilateral atresia is present with normal contralateral hearing, there is usually a normal development of speech and intelligence. For this reason, most patients with unilateral aural atresia have hitherto, in practice, not been provided with a hearing aid.

However, there is an obvious handicap in terms of spatial hearing and hearing with background noise (Niehaus et al. 1995; Sommer et al. 1998). Wazen et al. (2001) observed improved sound and speech recognition with regard to various hearing tests in treated patients with unilateral atresia following unilateral BAHA provision. Sommer et al. (2001) observed improved recognition for pure tones and speech without background noise in patients with unilateral atresia fitted with bone-conduction devices. In patients with unilateral aural atresia Snik et al. (2002) discovered an improvement of spatial hearing after provision of a BAHA during adulthood, which did not, however, result in a normalization of sound localization. In contrast, however, patients with acquired unilateral conductive hearing loss reached normal values in directive hearing tests perfectly well with a BAHA. It may be assumed that, in order to achieve optimal results in

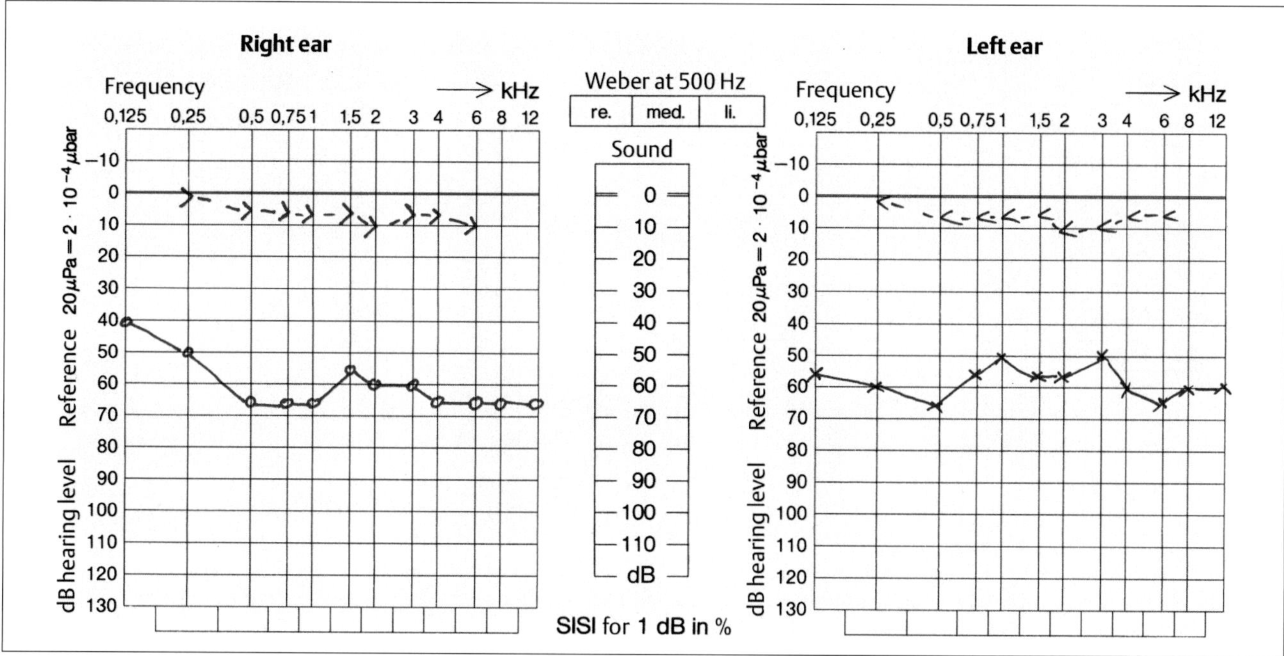

Fig. 6.**40** **Sound audiogram of a patient with bilateral congenital aural atresia and a subsequent bilateral sound conduction block of approximately 55–60 dB.**
Between the broken lines of the bone-conduction curve, which reflects the inner ear hearing ability, and the continuous air-conduction curve, which reflects the total hearing threshold, there is a maximal restriction of sound conduction in the middle ear secondary to the congenital atresia.

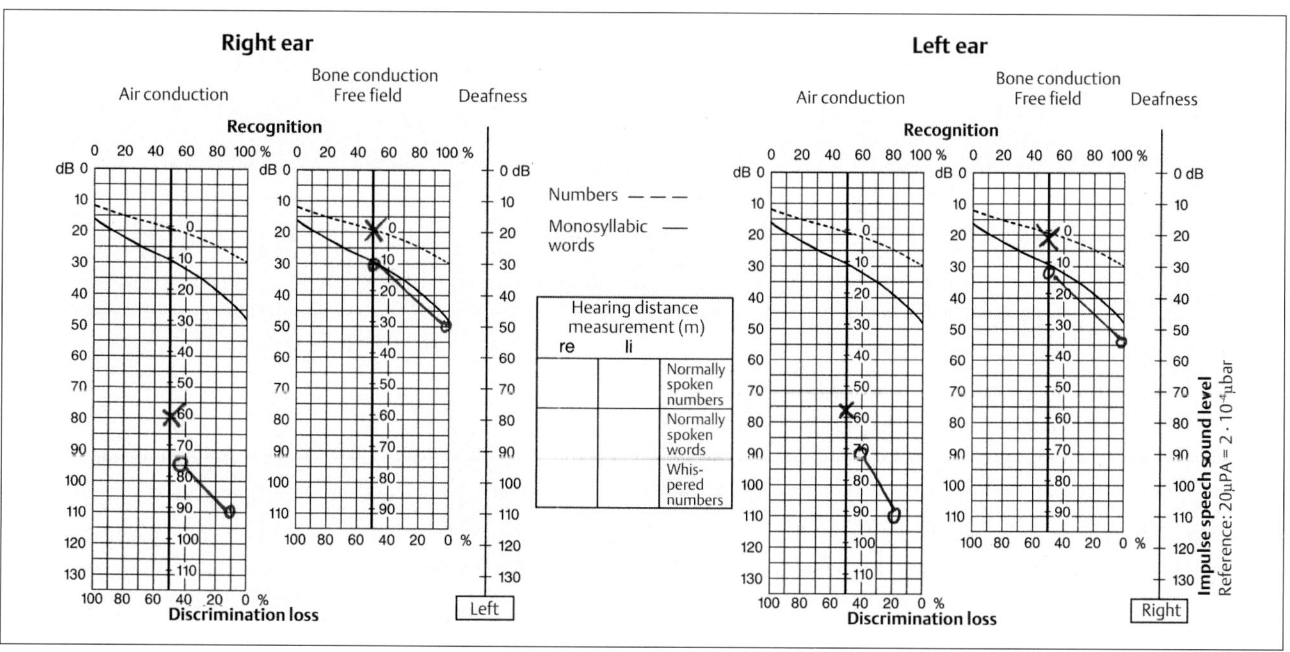

Fig. 6.**41** **Speech audiogram (Freiburg Speech Recognition Test) of a patient with bilateral aural atresia.**
In the air conduction test speech recognition for polysyllabic words (cross) and monosyllabic words (circle) is clearly limited. Recognition is normal in the bone-conduction test.

cases of unilateral atresia, provision of a hearing aid must be instigated before the central hearing pathways have completely matured. Early provision should be considered during the first year of life, as with bilateral atresia. Kiese-Himmel and Kruse (2001) postulated the general early provision of a hearing aid in early childhood for all forms of unilateral deafness, and thus also for unilateral aural atresia, in order to prevent secondary damage in the auditory, verbal-communicative, behavioral, and intellectual areas.

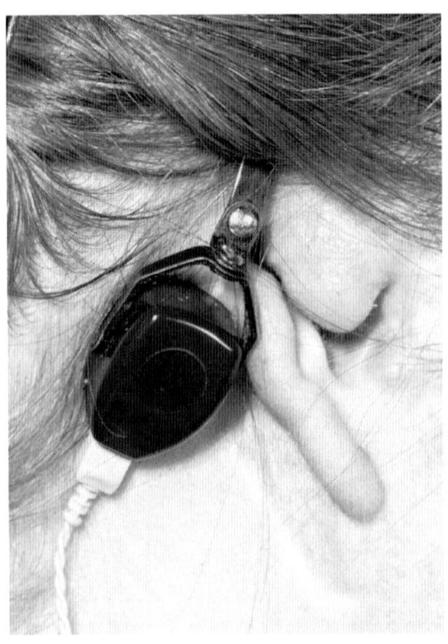
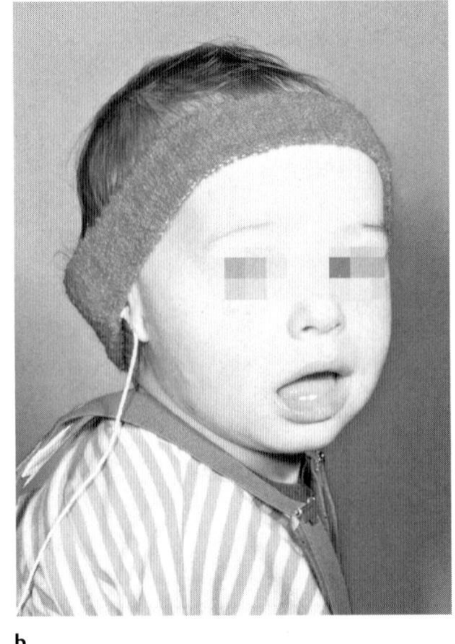
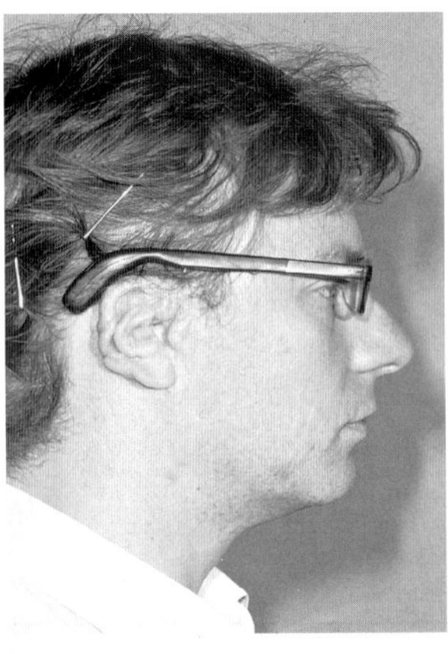

a b c

Fig. 6.**42** **Bilateral provision with a bone-conduction hearing aid: (a) bone-conduction receiver with clip, (b) bone-conduction receiver integrated in a headband, and (c) bone-conduction spectacles.**

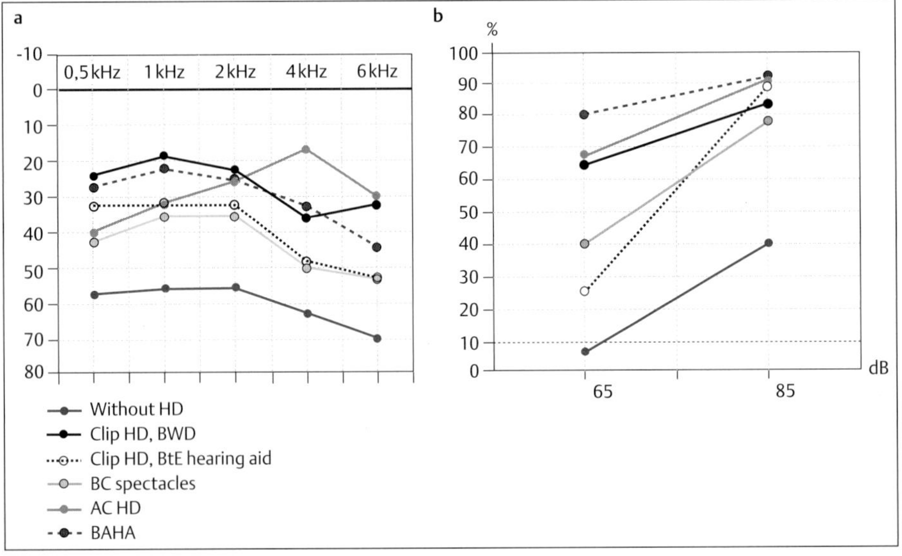

Fig. 6.**43** **Audiometry without and with provision with a hearing aid.**

a Hearing threshold in the unilateral free-field sound audiogram without and with hearing-aid provision, comparison of the various types of hearing aids.

b Comprehension for monosyllabic words in the unilateral Freiburg free-field speech recognition test without and with hearing aid.

HD: hearing aid; BWD: body-worn aid; BC: bone conduction; AC: air conduction; BtE: behind-the-ear hearing aid.

Bilateral Atresia of the Auditory Canal: Immediate Provision of a Hearing Aid

Immediate provision of a hearing aid in infancy is essential for bilateral aural atresia with bilateral conduction block, in order to guarantee normal speech development (Declau et al. 1999). Primary care in infancy is only possible with the aid of a bone-conduction device with a frame or preferably via a headband. Provision of bone-anchored systems, usually the BAHA, should be undertaken from the age of 3 years at the earliest. In cases of microtia, it is important to implant the screws outside the area where any later reconstruction of the external ear could take place (see Fig. 6.**47**). As alternatives to the bone-anchored devices, transcutaneous systems in the form of bone-conduction receivers and spectacles could, of course, still be prescribed. Numerous studies have, however, showed that both audiological results and patient acceptance are better in the long run and in most patients using percutaneous bone-anchored systems (Gangstrom and Tjellstrom 1997; Snik et al. 1998 b).

Regardless of the type of hearing aid, provision for bilateral atresia should, from the start, always be bilateral. Bilateral provision allows better spatial hearing and better speech recognition than unilateral provision, both in quiet surroundings and with background noise (Fig. 6.**43 a, b**; Hamann et al. 1991; Setou et al. 2001; Snik et al. 1998 a; van der Pouv et al. 1998; Bosmann et al. 2001).

6.5 Anchorage of Bone-Anchored Hearing Aids and Epitheses

S. Klaiber and H. Weerda

6.5.1 Bone-Anchored Hearing Aid (BAHA)

(See Fig. 6.48 b; p. 266)
The auditory organ is accessible via two routes: air conduction and bone conduction.

It is possible to provide a patient with a BAHA from the age of 3 years (Oppermann et al. 1996). In cases of congenital aural atresia (CAA), we recommend implantation at the age of 3–4 years. For provision of a hearing aid for bilateral CAA see p. 262; for unilateral CAA see p. 260.

Why Titanium?

In the late 1960s, Per-Ingvar Brånemark showed in animal and clinical studies that direct long-term contact between a titanium implant and bone tissue was possible (Tjellström 1989). According to Albrektsson (1987), osseointegration is a process by which a clinically asymptomatic rigid connection between an alloplastic implant and viable bone can be achieved and maintained under functional loading.

Demands for the Long-term Stability of Implants

The following requirements for the long-term stability of implants were proposed by Albrektsson et al. in 1987:

- Biocompatibility of the material
- Good design of the implant
- Good surface properties of the implant
- Optimal demands on the condition of the recipient area
- Sophisticated surgical implantation technique
- No premature functional loading

Type and Timing of Functional Loading

Premature loading can result in the formation of a fibrous capsule around the implants. A healing time of at least 3 months is therefore recommended (Kurt and Federspil 1994).

Indications for a Bone-Anchored Hearing Aid

If it is not possible to use an air-conduction hearing device, then provision of a bone-conduction hearing aid is necessary. Since conventional bone-conduction hearing aids have their disadvantages, as previously shown, the aim should be to provide a BAHA.

Exclusion Criteria

In order to achieve good therapeutic results, suitable patients must be selected with great care. Exclusion criteria (Tjellström and Hakansson 1995; Powell et al. 1996; Bejar-Solar et al. 2000) are:

- Perceptive deafness > 45 dB for the ear device and > 65 dB for the pocket device
- Speech discrimination < 60 %
- Poor personal hygiene
- Significant developmental retardation
- Age < 3 years

Patients or the parents of young patients must be thoroughly informed about the risks and the performance capacity of the hearing aids, in order to avoid any unrealistic expectations. Providing alcoholics and drug addicts with a BAHA also has its problems.

Preoperative Diagnostics

A thorough preoperative diagnostic work-up should be performed before provision of a BAHA:

- Comprehensive history taking (concomitant disorders, social history, medication, addictive drugs, etc.)
- Clinical and in particular ENT examination
- Pure-tone audiogram (see p. 261)
- Free-field audiogram with and without the fitted hearing device
- Test with a BAHA via a test rod
- If possible, uncomfortable loudness level and speech audiogram
- Radiological diagnostics
- Brainstem-evoked response audiometry (BERA) in infants

A radiological work-up should be performed, especially in small children, in order to obtain preoperative information about any difficulties that might be encountered (e. g., inadequate bone thickness).

A detailed discussion with the patient (or parents) about the advantages and disadvantages of this form of treatment is essential. Those involved should have realistic ideas about the BAHA. Support from family, school, and friends is essential. Consideration should also be directed to the anesthesiological difficulties involved with syndrome patients, such as difficult intubation and additional malformations.

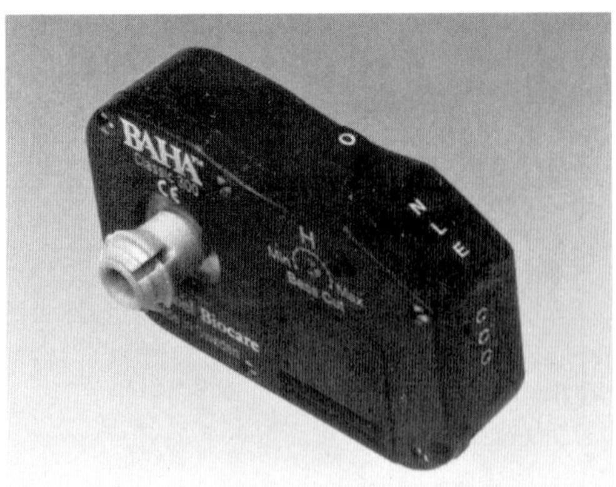

Fig. 6.**44** **BAHA Classic 300 (Entific Medical Systems).**

Available Hearing Aids

Currently four BAHA models are available (see www.entific.com):

BAHA Classic 300

The average bone-conduction threshold of the affected ear should be 45 dB or better (measured at 0.5, 1, 2, 3 kHz).

With the aid of a snap-on attachment, the device (Fig. 6.**44**) can be easily connected to the implant/abutment. For the safety of the patient, the device detaches itself when mechanically overloaded.

The unit is provided with a tone switch and an electrical input for connection with external devices. It is available in three colors (black, beige, gray) and is delivered as one set comprising hearing aid, abutment cover, battery, cleaning brush, safety lead, and user's manual. Several accessory parts are available, such a telecoil, audio-adapter, and directional microphone.

BAHA Compact

The audiological criteria for selecting patients are the same as for the BAHA Classic 300 (see above).

The BAHA Compact is 35% smaller that the Classic 300 and combines the most modern technology with many new designer features. As with the Classic 300, the BAHA Compact is supplied as a set. Available accessories include a telecoil and an audio-adapter.

BAHA Cordelle II

This device is intended for patients who suffer from a severe mixed form of deafness: patients with a bone-conduction threshold of up to 70 dB can be provided with it. The device comprises a head-worn transducer and a body-worn unit and is delivered as a set comprising the transducer and body-worn unit, a cover for the abutment, sound lead, rechargeable batteries, cleaning brush, and a user's manual.

BAHA Divino

The BAHA Divino is the first device in a new generation of BAHA sound processors. It is a digital sound processor with adjustable Automatic Gain Control Output compression (AGCO) for individual setting. AGCO limits distortion and the circuit has a dual time constant system, allowing for improved sound quality in loud environments. The Divino sound processor is available with a built-in directional microphone positioned on either the left or the right side. It was two programs: program 1 has an omnidirectional microphone, which means that the sound processor picks up sound regardless of the direction from which it comes; program 2 uses a directional microphone to emphasize sounds that come from the front and reduces the background noise. The Divino has an electrical input for connecting external equipment such as MP3 or FM hearing systems. It also has improved protection against mobile phone interference. The audiological indications are the same as for the BAHA Classic 300 and BAHA Compact.

For all BAHA models the head-worn transducer is secured by a screw, thus rendering head frame, headband, or hearing spectacles unnecessary. This lends the device greater cosmetic acceptance. The bone anchorage solves any pressure point problems, and the position of the hearing device is stable. There are no muffling tissues positioned between bone-conduction receiver and bone, thus rendering the sound conduction behavior for high frequencies particularly favorable and affording better speech recognition. Sound is experienced as more natural. Subjective acceptance is good and complications are rare. Handling is simple and can readily be learned by children (Bonding et al. 1992; Federspil 1994; Schorn and Stecker 1994; Tjellström and Halkansson 1995; Oppermann et al. 1996; Hartland and Proops 1996; Bejar-Solar et al. 2000; Arunachalam et al. 2001).

Hartland and Proops (1996) report that 69% of patients prefer the BAHA over their previous hearing devices. The reasons stated include fewer problems with ear infections, increased comfort, and an improved sound quality. Ninety-two percent of patients would opt for a BAHA again.

Surgical Procedure

In the early days of bone-anchored hearing devices and epitheses, the procedure was always a two-stage one. First, the titanium screw was implanted at the initial stage and about 3 months later it was exposed and the abutment was attached. The hearing aid was then attached a short time later. This **two-stage approach** is still indicated for children, patients who have undergone radiotherapy, or poor

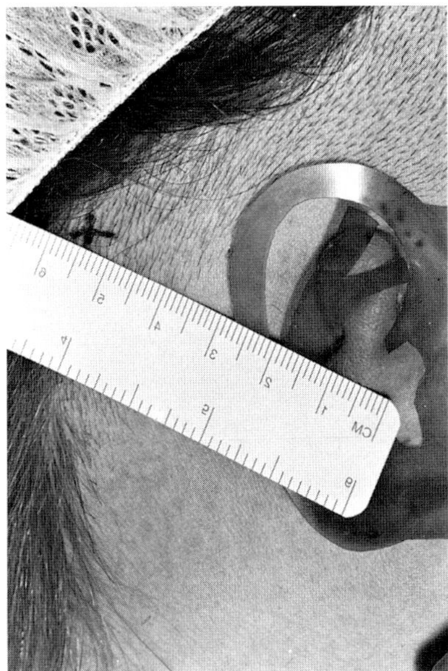

Fig. 6.**45** **Intraoperative planning of the implant site on the right side.**

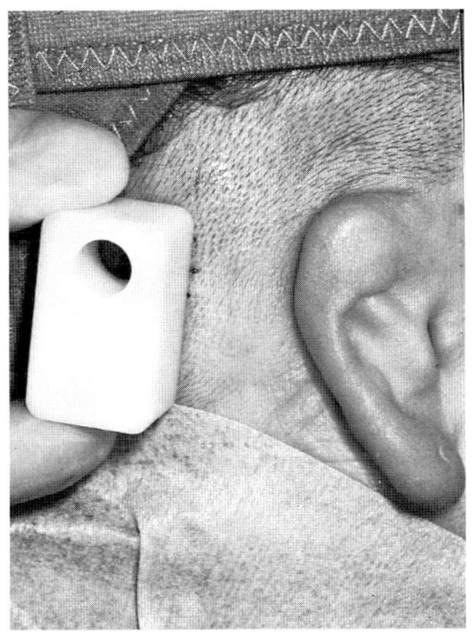

a

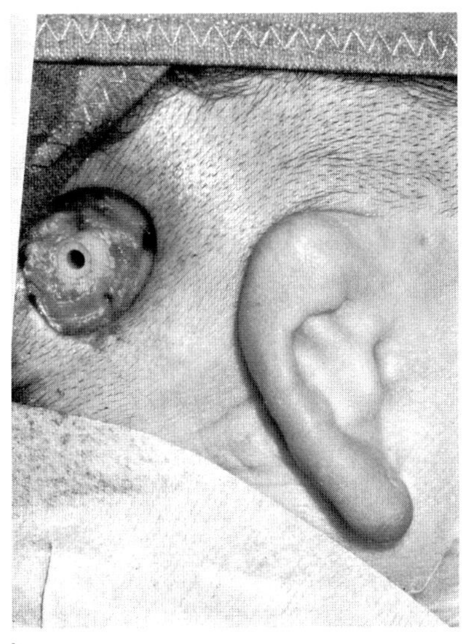

b

Fig. 6.**46** **Position of the bone screws (right ear).**
a Intraoperative planning of the implant site.
b Excised skin and drill hole placed; the periosteum should be preserved.

bone quality. The second operative stage is done after 3 months.

Since 1989 a **one-stage surgical procedure** has been favored (Tjellström 1989; Proops 1996; Mylamus and Cremers 1994) and is currently the method of choice for adults and for those patients who have not undergone radiotherapy.

Entific Medical Systems are the distributors for the parts required for implantation, the instruments for fixture installation and abutment connection, and the drilling equipment. Details of the surgical technique are also available from them. The following description is by Tjellström (1989).

Implantation Site

Careful planning for the location of the implants is necessary, especially in patients with malformations of the external ear. One implant is sufficient for the attachment of one hearing device. For patients with auricular malformations, we create a preoperative template of the external ear, about 65 × 35 mm, from an X-ray film (Fig. 6.**45**). During surgery the template is placed in the position where the reconstructed ear will come to lie (Fig. 6.**45**). The implant can then be placed about 2–3 cm from the external helical margin. The location should be at the 1- o'clock position on the left and at the 10-o'clock position on the right (Figs. 6.**45**, 6.**46**).

This method preserves the intact skin around the auricular remnant for later plastic reconstruction of the ear. The hearing aids come to lie in the hair-bearing region and are thus not noticeable, and the hearing device does not touch the ear on removal, thus avoiding feedback noise (Federspil and Federspil 2000).

Note. **A screw implanted in the region of the skin that will later be required for reconstruction of the external ear results in difficulty for, or even rejection of, any later auricular reconstruction (Fig. 6.47).**

One-stage Approach

After determining the site, the procedure is started by harvesting a 0.4 mm thick split-skin graft with a diameter of 2 cm from the implant site, or a curvilinear skin incision (diameter 2 cm) is placed. The subcutaneous tissue is removed down to the periosteum.

The operation then continues as for the two-stage procedure (see the Operating Manual at www.entific.com). Loading of the implant (Fig. 6.**48 a**) should be avoided for about 3 months to ensure a reliable osseointegration. The hearing device can then be attached (Fig. 6.**48 b**).

- The Brånemark technique requires a low drilling speed, intermittent pressure, and generous irrigation to maintain the temperature in the drilling region at only 34 °C.
- After removal from the packaging, the titanium implants should be held only with titanium instruments, according to the prescribed rules, in order not to reduce surface tension.

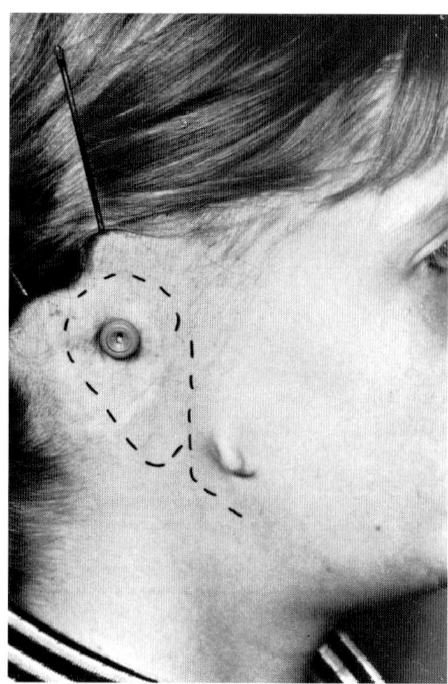

Fig. 6.**47** **Incorrect implant site: appearance after provision with a BAHA; child referred to us for auricular reconstruction.** The split-skin graft area and the implant are located too far anteriorly (see Figs. 6.**45**, 6.**46**). Auricular reconstruction is now only possible by using temporoparietal fascia (see p. 93 and Figs. 6.**48 a**,**b**).

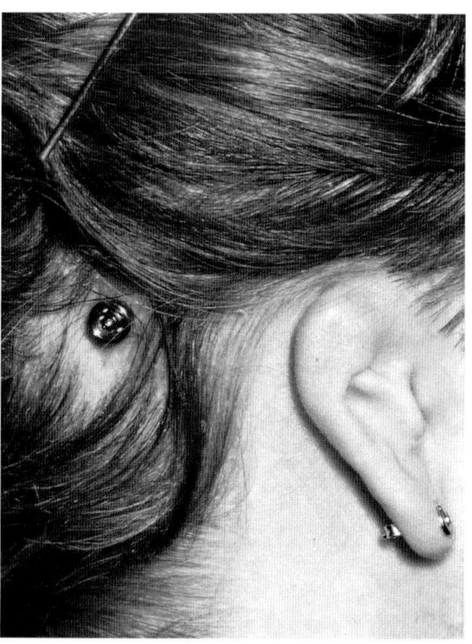

a

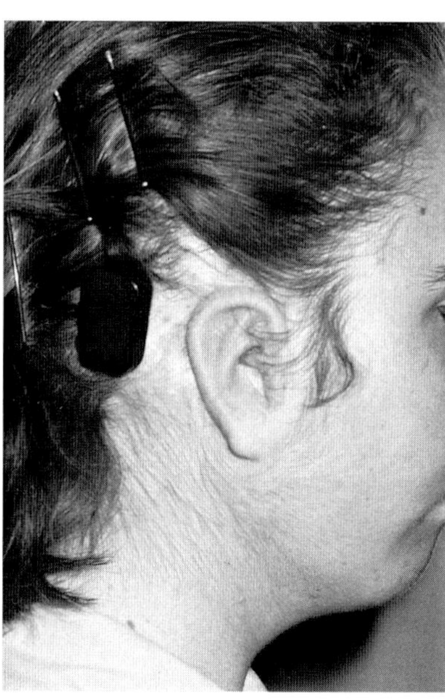

b

Fig. 6.**48** **Correct position of the bone screw and the BAHA in the hair-bearing region (s. Figs. 6.45, 6.46).**
a Abutment in situ (3 months after surgery; before auricular reconstruction).
b Hearing aid in situ, sufficient room behind the reconstructed ear.

- The drill canal should not be too wide because cortical bone cannot bridge a gap of more than 0.35 mm between titanium implant and bone.

Adherence to these guidelines is essential for successful osseointegration.

Complications

Intraoperative Complications

Perforation of the sinus or dura, for example, can occur during surgery. Emissary vessels can be damaged, resulting in considerable hemorrhage. The drill hole should be plugged with bone wax should significant hemorrhage occur, and a new site for the implantation should be used.

Postoperative Complications

There have been reports of paresthesias, which soon disappear; infections of the skin and bone, which may result in bone necrosis; as well as subdural hematomas, meningitis, and skin-graft and implant losses.

Infections call for specific antibiotic therapy. Subdural hematomas and bone necrosis may need surgical intervention. If graft loss occurs, a new graft can be placed, provided the wound conditions allow this. If the wound is infected, the infection will first require treatment. Good spontaneous epithelialization can occasionally occur. After implant loss and provided local conditions allow, a repeat implantation can be undertaken.

Skin Reactions

These are reported by various authors with a frequency of between 3.4 and 33% (Hakansson et al. 1990; Jacobsson et al. 1992; Bonding et al. 1992; Stevenson et al. 1993; Tjellström and Granström 1994; Tjellström and Hakansson 1995; Bejar-Solar et al. 2000).

The severity of the skin reactions and treatment recommendations have been reported by Holgers et al. (1984, 1994).

They distinguish five different types of skin reaction:

- **Type 0:** No evidence of a skin irritation.
  Therapy: Any epithelial debris should be removed.
- **Type 1:** Evidence of slight redness of the skin.
  Therapy: Local treatment with an ointment (e.g., containing povidone–iodine or antibiotic) should be undertaken until the irritation is resolved.
- **Type 2:** Red and slightly moist tissue, but no granulation tissue.
  Therapy: Local treatment with an ointment (e.g., containing povidone–iodine, antibiotic, or a steroid) should be undertaken until the irritation is resolved.
- **Type 3:** Evidence of redness and moist skin with areas of granulation tissue.
  Therapy: Initial attempt at conservative treatment using steroid ointments containing an additional antibiotic. If unsuccessful, surgical debridement of the granulation tissue.
- **Type 4:** Evidence of an extensive skin infection with skin defects.
  Therapy: Removal of the implant may be necessary, plus systemic antibiotics, topical cleansing, and disinfecting ointments.

To avoid skin reactions, careful thinning of the skin around the implant is necessary, as well as an intensive and regular care of the skin by the patient and/or carers.

Implant Loss

Implant loss can result from direct trauma, from poor hygiene resulting in infection, or from failed osseointegration. It is noteworthy that the skin of children that has primarily been thinned out can become thicker again during growth (Powell et al. 1996). The rate of implant loss in adults is reported to be between 3 and 10.7% (Stevenson et al. 1993; Kurt and Federspil 1994; Tjellström and Hakansson 1995; Federspil and Federspil 2000).

Postoperative Care

Two-stage Operation

The ointment-soaked gauze-strip pack is not removed until 1 week after the abutment operation and this region is cleaned with 3% hydrogen peroxide and a povidone–iodine solution. The gauze strip and ointment dressing should then be renewed for a further week. This should be followed by treatment with a steroid ointment until completion of would healing. The hearing device can be attached after the wound has completely healed.

One-stage Operation

The dressing is the same as for the two-stage operation. Loading of the fixture should be avoided until the osseointegration is complete. **Attachment of the hearing devices is only possible after 3 months at the earliest.**

Long-term Care

The skin surrounding the implant must be carefully cleaned every day, using dental floss, a soft (baby) toothbrush, or a water-jet cleaning set (as used for tooth cleaning) for poorly accessible areas. Any soiling within the abutment itself should be removed at least once a week. Occasionally loosening of the abutment can be the cause of skin reactions. The abutment can be retightened with a special screwdriver.

Should skin reactions still occur, further procedures should be considered in consultation with the surgeon. A renewed intensive topical ointment treatment is usually sufficient. Revision surgery is only rarely indicated. Experience with children has shown, however, that a primarily well-thinned-out skin graft thickens again as the child develops (Proops 1996).

Patients/parents must be carefully instructed about this type of care.

Acceptance/Quality of Life

The results of a questionnaire show that general improvements head the list, followed by social and physical improvements. Patients with congenital aural atresia report the most gain. The preconditions for these patients are very favorable, usually resulting in a normal inner-ear function and problems of sound conduction only. Patients with problems of the radical cavity also profit from a BAHA. They report the general and social improvements higher than the physical improvements.

- For accessories available to offer patients more comfort, see **www.entific.com**.
- For treatment plan in patients with auricular dysplasia and congenital aural atresia, see page 265.

Implants for Bone-Anchored Epitheses

If, for any reason, plastic surgical reconstruction is not possible or not desired by the patient, the provision of epitheses fastened to screw implants (see below) can be undertaken for purposes of rehabilitation.

Two to three screws are usually sufficient to guarantee secure fixation of the epitheses. The distance from the external auditory canal should be about 20 mm. The implants should be applied at the 8–11-o'clock position on the right side and 1–4-o'clock on the left. A distance of about 15 mm should be left between the implants to allow for careful cleaning (see pp. 269, 270).

6.6 Auricular Prostheses

6.6.1 The Development of Auricular Prostheses

H. Weerda and I. Greiner

Although, as we have already seen, reconstruction of the external ear was not undertaken until the end of the nineteenth century (see pp. 197 ff), surgeons had already made much earlier attempts to conceal loss of the ear with the aid of prostheses.

Ambroise Paré (1510–1590) had an ear prosthesis constructed using colored papier-mâché (Fig. 6.**49**; Paré 1579, cited in Roberts 1971). In the nineteenth century rubber prostheses colored with oil paint were used, and prostheses were also made of celluloid or enameled metal. Claude Martin (1889, cited in Strauss 1924) is said to have also made ear prostheses from porcelain. Strauss (1924) reports that the porcelain prostheses were painted in such a way that they could not be distinguished from the color of the face. Brandt (1904) reported anchoring a celluloid prosthesis to a wig using hooks and straps.

The gelatin prosthesis was developed by Hennigs and von Salomons in 1918 (cited in Strauss 1924). It was normally

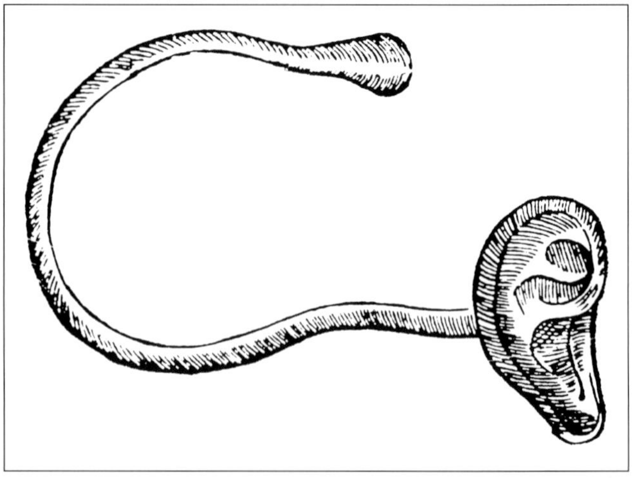

Fig. 6.**49** **Ear prosthesis made of painted papier-mâché and metal clips, dating from 1579 (taken from Roberts 1971).**

glued in place with mastic or gum arabic. In 1924 Strauss developed a special gelatin glue for soft-tissue prostheses.

In the 1950s rigid prostheses were constructed from acrylates, which were probably first introduced as a material for prostheses by Trittermann in 1927. Heinrich Paschke, a prosthesis constructor at the Maxillofacial Clinic in Erlangen, published 1957 a book on the manufacture of epitheses. He primarily describes rigid acrylate for the manufacturing of facial prostheses, followed by polyvinyl chloride with softeners and vinyl chloride acetate (Flexiderm) for soft prostheses. He describes the possibility of retention within the auditory canal and the gluing of the relatively soft, flexible epitheses. Furthermore, Roberts (1971) recommends the spectacle frame as a retention element and also describes the old spring clip as recommended by Paré.

In the 1960s the senior author worked as Paschke's pupil in his department, where he had a special interest in the production of epitheses and the possibilities of the retention of external ears (Weerda 1972; Fig. 6.**50 a–d**). All the attachments used in those days involved straps (Ombredanne 1956, cited in Weerda 1972). They had the disadvantage that the epitheses became loose after some time and, despite additional gluing, they no longer remained securely in place. The relatively heavy weight also contributed to our inability to offer satisfactory solutions for the fixation of auricular epitheses. It was not until the development of bone-anchored fixtures (Fig. 6.**51 a–c**) and the further development of a variety of silicone rubber epitheses (see p. 270) in various degrees of hardness that we attained the current position of manufacturing well-fitting and cosmetically faultless epitheses.

It is essential for the plastic surgeon to know that a prosthesis cannot dispel the feeling of being deformed. We therefore reject the idea of providing children with a defect prosthesis, and prefer surgical solutions with good results to allow them to forget that a malformation ever existed (see pp. 209, 210, 213–216, 259).

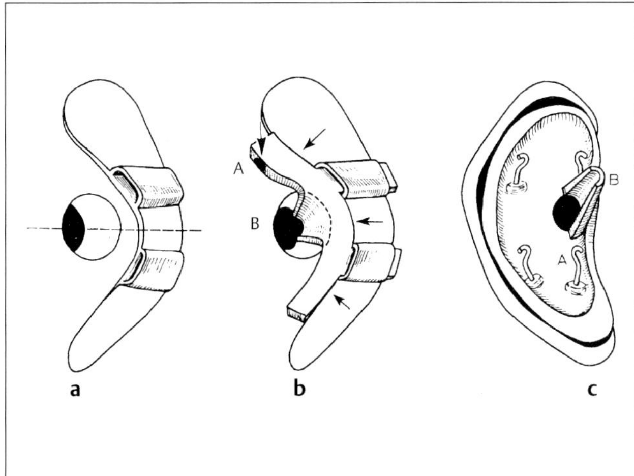

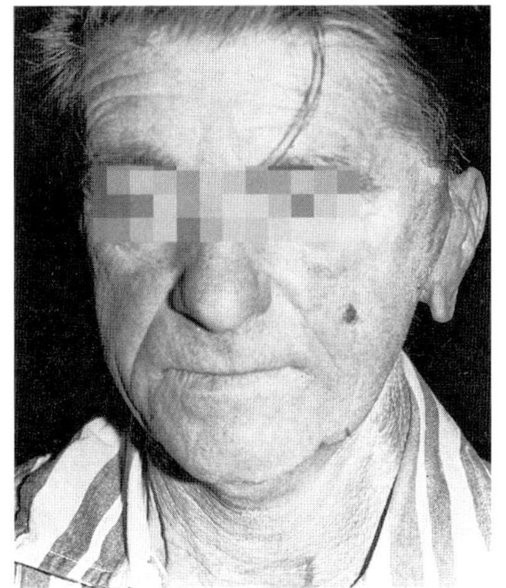

Fig. 6.**50 a–d** **An acrylate epithesis constructed by the senior author in 1970 with plastic retention elements fixed into skin loops (as described in Weerda 1972).**

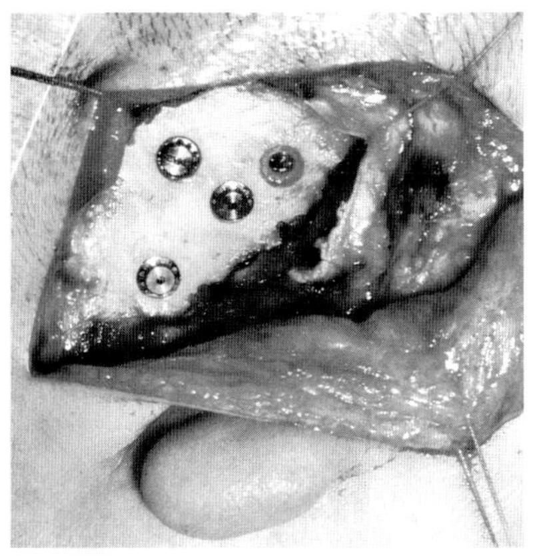

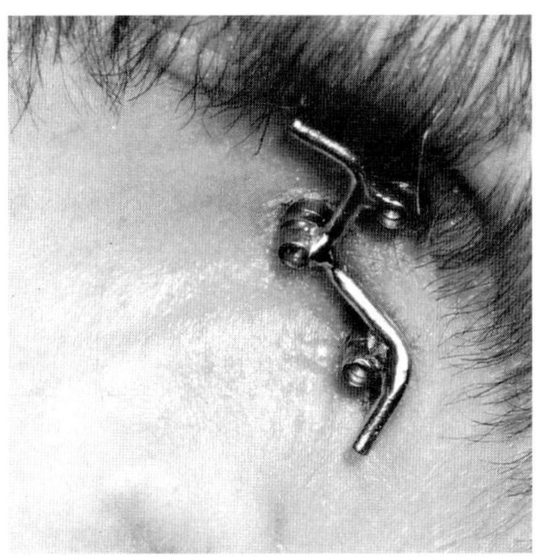

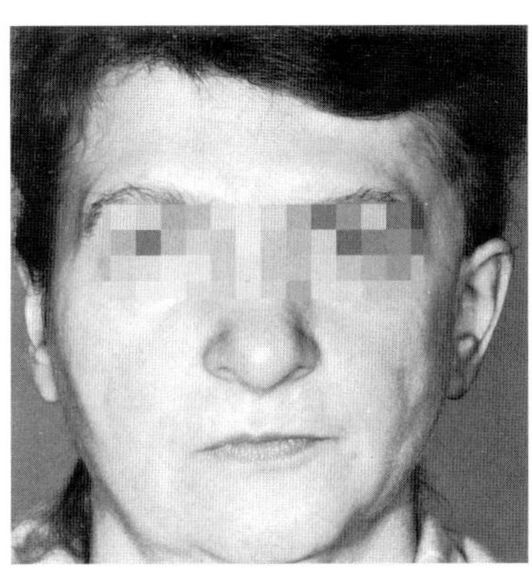

Fig. 6.**51** **Bone-anchored retention elements according to Brånemark, as used in our unit.**
a Insertion of the anchors in the bone.
b The bridging system as used in earlier times (see Fig. 6.**52 a**), shown here mounted.
c Silicone rubber prosthesis (left).

6.6.2 Provision of Prostheses for Defects of the Auricle

I. Greiner and H. Weerda

Introduction

If surgical reconstruction is not desired or not possible, we suggest the provision of epitheses for facial defects. These are reproductions of the facial structures using a suitable foreign material to correct the defect (also referred to as epiprostheses or extra-oral defect prostheses).

Rehabilitation with epitheses can be used either as an alternative to plastic surgical reconstruction, or in combination with it.

Aims

The provision of an epithesis serves primarily to reconstruct the natural form of the patient's face. This brings with it a new feeling of self-esteem, reintegration into society, and at the same time an easing of the mental and emotional repercussions of the defect. Furthermore, an ear epithesis can also have functional advantages: for example it can improve directional hearing or allow the wearing of a hearing aid or spectacles.

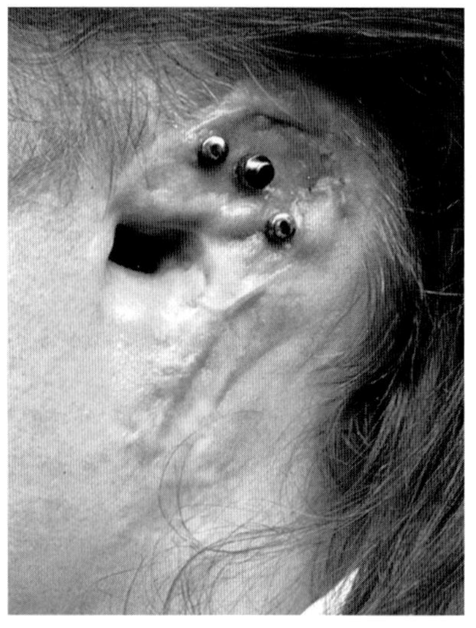

a

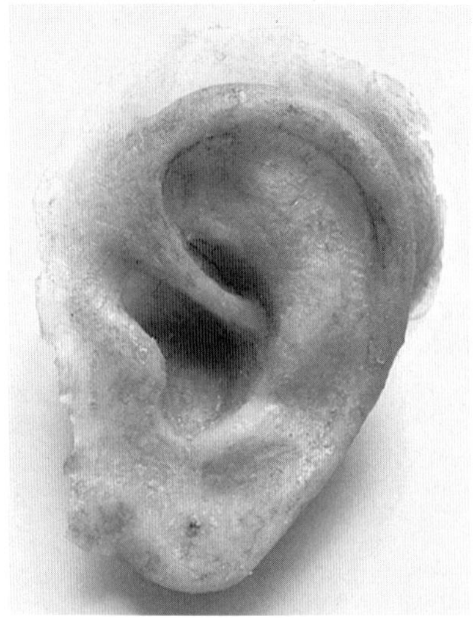

b

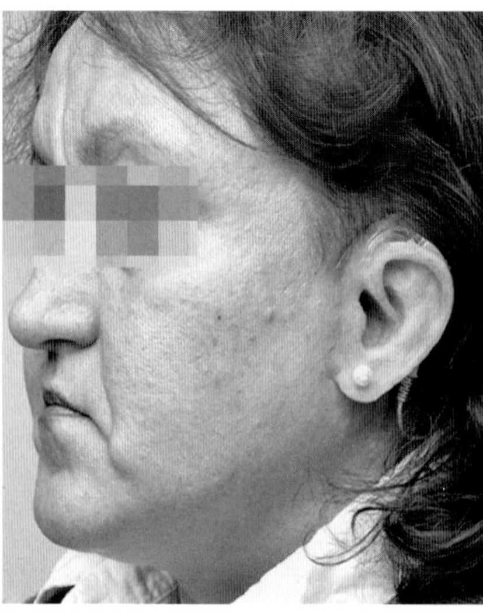

c

Fig. 6.**52** **Osseointegrated retention system and silicone rubber epithesis with hearing aid.**

a Retention elements.
b Silicone rubber epithesis.
c Epithesis with integrated hearing tube.

Advantages and Disadvantages of Modern Epitheses

The main advantage of an epithesis is quick and less troublesome coverage of facial defects. In addition, good esthetic results can be achieved with epitheses, especially with total defects. The further development of silicone has made a significant contribution to this. Silicone is a soft and pliable material, unlike traditional materials (acrylates). It is also possible to produce silicone in various degrees of hardness suitable for individual details of the epithesis. For example, soft and very thinly tapering margins allow the epithesis to lie flush with the skin (see Fig. 6.**52 c**).

One disadvantage is the aging of the material, especially if environmental effects are involved, e. g., air pollution, tobacco smoke, or lack of hygiene. Also, the repairability of silicone epitheses is limited.

Anchorage of Epitheses

Bone anchorage with titanium implants (see Figs. 6.**48**, 6.**51**) and magnetic attachments have proved to be the optimal methods of fixation. For this purpose the surgeon inserts three implants in a semicircle extending from above to behind the auditory canal (Fig. 6.**52 a**). This arrangement guarantees a snug fit of the epithesis to the ear. When using the magnetic system, the upper and lower implants are each provided with a round magnet, which protrudes about 0.5–1.5 mm above the skin. The central implant is fitted with a telescopic magnet which protrudes a further 4 mm. This prevents the epithesis from falling off during uncontrolled movements, while still allowing the epithesis itself to move within a region of about 3 mm.

Regular and careful hygiene is essential for maintaining the quality of the epithesis and for keeping the tissue healthy. The magnetic system is more easily cleaned.

Temporary Provision of an Epithesis

The provision of an epithesis secured with a special skin-friendly adhesive provides a temporary solution for children. The epithesis should be cleaned and refitted on a daily basis.

The temporary provision of an interim prosthesis is also an option immediately after wound healing following a surgical procedure. It can also provide a lasting solution for cases where fitting an implant or performing plastic surgical reconstruction is not possible.

Manufacture of Epitheses

A detailed discussion between the constructor of the epithesis, the doctor, and the patient forms part of the preliminary stages of manufacturing an epithesis.

Once any question of costs has been clarified with the funder, the epithesis is then produced in the course of several sessions. First, an imprint is made of the defect area with the purpose of later creating a positive mold of the face, including the defect area. A wax model of the epithesis is then formed by hand on this plaster face. After this, a plaster form is made from several components into which the implants are inserted for later anchorage. Next, the silicone, which is tinted in the patient's presence and matched to the color of his or her skin, is introduced into this mold in several layers. The mold is filled very carefully to avoid errors and to prevent the formation of air bubbles. Once the silicone has set, the ear is removed from the mold (deflasked) and the seams are removed from the form. The epithesis can then be tried on the patient and its correct fit verified.

At a second stage, the fine color shades of the skin surface are reproduced on the silicone model. Hairlines, beard, eyebrows, and lashes are now also stitched onto the silicone so that an epithesis evolves which is not recognizable as such to the observer. The transition from epithesis to skin (Fig. 6.**52 b**) should be extremely thin (paper thin), so that the reverse, which is covered with a layer of petroleum jelly, comes to lie on the surface of the skin without revealing the transition line (see Fig. 6.**51**).

After extensive instruction in the handling and care of the epithesis, the patient is thus provided for a period of 1–2 years, depending on any changes to the underlying tissue and any signs of wear of the epithesis (Fig. 6.**52 c**).

6.7 Maxillofacial Management of Hemifacial Microsomia

A. Hasse

Therapy of this complex facial malformation is always an interdisciplinary task.

6.7.1 Clinical Findings

Although the soft-tissue anomaly associated with hemifacial microsomia is usually obvious immediately after birth, especially in the region of the external ear, the skeletal malformation is only recognizable when markedly developed (Fig. 6.**53 a–d**). The shortened mandibular ramus and the malposition of the mentum dominate the external aspect. Nevertheless, the skull asymmetry is always complex, and can be traced back dorsally as far as the anterior and middle cranial fossae. Apart from the mandible, asymmetries of the malar prominence, orbital ring, and maxilla give the impression of a lopsided face. The unilateral hypoplastic muscles of mastication—especially the temporal and masseter muscles—underline this.

The clinically recognizable skeletal changes can be confirmed by radiology (Fig. 6.**54**).

Timely treatment in adolescence can reduce or prevent consecutive malformations of the neighboring structures which are not primarily damaged (Kaban et al. 1988; Murray et al. 1984).

6.7.2 Age for Treatment

The ideal time for treatment is during and after the second dentition period (Table 6.**3**; Moore et al. 1994). Whereas distraction treatment is most appropriate in childhood, traditional split osteotomies and transplantations are performed at the end of the growth phase. The high osteogenetic potency in infancy (Hollinger 1993 a, b; Reid et al. 1981), the avoidance of secondary growth deficits of adjacent structures, and the prevention of mental and emotional problems mitigate in favor of early surgical treatment (Murray et al. 1984).

Treatment delayed until the child is more mature (about 7–9 years of age), i. e., after the start of the second dentition, has the following advantages:

- The bone is more strongly mineralized and allows stable bone fixation.
- Some of the permanent teeth have already appeared in the oral cavity and are thus, on the one hand, less endangered from surgery than are the developing tooth buds in the depths of the mandible and, on the other hand, amenable for simultaneous orthodontic treatment.
- The degree of any necessary overcorrection can be better assessed, thanks to the advanced stage of development of the child, thus reducing the likelihood of further corrective surgery.
- The expected growth spurt is still sufficient for spontaneous correction of the adjacent structures.
- The patient's compliance is better.

For these, reasons, the author prefers to delay distraction treatment until the child is 7–9 years of ages.

6.7.3 Forms of Treatment

Transplantation

Surgery is currently the only possible option for replacing absent tissue.

Once correction of the mandible is complete, the **malar bone, orbital ring,** and **maxilla** are usually monitored with regard to their spontaneous development. Should they maintain a deficit requiring treatment by the end of the growth phase, they may be emphasized as required by using free grafts or augmentation.

Depending on the form required, the bone is harvested as a corticocancellous graft from the ribs, skull, or iliac crest and shaped with a scalpel and burr.

Determining the volume of augmentation is very important when reconstructing the midfacial region. Symmetry of

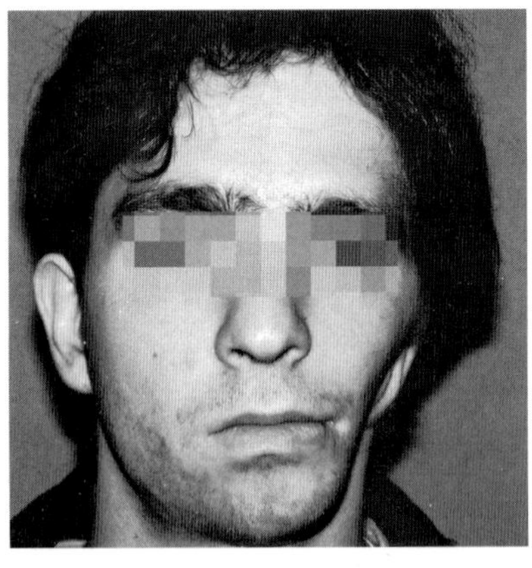

a

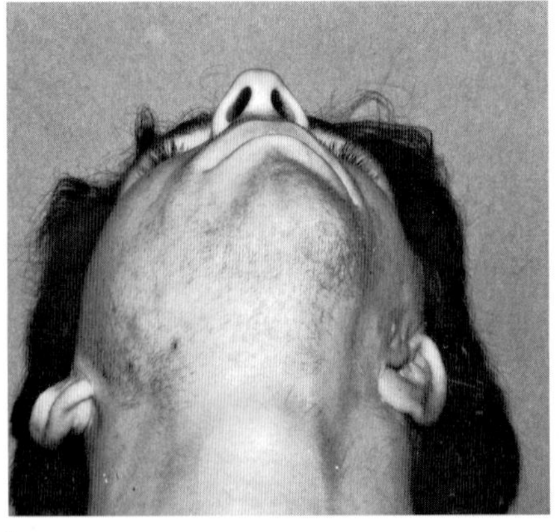

b

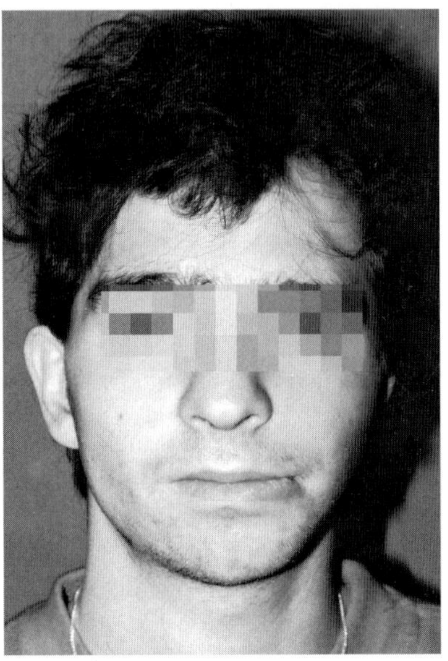

c

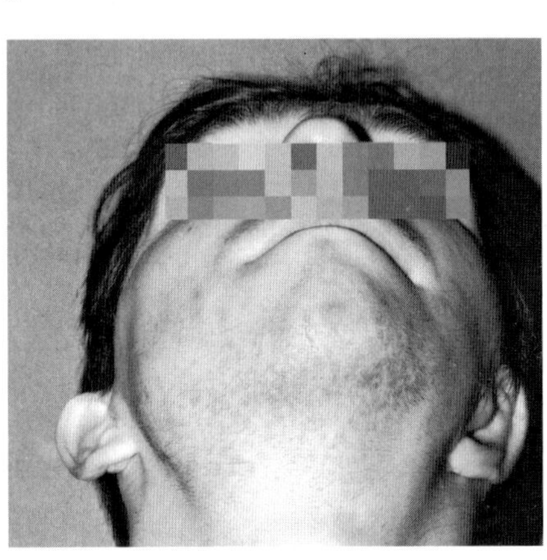

d

Fig. 6.**53 a–d** **Nineteen year-old youth with left hemifacial microsomia and grade III microtia before treatment (a, b) and after distraction treatment with a submucosal, unilateral distractor (c, d, s. Fig. 6.56).**
The position of the tip of the chin and the soft-tissue situation clearly improved, mild asymmetry of the corners of the mouth (congenital defect of 7 th cranial nerve) left unchanged; appearance after auricular reconstruction in the presence of grade III microtia at the ENT Clinic of the University of Lübeck, Germany.

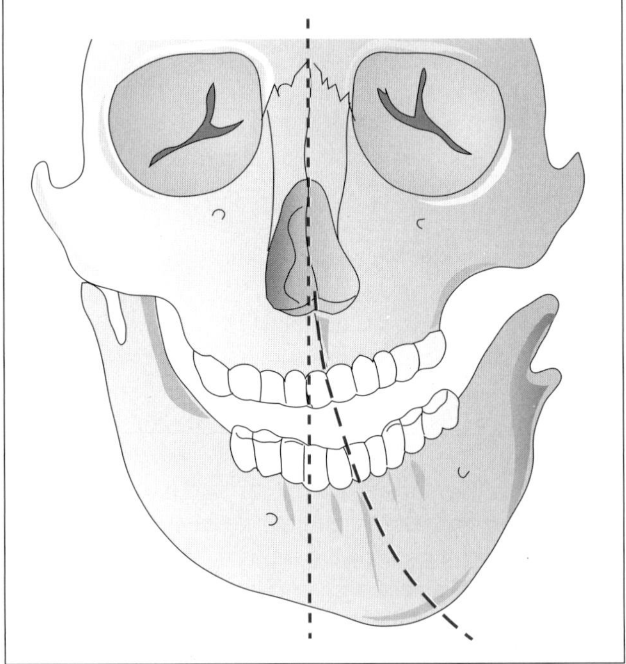

Fig. 6.**54** **Schematic presentation of the skeletal malformation (s. Fig. 6.53 a, b).**
Malformed, hypoplastic left temporomandibular joint head; mandibular ramus concave; diversion of the midline increases caudally; level of the alveolar processes lower on the left than on the right (including the maxilla).

Table 6.**3** Serial plan for the maxillofacial treatment of hemifacial microsomia

Type of treatment	Treatment age	Anatomical region	Duration	Indication
Distraction (extraoral)	1 year	Mandible	1 mm/day + consolidation time (~ 3 weeks)	Mandibular malformation obstructing airways
	3–4 years	Mandible	1 mm/day + consolidation time (~ 4 weeks)	Severe mandibular hypoplasia
Distraction (intraoral) + orthodontic treatment	7–9 years	Mandible	1 mm/day + consolidation time (~ 6 weeks)	Moderate to mild mandibular hypoplasia
Sagittal split osteotomy	> 17 years	Mandible	~ 2 weeks	1. Ramus shortening <10 % 2. Correction for reduced growth after distraction 3. Dysgnathias (with or without 1 and 2)
		Maxilla	~ 2 weeks	1. Inadequate spontaneous correction during growth after distraction 2. After maxillary distraction treatment of adults
Transplantation	5–8 years	Mandible	~ 2 weeks	Extreme hypo- and aplasia of the head of the temporomandibular joint or the mandibular ramus
	> 17 years	Maxilla	~ 2 weeks	For stabilization after sagittal split osteotomy with > 4 mm osteotomy gap
		Malar bone	~ 2 weeks	Partial or complete agenesis of the malar bone or malar arch
Augmentation	> 17 years	Malar bone, orbital ring	~ 2 weeks	Hypoplasic malar bone/orbital ring
Genioplasty	> 16 years	Chin	1 week	1. Malformation with dorsal or oblique chin position 2. Isolated progenia 3. As auxiliary measure for dysgnathias

the two halves of the face should not be forced at all costs by overcorrection, unlike with symmetry of the mandible. When malformation causes the eyeball to adapt a more dorsal and caudal position, this may lend the face a "dark" look and emphasize the asymmetry of the eye position even more. A restriction of the field of vision should also be avoided, especially in a lateral and caudal direction.

The author does not use alloplastic materials for augmentation.

Sagittal Split Osteotomies/Sandwich Plasties

A long-standing and proven method in plastic surgery is the redistribution of local tissue with the purpose of gaining length at the expense of width. Traditional mandibular osteotomy procedures can be traced back to the principles of extremity lengthening as performed in orthopedic surgery (Taylor 1916). After performing medial and lateral corticotomies on a bone at different levels, it is possible to split the intervening segment in a sagittal direction along its longitudinal axis. This procedure can help to balance out the loss of bone length found in hemifacial microsomia with a unilateral hypoplastic mandible.

In the author's experience, traditional mandibular osteotomies are indicated as supplementary procedures after a preparatory distraction, especially when treating adults. Although surgically induced retardation of growth is not necessarily expected when correctional osteotomies are performed before completion of growth, leaving surgery until the age of 16 or over has generally gained acceptance.

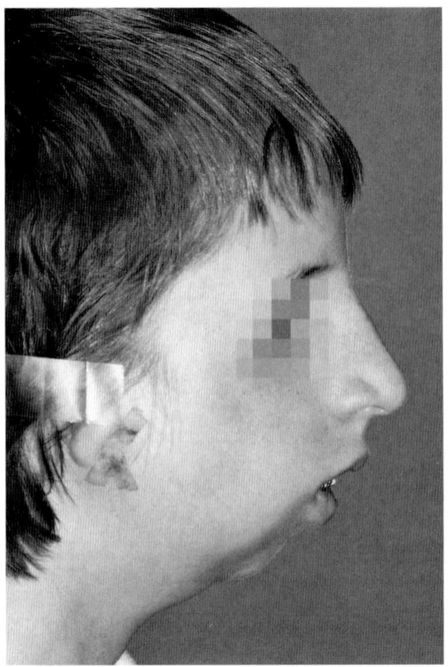

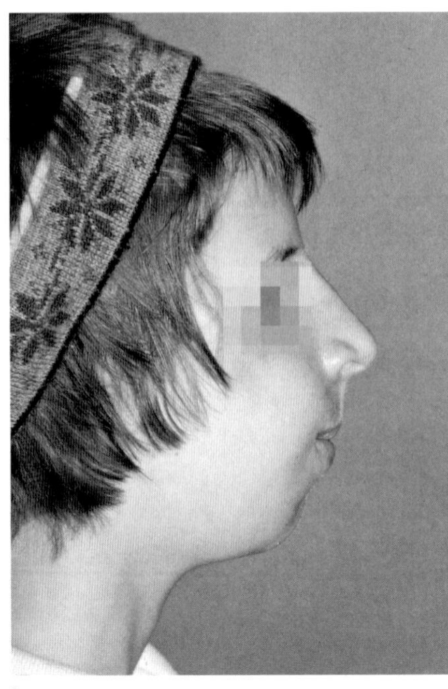

a b

Fig. 6.**55 a, b** **Craniofacial malformation (Treacher Collins syndrome).**
a Before commencement of the distraction treatment.
b After right-sided maxillary distraction, bimaxillary correctional osteotomy, malar augmentation, and genioplasty.

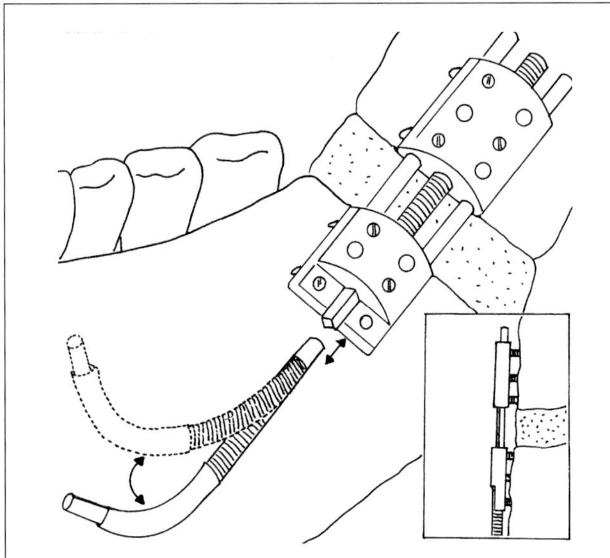

Fig. 6.**56** **Intraoral unidirectional distractor (as described by Hasse).**
The device is screwed directly onto the bone; the operating screw exits through the gums, and is removable on completion of distraction.

Genioplasty

Correctional osteotomy of the chin is mentioned here for the reason that, when performed properly, it is the simplest operation to improve the profile of the facial skull and also carries the lowest risk while providing the most stable results (Fig. 6.**55 a, b**).

Distraction Osteogenesis

Treatment Principle

The principle of distraction osteogenesis is based on the body's own ability to cause a fracture to heal. This procedure is derived from orthopedic surgery and traumatology and was introduced clinically after World War II by G. A. Ilizarov, becoming a routine method of lengthening tubular bones (Ilizarov 1971, 1989 a, b; Paley et al. 1991).

In 1992, McCarthy published the first clinical use of distraction osteogenesis for the mandible (McCarthy et al. 1992), and since then distraction has become the method of choice in the treatment of the hypoplastic mandible.

The great variety of distraction systems now available can be divided into devices for extra- and intra-oral fixation. The technical perfection of the intraoral devices has reduced the number of indications for **extra-oral distractor devices,** which function like an adjustable external fixator, to a small number of cases of very young patients with an extremely small bone stock.

An aesthetically advantageous result with fewer risks and little harm can be achieved by a two-dimensional correction with a unidirectional **intra-oral device** (Fig. 6.**56**), suitably aligned obliquely and with only one osteotomy.

Any form of distraction therapy can be divided into four clinical phases:

- Postoperative wound healing
- Distraction phase
- Consolidation phase
- Functional loading

For mandibular distraction, the mandible is exposed via an intra-oral approach, osteotomized, and then stabilized by the application of a distractor. It is not the osteotomy line, but rather the alignment of the distractor, which determines to what extent a ventral movement, in addition to a vertical elongation, is achieved. Precise preoperative planning is essential. The removal of sutures a week later completes the first phase. Distraction is initiated 5–7 days after surgery. The time as well as the distance to be distracted each day depends on the age of the patient. Optimal ossification is achieved when the daily distraction gap is distributed at regular intervals over as many distraction stages as possible (Ilizarov 1989 a, b), e. g., **0.3 mm three times a day** for 7–10 year olds. The duration of the second stage depends on the bone length to be achieved. After the calculated length of extension is obtained, a follow-up radiograph is performed. The distraction phase is completed once the actual length of distraction achieved corresponds to the calculated goal.

In modern distractors, the shaft for operating the distractor (connection with the milieu of the oral cavity, risk of infection) can be removed in this phase (see Fig. 6.**56**).

The subsequent functional loading of the distracted area causes the region to become reorganized, and it is macroscopically no longer different from the adjacent bone. Once the required bony consolidation has been achieved (approximately 6–10 weeks after the last distraction), the distractor can be removed. During the final phase, a **simultaneous functional orthodontic treatment** should be initiated to direct the adjustment of the regenerating alveolar process of the maxilla and to help the adaptation of the jaw muscles to the new situation.

Distraction treatment is also performed in the midfacial region. Distractor devices allow advancement of the malar bone and the maxilla as well as the entire midface complex by the formation of new bone after osteotomy (Klein 1998; Figueroa et al. 1999).

Disadvantages of distraction treatment as compared with bone grafting and traditional osteotomy include the longer duration of treatment and its reliance on the compliance of the patient and/or the parents. Its specific advantage is its affinity to physiological growth (Ilizarov 1989 a, b), which allows the adjacent tissue (muscles, nerves, skin, mucous membranes) the necessary time for simultaneous development. Fewer surgical risks and less traumatization are reasons for the current increasing use of this procedure. Hospitalization is shorter, and the patients are at work or school throughout the distraction period.

Course of Treatment

The most favorable age for treatment is between 7 and 9 years of age. Hospital stays are arranged in the school holidays whenever possible.

During the first hospital stay, a mandibular distractor is applied to the side of the malformation under general anesthetic. Daily distraction of 1 mm in three steps is initiated at a rate of 0.5–0.75 mm per day on the 5th postoperative day in children and 2 days later in adults. The patients can be discharged about 5 days after the operation, once the parents have mastered the use of the distractor device. During the consolidation phase, the distractor remains in place for about 10 weeks and can be removed during other operations, for example those on the ear. Any concomitant orthodontic treatment may already commence during the consolidation phase.

6.8 Methods of Epilation

M. B. Wimmershoff and M. Landthaler

(see also pp. 218, 220, 221)

Over time, a large number of laser and light systems have been developed for removing hair, in addition to conventional methods of hair removal, such as waxing, shaving, electroepilation, and chemical depilation. Wax epilation involves removing mainly the terminal hairs by applying warm wax and removing it with a sudden movement. This is a painful and temporary method which can result in inflammation and scars (Mimouni-Bloch et al. 1997).

6.8.1 Electroepilation

(see Fig. 5.**181 b**; p. 221)

A distinction is made between **electrolysis**, which entails the destruction of tissue by sodium hydroxide formed in a chemical reaction from sodium chloride and water at low electric currents, and **thermolysis**, which involves the destruction of the hairs by short, high-frequency electric currents and is clearly faster to perform. The combination of both procedures has also been successfully used (Olsen 1999).

6.8.2 Chemical Depilators

Chemical depilators (e. g., thioglycolate) work by splitting the disulfide bonds between the cysteine molecules in the hair shaft. After allowing the required time for the preparations to take effect on the skin, the hairs can be washed off without any problem. This can, however, result in skin irritations and allergic contact eczema (Kunte and Wolff 2001).

A further new procedure for treating hypertrichosis is medicinal therapy using eflornithine (DL-α-difluoromethyl ornithine; Kunte and Wolff 2001). This involves the inhibition of ornithine decarboxylase, which appears to be of importance for hair growth. A study was conducted to test the

Table 6.4 Methods of laser and light treatment for epilation

Method	Wave length (nm)	Impulse duration (ms)	Spot size (mm)
Ruby laser	694	0.5–5.0	2–10
Alexandrite laser	755	2–40	5–15
Diode laser	800	5–30	9 × 9
Nd:YAG laser	1064	0.01–4	4–7
Photoderm	515–1200	0.5–25	8 × 15, 8 × 35
Epilight	590–1200	2.5–7.0	8 × 35, 10 × 45

efficacy of 11.5% eflornithine cream. After 6 months, over 70% of the patients treated demonstrated a reduction in the amount of hairs. Acne-like skin reactions, pseudofolliculitis barbae (razor bumps), and burning and tingling sensations were reported as side effects. The effect is only temporary, so the treatment is lifelong or must be used in combination with laser or light systems.

6.8.3 Light-based Epilation

Light-based methods using lasers and pulsed light have recently enjoyed increasing and successful use for the removal of cosmetically troublesome hairs. These laser and light systems (Table 6.4; Olsen 1999; Raulin and Greve 2000), the effectiveness of which is based on the principle of selective photothermolysis, include:

- Long-pulsed ruby laser (694 nm)
- Long-pulsed alexandrite laser (755 nm)
- Nd:YAG laser (1064 nm)
- Diode laser (800 nm)
- High-energy pulsed light (515–1200 nm)

Mode of Action

Selective photothermolysis refers to the selective destruction of a targeted structure by adjusting the pulse time according to the thermal relaxation time (TRT) and adjusting the wave length according to its absorption maximum (Dierickx 1998). The ideal laser impulse length should lie between the thermal relaxation time of the epidermis (3–10 ms) and the TRT of the hair follicle (40–100 ms for terminal hair follicles with a diameter between 200 and 300 µm) (Dierickx 1998).

The melanin in the hair shaft of the hair follicle represents one of these target structures. Therefore, wave lengths between 700 and 1000 nm would appear to be ideal, since they are well absorbed by melanin. Follicle size and follicle depth vary, depending on the various regions of the body, which would imply the necessity of different laser-impulse lengths. A further difficulty in finding the ideal laser parameters is due to the fact that hair growth is a cyclic, multifactorial process, which has not yet been fully explained.

The dermal papilla and the bulb of the hair follicle at the insertion of the erector muscle are regarded as further target structures, given that this is where the stem cells are assumed to lie (Kunte and Wolff 2001). Destruction of these stem cells could result in permanent hair epilation. Here melanin functions as the target to absorb the light for the thermal destruction of the hair follicle. This could explain the better results after epilation of dark-haired patients in comparison with fair or gray-haired patients (Williams et al. 1998).

Adverse Reactions

Before initiating any epilation treatment, it is obligatory to obtain detailed informed consent from the patient, covering possible side-effects such as erythema, swelling, perifollicular purpura, eczema, the formation of blisters and crusts, disturbances of pigmentation, and scarring, as well as the possibility of no therapeutic success and the conduct of a trial treatment. Transient adverse reactions such as perifollicular edema, the formation of blisters and crusts, and hypo- and hyperpigmentation are not rare, and correlate directly with skin type and amount of sun exposure during the various seasons of the year (Nanni and Alster 1999). This type of side effect is thus encountered more frequently in darker skin types. Rare side effects such as small areas of atrophic scar formation (Nanni and Alster 1999), the triggering of an isomorphic irritating effect (Köbner phenomenon) in lichen planus after ruby laser treatment (Wimmershoff et al. 2000), and the development of urticaria vasculitis after treatment with a diode laser (Moreno-Arias et al. 2000) have also been reported in the literature. The use of appropriate cooling systems, e. g., transparent cooling gels or cold sapphire lenses, can noticeably reduce side effects. Depending on the duration of the growth cycle as a function of the region of the body, **repeating treatment at intervals of a few weeks is recommended.**

Treatment Results

Comparative results after treatment with long-pulsed ruby laser, long-pulsed alexandrite laser, the Nd:YAG laser, diode laser, and high-energy flash lamp with clearance rates of 20–75% after 1–6 months are reported in the literature (Olsen 1999).

The most detailed reports are on the use and efficacy of the ruby laser (Dierickx et al. 1998, Williams et al. 1998, Olsen 1999, Wimmershoff et al. 2000).

In a prospective study, Lorenz et al. (2002) report a reduction of hairs by more than 50% in a total of 44.9% of the volunteers 4 weeks after one treatment session with the Nd:YAG laser. After five treatment sessions, there was a **reduction of hair growth by 71.5%**. One year after completion of the treatment, there was still a reduction of the hairs by more than 50% in 40% of the volunteers.

Bäumler et al. (2003) found proof of the effect of different **spot sizes** on the efficacy of laser epilation in their work with the diode laser. They compared spot sizes of 8, 12, and 14 mm. One month after laser treatment, regrowth of hair was 23% (8 mm), 12% (12 mm), and 13% (14 mm). Three months after treatment, regrowth was found to be 67% (8 mm), 54% (12 mm), and 55% (14 mm). The depth of the dermal papilla of the developing hair follicle varies between 1 and 4.7 mm, depending on the size of the body region (Grossman et al. 1996). This confirmed improved efficacy after use of larger spot sizes because of the improved depth penetration.

6.8.4 Summary

In summary, a number of different therapies are currently available for the treatment of hypertrichosis. Short-term, but inexpensive, procedures include mechanical treatments such as wax epilation, shaving, and chemical epilation. Photoepilation is another innovative, quick, comfortable, nonpermanent method of hair removal with a low incidence of side-effects. Comparative studies with different types of laser show similarly good results with few side effects. Laser and light systems, however, should be generally used only by experienced doctors and after providing the patient with detailed information concerning potential side effects.

6.9 Tissue Engineering of Human Cartilage

A. Haisch

6.9.1 Introduction

In 1991, Vacanti at the Massachusetts Institute of Technology in Boston, USA, was the first to report the seeding of chondrocytes on a polymer fleece to provide a tissue scaffold for new cartilage formation.

6.9.2 Cartilage Morphology

Cartilage is an avascular, bradytrophic tissue comprising chondrocytes and an extracellular matrix, collagen, proteoglycans, and water. In nonarticulating regions, cartilage is enveloped by a thin, resistant layer of chondrogenic precursor cells and collagen fibers, the so-called **perichondrium**. The ability of cartilage to regenerate is low and originates from the perichondrium and the subchondral bone tissue. As dry substance, the intercellular substance of the basic cartilage framework contains approximately equal parts (about 40% each) of collagen fibers and chondroitin sulfate proteoglycan, and about 10% water-insoluble protein. Minerals account for almost 10% of the ground substance. A distinction is made between three different types of cartilage, depending on the composition and alignment of the collagen fibers: **hyaline cartilage**, **elastic cartilage**, and **fibrous cartilage**. Elastic cartilage is found in the auricular skeleton. Hyaline cartilage is easily cut and resilient to pressure.

6.9.3 Carrier Material

There are basically two groups of carrier materials, differently structured. Apart from porous, cross-linked fibrous structures, there are gel-like or even fluid carrier substances. In the group of fiber-like bioabsorbable materials, polymer fleece carrier materials made of polylactide and/or polyglycolide as well as hardened collagen have proved successful. These are similar in nature to the bioabsorbable suture materials that have been used for years, or collagen fleece for haemostasis (Haisch et al. 1966). In the other group, fluid and gel-like bioabsorbable materials such as hyaluronic acid, collagen, and fibrin, are competing for the favor of bioscientists. The advantages of both groups, however, can only be exploited for tissue engineering by the combination of gel-like and fibrous carrier materials, thus achieving both a homogenous three-dimensional cell distribution and sufficient ability to maintain its shape.

6.9.4 Review and Prospectives

"Tissue engineering" is a biotechnical discipline which opens the gate to new approaches and routes on the road to the optimal surgical care of patients with problems ranging from partial auricular defects to auricular dysplasia. Even today, grafts can be produced and formed in animal models from a small cartilage biopsy which are adapted to anatomical specifications and preformed in vitro, comprising chondrocytes and biocompatible and bioabsorbable carrier substances (Fig. 6.**57**). Provided the grafts are allowed to differentiate undisturbed, their biomechanical properties, which

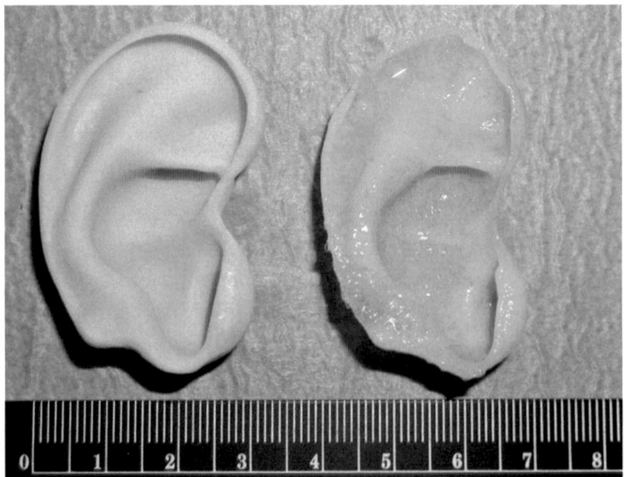

Fig. 6.57 **Comparison between a prototype taken from a mold of the patient's ear (left) and the human cartilage tissue preformed in vitro by tissue engineering (chondrocytes, polymer fleece, and fibrin gel).**

have been preformed in vitro, are comparable within 12 weeks to those biomechanical properties of human nasal septum cartilage. **Clinical use, however, remains ruled out for the present** until our current knowledge regarding immunological mechanisms of wound healing and their specific effect following subcutaneous implantation is improved. Despite strictly autologous transplantation using biocompatible and bioabsorbable carrier materials, damage to the tissue by surgery can trigger these mechanisms to interfere with graft differentiation in the organism, with the subsequent loss of form and function.

6.10 Psychosocial Aspects of Severe Microtia

R. Siegert

6.10.1 Introduction

The attractiveness of an esthetic body is a biological phenomenon found in every human culture. Even in the animal kingdom, the outward appearance represents for many species a criterion for partner selection. Darwin's theory of the survival of the fittest is thus given an additional dimension—the superiority of the attractive. This phenomenon has contributed to the evolutionary development of the blaze of color and wealth of form found in the animal kingdom, the teleological significance of which lies not in a survival advantage for the individual, but in the reproductive advantage which is enjoyed by the "conspicuous" or "impressive" individuals of a particular species.

In a large-scale study involving 376 male and 376 female 18-year-old first-year college students, Walster et al. (1966) examined the criteria of their dating behavior (i. e., their partner selection in the broadest sense). The only parameter that was of any significance for the "success" of the randomized assignment of a partner was that person's physical attractiveness.

The perception of physical attractiveness, the stereotyping of personality traits, and their effect on the selection of friendships start to develop between the ages of 3 and 6 years and correspond in their essential features to those of adults (Dion 1973, 1974; Lerner and Gellert 1969). It is also during this same age range that children with deformities begin to realize their outward divergence from the norm, regardless of any possible functional impairment (Straith and De Kleine 1938).

Malformations of the head represent an aesthetic impairment that is difficult to conceal. This may produce a significant psychosocial burden to children and adolescents during the development of their personalities.

Grades II and III microtia are severe forms of auricular dysplasia. Being malformations of the first two branchial arches, they are frequently combined to varying degrees with alterations of the lateral regions of the face and the middle ear (Siegert, Weerda, and Remmert 1994 c, s. pp. 271 ff, Figs. 6.**53 a, b**). In 5–10% of cases, microtia is part of a syndrome, such as for example the Goldenhar, Franceschetti, or Crouzon syndromes, or the consequence of an embryopathy, such as that resulting from measles or the thalidomide catastrophe of the 1960s (Mastroiacovo et al. 1995; Melnick and Myrianthopoulos 1979).

An isolated reconstruction of the external ear, without creation of the ear canal, or middle-ear reconstruction, serves in particular to improve the aesthetic appearance. In addition, it also improves support for spectacles or a hearing aid as well as auditive perception, such as improved directional hearing in cases where the middle ear is still functional.

6.10.2 Perceived Burden of Suffering Due to the Disorder

We conducted a study in Lübeck together with child and adolescent psychiatrists (Siegert et al. 1996 a), in which patients or the parents of affected young children with severe auricular deformities were interviewed before and after surgery with regard to their psychosocial situation. Their personality traits were also tested. The results of this study confirmed our impressions and experience gained over many years of caring for these patients.

Twenty-two percent of the children under 10 years old, or their parents, and 49% of the patients over 10 years old, reported that they had suffered teasing on account of their deformity. Eleven percent of the younger group and 52% of the older patients stated they were embarrassed about their ear. Fifteen percent and 55%, respectively, were afraid they might be rejected because of their malformation; 45% and 72%, respectively, always made a conscious effort to hide their malformation from others by their hairstyle, a hat, bathing cap, or similar headgear; and 32% of the children and 79% of the adolescents and adults had the opinion that "much in their lives would be easier without the ear deformity" (Fig. 6.58).

Some quotes may serve to illustrate these figures:

> Sometimes I reproach myself for ever having been born. I am afraid of having children myself with a deformity because I know how much one suffers from it (9-year-old girl).

> It very much got on my nerves to be repeatedly asked about my ear and I was often called the "one-eared boy," which very much upset me (13-year-old boy).

> My wish to become a banker was frustrated because I didn't get a training vacancy. The rejection was often justified with the comment that my appearance didn't meet the demands of the bank and I was therefore not suitable for working with customers (15-year-old boy).

> My thoughts very often revolved about whether others could see my deformity or whether my hair covered it well enough. This made me feel self-conscious. Some even called me "Spock ear" (25-year-old man).

> I didn't really feel any obvious limitation or burden because of the deformity, but I can imagine that it had an unconscious effect on me, as if I were driving a car with the handbrake on and didn't notice it (32-year-old male).

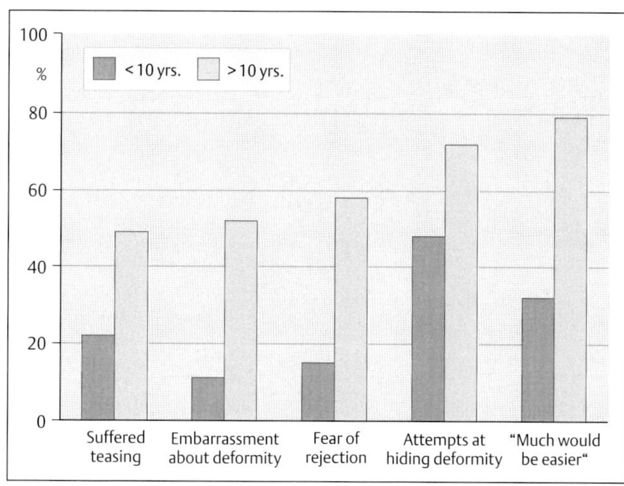

Fig. 6.58 **Perceived burden of suffering by patients with severe microtia.**

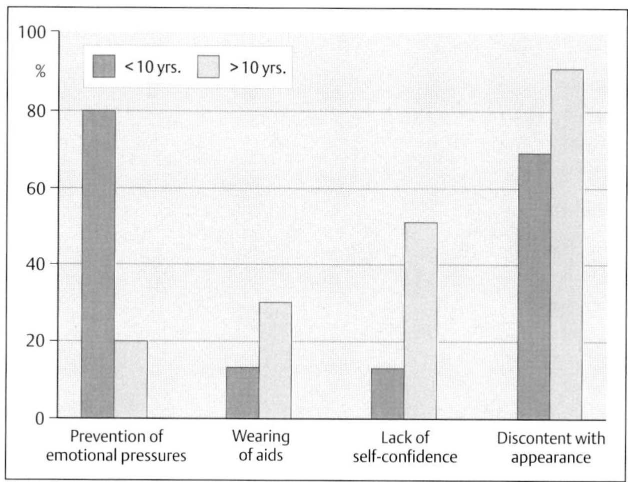

Fig. 6.59 **Motivation for auricular reconstruction.**

6.10.3 Motivation for Auricular Reconstruction

The motivation for auricular reconstruction derives from the perceived burden of suffering arising from the disorder and is summarized in Fig. 6.59. The prevention of emotional pressures was the main reason given by the parents of the younger patients. Adolescents and adults mainly reported their discontent with their own appearance. In addition, a large number of wider-reaching aspirations were associated with the desired operation, as illustrated in the following example:

> I hope to be able to cope with my emotional difficulties better and my greatest wish is to find a girlfriend after the ear reconstruction (31-year-old man).

Self-reproach or the personal experiences of the parents considerably influenced the decision for surgery, especially in the case of younger patients, as exemplified by the following two quotes:

> I was very shocked about the deformity during the first years after Tobias' birth. I myself suffered very much from teasing as a child because of my bat ears. I remember this time as being a very difficult period in which I often cried. I wanted to spare my child these problems, which is why I already decided in favor of surgical correction at an early stage (Mother of a 9-year-old patient).

> I suffered from very strong feelings of guilt because I took Novalgin [metamizole] tablets during the first six weeks of pregnancy. I wanted to make amends to Ralf and made the decision for an operation immediately after his birth (Mother of a 21-year-old patient).

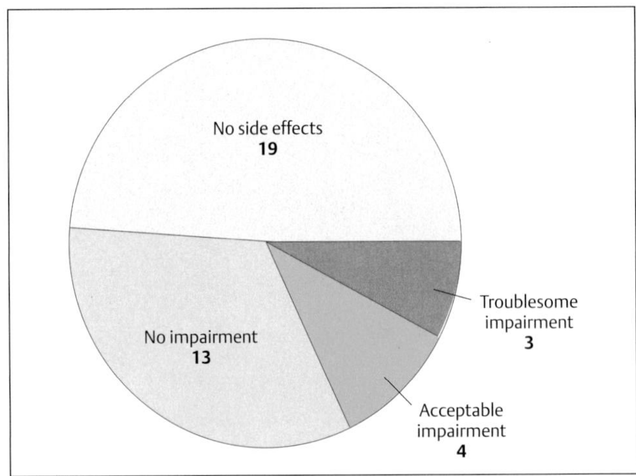

Fig. 6.**60** **Evaluation of side effects in relation to the operative result.**

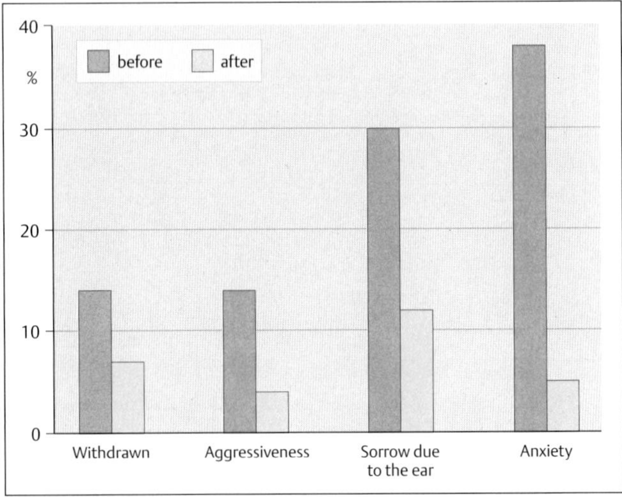

Fig. 6.**61** **Personality traits before and after surgery.**

6.10.4 Retrospective Assessment of the Operative Result

Thirty-six (92%) of the 39 patients felt the surgical result to be "better" or "much better" than the preoperative appearance. They were interviewed retrospectively and had all been operated on using the precursors of the techniques described in Chapter 5, which have meanwhile been developed further and improved. One patient believed that reconstruction of his ear had led to "no change" and two felt that the result was "worse" as compared with the unoperated state.

Thirty-four patients (87%) of the retrospective group would readily opt for the operation again, four would refrain from another operation, and one patient declined to comment.

Fifty-two percent of the patients reported that they were more satisfied with their appearance, 35% had gained more self-confidence as a result of the operation, and 33% mentioned that wearing spectacles had become less of a problem after reconstruction (multiple answers possible).

Here too, a few quotes may be enlightening:

> Jens is so proud of his new ear that he just has to show everybody (Parents of a 10-year-old patient).

> After the operation people no longer asked me about my ear so much, although others are more likely to see it now that I wear my hair shorter. I feel very much better. It's a good feeling to look in the mirror and to see something there that almost looks like a normal ear (19-year-old man).

> I would even have been happy had there had just been **something** there. But what appeared after the first dressing change was something I had never expected at all (29-year-old woman).

> The operation was very important for me and has considerably improved my self-confidence. I would advise anyone who was in the same mental state as I to have this operation done (29-year-old man).

> For me, I now feel positive towards every situation in life where I used to feel self-conscious and ill at ease. I now like it when it's windy, whereas I always used to be afraid that someone might see my ear. I now like going to events where there are a lot of people and I now lead quite a different emotional life (51-year-old woman).

Any overall assessment should also contain an appraisal of the disadvantages associated with the operation. These include hospital stays lasting many weeks, the emotional strain associated with the operations, and the surgical scars. The subjective appraisal of the side effects by the patients in relation to the surgical result is shown in Fig. 6.**60**. Ninety-one percent ticked the options ranging from "***no side effects***" to "***acceptable in relation to the surgical result.***"

6.10.5 Personality Traits Before and After Surgery

The personality trait "anxiety" had changed to a very significant extent and was identified in 35% of the patients interviewed prospectively and in only 5% of those interviewed retrospectively. These and other parameters are compared in Fig. 6.**61**.

6.10.6 Assessment

When assessing the psychosocial stress resulting from malformations, a basic distinction is made between the appraisals of parents of affected children and the appraisals of patients themselves.

Reactions of Parents

Their own mental stress resulting from the malformation of their children plays a significant role for parents. Parents who have a child with a deformity are initially shocked. The ideal conceptions which are projected into every planned child appear to recede into the unattainable distance. Irrational feelings of guilt are aroused, and one of the first questions during any counseling interview is about the causes. The way the parents then finally deal with their own mental stress has an effect on the children, especially during the preschool years, according to Lefebvre and Munro (1975).

Reactions of Children

Between **the ages of 3 and 6 years** the children start to incorporate their deformity into their own body image. They begin on the one hand to realize that they are different from others, while on the other hand the formation of their body image is dependent on the reactions they receive from their environment. The more parents try to protect their children in this phase from the offensive stares or even teasing of their peers, the more insecure will they become in dealing with their deformity (Lefebvre and Munro 1975).

At **school age**, peer pressure and the risk of isolation of a child with a deformity increase considerably. Many patients, especially the older ones, report in retrospect about very depressing episodes of teasing during this period.

With the onset of **puberty**, a phase commences in which body image, together with the significance of physical attractiveness, assumes an extremely high significance that lasts throughout life (Walster et al. 1966). This is the time in particular when dissatisfaction with their own appearance as a result of the malformation represents a heavy burden for the patients.

Nonsyndromic microtias do not represent by any means the severest forms of facial malformations. The assumption that their mental repercussions are therefore less serious is, however, unfounded, as studies by Macgregor (1974, 1975) involving 115 patients have shown. The typical reactions to the **type of deformity** are more decisive than to its severity. According to Macgregor's experience, patients with auricular malformations more often tend to be the target of provocative laughter, ridicule, and teasing and consequently to be emotionally more seriously affected than patients with malformations which tend to arouse compassion, such as cleft lip and palate.

In an earlier, yet still relevant, work, Macgregor et al. (1953) emphasize that there is still a considerable need for information, even among members of the health-care professions, with regard to the mental and emotional effects of facial malformations. Perhaps the present chapter can make a small contribution in this respect. Besides this, however, it is the vast majority of non-handicapped laypeople who create many difficulties in the first place, or intensify them for these patients by their prejudices and their thoughtless behavior.

The **motivation for auricular reconstruction** most frequently expressed by adolescent and adult patients is quite pragmatic and concerns their dissatisfaction with their own appearance. **None of the patients, however, reported that they wished to become "beautiful" as a result of the operation. It was not something positively special that was requested, but "social unobtrusiveness" in order to overcome the negative connotations of being different.**

The burden imposed by their unsatisfactory appearance was not stated as frequently, but was still one of the most important motivations for undergoing surgery for 77% of the patients with prominent ears who were examined in a study by Rasinger et al. (1983). In addition, the mental problems associated with the malformation played a decisive role in that study as well as in the present one. After all, 30% of our patients also expected advantages from surgery with regard to wearing aids such as spectacles or hearing devices.

Psychoprophylaxis is paramount for parents of those patients under 10 years old. Given the emotional stress already described previously for the older patients, this wish, together with the underlying assessment, appears realistic.

The vast majority of the patients interviewed were satisfied with their auricular reconstruction and would retrospectively opt for surgery again. This inevitably depends decisively on the quality of the operative result. Surgery lay many years in the past for most of the patients who were reviewed. They had not even benefited from the more recent experience and modified techniques (Siegert, Weerda et al. 1993; Siegert and Weerda 1994; Weerda 1997a, 2001) which are described in detail in Chapters 4 and 5.

One aspect, which was typical for the majority of the patients, was **the fact that the operation not only altered the external ear, but also their entire body image. They no longer felt themselves to be deformed.** This effect is beyond comparison with any psychological counseling, an appropriate hairstyle—no matter how well it covers the deformity—or an epithesis, however artistically well it has been designed. According to Arndt et al. (1956) and Lefebvre and Munro (1975), it is the feeling of self-esteem that has been raised by the operation and contributes to the improved quality of life, thus allowing the patient to overcome social barriers.

Apart from any possible optimal restoration of hearing by tympanoplasty (see Chapter 6.2; p. 245, 6.3; p. 255), or by the provision of a hearing aid (see Chapter 6.4; pp. 260 ff), the **therapeutic goal** when dealing with patients with severe microtia must take the following aspects into consideration:

- The creation of their **"own"** auricle, i. e., not an epithesis, to produce the preconditions for altering their own self-esteem
- The creation of an auricle which appears **as natural as possible**, so that it is not recognized at first sight by the patient's peers as being the work of surgery (see pp. 188, 190, 230, 259).

The described phases of development of an individual's perception of their own body and the subsequent pressures resulting from deformities, which are apparent to the outside world, have led many to demand that surgical corrections be performed as soon as possible (Lefebvre and Munro 1975; Macgregor et al. 1953). Auricular reconstruction at an age before the children have even started to realize they have a deformity (Straith and De Kleine 1938; MacGregor 1974), i. e., before kindergarten age, is not technically possible because insufficient autologous costal cartilage is available. Brent recommended reconstruction before children start school (Brent 1992), but this is only possible using the expansile framework technique.

Only after the age of 10 is there sufficient costal cartilage for the "three-dimensional," i. e., more stable and higher, form of framework proposed by Nagata (see Chapter 5). According to Macgregor et al. (1953), the operations should be done, if not during infancy, then if at all possible before puberty. It is for this reason that we recommend a suitable time for auricular reconstruction to be between the ages of 8 and 14 years, which is a compromise between surgical necessity and psychosocial rehabilitation.

In order to prepare the patient optimally for the operation, detailed counseling with regard to the risks and benefits is necessary, as with any elective surgery. In addition, talks with other affected patients and, in particular, the supplementary work done by support groups, such as the Goldenhar **support groups** or the Let's Face It organization in Britain and the USA, have proved to be of considerable assistance (see Appendix 3 for details).

7 Epilogue

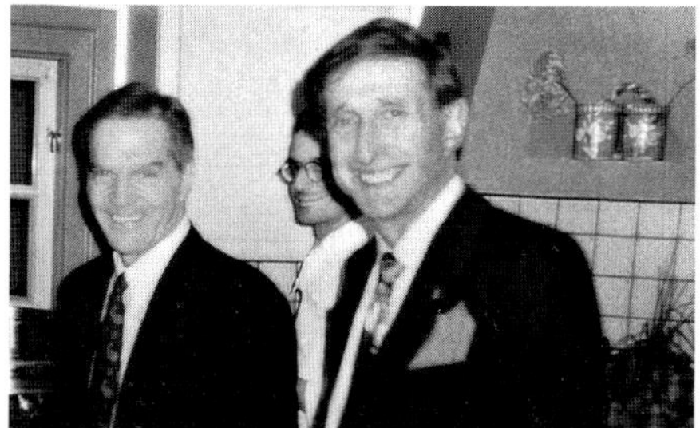

Fig. 7.1 **Burt Brent (right) and Bob Jahrsdoerfer at our symposium in Lübeck, Germany, in 1997.**

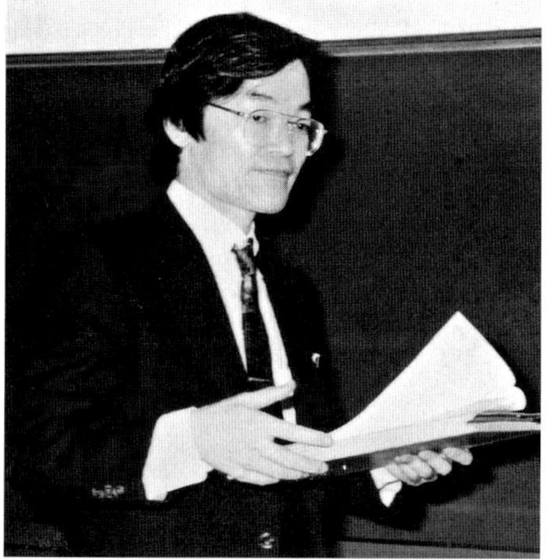

Fig. 7.2 **Satoru Nagata in Lübeck, Germany, in 1997.**

I completed the German edition of this book in the summer of 2002. The revised and updated English edition was completed in 2006. This book comprises the sum of my experience and the experiences of my team in Lübeck in a speciality to which I devoted myself for almost 35 years.

I should like to thank my role models and tutors:

- Professor Fritz Zöllner
- Professor Chlodwig Beck
- Professor Gert Lange

Books by Tanzer, Converse, and Brent provided me with my first inspirations.

I was particularly inspired by Burt Brent (Fig. 7.1) whom I visited in California and whom I accompanied to his operations in various clinics. Most memorable occasions also included my visit to Satoru Nagata (Fig. 7.2) in Japan in 1995 and the symposium with a live operation course held in Lübeck, Germany, in 1997. Together with Bob Jahrsdoerfer, currently the best-known surgeon for middle-ear malformations (Fig. 7.1), the leading surgeons for auricular malformations reported on their experience and demonstrated their subtle surgery in our operating theatre (Weerda H, Siegert R 1998g).

May I particularly express my thanks for the encouraging words about this book and the support reflected in the texts of the forewords and contributions.

Freiburg, Germany 2007 — Hilko Weerda

8 References

Abul-Hassan HS, Ascher G von, Aceland R. Surgical Anatomy and Blood Supply of the Facial Layers of the Temporal Region. Plast Reconstr Surg. 1986;77:17–24.

Adamson PA. Otoplasty: Critical review of clinical results. Laryngoscope. 1991;101:883–888.

Afzelius LE, Gunnarson M, Nordgreen H. Guidelines for prophylactic radical lymph node dissection in cases of carcinoma of the external ear. Head Neck Surg. 1980;2:361–365.

Afzelius LE, Nordgreen H. Histologische Punktesysteme bei verschiedenen Karzinomen des äußeren Ohres. HNO. 1984;32:63.

Agrawal K, Mishra S, Panda K. Primary reconstruction of major human bite wounds of the face. Plast Reconstr Surg. 1992;90:394.

Aguilar E, Jahrsdoerfer RA. The Surgical Repair of Congenital Microtia and Atresia. Otolaryngol. 1988;98:600–606.

Aguilar EF. Auricular reconstruction of congenital microtia (grade III). Laryngoscope. 1996;82:1–26.

Alanis SZ. A new method for earlobe reconstruction. Plast Reconstr Surg. 1970;45:254–257.

Albrektsson T, Albrektsson B. Osseointegration of bone implants. Acta Orthop Scand. 1987;58:567–577.

Aleksandrov NM. A method of plastic repair with the aid of Filatov's tubed flap in the formation of the external ear. Vestn Otorhinolaryngol. 1963;25:24–29.

Alexander AE Jr, Caldemeyer KS, Rigby P. Clinical and surgical application of reformatted high-resolution CT of the temporal bone. Neuroimaging Clin N Am. 1998;8:631–50.

Alexander G. Eine neue Helikoplastik zur Stellungskorrektur und Vergrößerung der Ohrmuschel bei relativer Mikrotie. Mschr Ohrenheilk und Laryngol Rhinol. 1919;53:113–116.

Alexander G. Zur plastischen Korrektur abstehender Ohren. Wien Klin Wschr. 1928;41:1217.

Alexandrov NM. Traumatic defects of the auricle and methods of their repair. Acta Chir Plast. 1964;6:302–312.

Al-Quattan M, Cosman B. Question mark ear. Congenital auricular cleft between the fifth and sixth hillock. Plast Reconstr Surg. 1998;102:439–441.

Altmann F. Malformations of the auricle and external auditory meatus. Arch Otolaryngol. 1951;54:115–139.

Altmann F. Mißbildungen des Ohres. In: Berendes, Link, Zöllner. Hals-Nasen-Ohren-Heilkunde. Band III/1. Stuttgart: Thieme; 1965.

Altmeyer P, Luther H, Koffmann K, El-Gammal S, Bacharach-Buhles M. Möglichkeiten und Grenzen neuerer Verfahren in der Diagnostik des malignen Melanoms. Hautarzt. 1991;41(Suppl. X):83–87.

Alvares Cruz N, da Sieva Castro D, Luis A. Carcinomes primitifs de l'oreille externe et de l'oreille moyenne. Ann Otolaryngol. 1981;98:613.

Andes C, Koch A. Die Ohrmuschelplastik – Ergebnisse und Komplikationen mit einer abgewandelten Technik nach Mustardé. Laryngo Rhino Otol. 1991;70:620–624.

Anthony J, Lineaweaver W, Davis J, Buncke H. Quantitative fluorimetric effects of leeching on a replanted ear. Microsurgery. 1989;10:167–169.

Antia N, Buch V. Chondrocutaneous advancement flap for the marginal defects of the ear. Plast Reconstr Surg. 1967;39:472–477.

Antia N. Repair of segmental defects of the auricle in mechanical trauma. In: Tanzer R, Edgerton M. Symposium on reconstruction of the auricle. St Louis: CV Mosby & Co; 1974:213–220.

Argamaso RV, Lewin M. Repair of partial ear loss with local composite flap. Plast Reconstr Surg. 1968;42:437–441.

Argamaso RV, Lewin M. The lateral transhelical approach for correction of deformities of the external ear. Aesth Plast Surg. 1978; 2:357–362.

Argamaso RV. Ear reduction with or without setback otoplasty. Plast Reconstr Surg. 1989;83:967–975.

Ariyan S, Chicarilli Z. Replantation of a totally amputated ear by means of a platysma musculocutaneous "sandwich" flap. Plast Reconstr Surg. 1986;78:385–389.

Arndt EM, Travis F, Lefebvre A, Niec A, Munro IR: Beauty and the eye of the beholder: Social consequences and personal adjustments for facial patients. Br J Plast Surg 39 (1956) 51–54

Aronson RS, Batsakis JG, Rice DH, Work W. Anomalies of the First Branchial Cleft. Arch Otolaryngol 1976;102:737–741.

Arunachalam PS, Kilby D, Meikle D, Davison T, Johnson IJM. Bone-anchored hearing aid quality of life assessed by Glasgow benefit inventory. Laryngoscope. 2001;111:1260–1263.

Atilla S, Akpek S, Uslu S, Ilgit ET, Isik S. Computed tomographic evaluation of surgically significant vascular variations related with the temporal bone. Eur J Radiol. 1995;20:52–56.

Avila J, Bosch A, Aristizabal S, Frias Z, Marcial V. Carcinoma of the Pinna. Cancer. 1977;40:291–295.

Bäckdahl M, Consiglio V, Falconer B. Reconstruction of the external ear with the use of maternal cartilage. A follow up investigation of twenty-five cases. Br J Plast Surg. 1954;7:263–274.

Bahmer F. Keloid der hinteren Ohrmuschel: Therapie mittels Laser und "Austernschale". Z Hautkrh. 1997;72:785.

Bailin PL, Levin H, Wood B, Tucker H. Cutaneous carcinoma of the auricular and periauricular region. Arch Otorhinolaryngol Head Neck Surg. 1980;106:692.

Bardsley A, Mercer D. The injured ear: a review of 50 cases. Br J Plast Surg. 1983;36:466–469.

Barron J, Emmet A. Subcutaneous pedicled flap. Br J Plast Surg. 1965;18:51–56.

Barsky AJ, ed. Plastic Surgery. Philadelphia: WW Saunders; 1938.

Barsky AJ. Priciples and practice of plastic surgery. Baltimore: Williams & Williams Co; 1950:203–205.

Barsky AJ, Kahn S, Simon BE . Principles and practice of plastic surgery. New York: McGraw-Hill Book Co; 1964;303–307.

Batisse R, Mahe E, Camblin J. Technique de striation cartilagineuse antèrieure dans la correction des oreilles décollèes. Ann Otol Laryngol. 1973;90:389–396.

Baudet J. La réimplantation du pavillon de l'oreille mutilé. La Nouvelle Presse Médicale. 1972;5:344–346.

Baudet J, Tramond P, Gonmain A. A propos d'un procédé original de réimplantation d'un pavillon de l'oreille totalement séparé. Ann Chir Plast Esthet. 1972 a;17:67–72.

Baudet J, Tramond P, Massard J, Goumain A. Les reimplantations du pavillon de l'oreille mutilee. Rev Laryngol Otol Rhinol. 1972 b;93:241–256.

Bauer BS. Reconstruction of the Microtic Ear. J Ped Surg. 1984; 19:440–445.

Bauer BS. The role of tissue expansion in reconstruction of the ear. Clin Plast Surg. 1990;17:319–325.

Bauer E, Wodak E. Spätergebnisse nach Ohrmuschelplastiken. Mschr Ohrenheilk und Laryngol Rhinol. 1968;102:468–477.

Bauer M, Loosely RM, Anders H, Wilfingseder P. Operative Behandlung maligner Epitheliome der Haut. Chirurg. 1977;48:170.

Bäumler W, Scherer K, Abels C, Neff S, Landthaler M, Szeimies RM. The effect of different spotsizes of the efficacy of hair removal using a long-pulsed diode laser. Derm Surg. 2002;28:118–121.

Beck J. Über die plastischen Operationen an Nase und Ohr. Internat Zbl Ohrenhlkd. 1923;21:134.
Becker O. Surgical correction of the abnormally protruding ear. Arch Otol. 1949;50:541.
Becker O. Correction of the protruding ear deformity. Br J Plast Surg. 1952;5:187–196.
Beek van A. Invited comment. Ann Plast Surg. 1988;21:178–179.
Bejar-Solar I, Rosette M, De Jesus Madrazo M, Baltierra C. Percutaneous bone-anchored hearing aid at a pediatric institution. Otolaryngol Head Neck Surg. 2000;122:887–891.
Belenky W, Medina J. First Branchial Cleft Anomalies. Laryngoscope. 1980;90:28–39.
Bennett ME: Psychologic and Social Consequences of Craniofacial Disfigurement in Children. Facial Plast Surg 11 (1995) 76–51
Benton C, Bellet PS. Imaging of congenital anomalies of the temporal bone. Neuroimaging Clin N Am. 2000;10:35–53.
Berghaus A. Surgical concepts for reconstruction of the auricle. History and current state of the art. Arch Otolaryngol Head and Neck 1986;112:388–397
Berghaus A. Porecon implant and fan flap: a concept for reconstruction of the auricle. Fac Plast Surg. 1988;5:399–340
Bernstein L, Nelson R. Replanting the severed auricle. Arch Otolaryngol Head Neck Surg. 1982;108:587–590.
Berson MI. Complete reconstruction of auricle. Berson technic. In: Morton I, Berson I. Atlas of Plastic Surgery. New York: Grune & Stratton; 1948:188–196.
Bethmann W, Zoltan J. Operationen an der Ohrmuschel. In: Bethmann W. Methoden der plastischen Chirurgie. Jena: Fischer; 1968;267–282.
Biesenberger H. Plastische Operationen abstehender Ohren nach Gersuny. Zbl Chir. 1924;51:1126–1127.
Black P. Correction of the flap-folded helix. Plast Reconstr Surg. 1971;48:86–87.
Blake GB, Wilson JSP. Malignant tumours of the ear and their treatment. Br J Plast Surg. 1974;27:67–76.
Blass K, Bartholemé W. Echte Polyotie, eine seltene frühembryonale Entwicklungsstörung. HNO. 1976;24:309–310.
Blondell JH, Lelion PH. Ossification des cartilages auriculaires. J F Oto-Rhino-Laryngol. 1991;40:475–476.
Bockenheimer S, Weerda H, Hartenstein V. Die hochauflösende Computertomographie des Felsenbeines bei Ohrmuschelmißbildungen (Ein Vergleich mit der normalen Felsenbeinanatomie). Arch Otorhinolaryngol Teil II. 1984;211.
Boenninghaus HG. Beitrag zur Verhütung einer Ohrmuschelschrumpfung nach Perichondritis durch Einsetzen einer Supramidstütze. Zschr Laryngo Rhinol Otol. 1952;31: 287–289.
Boenninghaus HG. Ohrverletzungen. In: Berendes, Link, Zöllner. HNO-Heilkunde, Bd. III/1, 2.Aufl. Stuttgart: Thieme; 1979; 833–839.
Bogdasarian R, Baker S. Surgery for the congenitally malformed external ear. Ear, Nose, Throat 1983;62:635–643.
Bonding P, Holm Jonsson M, Salomon G, Ahlgren P. The bone-anchored hearing aid. Acta otolaryngol suppl (Stockh).1992;492: 42–45.
Boo-Chai K. The pixie earlobe: A method of correction. Plast Reconstr Surg. 1985;76:636–638.
Borges AF. Prominent ears: Modification of Dr. Forrest Young's technique. Plast Reconstr Surg. 1953;12:208.
Bosmann AJ, Snik AF, van der Pouw CT, Mylanus EA, Cremers CW. Audiometric evaluation of bilaterally fitted bone-anchored hearing aids. Audiology. 2001;40:158–167.
Boudard P, Portmann M. Technique chirurgicale de reconstruction totale du pavillon de l'oreille dans les cas d'agénésie majeure: utilisation d'un greffon cartilagineux costal. Rev Laryngol. 1987;108:507–513.
Boudard P, Benassayagi C, Dhillon R et al. Aesthetic surgery of microtia. Arch Otorhinolaryngol. 1989;46:349–352.
Brandt F. Human bites of the ear. Plast Reconstr Surg. 1969;43: 130–134.
Braun-Falco O, Plewig G, Wolff H. Dermatologie und Venerologie, 3. Aufl. Berlin: Springer; 1983.
Braun-Falco O, Plewig G, Wolff H, Winkelmann RK. Dermatology. Berlin: Springer; 1991.
Brent B. Ear reconstruction with an expansile framework of autogenous rib cartilage. Plast Reconstr Surg. 1974;53:619–628.
Brent B. Reconstruction of ear, eyebrow and sideburn in the burned patient. Plast Reconstr Surg. 1975;55:312–317.
Brent B. Earlobe construction with an auriculo-mastoid flap. Plast Reconstr Surg. 1976;57:389–391.
Brent B. The acquired auricular deformity. Plast Reconstr Surg. 1977;59:475–485.
Brent B. The correction of microtia with autogenous cartilage grafts: Part I. The classic deformity. Part II Atypical and complex deformities. Plast Reconstr Surg. 1980;66:1–12;13–22.
Brent B. A personal approach to total auricular construction. Clin Plast Surg. 1981;8:211–222.
Brent B. An improved one-stage total ear reconstruction procedure (Discussion). Plast Reconstr Surg. 1983;71:623.
Brent B, Byrd HS. Secondary ear reconstruction with cartilage grafts covered by axial, random, and free flaps of temporoparietal fascia. Plast Reconstr Surg. 1983;72:141–151.
Brent B, Upton J, Acland RD, Shaw WW, Finseth FJ, Rogers C, Pearl RM, Hentz VR. Experience with the temporoparietal fascial free flap. Plast Reconstr Surg. 1985;76:177–188.
Brent B. Auricular repair with a conchal cartilage graft. In: Brent B, ed. The artristry of reconstructive surgery. St Louis: CV Mosby & Co; 1987 a:107–112.
Brent B. Total auricular construction with sculpted costal cartilage. In: Brent B, ed. The artistry of reconstructive surgery. St Louis: CV Mosby & Co; 1987 b:113–127.
Brent B: Auricular repair with autogenous rib cartilage grafts: Two decades of experience with 600 cases. Plast Reconstr Surg. 1992;90:355–374.
Brent B. Modification of the stages in total reconstruction of the auricle (Discussion). Plast Reconstr Surg. 1994;93:267.
Brent B. Personal communication at the "Symposium on Auricular and Middle Ear Malformations, Ear Defects and their Reconstruction." Lübeck. Sept. 1997.
Brent B. Auricular repair with sculpted autogenous rib cartilage. In: Weerda H, Siegert R, eds. Auricular and Middle Ear, Malformations, ear Defects and their Reconstruction. The Hague/The Netherlands: Kugler Publications; 1998 a:17–29.
Brent B. Development of ear reconstruction: the past, present und future. Keynote address presented at ear reconstruction. Choices for the future. Chateau Lake Louise, Canada. 1998 b.
Brent B. The pediatrician's role in caring for patients with congenital microtia and atresia. Pediatr Ann. 1999 a;28:374.
Brent B. Technical advances in ear reconstruction with autogenous rib cartilage grafts: Personal experience with 1200 cases. Plast Reconstr Surg. 1999 b;104:319–334.
Broadbent TR, Mathews VL. Artistic relationship in surface anatomy of the face: application to reconstructive surgery. Plast Reconstr Surg. 1957;20:1–17.
Brodovsky S, Westreich M. Question Mark Ear: Method for Repair. Plast Reconstr Surg. 1997;100:1254–1257.
Brown JB, Cannon B. Composite free graft of two surfaces of skin and cartilage from the ear. Ann Surg. 1946;124:1101–1107.
Brown JB, Cannon B, Lischer C, Davis WB, Moore A, Murray J. Further reports on the use of composite free grafts of skin and cartilage from the ear. Plast Reconstr Surg. 1946;1:130–134.
Brown JB, Cannon B, Lischer C, Davis W, Moore A. Surgical substitution for cases of the external ear. Simplified local flap method of reconstruction. Surg Gynecol Obstet. 1947;84:192.
Brown JB, Freyer MP, Morgan LR. Problems in reconstruction of the auricle. Plast Reconstr Surg. 1969;43:597–604.

Brown W. Extraordinary case of horse bite: the external ear completely bitten off and successfully replaced. Lancet. 1898;1: 1533–1534.

Bruck HG, Gisel I. Ästhetische Gesichtschirurgie. Leipzig: Barth; 1976.

Brusis T. Die Behandlung des Otseroms mit Fibrinkleber. HNO. 1982;30:272–274.

Bukal J, Fries R, Engleder R, Platz H. Zur Klinik der Basaliome, Plattenepithelkarzinome und Keratoakanthome der Gesichts- und Halshaut. In: Pfeifer G, Schwenzer N, Hrsg. Fortschritte der Kiefer- und Gesichtschirurgie. 1982; XXVII.

Bull T, Mustardé JC. Mustardé Technique in Otoplasty. Facial Plast Surg. 1985;2:101–108.

Buncke H, Schulz W. Total ear reimplantation in the rabbit utilising microminiature vascular anastomoses. Br J Plast Surg. 1966;19: 15–22.

Burgess PA, Novia M, Frankel S, Hicks J, Yim D. Avulsions of the Auricle. Ear Nose Throat 1985;61:546–548.

Burnett W. Yank meets native. National Geographic Magazine. 1945;88:105–128.

Byers RM. Squamous Cell Carcinoma of the External Ear. Amer J Surg. 1983;146:447.

Caldas JG, Iffenecker C, Attal P, Lasjaunias P, Doyon D. Anomalous vessel in the middle ear: the role of CT and MR angiography. Neuroradiology. 1998;40:748–751.

Caldemeyer KS, Mathews VP, Azzarelli B, Smith RR. The jugular foramen: a review of anatomy, masses, and imaging characteristics. Radiographics. 1997;17:1123–1139.

Cannive B. Histopathologische Aspekte einer tierexperimentellen Studie zum Ohrmuschelabriß [Dissertation]. Universität Freiburg; 1985.

Caputo R. Ethiopia. Revolution in an ancient empire. National Geographic Magazine. 1983;163:614–644.

Casselman JW, Kuhweide R, Ampe W, Meeus L, Steyaert L. Pathology of the membranous labyrinth: comparison of T1- and T2-weighted and gadolinium-enhanced spin-echo and 3DFT-CISS imaging. AJNR Am J Neuroradiol. 1993;14:59–69.

Cavanaugh EB. Management of lesions of the helical rim using a chondrocutaneous advancement flap. J Dermatol Surg Oncol. 1982;8:691–696.

Ceilley R, Bumsted R, Smith WH. Malignancies on the external ear: methods of ablation and reconstruction of defects. J Dermatol Surg Oncol. 1979;5:762–767.

Chami RG, Apesos J. Treatment of Asymptomatic Preauricular Sinuses: Challenging Conventional Wisdom. Ann Plast Surg. 1989;5:406–411.

Chen KT, Dehner L. Primary tumours of the external and middle ear. Arch Otolaryngol Head Neck Surg. 1978;104:247.

Chen ZJ, Chen C. Earlobe reconstruction using island flap with postauricular blood vessels. Facial Plast Surg. 1990;5:426–430.

Chen ZJ. Improved technique for a one-stage repair of significant defects of the ear. Plast Reconstr Surg. 1990;86:987–990.

Chilla R, Miehlke A. Zur Klinik und Topographie des "doppelten Gehörgangs". 1984;63:229–232.

Chmyrev VS. Plastic restauration of the auricular concha with the use of a carcass woven from polyamide thread. Vestn Otorinolaryngol. 1967;29:26–29.

Choi S, Lam V, Chan V, Ghadially F, Ng A. Endchondral pseudocyst of the auricle in chinese. Arch Otolaryngol. 1984;110:792–796.

Chongchet V. A Method of anthelix reconstruction. Br J Plast Surg. 1963;16:268–272.

Clemons J, Connelly M. Reattachment of a totally amputated auricle. Arch Otolaryngol Head Neck Surg. 1973;97:269–272.

Clodius L. Local hypothermia for the avulsed external ear. Br J Plast Surg. 1968;21:250–252.

Cloutier AM. Correction of outstanding ears. Plast Reconstr Surg. 1961;28:412–416.

Cloutier AM. Total ear reconstruction. Arch Otolaryngol. 1968;88: 95–100.

Cole RR, Jahrsdoerfer RA. The risk of cholesteatoma in congenital aural stenosis. Laryngoscope 1990; 100: 576–8.

Conley J, Pack GT. Melanoma of the Mucous Membranes of the Head and Neck. Arch Otolaryngol. 1974;99:315.

Conroy W. Letter to the editor: Salvage of an amputated ear. Plast Reconstr Surg. 1972;49:564.

Converse JM. Reconstruction of the external ear by prefabricated framework of refridgerated bone and cartilage. Plast Reconstr Surg. 1950;5:148–156.

Converse JM, Nigro A, Wilson F, Johnson N. A technique for surgical correction of lop ears. Plast Reconstr Surg. 1955;15:411–418.

Converse JM. Reconstruction of the auricle, Part 1 und 2. Plast Reconstr Surg. 1958;22:150–163 u. 230–249.

Converse JM. Construction of the auricle in congenital microtia. Plast Reconstr Surg. 1963;32:425–438.

Converse JM. Traumatic deformities of the auricle. In. Kazanjian M, Converse JM, eds. Surgical treatment of facial injuries. Baltimore: Williams & Wilkins; 1974:1289–1299.

Converse JM. Reconstructive plastic surgery. 2nd ed. Philadelphia: Saunders; 1977.

Converse JM, Brent B. Acquired deformities. In: Converse JM, ed. Reconstructive plastic surgery. Vol. III, 2nd ed. Philadelphia: Saunders; 1977:1724–1733.

Converse JM, Wood-Smith D. Techniques for the repair of defects of the lip and cheeks. In: Converse JM, ed. Reconstructive Plastic Surgery. 2nd ed. Philadelphia: Saunders; 1977:1544–1594.

Conway H, Neumann CG, Gelb J, Leveridge LL, Joseph JM. Reconstruction of the external ear. Ann Surg. 1948;128:226–238.

Conway H, Wagner K. Congenital Anomalies of the Head and Neck. Plast Reconstr Surg. 1965;36:71–79.

Cosman B et al. The surgical treatment of keloids. Plast Reconstr Surg. 1961;27:335–358.

Cosman B, Crikelair GF. The composed tube pedicle in ear helix reconstruction. Plast Reconstr Surg. 1966;37:517–522.

Cosman B, Bellin H, Crikelair GF. The question mark ear. Plast Reconstr Surg. 1970;46:454–457.

Cosman B. Repair of moderate cup ear deformities. In: Tanzer R, Edgerton M, eds. Symposium on reconstruction of the auricle. St Louis: Mosby & Co; 1974:X:118–139.

Cosman B. The question mark ear: an unappreciated major anomaly of the auricle. Plast Reconstr Surg. 1984;73:572–576.

Cremers C, Oudenhofen, Marres E. Congenital Aural Atresia. A New Subclassification and Surgical Managment. Clin Otolaryngol. 1984;9:119–127.

Crikelair G. A Method of partial ear reconstruction for avulsion of the upper portion of the ear. Plast Reconstr Surg. 1956;17: 438–443.

Crikelair GF. Another solution for the problem of the prominent ear. Ann Surg. 1964;160:314–324.

Cronin TD. One-stage reconstruction of the helix: two improved methods. Plast Reconstr Surg. 1952;9:546–556.

Cronin TD. The use of a silastic frame for total and subtotal reconstruction of the external ear: preliminary report. Plast Reconstr Surg. 1966;37:399–405.

Cronin TD, Greenberg GL, Brauer OR. Follow-up study of silastic frame for reconstruction of external ear. Plast Reconstr Surg. 1968;42:522–529.

Cronin TD. Use of a silastic frame for construction of the auricle. In: Tanzer R, Edgerton MT, eds. Symposium on reconstruction of the auricle. St Louis: CV Mosby & Co; 1974:33–45.

Curtis H. A plastic operation to restore part of the ear. Lancet. 1920;98:1094–1095.

Czarnetzki B, Kerl H, Sterry W. Dermatologie und Venerologie. Berlin: deGruyter; 1992.

Czarnetzki B, Macher E, Sucius et al. Long-term adjuvant immunotherapy in stage I high risk malignant melanoma. Eur J Cancer. 1993;29A:1237–1242.

Danter J, Weerda H, Semeradt A, Siegert R. Results of middle Ear Surgery in Patients with Auricular Dysplasias and Congenital Aural Atresias: An Analysis of 58 Operations in other Institutions. Eur Arch Oto Rhino Laryng. 1997;254:26.

Davis AD. Plastic surgery of the ear, nose and face. Arch Otolaryngol Head Neck Surg. 1929;10:575–584.

Davis J. Auricle reconstruction. In: Saad MN, Lichtveld P, eds. Reviews in plastic surgery. Amsterdam: Exerpta Medica; 1974 a: 109–140.

Davis J. Repair of severe cup ear deformities. In: Tanzer R, Edgerton M, eds. Symposium on reconstruction of the auricle. St Louis: CV Mosby & Co; 1974 b.

Davis J. Prominent ear. In: Aesthetic and Reconstructive Otoplasty. Berlin: Springer; 1987.

Davis J. (Ed.) Aesthetic and Reconstructive Otoplasty. Berlin: Springer; 1987

Davis J. Otoplasty: Aesthetic and Reconstructive Techniques. Berlin: Springer; 1997.

Davis JE. Aesthetic Otoplasty. In: Lewis J, ed. The art of aesthetic plastic surgery. Boston: Little Brown; 1989:I.

Davis JS, Kitlowski EA. Abnormal prominence of the ears: A method of readjustment. Surgery. 1937;2:835–847.

Day HF. Reconstruction of ears. Boston Med Surg J. 1921;185: 146–147.

Declau F, Cremers C, Van-de-Heyning P. Diagnosis and management strategies in congenital atresia of the external auditory canal. Br J Audiol. 1999;33:313–327.

Destro M, Speranzini M. Total reconstruction of the auricle after traumatic amputation. Plast Reconstr Surg. 1996;94:859–864.

Di Martino G. Anomalie de pavillon d'oreille. Bull Acad Natl Med. 1856/1857;22:17.

DiBartolomeo JR. The Petrified Auricle: Comments on ossification, calcification and exostoses of the external ear. Laryngoscope. 1985;95:566–576.

Dieffenbach JF. Von dem Wiederersatze des äußeren Ohres. In: Dr. JF Dieffenbach. Chirurgische Erfahrungen, besonders über die Wiederherstellung zerstörter Teile des menschlichen Körpers nach neuen Methoden. Berlin: Enslin; 1830:115–189.

Dieffenbach JF. Die Ohrbildung, Otoplastik. In: Dieffenbach JF. Die operative Chirurgie. Leipzig: Brockhaus; 1845 a:395–397.

Dieffenbach JF. In: Fritze HE, Reich OF, Hrsg. Die Plastische Chirurgie in ihrem weitesten Umfange dargestellt und durch Abbildungen erläutert. Berlin: Hirschwald; 1845 b.

Dierickx CC, Grossmann MC, Farinelli WA, Anderson RR. Permanent hair removal by normal-mode ruby laser. Arch Dermatol. 1998;134:837.

Dion K: Young children's stereotyping of facial attractiveness. Develop Psychol 1973;9:153–155

Dion K, Berscheid E: Physical attractiveness and peer perception among children. Sociometry 1974;37:1–12

Dirks DD. Bone conduction threshold testing. In: Katz J, Gabbay WL, Gold S, Medwetsky L, Ruth RA, editors. Handbook of clinical audiology. Baltimore: William and Wilkins, 1994: 132–45.

Dongen van R. Geschichte der Gefäßchirurgie. In: Heberer G, van Dongen R, Hrsg. Gefäßchirurgie. Berlin: Springer; 1987.

Draf W. Zur Frage der Rekonstruktion und Lymphknotenausräumung bei Malignomen der Ohrmuschel. In: Müller P, Friedrich H, Petres J, Hrsg. Operative Dermatologie im Kopf-Hals-Bereich. Berlin: Springer; 1984.

Dufourmentel C. Chirurgie réparatrice et correctrice, 2e ed. Paris: Masson & Cie; 1950:325–329.

Dufourmentel C. Chirurgie plastique de l'oreille externe. La Revue du Pratitien. 1958 a;8:3097–3107.

Dufourmentel C. La greffe cutanée libre tubulée. Nouvel artifice technique pour la réfection de l'helix àu cours de la reconstruction du pavillon de l'oreille. Ann Chir Plast Esthet. 1958 b;3: 311–315.

Dufourmentel C. Reconstitution du pavillon de l'oreille. Rev Laryngol Otol Rhinol. 1958 c;59:517–518.

Dufourmentel C, Mouly R. Chirurgie plastique. Editions Medicale Flammarion Paris. 1959;806–808.

Dujon D, Bowditch. The thin tube pedicle: A valuable technique in auricular reconstruction after trauma. Br J Plast Surg. 1995;48: 35–38.

Dupertius SM, Musgrave RH. Experiences with the reconstruction of the congenitally deformed ear. Plast Reconstr Surg. 1959;23: 361–373.

Earley MJ, Bardsley AF. Human bites: a review. Br J Plast Surg. 1984;37:458–462.

Eavey RD. Microtia and Significant Auricular Malformation. Arch Otolaryngol. 1995;121:57–62.

Edgerton MT. Ear construction on children with congenital atresia and stenosis. Plast Reconstr Surg. 1969;43:373–380.

Edgerton MT, Bacchetta CA. Principles in the use and salvage of implants in ear reconstruction. In: Tanzer R, Edgerton MT, eds. Symposium on reconstruction of the auricle. St Louis: CV Mosby & Co; 1974:58–68.

Eisenklam J. Plastische Verkleinerung großer Ohren. Wien Klin Wschr. 1930;38:1176–1178.

Eitner E. 2 Auroplastiken. Münch Med Wschr. 1914;30:1681–1682.

Eitner E. Ohrmuschelersatz. Dtsch Zschr Chir. 1934;242:797–801.

Eitner E. Eine einfache Methode zur Korrektur abstehender Ohren. Wien Klin Wschr. 1937;50:1206.

Elsahy N. Ear replantation combined with local flaps. Ann Plast Surg. 1986 a;77:102–111.

Elsahy N. Reconstruction of the cleft earlobe with preservation of the perforation for an earring. Plast Reconstr Surg. 1986 b;77: 322–324.

Elsahy N. Technique for correction of lop ear. Plast Reconstr Surg. 1990;85:615–620.

Ely ET. An Operation for prominence of the auricle. Arch Otolaryngol. 1881;10:97.

Erich JB. Plastic correction of the lop ear. Proc Staff Meet Mayo Clinic. 1963;38:38–96.

Erich JB. Congenital cup-shaped deformity of the ears transmitted through four generations. Mayo Clin Proc. 1965;40:597.

Ernst H, Besserer A, Flemming J. Strahlenprophylaxe von Keloiden und Narbenhypertrophien. Strahlentherapie. 1979;155:614–617.

Erol Ö, Don Parsa F, Spira M. The use of the secondary island graft flap in reconstruction of the burned ear. Br J Plast Surg. 1981;34:417–421.

Esser J. Methode nouvelle et simple pour resoudre le probleme le plus difficile de la chirurgie plastique facial. La Presse Med. 1935;17:325–326.

Esser JFS. Totaler Ohrmuschelersatz. Münch Med Wschr. 1921; 36:1150–1151.

Esser JFS, Aufricht G. Operativer Ersatz der Ohrdefekte durch "Epithel-Einlage". Arch Klin Chir. 1922;120:518–525.

Farkas LG. Growth of the normal and reconstructed auricles, In: Tanzer RC, Edgerton MT, eds. Symposium on the auricle. St Louis: CV Mosby & Co; 1974:X/24–31.

Farkas LG. Anthropometry of the head and face in medicine. New York: Elsevier; 1981.

Fatah MF. L-plasty technique in the repair of split ear lobe. Br J Plast Surg. 1985;38:410–414.

Federspil P, Welke S. Entzündliche Erkrankungen des äußeren Ohres. Dtsch Ärztebl. 1977;43:2567–2572.

Federspil P. Knochenverankerte Hörgeräte. HNO aktuell. 1994;2: 91–98.

Federspil P. Moderne HNO-Therapie, 2.Aufl. Landsberg: Ecomed; 1987.

Federspil P, Federspil PA. Knochenverankerte aktive Hörimplantate. Dt Ärztebl. 2000;97:528–533.

Feneis H. Anatomisches Bildwörterbuch, 5. Aufl. Stuttgart: Thieme; 1982.

Feuerstein SS. Complications and revisions in otoplasty. Fac Plast Surg. 1985;2:141–151.

Figueroa AA, Polley JW, Ko EW. Maxillary distraction for the management of cleft maxillary hypoplasia with a rigid external distraction system. Semin Orthod Mar. 1999; 5;46–51.

Firmin F. La reconstruction secondaire du pavillon auricular de fruit par bruhure. Ann Chir Plast Esthet. 1995;40:252–263.

Fissette J, Nizet JL. Evaluation de la technique de "Mustardé" dans le traitement des oreilles décollés. Ann Chir Plast Esth. 1992;37: 189–193.

Fitzpatrick IJ. Malignant Melanoma of the Head and Neck – a Clinicopathological Study. Canad J Surg. 1972;15:90.

Fox WJ, Edgerton MT. The fan flap: an adjunct to ear reconstruction. Plast Reconstr Surg. 1976;58:663–667.

Freedlander E, Chung F. Squamous cell carcinoma of the pinna. Br J Plast Surg. 1983;36:171.

Fregenal F, Garcia-Morato V, Salinas V. Surgical correction of lop and cup ear deformities. Eur J Plast Surg. 1992;15:90–93.

Friedmann HS. Otoplasty. Arch Otolaryngol. 1959;70:454–458.

Fritsch MH: Incisionless otoplasty. Laryngoscope. 1995;105:1–11.

Fritze HE, Reich OFG. Von der Otoplastik (Ohrbildung). In: Fritze HE, Reich OFG. Die plastische Chirurgie, in ihrem weitesten Umfange dargestellt und durch Abbildungen erläutert. Berlin: Hirschwald; 1845:110–111.

Fukuda O. The microtic ear: survey of 180 cases in 10 years. Plast Reconstr Surg. 1974;53:458–463.

Fukuda O. Complications and postoperative problems in reconstruction of the microtic ear. Transactions of the Internat Congress of Plastic and Reconstr Surg Sydney; 1988.

Fukuda O. Long-term Evaluation of Modified Tanzer Ear-Reconstruction. Clin Plast Surg. 1990; 17:241–249.

Fuleihan N, Natout M, Webster R, Hariri N, Samara M, Smith R. Successful replantation of amputated nose and auricle. Arch Otolaryngol Head Neck Surg. 1987;97:18–23.

Fumiiri M, Hyakusoku H. Congenital auricular cleft. Plast Reconstr Surg. 1983;70:249–250.

Furnas D. Correction of prominent ears by concha mastoid sutures. Plast Reconstr Surg. 1968;42:189.

Furnas D. Complications of surgery of the external ear. Clin Plast Surg. 1990;17:305–318.

Furnas D. Microtia. In: Vistnes L, ed. Procedures in plastic and reconstructive surgery. How they do it. Boston: Little Brown; 1991:365.

Furukawa M, Mitzutani Z. Hamada T. A simple operative procedure for the treatment of the Stahl's ear. Br J Plast Surg. 1985;38: 544–545.

Gangstrom G, Tjellström A. The bone-anchored hearing aid (BAHA) in children with auricular malformations. Ear Nose Throat J. 1997;76:238–240, 242, 244–247.

Garbe C, Orfanos CE. Epidemiologie des malignen Melanoms – Aktueller Stand in der Bundesrepublik Deutschland. Hautarzt. 1991;41 (Suppl. X):71–79.

Garbe C. Basaliome und Plattenepithelkarzinome der Haut. Forum DKG. 1995;10:285–291.

Gault D, Clement M. Trow R, Kierman M. Removing unwanted hairs by lasers. In: Weerda H, Siegert R, eds. Auricular and Middle Ear Malformations, Ear Defects and their Reconstruction. The Hague/ The Netherlands: Kugler Publications; 1998:129–130.

Gemperli R, Neves R, Ferreira M. Traumatismos extensos do pavilhao auricular: conduta cirurgica. Rev Paul Med. 1991;109:19–23.

Gerow EJ, Spira M, Baron-Hardy S. Plastic surgery applications of synthetic implants. Medical Instrumentation. 1973;7:96–99.

Gersuny R. Über einige kosmetische Operationen. Wien Med Wschr. 1903;48:2253–2257.

Gibson T, Davis WB. The distortion of autogenous cartilage grafts: Its cause and prevention. Br J Plast Surg. 1958;10:257.

Giesen van P, Seaber A, Urbaniak J. Storage of amputated parts prior to replantation – an experimental study with rabbit ears. J Hand Surg. 1983;8:60–65.

Giffin Ch. Wrestler's ear (acute auricular haematoma). Arch Otolaryngol. 1985;111:161–164.

Giffin Ch. Wrestler's ear: pathology and treatment. Ann Plastic Surg. 1992;28:131–139.

Gifford G. Letters to the Editor: Replantation of severed part of an ear. Plast Reconstr Surg. 1972;49:202–203.

Gillies HD. Injuries to the pinna. In: Gillies HD, ed. Plastic surgery of the face. London: Frowde, Hodder and Stoughton Oxford, University Press 1920 a:381–387.

Gillies HD. Plastic surgery of facial burns. Surg Gynecol Obstet. 1920 b;15:121–134.

Gillies HD. Reconstruction of the external ear with special reference to the use of maternal ear cartilage as the supporting structure. Rev Chir Structive. 1937;7:169–179.

Ginestet G, Frézières H, Dupuis A, Pons J. Chirurgie plastique et reconstructive de la face. Éditions Médicales Flammarion Paris; 1967.

Gingrass RP, Pickrell KL. Techniques for closure of conchal and external auditory canal defects. Plast Reconstr Surg. 1968;41:568–571.

Ginsbach G, Busch LC, Kühnel W: The nature of the collagenous capsules around breast implants. Plast Reconstr Surg. 1979,64: 456–464.

Giraldo-Ansio F, Bueno C, Montes J. Butterfly Winged Island Temporoparietal Fascial Flap for Secondary Auricular Reconstruction. Plast Reconstr Surg. 1998;102:831–834.

Goedecke CH. Geschichte der plastisch-rekonstruktiven Chirurgie von erworbenen Ohrmuscheldefekten [Dissertation]. Medizinische Universität zu Lübeck; 1995.

Gohary A, Rangecroft L, Cook R. Congenital Auricular and Preauricular Sinuses in Childhood. Z Kinderchir. 1983;38:81–82.

Goldberg DJ, Littler DM, Wheeland RG. Suspension-assisted Q-switched ND:YAG Laser Hair Removal. Dermatol Surg. 1997, 741–745.

Goldstein MA. The cosmetic and plastic surgery of the ear. Laryngoscope. 1908;18:826–851.

Gonzalez-Ulloa M. An easy method to correct prominent ears. Br J Plast Surg. 1951;4:207–209.

Goodyear HM. Plastic operations for protruding ears. Arch Otolaryngol. 1933;18:527–530.

Gordon SD. "Button" skin repair of an ear defect. Plast Reconstr Surg. 1971;48:190–191.

Gorney M, Falces E, Shapiro R. Spliced autogenous conchal cartilage in secondary ear reconstruction. Plast Reconstr Surg. 1971;47: 432–437.

Grant D, Finlay M, Coers C. Early Management of the Burned Ear. Plast Reconstr Surg. 1969;44:161–166.

Greeley PW. Reconstructive otoplasty, further observations of tantalum wire mesh support. Arch Surg. 1946;53:24–31.

Grossman MC, Dierickx C, Farinelli BS, Flotte A, Anderson RR. Damage to the hair follicles by normal mode ruby laser pulses. J Am Acad Dermatol. 1996;35:889–894.

Grotting J. Otoplasty for congenital cupped and prominent ears using a postauricular flap. Plast Reconstr Surg. 1958;22:164.

Grüner R. Tierexperimentelle Untersuchungen zur Einheilung großer, frei transplantierter composite grafts der Ohrmuschel. [Dissertation] Universität Freiburg; 1985

Gurr E, Yeung A, Al-Azzawi M, Thomson H. The Excised Preauricular Sinus in 14 Years of Experience: Is there a Problem? Plast Reconstr. Surg. 1998;105:1405–1408.

Guyla AJ, Stach B. Hearing aids II. Implantable hearing aids. Arch Otolaryngol Head Neck Surg 1996;122.

Haas E, Meyer R. Composite grafts. In: Gohrbrandt E, Gabka J, Berndorfer A, Hrsg. Handbuch der plastischen Chirurgie, Band II. Berlin: De Gruyter; 1973 a:33/3–33/4.

Haas E, Meyer R. Konstruktive und rekonstruktive Chirurgie der Nase. In: Gohrbrandt E, Gabka J, Berndorfer A, Hrsg. Handbuch der plastischen Chirurgie, Band II/2. Berlin: De Gruyter;1973 b.

Haas E. Oncological principles of the treatment of malignoma of the facial area (in German). Laryngo Rhino Otol. 1982;61:611.

Haas E. Plastische Gesichtschirurgie. Stuttgart: Thieme; 1991.

Hage J. Transposition of the congenital displaced auricle in the first and second branchial arch syndrome. Amsterdam: Excerpta Medica, 1967

Haisch A, Schultz O, Perka C, Jahnke V, Burmester GR, Sittinger M. Tissue engineering of human cartilage tissue for reconstitutive surgery using resorbable fibrin gel and polymer carriers. HNO. 1996;44:624–629.

Haisch A, Kläring S, Gröger A, Gebert C, Sittinger M. A tissue-engineering model for the manufacture of auricular-shaped cartilage implants. Eur Arch Otorhinolaryngol. 2002;259:316–321.

Hakansson B, Liden G, Tjellström A, Ringdahl A, Jacobsson M, Carlsson P, Erlandson BJ. Ten years of experience with the Swedish bone-anchored hearing system. Ann Otol Rhinol Laryngol Suppl. 1990;151:1–16.

Hall JD, Stevenson TR. Congenital ear deformity: reconstruction using composite graft. Ann Plast Surg. 1988;21:145–148.

Hamann C, Manach Y, Roulleau P. Bone anchored hearing aid: Results of bilateral applications. Rev Laryngol Otol Rhinol (Bord). 1991;112:297–300.

Hamblen-Thomas C. Repair for partial loss of the auricle. J Laryng Otol. 1938;53:259–260.

Hammond V. Diseases of the external ear. In: Booth J, ed. Otology, Vol III. 5th ed. London: Butterworth; 1987:156–171.

Hansen PB, Jensen SM. Late results following radiotherapy of skin cancer. Acta Radiol. 1968;7:307–319.

Hartland SH, Proops DW. Bone anchored hearing aid wearers with significant sensorineural hearing losses (borderline candidates): patients' results and opinions. J Laryngol Otol Suppl. 1996;41–46.

Hartmann A, Brunner FX, Burg G, Höhmann D. Tumoren des äußeren Ohres. In: Naumann HH, Helms J, Herberhold C, Kastenbauer E, Hrsg. Band 3: Otologie. Stuttgart: Thieme; 1994:518–544.

Hartman DF, Goode RL. Pharmacologic Enhancement of Composite Graft Survival. Arch Otolaryngol. 1987;133:720–723.

Hasse A, von Domarus H. Reconstruction of midfacial and mandibular complex in cases of hemifacial microsomia. In: Weerda H, Siegert R, eds. Auricular and Middle Ear Malformations, Ear Defects and their Reconstruction. The Hague/The Netherlands: Kugler; 1998:131–137.

Hauben D, Zirkin H, Mahler D, Sacks M. The biologic behavior of basal cell carcinoma: analysis of recurrence in excised basal cell carcinoma Part II. Plast Reconstr Surg. 1982;69:110.

Haug R. Eine Einführung neuer Methoden zur Rücklagerung hochgradig abstehender Ohrmuscheln. Dtsch Med Wschr. 1894;20:776.

Hausamen J, Reuther J, Stoffel J. Experimental reimplantation utilizing microvascular anastomosis in animals. J Maxillofac Surg. 1977;5:203–207.

Hausschild A, Tronier M, Möller M, Achtelik WV, Wolff HH, Christophers E. Aktuelle operative und adjuvante Therapie des Melanoms. Ärztebl SH. 1998;8:6–8.

Hayashi R, Matsuo K, Hirose T. Familial cryptotia. Plast Reconstr Surg. 1993;91:1337–1339.

Hedington JT. Epidermal Carcinomas of the Integument of the Nose and Ear. In: Batsakis JG. Tumors of the Head and Neck, Clinical and Pathological Considerations. Baltimore: Williams & Williams; 1974.

Helms J: Ergebnisse der Mikrochirurgie bei Ohrmissbildungen. Laryngorhinootol. 1987,66:16–18.

Helms J, Knaus C. Techniques and results of reconstrction in malformed middle ears. In: Weerda H, Siegert R, eds. Auricular and Middle Ear Malformations, Ear Defects and their Reconstruction. The Hague/The Netherlands: Kugler; 1998:199–201.

Henrich DE, Logan TC, Lewis RS, Shockly WW. Composite Graft Survival. Arch Otolaryngol. 1995;121:1137–1142.

Heppt W, Trautmann Y. Otoplastik zur Korrektur abstehender Ohrmuscheln. HNO. 1999;47:688–694.

Herrmann A. Fehler und Gefahren bei Operationen am Hals, Ohr und Gesicht. Berlin: Springer; 1968:197.

Hertig P. Les vasocelallulaires de la face et leur traitment. ORL.1978;66–75.

Hildmann H, Rauchfuß A, Hildmann A: Indikation und chirurgische Behandlung der großen Mittelohr-Missbildung. HNO. 1992;40:232–235.

Himi T, Sakata M, Shintani T, Mitsuzawa H, Kamagata M, Satoh J, Sugimoto H. Middle ear imaging using virtual endoscopy and its application in patients with ossicular chain anomaly. ORL J Otorhinolaryngol Relat Spec. 2000;62:316–320.

Hinderer UT. Cirurgia plastica de las deformidades de la oreja. Abstract Book (Film). III Congresso Nacional de Cirurgia Plastica Valencia; 1972.

Hinderer UT, Rio del J, Fregenal F. Otoplasty for lop ear. Aesth Plast Surg. 1987 a;11:75–80.

Hinderer UT, Rio del J, Fregental F. Macrotia. Aesth Plast Surg. 1987 b;11:81–85.

Hirose T, Tomono T, Matsuo K. Cryptotia: Our classification and treatment. Br J Plast Surg. 1985;98:352–360.

His W. Anatomie menschlicher Embryonen. Band III. Leipzig: FCW Vogel; 1885.

Hohan M, Appukuttan P, Skinivasan A. Earlobe Reconstruction with a Preauricular Flap. Past Reconstr Surg. 1978;62:267–270.

Holgers KM, Tjellström A, Bjursten LM, Erlandsson BE. Soft tissue reactions around percutaneous implants: a clinical study of soft tissue conditions around skin-penetrating titanium implants for bone- anchored hearing aids. Am J Otol. 1988; 9:56–59.

Holgers KM, Thomsen P, Tjellström A, Ericson LE, Bjursten LM. Morphologic evaluation of clinical long- term percutaneous titanium implants. Int J Oral Maxillofac Implants. 1994;9:689–696.

Hollinger J. Factors of osseous repair and delivery: part I. J Craniofac Surg. 1993 a;4;102–108.

Hollinger J. Factors of osseous repair and delivery: part II. J Craniofac Surg. 1993 b;4;135–141.

Holmes EM. The microtic ear. Arch Otolaryngol. 1949;49:243–265.

Horlock N, Grobbelaar A, Gault D. 5-year series of constricted (lop and cup) ear correction. Development of the mastoid hitch as an adjunctive technique. Plast Reconstr Surg. 1998;102:2325–2332.

Husstedt HW, Prokop M, Dietrich B, Becker H. Low-dose high-resolution CT of the petrous bone. J Neuroradiol. 2000;27:87–92.

Ilizarov GA. Basic principles of transosseous compression and distraction osteosynthesis. Ortop Travmatol Protez. 1971;32;7–15.

Ilizarov GA. The tension-stress effect on the genesis and growth of tissues. part I. The influence of the stability of fixation and soft tissue preservation. Clin Orthop. 1989 a;238;249–281.

Ilizarov GA. The tension-stress effect on the genesis and growth of tissues. part II: The influence of the rate and frequency of distraction. Clin Orthop. 1989 b;239;263–285.

Jackson IT. Local flaps in head and neck reconstruction. St Louis: CV Mosby & Co; 1985 a:251–272.

Jackson IT. Local flaps in head and neck reconstruction. St Louis: CV Mosby & Co; 1985 b;327–412.

Jacobsson M, Albrektsson T, Tjellstöm A. Tissue-integrated implants in children. Int J Pediatr Otorhinolaryngol. 1992;24:235–243.

Jahrsdoerfer RA. Congenital Ear Atresia. In Tanzer RC, Edgerton MT, eds. Symposium on reconstruction of the auricle. St Louis C. V. Mosby. 1974;150–160.

Jahrsdoerfer RA: Congenital Atresia of the Ear. Laryngoscope. 1978;88:1–48.

Jahrsdoerfer RA: Surgical correction of congenital malformations of the sound-conducting system. In: Shambaugh G, Glosscock M, eds. Surgery of the ear. Philadelphia: Saunders; 1980:380–407.

Jahrsdoerfer RA, Cole RR, Gray LC. Advances in congenital aural atresia. Adv Otolaryngol. 1991;5:1–15.

Jahrsdoerfer RA, Yeakley JW, Aguilar EA et al. Grading System for the Selection of Patients with Congenital Aural Atresia. Amer J Otol. 1992;13:6–12.

Jahrsdoerfer RA. Transposition of the facial nerve in congenital aural atresia. Am J Otol. 1995;16:290–294.

Jahrsdoerfer RA, Lambert PR. Facial nerve injury in congenital aural atresia surgery. Am J Otol. 1998;19:283–287.

Jahrsdoerfer RA, Yeakley JW, Hall JW, Robbins KT, Gray LC. High resolution CT scanning and auditory brainstem response in aural atresia: patient selection and surgical correlation. Otolaryngol Head and Neck Surgery 1985; 93: 292–8.

Jayes PH. The treatment of prominent ears. Br J Plast Surg. 1951;4:193–201.

Jörgensen G. Mißbildungen im Bereich der Hals-Nasen-Ohrenheilkunde. Arch Otorhinolaryngol. 1972;202:1–50.

Joseph J. Demonstration operierter Eselsohren. Verl Berl Med Ges; 1896:I/206.

Joseph J. Die Gestaltungsfehler der Ohren. In: Katz L, Preysing H, Blumenfeld F, Hrsg. Handbuch der speziellen Chirurgie des Ohres. Würzburg; Kabitzsch; 1912 a:167.

Joseph J. Korrektive Nasen- und Ohrenplastik. In: Katz L, Preysmy, Blumenfeld F, Hrsg. Handbuch der speziellen Chirurgie des Ohres und der oberen Luftwege. Würzburg: Kabitzsch; 1912 b.

Joseph J. Ohrdefekte (Otoneoplastik). In: Joseph J. Nasenplastik und sonstige Gesichtsplastik. 3. Abteilung. Leipzig: Kabitzsch; 1931:717–736.

Joseph V, Jacobsen A. Single Stage Excision of Preauricular Sinus. Aus NZ J Surg. 1995;65:254–256.

Jost G, Danon J, Hadjean E, Mahe E, Vertut J. Reparations plastiques des pertes de substances cutanées de la face. Paris: Librairie Arnette; 1977 a.

Jost G, Legent F, Meresse B, Ocker K. Atlas der ästhetischen plastischen Chirurgie. Stuttgart: Schattauer; 1977 b.

Ju DMC. The psychological effect of protruding ears. Plast Reconstr Surg. 1963 a;31:424–427.

Ju DMC, Li C, Crikelair GF. The surgical correction of protruding ears. Plast Reconstr Surg. 1963 b;32:283–293.

Jung EG. Lichtbiologie der Melanome. Hautarzt. 1991;41 (Suppl. X): 79–80.

Juri J, Irigaray A, Juri C, Grilli D, Blanco C, Vazquez G. Ear replantation. Plast Reconstr Surg. 1987;80:431–435.

Kaban LB, Moses MH, Mulliken JB. Surgical correction of hemifacial microsomia in the growing child. Plast Reconstr Surg. 1988; 82; 9–19.

Kaeseman L. Feststellung von Normwerten der Ohrmuschel der Mitteleuropäer mittels kephalometrischer computergestützer Messverfahren [Dissertation]. Lübeck 1991.

Kaplan H, Hudson D. A novel surgical method of repair for STAHL's ear: A case report and review of current treatment modalities. Plast Reconstr Surg. 1999;103:566–569.

Kaps C, Bramlage C, Smolian H, Haisch A, Ungethum U, Burmester GR, et al. Bone morphogenetic proteins promote cartilage differentiation and protect engineered artificial cartilage from fibroblast invasion and destruction. Arthritis Rheum. 2002;46: 149–162.

Karhuketo TS, Ilomaki JH, Dastidar PS, Laasonen EM, Puhakka HJ. Comparison of CT and fiberoptic video-endoscopy findings in congenital dysplasia of the external and middle ear. Eur Arch Otorhinolaryngol. 2001;258:345–348.

Kastenbauer E. Spezielle Rekonstruktionsverfahren im Gesichtsbereich. Arch Otorhinolaryngol. 1977;216:123–250.

Katsaros J, Tan E, Sheen R. Microvascular ear replantation. Br J Plast Surg. 1988;41:496–499.

Kaufmann R, Landes E. Dermatologische Operationen – Farbatlas und Lehrbuch der Hautchirurgie. Stuttgart: Thieme; 1987.

Kaufmann R, Weber L, Rodermund OE. Kutane Melanome – Klinik und Differentialdiagnose. Basel: Editiones Roche; 1989.

Kaye L. A simplified method for correcting the prominent ear. Plast Reconstr Surg. 1967;40:44–48.

Kazanjian V. Surgical treatment of congenital deformities of the ears. Am J Surg. 1958;95:185–188.

Kazanjian V, Converse J. Traumatic deformities of the auricle. In: Reconstructive Plastic Surgery. 3rd Edition. Philadelphia: Saunders Co; 1959 a;1289–1298.

Kazanjian V, Converse J. Traumatic amputation of eyelid, nose or ear. In: Kazanjian V, Converse J, eds. Surgical Treatment of Facial Injuries. 3rd Edition. Baltimore Maryland: Williams & Wilkins Co; 1959 b;121–122.

Keen W. New method of operating for relief of deformity from prominent ears. Ann Surg. 1890;49.

Kelleher JC, Sullivan JG, Baiba KGJ, Dean KK. The wrestler's ear. Plast Reconstr Surg. 1967;40:540–546.

Kiese-Himmel C, Kruse E. Unilateral hearing loss in childhood. An empirical analysis comparing bilateral hearing loss. Laryngo Rhino Otol. 2001;80:18–22.

Kimmelmann C, Lucente F. Use of ceftazidine for malignant external otitis. Ann Otol. 1989;98:721–725.

Kirkham HLD. The use of preserved cartilage in ear reconstruction. Ann Surg. 1940;111:896–902.

Kirschner M. Allgemeine und spezielle chirurgische Operationslehre. Band III/1. Berlin: Springer; 1935.

Kischer CW et al. Hypertrophic Scars and Keloids: A Review and New Concept Concerning their Origin. Scan Electon Microsc 1982;4:1699–1713.

Kislov R. Surgical correction of the cupped ear. Plast Reconstr Surg. 1971;48:121–125.

Klein C. Mittelgesichtsdistraktion bei einem Patienten mit Crouzon-Syndrom. Mund Kiefer Gesichts Chir. 1998;2 (Suppl 1);52–57.

Koll Y, Ernst K, Hundeiker M. Keratoakanthosis der Ohmuscheln. HNO. 1993;41:532–535.

Kon M. Fascia lata suspension of malpositioned ear. Plast Reconstr Surg. 1996; 98: 167

König F. Die Krankheiten des äusseren Ohres. In: König F. Lehrbuch der speziellen Chirurgie für Ärzte und Studierende. Band I. Berlin: Hirschwald; 1885;475–476.

König F. Zur Deckung von Defekten der Nasenflügel. Berl Klin Wochenschr. 1902;39:137–138.

Koonin AJ. The Aetiology of Keloids: A Review of the Literature and a New Hypothesis. S Afr Med J. 1964;38:913–916.

Koopman CF, Coulthard SW. A postauricular muscle-skin flap for conchal defects. Laryngoscope. 1982;92:596–598.

Koplin L, Zarem H. Recurrent basal cell carcinoma. Plast Reconstr Surg. 1980;65:656.

Körner O. Mechanische Verletzungen. Kontinuitätstrennung an der Ohrmuschel. In: Körner O. Lehrbuch der Ohren-, Nasen- und Kehlkopfheilkunde. Wiesbaden: Bermann; 1918;395.

Körte W. Fall von Ohrenplastik. Sitzung am 13.11 1905. Verh Fr Vrgg Chir Berlins. 1905;18:91–92.

Kotthaus E, Blatt HJ, Schröder F. Freie autologe Transplantation von composite grafts unter Veränderung physikalischer Bedingungen. In: Schuchardt K, Schilli W, Hrsg. Fortschritte Kiefer- und Gesichtschirurgie. Stuttgart: Thieme; 1978;Bd.XIII/9–11.

Kountakis SE, Helidonis E, Jahrsdoerfer RA. Microtia grade as an indicator of middle ear development in aural atresia. Arch Otolaryngol Head and Neck Surgery 1995;121:885–886.

Krespi YP, Ries WR, Shugar JMA, Sisson GA. Auricular reconstruction with postauricular myocutaneous flap. Otolaryngol Head Neck Surg. 1983;91:193–196.

Krüger E. Die Knorpeltransplantation. Anwendung in der Kiefer- und Gesichtschirurgie. München: Hanser; 1964.

Krummel F. Korrektur angeborener Ohrmuscheldeformitäten. Arch Otorhinolaryngol. 1986;Suppl II:130–131.

Kunte C, Wolff H. Aktuelle Therapie der Hypertrichosen. Hautarzt. 2001;52:993–997.

Kurt P, Federspil P. Knochenverankerte Epithesen und Hörgeräte. Eine Übersicht. In: Ganz H, Schätzle W, Hrsg. HNO Praxis Heute. Berlin: Springer; 1994;157–77.

Lackmann GM, Draf W, Isselstein G, Töllner U. Surgical treatment of facial dogbite injuries in children. J Cran Max Surg. 1992;20: 81–86.

Lam HCH, Soo G, Wormald PJ. Excision of the Preauricular Sinus: A Comparison of two Surgical Techniques. Laryngoscope. 2001;111:317–319.

Lambert PR. Congenital aural atresia: stability of surgical results. Laryngoscope. 1998;108:1801–1805.

Landthaler M, Hohenleutner U, Abdel-Raheem I. Laser therapy of childhood haemangiomas. Br J Dermatol. 1995;133:275–281.

Landthaler M, Hohenleutner U. Lasertherapie in der Dermatologie. Berlin: Springer; 1999:110.

Langrana NA et al. Effect of mechanical load in wound healing. Ann Plast Surg. 1983;10:200–208.

Larsen J, Pless J. Replantation of severed ear parts. Plast Reconstr Surg. 1976;57:176–179.

Lasjaunias P, Berenstein A. Surgical Neuroangiography. Berlin: Springer; 1987:84–96.

Lask G, Elman M, Slatkine M. Laser-assisted hair removal by selective photothermolysis: preliminary results. Dermatol Surg. 1997;23:737.

Laskin D, Donohue W. Treatment of human bites of the lip. J Oral Surg. 1958;16:236.

Lautenschlager S, Etin PH, Rufti T. The petrified ear. Dermatology. 1994;189:435–436.

Lawrence WT. In Search of the Optimal Treatment of Keloids: Report of a Series and a Review of the Literature. Little Brown Ca, 1991.

Ledermann M. Malignant tumours of the ear. J Laryngol Otol. 1965;71:85.

Lee D, Nash M, Har-El G. Regional Spread of Auricular and Periauricular Cutaneous Malignancies. Laryngoscope. 1996;106:998–1001.

Lee K, MacKeen ME, McGregor EA. Metastatic Patterns of Squamous Carcinoma in the Parotid Lymph Node. Brit J Plast Surg. 1985;38:6.

Lee Y and Lee E. Correction of low-set ears. Plast Reconstr Surg. 1999; 104: 1982

Leemans R, Middelweerd R, Vuyk H. Facial Reconstructive Surgery. Academic Report Wageningen; Pousen & Loojen: 2000.

Lefebvre A, Munro I: The role of psychiatry in a craniofacial team. Plast Reconstr Surg 61 (1978) 564–569

Lehmann J, Cervino L. Replantation of the severed ear. J Trauma. 1975;15:929–930.

Lehmuskallio E, Lindholm H, Koskenvuo K et al. Frostbite of the face and ears: epidemiological study of risk factors in Finnish conscripts. BMJ. 1995;311:1661–1663.

Lehnhardt E. Die operative Korrektur der abstehenden Ohrmuschel. Laryngorhinootol. 1959;38:316–319.

Leiber B. Ohrmuscheldystopie, Ohrmuscheldysplasie und Ohrmuschelmißbildung – klinische Wertung und Bedeutung als Symptom. Arch Otorhinolaryngol. 1972;202:51–84.

Lejour M. The cheek island flap. In: Bohnert H, Hrsg. Plastische Chirurgie des Kopf- und Halsbereichs und der weiblichen Brust. Stuttgart: Thieme; 1975.

Lemmen M. Exzision von Keloiden nur in Ausnahmefällen. Dt Ärztebl. 1995;92:B-1466.

Lerner RM, Gellert E: Body build identification. Preference and aversion in children. Develop Psychol 1 (1969) 456–462

Lettermann GS, Harding RL. The management of the hairline in ear reconstruction. Plast Reconstr Surg. 1956;18:199–207.

Lever WF, Schaumburg-Lever G. Histopathology of the Skin. 7th ed. Philadelphia: Lipp u. Cott; 1999.

Levin BC, Adams CA, Becker GD. Healing by Secondary Intention of Auricular Defects After Mohs Surgery. Arch Otolaryngol. 1996;122:59–67.

Lewis E, Fowler J. Two replantations of severed ear parts. Plast Reconstr Surg. 1979;64:703–705.

Lexer E. Ersatz der Ohrmuschel. In: König F, von Eiselsberg A, Körte W, Hildebrand O. Arch Klin Chir. 1910 a;3:774–778.

Lexer E. Zur Gesichtsplastik. III. Ersatz der Ohrmuschel. Arch Klin Chir. 1910 b;92:774–793.

Lexer E. Otoplastik, Ohrbildung. In: Coenen et al, Hrsg. Chirurgie des Kopfes. Stuttgart: Enke; 1921:731–735.

Lexer E. Die gesamte Wiederherstellungschirurgie. Bd. I. Leipzig: Barth; 1933:441.

Liew SH, Ladhani K, Grobelaar AO, Gault DT et al. Ruby Laser-Assisted Hair Removal: Success in Relation to Anatomic Factors and Melanin Content of Hair Follicles. Plast Reconst Surg. 1999; 103:1736–1743.

Limberg A. Planimetrie und Stereometrie der Hautplastik. Jena: Fischer; 1967.

Lindig M, Weerda H, Siegert R. Postoperative Schmerztherapie mittels on-demand-Analgesie nach Ohrmuschelaufbau mit Rippenknorpel. Laryngo Rhino Otol. 1997;76:379–383.

Lockwood CD. Plastic surgery of the ear. Surg Gynecol Obstet. 1929;49:392–394.

Löffler JA, Siegert R, Bruker D, Jäger H, Weerda H. Use of Electroepilation for Removing Unwanted Hair. In: Weerda H, Siegert R, eds. Auricular and Middle Ear Malformations, Ear Defects and their Reconstruction. The Hague/The Netherlands: Kugler; 1998 a:45–58.

Löffler JA, Siegert R, Bruker D, Landwehr FJ, Jäger H, Weerda H. Use of Electroepilation for Removing Unwanted Hair. Face. 1998 b;6:45–50.

Lorenz S, Brunnberg S, Landthaler M, Hohenleutner U. Hair removal with the long pulsed Nd:YAG Laser: a prospective study with one year follow-up. Lasers in Surg Med. 2002;1–8.

Lowe LH, Vezina LG. Sensorineural hearing loss in children. Radiographics. 1997;17:1079–1093.

Luckett H. A new operation for prominent ears based on the anatomy of the deformity. Surg Gynecol Obstet. 1910;10:635.

Lueders HW. One-stage enlargement of the burned ear. Plast Reconstr Surg. 1966;37:512–516.

Lundt HZ, Greensborough. How often does squamous cell carcinoma of the skin metastasize? Arch Dermatol. 1965;92:635.

Lüthi A. Eine einfache Methode zur Korrektur abstehender Ohren. Zbl Chir. 1930;801.

Lynch JB, Pousti A, Doyle JE, Lewis SR. Our experiences with silastic ear implants. Plast Reconstr Surg. 1972;49:283–285.

Macgregor FC, Abel TM, Bryt A, Lauer E, Weissman S. Facial deformities and plastic surgery. Charles C Thomas Publisher, Springfield, Illinois (1953)

Macgregor FC: Transformation and Identity: The face and plastic surgery. The New York Times Book Company (1974)

Macgregor FC: Ear deformities: Social and psychological implications. Clin Plast Surg 5 (1975) 347–350

Mack MG, Vogl TJ, Dahm MC, Pegios W, Balzer JO, Hammerstingl R, Söllner O, Felix R. Wertigkeit der hochauflösenden MRT für die Darstellung normaler und pathologischer Strukturen des Innenohrs. Klinische Neuroradiologie. 1997;7:77–82.

Macomber DW. Plastic mesh as a supporting medium in ear construction. Plast Reconstr Surg. 1960;25:248–252.

Malbec EF, Beaux AR. Reconstruccion del pabellon auricular. Prensa Méd Argent. 1952;39:3301–3304.

Mall R. Der Einfluß der Ischämiedauer von 2, 5 und 10 Stunden bei Raumtemperatur auf die Einheilung als freies Composite graft [Dissertation]. Freiburg: Universität Freiburg 1989.

Manach Y, Perrin A, Depondt J, Hamann C. La chirurgie plastique des aplasies du pavillon. A propos de 65 cas. Ann Otolaryngol. 1987;104:599–605.

Maniglia A, Maniglia J, Witten B. Otoplasty – an elective technique. Laryngoscope. 1977;87:1359–1368.
Maniglia A, Maniglia J. Kongenitale Fehlbildungen des äußeren Ohres. Extracta Otorhinolaryngol. 1981;3:415–425.
Manktelow RT. Mikrovaskuläre Wiederherstellungschirurgie. Berlin: Springer; 1986.
Martin G. Operationsresultate nach Ohrmuschelanlegeplastiken. HNO. 1976;24:134–137.
Marx H. Die Mißbildungen des Ohres. In: Denker-Kahler, Hrsg. Handbuch der HNO-Heilkunde. Bd. 6/1. Berlin: Springer; 1926.
Marx H. Kurzes Handbuch der Ohrenheilkunde. Jena: Fischer; 1938; 807.
Masson J. A simple island flap for reconstruction of concha-helix defects. Br J Plast Surg. 1972;25:399–403.
Mastroiacovo P, Corchia C, Botto LD, Lanni R, Zampino G, Dusco D: Epidemiology and genetics of microtia-anotia: A registry based study on over one million births. J Med Genet 32 (1995) 453–457
Matsuo K, Hiroje T, Tomono T, Iwasawa M et al. Nonsurgical correction of congenital auricular deformities in the early neonat: a preliminary report. Plast Reconstr Surg. 1984;73:38–50.
Matsuo K, Hirose T. A splint for nonsurgical correction of cryptotia. Eur J Plast Surg. 1989;12:186–187.
Matsuo K. Nonsurgical correction of congenital auricular deformities. Clin Plast Surg. 1990;17:383–395.
Matsuo K, Hirose T. Reconstruction of the crus helicis in mild microtia using a preauricular tag. Plast Reconstr Surg. 1991;88:890–894.
Matthews D. Storage of skin for autogenous grafts. Lancet. 1945;23:775–778.
Matthews D. Reconstruction of the ear. Fortschr Kiefer Gesichtschir. Bd.VII. Stuttgart: Thieme. 1961;96–101.
Maurer J, Mann W, Welkobosky H-J. Zur Therapie des Othämatoms und des Otseroms. HNO. 1990;38:214–216.
Mavili ME, Safak T, Özgür F, Erk S. Correction of congenital constricted ears using a chondrocutaneous postauricular flap. Eur J Plast Surg. 1996;16:177–179.
Mc Collough G, Hom D. Correction of the enlarged earlobe: Auricular lobuloplasty – an adjunictive face-lift procedure. Laryngoscope. 1989;99:1193–1194.
Mc Coy F. Macrotia. In: Aesthetic surgery of the ear. 1972.
Mc Evitt WG. The problem of the protruding ear. Plast Reconstr Surg. 1947;2:481–497.
Mc Laren LR. Surgery of the external ear. J Laryngol Otol. 1974;88:23–38.
Mc Nichol JW. Total helix reconstruction with tubed pedicles following loss by burns. Plast Reconstr Surg. 1950;6:373–386.
McCarthy JG, Schreiber J, Karp N, Thorne TH, Grayson BH. Lengthening the human mandible by gradual distraction. Plast Reconstr Surg. 1992;89; 1–8.
Mehra Y, Dubey S, Mann S, Suri S. Correlation between High-resolution Computed Tomography and Surgical Findings in Congenital Aural Atresia. Arch Otolaryngol. 1988;114:137–141.
Mellette R. Ear reconstruction with local flap. J Dermatlog Surg Oncol. 1991;17:176–182.
Melnick M,Myrianthopoulos NC: External ear malformations: Epidemiology, genetics, and natural history. Birth Defects: Original Article Series, Alan Liss, New York 15 (1979)
Mercer DM, Studd DM. "Oyster-splint": a new compression device for the treatment of keloid scars of the ear. Br J Plast Surg. 1983;36:75–78.
Messner AH, Crysdale WS. Otoplasty: Clinical Protocol and Long-term Results. Arch Otolaryngol. 1996;122:773–777.
Meyer R. Rekonstruktion der Ohrmuschel mit Nylonimplantat bei kongenitaler Aplasie. Mschr Ohrenheilk. 1955 a;89:18.
Meyer R. Über Ohrmuscheltransplantate. Pract Oto-Rhino-Laryng. 1955 b;17:440–447.
Meyer R, Sieber H. Konstruktive und rekonstruktive Chirurgie des Ohres. In: Gohrbrandt, Gabka, Berndorfer, Hrsg. Handbuch der Plastischen Chirurgie. Bd.II/3. Berlin: De Gruyter; 1973:1–62.
Millard DR. The chondrocutaneous flaps in partial auricular repair. Plast Reconstr Surg. 1966;37:523.
Millard DR, McCafferty LR, Prado A. A simple direct-correction of the constricted ear. Br J Plast Surg. 1988;41:619–623.
Millay DJ, Larrabee F, Dion T. Nonsurgical correction of auricular deformities. Laryngoscope. 1990;100:910–913.
Mimouni-Bloch A, Metzker A, Mimouni M. Severe folliculitis with keloid scars induced by wax epilation in adolescents. Cutis 1997;59: 41–42.
Minderjahn A, Hüttl WJ, Hildmann H. Früh- und Spätergebnisse nach Ohrmuschelreliefplastik, In: Schuchardt K, Hrsg. Fortschritte der Kiefer- und Gesichtschirurgie. Bd. XXIV. Stuttgart: Thieme; 1979.
Mir y Mir L. The role of the meniscus of the knee in plastic surgery. Plast Reconstr Surg. 1952;10:431–443.
Mladick R, Horton C, Adamson J, Cohen B. The pocket principle. Plast Reconstr Surg. 1971;48:219–223.
Mladick R, Curraway J. Ear reattachment by the modified pocket principle. Plast Reconstr Surg. 1973;51:584–587.
Mohan M, Appukuttan P, Srinivasan A. Earlobe reconstruction with a preauricular flap. Plast Reconstr Surg. 1978;62:267–270.
Mohs F. Chemosurgery, a microscopically controlled method of cancer excision. Arch Surg. 1941;42:279.
Mohs F. Chemosurgical Treatment of Cancer of the Ear: A Microscopically Controlled Method of Excision. Surgery. 1947;21:605.
Mohs F. Fixed tissue micrographic surgery for melanoma of the ear. Arch Otolaryngol Head Neck Surg. 1988;114:625.
Monks GH. Operations for correcting the deformity due to prominent ears. Boston Med Surg. 1891;124:84–86.
Moore GF, Moore IJ, Yonkers AJ, Nissen AJ: Use of full thickness skin grafts in canalplasty. Laryngoscope 1984;94:1117–1118.
Moore JR. Correction of congenital cupping of the ear. Chir Plast. 1977;4:57–62.
Moore MH, Guzmann-Stein G, Proudman TW, Abbott AH, Netherway DJ, David DJ. Mandibular lengthening by distraction for airway obstruction in Treacher-Collins Syndrome. J Craniofac Surg. 1994;5;22–25.
Moreno-Arias GA, Tiffon T, Marti T, Campos-Fresneda A. Urticaria vasculitis induced by diode laser photo-epilation. Dermatol Surg 2000;26:1082–1083.
Morestin MH. Reposition et dur plissement cosmétique du pavillon de l'oreille. Rev Orthop. 1903;4:289.
Moser A, Wespi HH. Korrektur abstehender Ohrmuscheln: Eine Verlaufskontrolle. Aktuelle Probleme der Otorhinolaryngologie. 1991;95:97–105.
Muck O. Mechanische und psychisches Trauma. In: Denker A, Kahler O, Hrsg. Handbuch der Hals-Nasen-Ohrenheilkunde. Die Krankheiten des Gehörganges III. Band III. Berlin: Springer, München: Bergmann; 1927:321–325.
Müller R, Petres J. Semimaligne und maligne Tumoren der Haut im Kopf-Hals-Bereich (semimalignant and malignant tumours in the head and neck region, in German). In: Müller R, Friedrich H, Petres J, Hrsg. Operative Dermatologie im Kopf-Hals-Bereich. Berlin: Springer; 1984.
Mündnich K. Die wiederherstellende Ohrmuschelplastik. In: Sercer A, Mündnich K. Plastische Operationen an der Nase und an der Ohrmuschel. Stuttgart: Thieme; 1962 a:325–382 u. 411–451.
Mündnich K. Stellungs- und Formanomalien der Ohrmuschel (einschl. Ohrmißbildungen) und ihre operative Behandlung. Arch Ohr-Nas-Kehlk-Heilk. 1962 b;180:395–402.
Mündnich K, Terrahe K. Mißbildungen des Ohres. In: Berendes J, Link R, Zöllner F, Hrsg. Hals-Nasen-Ohrenheilkunde. Bd. V. 2.Aufl. Stuttgart: Thieme; 1979.
Muraoka M, Nakai Y, Ohashi Y, Furukawa M. A simple prosthesis for correction of cryptotia. Laryngoscope. 1984;94:243–248.
Muraoka M, Nakai Y, Ohashi Y, Sasaki T et al. Tape attachment for corrections of congenital malformations of the auricle, clinical and experimental studies. Laryngoscope. 1985;95:167–175.

Murray JE, Kaban LB, Mulliken JB. Analyses and treatment of hemifacial microsomia. Plast Reconstr Surg. 1984;74;186–99.

Müsebeck K, Knorpelbrückenplastik bei Katzenohrmißbildungen. Laryngo Rhino Otol. 1970;49:20–25.

Musgrave RH. A variation on the correction of the congenital lop ear. Plast Reconstr Surg. 1966;37:394–398.

Musgrave RH, Garret WS. Management of avulsion injuries of the external ear. Plast Reconstr Surg. 1967;40:534–539.

Mustardé JC. Effective formation of antihelix fold without incising the cartilage. In: Transactions of the International Society of Plastic Surgeons, Second Congress, AB Wallace. Baltimore: Williams & Wilkens; 1960.

Mustardé JC. The correction of prominent ears. Using simple mattress sutures. Br J Plast Surg. 1963;16:170–176.

Mustardé JC. The treatment of prominent ears by buried mattress sutures: a ten-year survey. Plast Reconstr Surg. 1967;39:382–386.

Mutimer K, Banis J, Upton J. Microsurgical reattachment of totally amputed ears. Plast Reconstr Surg. 1987;79:535–540.

Mylanus EA, Cremers CW. A one-stage surgical procedure for placement of percutaneous implants for the bone-anchored hearing aid. J Laryngol Otol. 1994;108:1031–1035.

Nagata S. A new method of total reconstruction of the auricle for microtia. Plast Reconstr Surg. 1993;92:187–201.

Nagata S. Modification of the stages in total reconstruction of the auricle: Part I. Grafting the three-dimensional costal cartilage framework for lobule-type microtia. Past Reconstr Surg. 1994a, 221–230.

Nagata S. Modification of the stages in total reconstruction of the auricle. Part II: Grafting the three-dimensional costal cartilage framework for concha type microtia. Plast Reconstr Surg. 1994b;93:231–242.

Nagata S. Modification of the stages in total reconstruction of the auricle: Part III. Grafting the three-dimensional costal cartilage framework for small concha type microtia. Plast Reconstr Surg. 1994c;93:243–253.

Nagata S. Modification of the stages in total reconstruction of the auricle: Part IV: Ear elevation for the constructed auricle. Plast Reconstr Surg. 1994d;93:254–266.

Nagel F. The reconstruction of partial auricular loss. Plast Reconstr Surg. 1972;49:340.

Nagel F. Die Wiederherstellung der menschlichen Ohrmuschel im Tierversuch. Arch klin exp Ohr-Nas-Kehlk-Heilk. 1973;205: 166–170.

Nagel F. Fehler bei der Otoplastik – ihre Verhütung nach Korrektur. In: Düben H et al, Hrsg. Fehler und Gefahren in der plastischen Chirurgie. Stuttgart: Thieme; 1978.

Nahai F, Hyhurst J, Saliblin A. Microvascular surgery in avulsive trauma to the external ear. Clin Plast Surg. 1976;5:423–426.

Nakai H, Ishii Y, Ozaki S, Sezai Y. Use of resurfaced temporoparietalis flap in total ear reconstruction with less-than-favorable skin coverage. Aesth Plast Surg. 1984;8:253–258.

Nakajima T, Yoshimura Y, Kami T. Surgical and Conservative Repair of Stahl's Ear. Aesth Plast Surg. 1984;8:101–107.

Nanni CA, Alster TS. Optimizing treatment parameters for hair removal using a topical carbon-based solution and 1064-nm Q-switched neodymium: YAG-laser energy. Arch Dermatol. 1997;133:1546.

Nanni CA, Alster T. Laser-assisted hair removal:side effects of Q-switched Nd:YAG, long-pulsed ruby and alexandrite lasers. J Am Acad Dermatol. 1999;41:165–171.

Navabi A. One-stage reconstruction of partial defect of the auricle. Plast Reconstr Surg. 1964;33:77–79.

Nelaton C, Ombredanne L. Troisième partie otoplastie. In: Nelaton C, Ombredanne L. Les Autoplasties. Paris: Steinheil; 1907:125–198.

Neumann CG. The expansion of an area of skin by progressive distension of a subcutaneous balloon. Plast Reconstr Surg 1957;19:124–130.

Niehaus HH, Olthoff A, Kruse E. Early detection and hearing aid management of pediatric unilateral hearing loss. Laryngo Rhino Otol. 1995;74:657–662.

Nielsen F, Kristensen S, Crawford M. Prominent Ears: A follow-up study. J Laryngol Otol. 1985;95:221–224.

Niparko J, Swanson N, Baker S, Telian St, Sullivan M, Kemink J. Local control of auricular, preauricular, and external canal cutaneous malignancies with Mohs surgery. Laryngoscope. 1990;100:1047.

Nolst-Trenite GJ. A Modified Anterior Scoring Technique. Facial Plastic Surg. 1994;10:255–266.

Nomura Y, Nagao Y, Fukaya T. Anomalies of the middle ear. Laryngoscope 1988; 98: 390.

Nordström R, Salo H, Rintala A. Auricle Reconstruction with the Help of Tissue Expansion. In: Nordström R, ed. Tissue Expansion in Facial Plastic Surgery 1988; 5:338–346.

Norris JE. Superficial X-Ray-Therapy in Keloid Management: A Retrospective Study of 24 Cases and Literature Review. Plast Reconstr Surg. 1995;95:1051–1056.

O'Connor GB, Pierce GW. Refrigerated cartilage isografts. Surg Gynecol Obstet. 1938;67:796.

Ohlsen L. Reconstructing the antihelix of protruding ears by perichondrioplasty: A modified technique. Plast Reconstr Surg. 1980;92:753–762.

Olsen EA. Methods of hair removal. J Am Acad Dermatol. 1999;40:143–155.

Ombredanne L. Reconstruction autoplastique de la moitié du pavillon de l'oreille. La Presse Medicale. 1931;53:982–983.

Ono I, Gunji H, Sato M, Kaneko F. A method of treatment for constricted ears with a conchal cartilage graft to the posterior auricular plane. Plast Reconstr Surg. 1993;92:621–627.

Oppermann P, Siegert R, Weerda H. Knochenverankerte Hörgeräte in der plastischen und funktionellen Rehabilitation von Kindern mit Fehlbildungen des Ohres. In: Gross M, Hrsg. Aktuelle phoniatrisch-pädaudiologische Aspekte. Bd. 3. Berlin. 1996.

Osguthorpe JP. Head and neck burns. Arch Otolaryngol. 1991;117:969–974.

Otto HD. Pathologie der Aurikularanhänge, Melotie und Polyotie. Arch Otorhinolaryngol. 1979;225:45–56.

Otto HD. Pathogenese der branchiogenen Überschußbildungen. HNO-Praxis. 1983;8:161–169 u. 247–257.

Padgett EC. Total reconstruction of the auricle. Surg Gynecol Obstet. 1938;67:761–768.

Paley D, Rumley TO, Kovelmann H. The Ilizarov technique: A method to regenerate bone and soft tissue. In: Habal MB, Levin ML, Morain WD, eds. Advances in Plastic and Reconstructive Surgery. Chicago: Mosby; 1991:1–40.

Pardue AM. Repair of torn earlobe with preservation of the perforation for an earring. Plast Reconstr Surg. 1973;51:472–473.

Park Ch, Shin K, Kang H et al. A new arterial flap form the postauricular surface. Plast Reconstr Surg. 1988;82:498–504.

Park Ch, Chung S. Reverse-flow postauricular arterial flap for auricular reconstruction. Ann Plast Surg. 1989;23:369.

Park Ch, Lineaweaver WC, Rumley TO, Buncke HJ. Arterial supply of the anterior ear. Plast Reconstr Surg. 1992;90:38–44.

Park Ch, Roh T. Button-down procedure for correction of cleft earlobe malformation. Plast Reconstr Surg. 1997;99:1429–1432.

Park Ch. Lower Auricular Malformations: Their Representation Correction, and Embryologic Correlation. Plast Reconstr Surg. 1999;104:29–40.

Park Ch, Dae-Hyun L, Won-Min Y. An Analysis of 123 Temporoparietal Fascial Flaps: Anatomy and Clinic in Total Auricular Reconstruction. Plast Reconstr Surg. 1999;104:1295–1306.

Park Ch, Roh TS. Total Ear Reconstruction in the Devascularized Temporoparietal Region: I. Use of the Contralateral Temporoparietal Fascial Free Flap. Plast Reconstr Surg. 2001;108: 1145–1153.

Park Ch. Balanced auricular reconstruction in dystopic microtia with the presence of the external auditory canal. Plast Reconstr Surg. 2002; 109: 1489

Passow A. Die Operationen am Gehörgang: Othämaton. In: Bier, Braun, Kümmel, Hrsg. Chirurgische Operationslehre. Band II. Leipzig: Barth; 1923:7.

Paver K, Poyzen K, Burry et al. The Incidence of Basal Cell Carcinoma and their Metastasis in Australia and New Zealand. Aust J Dermatol. 1977;14:53.

Peer LA. The fate of living and dead cartilage transplanted in humans. Surg Gynecol Obstet. 1939;68:603–609.

Peer LA. Diced cartilage grafts. Arch Otolaryngol. 1943;38:156–165.

Peer LA, Walker JC. Plastic surgery summaries of the bibliographic material available in the field of otolaryngology. Arch Otolaryngol. 1955;61:664.

Peer LA, Walker JC. Total reconstruction of the ear. J Int Coll Surg. 1957;27:290–304.

Pegram N, Peterson R. Repair of partial defects of the ear. Plast Reconstr Surg. 1956;18:305.

Pellnitz D. Über das Wachstum der menschlichen Ohrmuschel. Arch Ohrenheilk Z Halsheilk. 1958;171:334–340.

Pennington D, Lai M, Pelly A. Successful replantation of a completely avulsed ear by microvascular anastomosis. Plast Reconstr Surg. 1980;65:820–823.

Pennisi VR, Klabunde EH, McGregor M, Brown O, Connor G, Pierce GW, Fagella R. The use of MARLEX 50 in plastic and reconstructive surgery. Plast Reconstr Surg. 1962;30:254–262.

Pennisi VR, Klabunde EH, Pierce G. The preauricular flap. Plast Reconstr Surg. 1965;35:552--556.

Petres J, Rompel R. Operative Dermatologie. Berlin: Springer; 1996.

Pierce GW. Reconstruction of the external ear. Surg Gynecol Obstet. 1930;50:601–605.

Pierer H. Rekonstruktion und Replantation der Ohrmuschel. Chir Plast Reconstr. 1967;3:112–124.

Pitanguy I: Consideracoes sobre a cirurgia reconstructora da orelha. Rev Brasil Chir. 1958;36:258–266.

Pitanguy I. Ansiform ear-correction by "island" technique. Acta Chir Plast. 1962;4:267–277.

Pitanguy I, Flemmings I. Plastische Eingriffe an der Ohrmuschel. In: Naumann HH, Hrsg. Kopf- und Halschirurgie. Band 3. Stuttgart: Thieme; 1976 a;1–69.

Pitanguy I, Flemmings I. Ohrmuschelrekonstruktion. In: Naumann HH, Hrsg. Kopf- und Halschirurgie. Band 3. Stuttgart: Thieme; 1976 b;31–48.

Pitanguy I. Ear reconstruction. In: Pitanguy I. Aesthetic plastic surgery of head and body. Berlin: Springer; 1981;323–341.

Plester D, Katzke D. The promontorial window technique. Laryngoscope 1983;93:824.

Pollet J, Mahé E. Contribution a l'étude de la chirugie reconstructive dans les aplasies d'oreille unilaterales. Ann Chir Plast. 1964;9: 35–44.

Pollet J. Chirurgie plastique et reconstructive du pavillon de l'oreille. Arnette Medicale de France. 1966 a;73:535–539.

Pollet J. Résultats des reconstitutions du pavillon de l'oreille par des greffes composées. Ann Chir Plast. 1966 b;11:270–274.

Postnick JC, Al-Quatta MM, Whitaker LA. Assessment of the preferred vertical position of the ear. Plast Reconstr Surg. 1993;91:1198.

Potsic W, Naunton R. Reimplantation of an amputated pinna. Arch Otolaryngol Head Neck Surg. 1974;100:73–75.

Powell RH, Burrell SP, Cooper HR, Proops DW. The Birmingham bone anchored hearing aid programme: paediatric experience and results. J Laryngol Otol Suppl. 1996;21:21–29.

Prasad S, Grundfast K, Milmoe G. Management of Congenital Preauricular Pit and Sinus Tract in Children. Laryngoscope. 1990;100:320–321.

Proops DW. The Birmingham bone anchored hearing aid programme: surgical methods and complications. J Laryngol Otol Suppl. 1996;21:7–12.

Psillakis JM. Prominent ears: evolution of a surgical technique. Aesthetic Plast Surg. 1979;3:147–152.

Purcell F. Two cases of the external ear completely cut off and successfully replanted. Lancet. 1898;6:1616–1617.

Quatela V, Cheney M. Reconstruction of the auricle. In: Baker SH, Swanson N, eds. Local flaps in facial reconstruction. St Louis: CV Mosby & Co; 1995:443–479.

Radovan C. Advantages and complications of breast reconstruction using temporary expander. Plast Surg Forum. 1980;3:63.

Ragnell A. A new method of shaping deformed ears. Br J Plast Surg. 1951;4:202.

Rapaport D, Breitbart A, Karp N, Siebert J. Successful microvascular replantation of a completely amputated ear. Microsurgery. 1993;14:312.

Rasinger GA, Arnoldner M, Wicke W. Spätergebnisse der Korrektur abstehender Ohrmuscheln. Laryngorhinootol. 1983;62:328–330.

Rassner G, d'Hoedt B, Stroebel W, Stutte H. Melanomnachsorge – Integriertes Nachsorgekonzept der Tübinger Hautklinik sowie Ergebnisse einer Umfrage zur Melanomnachsorge an deutschen Hautkliniken. Hautarzt. 1991;41 (Suppl. X) :94–97.

Rauber-Kopsch. Lehrbuch und Altas der Anatomie des Menschen. Band I. 19. Aufl. Stuttgart: Thieme;1955;138.

Rauber-Kopsch. Lehrbuch und Atlas der Anatomie des Menschen, Band III. Nervensystem und Sinnesorgane. Leonhardt H, Töndury G, Zilles K, Hrsg. Stuttgart: Thieme; 1987.

Raulin C, Greve B. Aktueller Stand der Photoepilation. Hautarzt 2000;51:809–817.

Reichert H. Moderne Operationsverfahren zur plastischen Wiederherstellung und Korrektur der Ohrmuschel. Aesthet Med. 1963;1:18–28.

Reichert H. Konturverbessernde Operationen an der Ohrmuschel durch gezielte Veränderung des Spannungsgefüges im Knorpelgerüst. Fortschr Kiefer-Gesichts-Chir. 1979;24:140–143.

Reid CA, McCarthy JG, Kolber AB. A study of regeneration in parietal defects in rabbits. Plast Reconstruct Surg. 1981;67;591–596.

Remmert S, Sommer K, Weerda H. Freie Transplantate. In: Weerda H. Plastisch-rekonstruktive Chirurgie im Gesichtsbereich. Stuttgart: Thieme; 1999;125–136.

Remmert S, Sommer K, Weerda H. Free Flaps. In: Weerda H. Reconstructive Facial Plastic Surgery. Stuttgart; Thieme; 2001;125–136.

Renard A. Postauricular flaps based on a dermal pedicle for ear reconstruction. Plast Reconstr Surg. 1981;68:159–165.

Rhys-Evans PH. Prominent ears and their surgical correction. J Laryngootol. 1981;95:881–892.

Rhys-Evans PH. The anterior scoring technique. Fac Plast Surg. 1985;2:93.

Rich J, Gottlieb V, Shesol BF. A simple method for correction of the pixie earlob. Plast Reconstr Surg. 1982;69:136–138.

Richter E, Feyerabend T. Normal lymphnode topography: CT-Atlas. Berlin: Springer; 1991.

Richter E. Feyerabend T. Grundlagen der Strahlentherapie. Berlin: Springer; 1996.

Rigg BM. Future Material in Otoplasty. Plast Reconstr Surg. 1979;63:409–410.

Roberts AC. Facial Prostheses. London: Henry Kimpton Publishers; 1971:2.

Rodgers GK, Applegate L, De la Cruz A, Lo W. Magnetic resonance angiography: analysis of vascular lesions of the temporal bone and skull base. Am J Otol. 1993;14:56–62.

Rogers BO. Microtic, lop, cup and protruding ears: four directly inheritable deformities. Plast Reconstr Surg. 1968;41:208–231.

Rogers BO. Anatomy, Embryology and Classification of Auricular Deformities. In: Tanzer R, Edgerton M, eds. Symposium on reconstruction of the auricle. St Louis: CV Mosby & Co; 1974:3–11.

Romo T. Otoplasty using the postauricular skin flap technique. Arch Otolaryngol Head Neck Surg. 1994;120:1146–1150.

Roosa DB. Lehrbuch der praktischen Ohrenheilkunde. Berlin: Hirschwald; 1889.

Russ JE. Aspiration Cytology of Head and Neck Masses. Amer Surg. 1978;136:342.

Ruttin E. Eine Methode zur Korrektur abstehender Ohren. Monatsschr Ohrenheilk. 1910;44:196–199.

Sadove R. Successful replantation of a totally amputated ear. Ann Plast Surg. 1990;24:366–370.

Safak T, Özcan G, Kecik A, Gürsu G. Microvascular ear replantation with no vein anastomosis. Plast Reconstr Surg. 1993;92:945–950.

Salyapongse A, Lorenzo P, Suthunyarat P. Successful replantation of a totally severed ear. Plast Reconstr Surg. 1979;64:706–707.

Sanders B, McKelvy B: Split-thickness skin grafts transplanted over exposed maxillary bone in dogs. J Oral Surg. 1976,34:510–513.

Sanvero-Rosselli G. La chirurgie plastique du pavillon de l'oreille. Rev Chir Plast. 1932;2:27–53.

Schanz F. Wiederersatz einer verlorengegangenen Ohrmuschel. Korrespondenz-Blätter des allgem Ärztl Vereins von Thüringen. 1890;19:288–293.

Schewior S. Die Behandlung des Ohrmuschelabrisses. Ein geschichtlicher Überblick [Dissertation]. Medizinische Universität zu Lübeck; 1995.

Schiffmann NJ. Squamous cell carcinoma of the skin of the pinna. Can J Surg. 1975;18:279–283.

Schmidt H. Die Ohrmuschel in der Medizin des 19. und 20. Jahrhunderts und die Entwicklung der Anlegeplastik [Dissertation]. Medizinische Universität zu Lübeck; 2000.

Schmieden L. Ohrverletzungen. Berl Klin Wschr. 1908;81:1433–1435.

Schmieden V. Der plastische Ersatz von traumatischen Defekten der Ohrmuschel. Berl Klin Wschr. 1908;45:1433–1435.

Schoeneich H, Biemer E. Versorgung akuter Gesichtsverletzungen in mikrochirurgischer Technik. Langenbecks Arch Chir. 1987;372:697–699.

Schorn K, Stecker M. Hörgeräteanpassung im Kindesalter. In: Naumann HH, Helms J, Herberhold C, Kastenbauer E, Hrsg. Oto-Rhino-Laryngologie in Klinik und Praxis. Band I. Stuttgart: Thieme. 1994;835–836.

Schrader B, Chilla R, Lawory S, Brandt G. Zur Metastasierung der Ohrmuschelkarzinome. HNO. 1988;36:84–87.

Schrode K, Huber F, Staszak J, Altman DJ, Shander D, Morton J. Randomized, double-blind, vehicle-controlled safety and efficacy evaluation of eflornithine 15% cream in the treatment of women with exessive facial hair. Poster presented at the 58th annual meeting of the American Academy of Dermatology.

Schuchardt K. Grundsätzliches zur primären und sekundären Defektdeckung nach der Operation von gutartigen und bösartigen Gesichtstumoren. Chir Plast Rekonstr. 1967;3:180.

Schuffenecker J. Conduite à tenir vis-à-vis de la réimplantation post-traumatique du pavillon de l'oreille. Ann Chir Plast Esthet. 1991;36:353–359.

Schuknecht HF: Congenital aural atresia. Laryngoscope 1989;99: 908–917.

Schulz H. Operative Eingriffe im Gesicht. Praxisfähige Eingriffe. Berlin: Diesbach; 1988.

Schütze E. Zur Korrektur abstehender Ohrmuscheln. Chirurg. 1956;27:273.

Schwager K, Helms J. [Facial nerve abnormalities in malformed temporal bone] (in German). Laryngorhinootologie. 1995;74:549–552.

Schwartz PW. Maßnahmen zur Früherkennung von Hautkrebs in der Bundesrepublik Deutschland. Dtsch Ärztebl. 1980;3:123.

Schwartze H. Handbuch der Ohrenheilkunde. Band I. Leipzig: FCW Vogel; 1892.

Scott M, Klaasen M. Immediate reconstruction of the helical skin after bite injury using the posterior auricular flap. Injury. 1992;23:333–335.

Seemann MD, Seemann O, Bonel H, Suckfull M, Englmeier KH, Naumann A, Allen, CM, Reiser MF: Evaluation of the middle and inner ear structures: comparison of hybrid rendering, virtual endoscopy and axial 2D source images. Eur Radiol. 1999;9: 1851–1858.

Sefrin P. Notfalltherapie im Rettungsdienst. 3. Aufl. München: Urban & Schwarzenberg; 1991.

Seltzer AP. Plastic surgery of prominent auricle. Arch Otolaryngol. 1954;60:316.

Sénéchal G, Pech A. Chirurgie du pavillon de l'oreille. Texte und Atlas. Paris: Librairie Arnette; 1970.

Sercer A, Mündnich A. Plastische Operationen an der Nase und an der Ohrmuschel. Stuttgart: Thieme; 1962.

Setou M, Kurauchi T, Tsuzuku T, Kaga K. Binaural interaction of bone-conducted auditory brainstem responses. Acta Otolaryngol. 2001;121:486–489.

Sexton RP. Utilization of the amputated ear cartilage. Plast Reconstr Surg. 1955;15:419–422.

Siegert R. Synopsis of Otoplasty. Facial Plast Surg. 2004;20:299–230.

Siegert R, Weerda H, Hoffmann S, Mohadjer C. Klinische und experimentelle Untersuchungen zur intermittierenden, intraoperativen Kurzzeitexpansion. Arch Ohren-, Nasen- und Kehlkopfheilkunde Suppl. II. 1991 a;223–224.

Siegert R, Weerda H, Hoffmann S, Mohadjer C. Clinical and experimental evaluation of intermittent intraoperative short-term-expansion. Plast Reconstr Surg. 1991 b;92:248–254.

Siegert R, Weerda H, Löffler JA, Gromoll B. Subkutane Hautexpansion im Hundemodell – Beeinflussung der epidermalen Mitoserate und dermalen Vaskulation. HNO-Information. 1993;18:107.

Siegert R, Weerda H. Die Hautexpansion. Teil 1: Technische und physiologische Grundlagen. HNO. 1994 a;42:124–137.

Siegert R, Weerda H. Die Hautexpansion. Teil 2: Klinische Anwendung und Komplikationen. HNO. 1994 b;42:182–194.

Siegert R, Weerda H, Löffler J. Baretton G. Die epidermale Proliferationsrate nach Hautexpansion im Hundemodell. Laryngol Rhinol Otol. 1994 a;73:206–208.

Siegert R, Weerda H, Remmert S. Die Rekonstruktion der teilamputierten Ohrmuschel. In: Zilch H, Schumann E, Hrsg. Plastisch-rekonstruktive Maßnahmen bei Knochen- und Weichteildefekten. Stuttgart: Thieme, 1994 b:59–60.

Siegert R, Weerda H, Remmert S. Embryology and Surgical Anatomie of the Auricle. Fac Plast Surg. 1994 c;10:232–243.

Siegert R, Weerda H, Mayer T, Brückmann H. Bildgebende Verfahren: Hochauflösende Computertomographie fehlgebildeter Mittelohren. HNO-Informationen. Mitteilungen der DG für HNO-Heilkunde, Kopf- und Hals-Chirurgie. 1995 a;1:101.

Siegert R, Wössmann D, Weerda H. Untersuchungen zur technischen Sicherheit von Expanderventilen. HNO. 1995 b;43:654–663.

Siegert R, Knölker U, Konrad E. Psychosoziale Aspekte der totalen Ohrmuschelrekonstruktion bei Patienten mit schwerer Mikrotie. Laryngo Rhino Otol. 1996 a;75:155–161.

Siegert R, Weerda H, Mayer T, Brückmann H. Hochauflösende Computertomographie fehlgebildeter Mittelohren. Laryngo Rhino Otol. 1996 b;75:187–194.

Siegert R, Weerda H. Die Technik nach Crikelair und der abstehende Lobulus. Laryngo Rhino Otol. 1997;76:715.

Siegert R, Rohweder J, Witte J, Weerda H. Knochenleitungshörgerät mit Flüssigkeitsankopplung. WMW 147. 1997;10:244–248.

Siegert R, Weerda H. The Crikelair Technique for Correction of the Protruding Lobule. Eur Arch Otorhinolaryngol. 1998;255:88.

Siegert R, Danter J, Löffler A, Jurk V, Eggers R, Weerda H. Tissue selective thining of short-term expanded skin with ultrasound and powerful water-jet. An animal study. Face. 1998 a;6:51–58.

Siegert R, Krappen S, Kaesemann L, Weerda H. Computer-assisted anthropometry of the auricle. Face. 1998 b;6:1–6.

Siegert R, Weerda H: Two step external ear canal construction in atresia as part of auricular reconstruction. Laryngoscope 2001,111:708–714.

Silbergleit R, Quint DJ, Mehta BA, Patel SC, Metes JJ, Noujaim SE. The persistent stapedial artery. AJNR Am J Neuroradiol. 2000;21: 572–577.

Simo R. Jones NS. Head bandaging following otoplasty – how we do it. J Laryngol Otol. 1994;108:410–412.

Simons J. Cryptotia. The role of the prosthesis in correction of the ear deformities. In: Tanzer R, Edgerton MT, eds. Symposium on reconstruction of the auricle. St Louis: CV Mosby & Co; 1974:X.

Smahel J, Converse JM. Anatomical Features of Auricular and Retroauricular Skin. Chir Plastica. 1980;5:1139–1145.

Smith F. Plastic and reconstructive surgery: a manual of management. Philadelphia: Saunders & Co; 1950:468.

Smith H. Plastic operation for restauration of the auricle, following injury from an explosion. Ann Otol Rhinol Laryng. 1917;26: 831–833.

Smith HW. Calibrated otoplasty. Laryngoscope. 1979;89:657–665.

Smith R, Dickinson J, Cipcic J. Composite grafts in facial reconstructive surgery. Arch Otolaryngol Head Neck Surg. 1972;95:252–264.

Smith RA. The free fascial scalp flap. Plast Reconstr Surg. 1980;66:204.

Snik AF, Dreschler WA, Tange RA, Cremers CW. Short and long-term results with implantable transcutaneous and percutaneous bone conductive devices. Arch Otolaryngol Head Neck Surg. 1998;124:265–268.

Snik AF, Mylanus EA, Cremers CW. The bone-anchored aid in patients with a unilateral air-bone gap. Otol Neurotol. 2002;23:61–66.

Snik FM, Beynon AJ, van der Pouw CTM, Mylanus EAM, Cremers WRJ. Binaural application of the bone-anchored hearing aid. Ann Otol Rhinol Laryngol. 1998;107:187–193.

Snik FM, Teunissen B, Cremers WRJ. Speech recognitation in patients after successful surgery for unilateral congenital ear anomalies. Laryngoscope. 1994;104:1029–1034.

Sobin LH, Wittekind Ch, eds. UICC TNM Classification of Malignant Tumours, 6th ed. Chichester:Wiley;2002

Sommer H, Kux A, Siegert R, Weerda H, Schmielau F, Eder R. Richtungshörvermögen von Patienten mit unilateraler Atresia auris congenita. HNO. 1998;46:460.

Sommer H, Siegert R, Weerda H: Möglichkeiten der Hörgeräteversorgung bei ausgeprägter Schalleitungsschwerhörigkeit. Bone Anchored Applications. 2001;1:12–14.

Song R, Chen Z, Yang P, Yue J. Reconstruction of the external ear. Clin Plast Surg. 1982 a;9:49–52.

Song R, Gad Y, Song Y et al. The forearm flap. Clin Plast Surg. 1982 b;9:21.

Spira M, Hardy. Management of the injured ear. Am J Surg. 1963;106:678–684.

Spira M. Correction of the principal deformities causing protruding ears. Plast Reconstr Surg. 1969;44:150–154.

Spira M. Early care of deformities of the auricle resulting from mechanical trauma. In: Tanzer RC, Edgerton MT, eds. Symposium on reconstruction of the auricle. St Louis: CV Mosby & Co; 1974;X:204–217.

Stadler R, Orfanos CE. Neue Chemotherapien und kombinierte immunochemotherapeutische Verfahren beim malignen Melanom. Hautarzt. 1991;41 (Suppl X):87–94.

Staindl O. Über Misserfolge und Komplikationen nach Ohrmuschelanlegeplastiken. Laryngo-Rhino-Otol. 1986;65:646–657.

Staindl O. Zur Korrektur der abstehenden Ohrmuschel. HNO. 1980;28:234–240.

Stal S, Spira M. Long-term results in otoplasty. Fac Plast Surg. 1985;2:153–165.

Stark RB, Saunders DE. Natural Appearance Restored to the Unduly Prominent Ear. Br J Plast Reconstr Surg. 1962;15:385–397.

Steffanoff DN. Auriculo-mastoid tube pedicle for otoplasty. Plast Reconstr Surg. 1948;3:352–360.

Steffen A: Die Verletzungen der Ohrmuschel – eine retrospektive Analyse von Ursachen und Behandlungskonzepten (Dissertation), Medical Faculty of the University of Lübeck, Germany, 2004.

Steffensen WH. Comments on total reconstruction of the ear. Plast Reconstr Surg. 1952;10:186–190.

Steigleder GK. Therapie der Hautkrankheiten. 3. Aufl. Stuttgart: Thieme; 1986.

Stenström SJ. A "Natural" technique for correction of congenitally prominent ears. Plast Reconstr Surg. 1963;32:509–518.

Stenström SJ. Cosmetic deformities of the ears. In: Graff WC, Smith JW, eds. Plastic surgery: a concise guide to clinical practice. Boston: Little Brown & Co; 1968;522.

Stenström SJ. Cosmetic deformities of the ear. In: Graff WC, Smith JW, eds. Plastic surgery: a concise guide to clinical practice. 2nd Ed. Boston: Little Brown & Co; 1973;603–604.

Stephenson K. Correction of a lop ear type deformity. Plast Reconstr Surg. 1960;26:540.

Stern J, Lucente F. Carbon Dioxide Laser Excision of Earlobe Keloids. Arch Otolaryngol. 1989;155:1107–1111.

Steuer G. Erfahrungen mit Ohrmuschelkorrekturen [Dissertation]. Berlin: 1979.

Stevenson DS, Proops DW, Wake MJC, Deadman MJ, Worollo SJ, Hobson JA. Osseointegrated implants in the management of childhood ear abnormalities: the initial Birmingham experience. J Laryngol Otol. 1993;107:502–509.

Straith CL, De Kleine EH: Plastic surgery in children: The medical and psychologic aspects of deformity. J Am Med Ass 1938;111: 2364–2370

Strauch B, Sharzer L, Petro J, Greenstein B. Replantation of amputated parts of the penis, nose, ear and scalp. Clin Plast Surg. 1983;10:115–124.

Strauss J. Über Weichteilprothesen. Zürich: Berichthaus; 1924.

Streeter GC. Devolopment of the auricle in the human embryo. Contrib Embryol. 1922;95:300–303.

Streit R. Einige plastische Operationen an der Ohrmuschel. Arch Ohrenheilk; 1914:95:300–303.

Strutz J, Mann W. Die Duplikatur des Gehörganges. Laryng Rhinol Otol. 1989;68:694–697.

Stucker F, Shaw G, Boyd S, Shockley W. Management of Animal and Human Bites in Head and Neck. Arch Otolaryngol Head Neck Surg. 1990;116:789–793.

Sudhoff H. Untersuchungen zur nicht operativen Verformbarkeit der Ohrmuschelform des Kaninchens [Dissertation]. Bochum: 1996.

Sultan G. Chirurgie des Ohres. In: Sultan G. Grundriss und Atlas der speziellen Chirurgie. Teil I. München: JF Lehmann's; 1907: 238–240.

Swartz JD. Sensorineural hearing deficit: a systematic approach based on imaging findings. Radiographics. 1996;16:561–574.

Sylven B, Hamberger CA. Malignant Melanoma of the External Ear. Ann Otol Rhinol Laryngol. 1950;59:631.

Szymanowski von J. Ohrbildung, Otoplastik. In: Szymanowski von J. Handbuch der operativen Chirurgie. Braunschweig: F Vieweg & Sohn; 1870;303–306.

Tagliacozzi T. De curtorum chirurgia per insitionem. Libri duo, Venetia 1597, Berlin: Recognovit et editit Max Troschel, G. Reimer; 1931.

Tan S. Shibu M, Gault D. A splint for correction of congenital ear deformities. Br J Plast Surg. 1994;47:575–578.

Tanaka Y, Tajima S. Completely successful replantation of an amputated ear by microvascular anastomosis. Plast Reconstr Surg. 1989;84:665–668.

Tanzer RC. Total reconstruction of the external ear. Plast Reconstr Surg. 1959;23:1–15.

Tanzer RC. Total reconstruction of the external auricle. Arch Otolaryngol. 1961;73:64–68.

Tanzer RC. The correction of prominent ears. Plast Reconstr Surg. 1962;30:236–246.

Tanzer RC. An analysis of ear reconstruction. Plast Reconstr Surg. 1963 a;31:16–30.
Tanzer RC. Ear reconstruction – an exercise in design. Surg Clin North Am. 1963 b;43:1271–1276.
Tanzer RC. Ear reconstruction – a progress report. Trans Third Internat Cong Plast Surg Washinton. 1963 c;480–487.
Tanzer RC. The reconstruction of acquired defects of the ear. Plast Reconstr Surg. 1965;35:355–365.
Tanzer RC. Total reconstruction of the auricle: a ten-year report. Plast Reconstr Surg. 1967 a;40:547–550.
Tanzer RC. Ear reconstruction. A second progress report. Trans Fourth Internat Cong Plast Surg Rome. 1967 b;644–646.
Tanzer RC. Secondary reconstruction of microtia. Plast Reconstr Surg. 1969;43:345–350.
Tanzer RC. Total reconstruction of the auricle. The evolution of a plan of treatment. Plast Reconstr Surg. 1971;47:523–533.
Tanzer RC. Reconstruction of the auricle. In: Goldwyn RM, ed. The unvavorable result in plastic surgery. Boston: Little Brown; 1972:147–157.
Tanzer RC, Rueckert F. Reconstruction of the ear. In: Grabb W, Smith J. Plastic Surgery, Boston: Little Brown; 1973;494.
Tanzer RC. Correction of the microtia with autogenous costal cartilage. In: Tanzer RC, Edgerton MT, eds. Symposium on reconstruction of the auricle. St Louis: CV Mosby & Co; 1974 a;X:46–57.
Tanzer RC. Secondary reconstruction of the auricle. In: Tanzer RC, Edgerton MT, eds. Symposium on reconstruction of the auricle. St Louis: CV Mosby & Co; 1974 b;X:238–247.
Tanzer RC. Correction of microtia with autogenous costal cartilage. In: Tanzer RC, Edgerton MT, eds. Symposium on reconstruction of the auricle. St Louis: CV Mosby & Co; 1974 c;X.
Tanzer RC. Discussion to Davis J: Repair of severe cup ear deformities. In: Tanzer RC, Edgerton MT, eds. Symposium on reconstruction of the auricle. St Louis: CV Mosby & Co;1974 d;X:134–142.
Tanzer RC. The constricted cup and lop ear. Plast Reconstr Surg. 1975;55:406–415.
Tanzer RC. Congenital deformities. In: Converse JM, ed. Reconstructive plastic surgery. Philadelphia: Saunders; 1977:1671–1719.
Tanzer RC, Bellucci RJ, Convers JM, Brent B. Deformities of the auricle. In: Converse JM, ed. Reconstructive plastic surgery. Philadelphia: Saunders; 1977:1671–1719.
Tanzer RC. Microtia – a long-term follow-up of 44 reconstructed auricles. Plast Reconstr Surg. 1978 a;61:161–166.
Tanzer RC. Microtia. Clin Plast Surg. 1978 b;5:317–336.
Tanzer RC. Total reconstruction on the external ear. Ann Plast Surg. 1983;10:76–85.
Tanzer RC. Discussion to Matsuo K, Hirose T et al. Plast Reconstr Surg. 1984:73.
Tanzer RC. Discussion to Brent B. Technical advances in ear reconstruction. Personal experience with 1200 cases. Plast Reconstr Surg. 1999;104:335–338.
Tarabey F. Remise en place de deux pertes de substance importantes du pavillon de l'oreille. Ann Chir Plast Esteht. 1981;26:380–382.
Tateshita T, Ono I. One-stage reconstruction of microtia in microform. Plast Reconstr Surg. 1999;103:179–185.
Taylor R. Shortening long legs and lengthening short legs: a new surgical procedure. Am J Orth Surg. 1916;14;598–606.
Tebbetts J. Auricular reconstruction: selected single-stage techniques. J Dermatol Surg Oncol. 1982;8:557–566.
Tegtmeier R, Gooding R. The use of a fascial flap in ear reconstruction. Plast Reconstr. Surg. 1977;60:406–411.
Templer J, Davis WE, Thomas JR. A rotation flap for low posterior auricular defects. Laryngoscope. 1981;91:826–828.
Tenta LT, Keyes GR. Reconstructive surgery of the external ear. Otolaryngol Clin North Am. 1981;14:917–938.
Thomson H, Kim TY, Ein SH. Residual problems in chest donor sites after microtia reconstruction: a long-term study. Plast Reconstr Surg. 1995;95:961.
Tilgen W. Kaufmann R. Malignes Melanom. Forum DKG. 1995;10:310–323.
Tilkorn H, Lüerssen W, Ernst K. Keloide und hypertrophe Narben, Vortrag Berlin 1990.
Tjellstrom A, Yontchev E, Lindström J, Branemark PJ. Five years experience with bone anchored auricular prostheses. Otolaryngology Head Neck Surg. 1985;93:366–372.
Tjellström A. Titanimplantate in der Hals- Nasen- Ohren- Heilkunde. HNO. 1989;37:309–314.
Tjellström A, Granström G. Long-term follow-up with the bone-anchored hearing aid: a review of the first 100 patients between 1977 and 1985. Ear Nose Throat J. 1994;73:21–23.
Tjellström A, Hakansson B. The bone-anchored hearing aid. Design principles, indications and long-term clinical results. Otolaryngol Clin North Am. 1995;28:53–72.
Tolleth H. Artistic anatomy, dimensions and proportions of the external ear. Clin Plast Surg. 1978;5:337–345.
Tolsdorff P, Walter C. Technik und Anwendungsbereich des retroaurikulären Insellappens. Laryngo Rhino Otol. 1974;53:887.
Toplak FH. Die Totalrekonstruktion der Ohrmuschel (the total reconstruction of the auricle, in German) [Dissertation]. Berlin: Universitätsklinikum Steglitz; 1986.
Tramier H. Personal Approach to Treatment of Prominent Ears. Plast Reconstr Surg. 1995;99:562–565.
Trendelenburg 1886, cit. after Joseph 1931.
Troha FV, Baibak GJ, Kelleher JC. Auriculo-mastoid tube pedicle for partial ear reconstruction. Plast Reconstr Surg. 1990;86: 1037–1038.
Tsai T. Experimental and clinical application of microvascular surgery. Ann Surg. 1975;181:169–171.
Turpin I. Ear replantation: a case report. J Reconstr Microsurg. 1987;4:39–41.
Turpin I, Altman D, Cruz H, Achauer B. Salvage of the Severely Injured Ear. Clin Plast Surg. 1988;17:397–403.
Uysal O, Kecik A. Gürsu G. Congenital auricular clefts. Eur J Plast Surg. 1990;13:178–181.
Vacanti CA, Langer R, Schloo JP. Synthetic polymers seeded with chondrocytes provide a template for new cartilage formation. Plast Reconstr Surg 1991;88:753–759.
Van der Pouw KT, Snik AF, Cremers CW. Audiometric results of bilateral bone-anchored hearing aid application in patients with bilateral congenital aural atresia. Laryngoscope 1998;108:548–553.
Vecchione TR. Needle scoring of the anterior surface of the cartilage in otoplasty. Plast Reconstr Surg. 1979;64:568.
Vogel K. Operative subcutane Verkleinerung der Ohrmuschel. 15. Jhr-Vers Ges Dt HNO. Bonn. 1938;366–367.
Vogl A. Abstehende Ohren. Aesthet Med. 1961;10:149–151.
Wachsberger A. Successful auricular autotransplantation. Arch Otolaryngol. 1947;46:549–551.
Walster E, Aronson V , Abrahams D, Rottman L: Importance of physical attractiveness in dating behavior. J Personal Soc Psychol 1966;4:508–516
Walter C. Die Anwendung der sogenannten composite grafts in der plastischen Chirurgie im Hals-, Nasen- und Ohrbereich. In: HNO-Wegweiser für die fachärztliche Praxis. Berlin: Springer: 1966;7:200–205.
Walter C. Die Probleme der Rekonstruktion der Ohrmuschel. HNO. 1969;17:301–305.
Walter C. Cartilage incision and excision technique. Fac Plast Surg. 1994 a;10:277–286.
Walter C. Revision otoplasty and special problems. Fac Plast Surg. 1994 b;10:298–308.
Wazen JJ, Spitzer J, Ghossaini SN, Kacker A, Zschommler A. Results of the bone-anchored hearing aid in unilateral hearing loss. Laryngoscope 2001;111:955–958.
Webster JP. Refrigerated skin grafts. Am Surg. 1944;120:431.
Weerda H. Retentionselemente für Ohrmuschelepithesen (Attachments for Auricular Prostheses). HNO. 1972;20:83–86.

Weerda H. Attachements for facial prostheses. Sonderheft des First International Symposium on Facial Prosthetics. Arnheim/NL. 1976:43.

Weerda H. Die Defektdeckung mit Nahlappen nach Exstirpation von Tumoren in der Ohrregion. Laryngo Rhino Otol 1978;57:93–98.

Weerda H. Bemerkungen zur Ohrmuschelplastik und zum Ohrmuschelabriß. Laryngo Rhino Otol 1979 a;53:242–251.

Weerda H. Covering Defects after Exstirpation of Tumours in the Ear Region. ORL. 1979 b;4:33.

Weerda H. Das Ohrmuscheltrauma. HNO. 1980 a;28:209–217.

Weerda H. Plastisch-rekonstruktive Chirurgie im Hals-Nasen-Ohrenbereich, Hamburg-Norderstedt: Ethicon; 1980 b:2–13.

Weerda H. Bemerkungen zur Chirurgie der Ohrmuschelmißbildung. Arch Otorhinolaryngol. 1981;231;606–609.

Weerda H, Münker G. Einzeitige Rekonstruktion von Ohrmuscheldefekten mit einem Transpositions-Rotations-Lappen. Laryngo Rhino Otol. 1981;60:312–317.

Weerda H. Unsere Erfahrungen mit der Chirurgie der Ohrmuschelmißbildungen. Teil I: Die Chirurgie einfacher Missbildungen. Laryngo Rhino Otol. 1982 a;61: 346–349

Weerda H. Unsere Erfahrungen mit der Chirurgie der Ohrmuschelmißbildungen. Teil II: Die Chirurgie der Makrotie und des Tassenohres. Larygo Rhino Otol. 1982 b;350–353.

Weerda H. Unsere Erfahrungen mit der Chirurgie der Ohrmuschelmißbildungen. Teil III: Das "Miniohr" und das stark deformierte Tassenohr. Laryngo Rhino Otol. 1982 c:493–496.

Weerda H. Unsere Erfahrungen mit der Chirurgie der Ohrmuschelmißbildungen., Teil IV: Die Mikrotie. Laryngo Rhino Otol. 1982 d:497–500.

Weerda H, Münker G. Der "Bi-lobed flap" in der Rekonstruktion von Defekten der Ohrmuschel. In: Scheunemann H, Schmidseder R, Hrsg. Sonderband der Deutschen Gesellschaft für Plastische Chirurgie. Heidelberg; 1982.

Weerda H. Bi-lobed and Tri-lobed flaps in Head and Neck Defect Repair. Fac Plast Surg. 1983 a;1:51–60.

Weerda H. Die Onkochirurgie der Ohrmuschel. Langenbeck's Arch. 1983 b;361:742.

Weerda H. Die Chirurgie der kindlichen Ohrmuschelmißbildung. Laryngo Rhino Otol. 1984 a;63:120–122.

Weerda H. Die Chirurgie der Ohrmuschel nach Unfallverletzungen. In: Jungbluth K, Mommsen U, Hrsg. Plastische und wiederherstellende Massnahmen bei Unfallverletzungen. Berlin: Springer; 1984 b.

Weerda H. Probleme der operativen Therapie der Ohrmuschel-Malignome (Problems of surgery on malignancies of the auricle, in German). In: Müller R, Friedrich H, Peters J, Hrsg. Operative Dermatologie im Kopf-Hals-Bereich. Berlin: Springer;1984 c.

Weerda H, Walter C. Surgery of the pinna and surrounding area. In: Ward PH, ed. Plastic and reconstructive surgery of the head and neck. St Louis: CVMosby & Co; 1984:827–846.

Weerda H. Embryology and structural anatomy of the external ear. Fac Plast Surg. 1985 a;2:85–91.

Weerda H. Fehler und Gefahren bei der Rippenknorpel- und Rippenentnahme. Laryngo Rhino Otol. 1985 b;64:221–222.

Weerda H. Die Chirurgie der Mißbildungen der Ohrmuschel und des Mittelohres. In: Pfeifer G, Hrsg. Die Ästhetik von Form und Funktion in der Plastischen und Wiederherstellungschirurgie. Berlin: Springer; 1985 c.

Weerda H, Bockenheimer S, Trübi M. Gehörverbessernde Operationen bei Ohrmuschelmißbildungen. HNO. 1985;33:449–452.

Weerda H. Fibrinkleber in der Ohrmuschelchirurgie. In. Reifferscheid M, Hrsg. Neue Techniken in der operativen Medizin. Berlin: Springer; 1986 a.

Weerda H. The use of fibrin glue in auricular surgery. In: Schlag G, Redl H, eds. Fibrin sealant in operative medicine. Otorhinolaryngol. 1986 b;1:133.

Weerda H. Die Rekonstruktion der Ohrmuschel mit Knorpeltransplantaten. In: Kastenbauer E, Wilmes E, Mees K, Hrsg. Das Transplantat in der Plastischen Chirurgie. Deutsche Gesellschaft für Plastische und Wiederherstellungschirurgie; 1986 c.

Weerda H, Zöllner C. Chirurgie der Tumoren an der alternden Haut der Ohrregion. In: Neubauer H, Hrsg. Plastische und Wiederherstellungschirurgie. Berlin: Springer, 1986.

Weerda H, Grüner R, Cannive B. Die Einheilungsrate frei transplantierter, großer "Composite grafts". Arch Otorhinolaryngol. 1986;Suppl II/129.

Weerda H. Plastic surgery of the ear. In: Kerr AG, ed. Scott Brown's diseases of the ear, nose and throat. 5th ed. London: Butterworth; 1987:3.

Weerda H. Classification of congenital deformities of the auricle. Fac Plast Surg. 1988 a;5:385–388.

Weerda H. Reconstructive surgery of the auricle. Fac Plast Surg. 1988 b;5:399–410.

Weerda H. Helixgleitlappen in der Ohrmuschelrekonstruktion. In: Samii M, Rudolph H, Hrsg. Moderne Verfahren der Rekonstruktion von Knochenstrukturen, Gefäß- und Nervennaht sowie Transplantation in der Plastischen und Wiederherstellungschirurgie; 1988 c.

Weerda H. Trauma of the auricle: late repair. Fac Plast Surg. 1989 a;6:60–66.

Weerda H. Chirurgie der Ohrmuschelmißbildungen. In: Keßler L, Hrsg. Fehlbildungen in der Otorhinolaryngologie – Ätiologie, Diagnostik, Therapie. Leipzig: Barth; 1989 b.

Weerda H. Hals-, Nasen-, Ohrenheilkunde. Stuttgart: Enke; 1989 c.

Weerda H. Rekonstruktion der Ohrmuschel nach Tumorresektion, Unfall und Mißbildungen. In: Odar J, Hrsg. Techniken und Methoden der modernen Medizin. Darmstadt: Steinkopff; 1990 a.

Weerda H. Weichteilverletzungen im Ohrbereich und ihre Versorgung. Arch Otolaryngol. 1990 b;Suppl.II/101–103.

Weerda H. Das Ohrmuscheltrauma. In: Ganz H, Schätzle W, Hrsg. HNO-Praxis Heute. Berlin: Springer; 1991 a:11.

Weerda H. The Surgical Treatment of First and Second Degree Auricular Dysplasies. In: Stucker FJ, ed. Plastic and reconstructive surgery of the head and neck. Philadelphia: Decher; 1991 b.

Weerda H. Reproducing a Near-Normal Pinna Anatomy. In: Stucker FJ, ed. Plastic and reconstructive surgery of the head and neck: Philadelphia: Decher; 1991 c.

Weerda H. Indikation und Technik zu plastischen Eingriffen am kindlichen Gesicht einschließlich der Ohrmuschel. Abstracts, 74. Jahrestagung der Nordwestdeutschen Vereinigung der Hals-Nasen-Ohrenärzte, 1991 d.

Weerda H. Ausgesuchte Beispiele der rekonstruktiven Praxis im Kopf-Halsbereich, Schwerpunkt: Ohrmuschelrekonstruktion. In: Freigang B, Weerda H, Hrsg. Fibrinklebung in der Otorhinolaryngologie. Berlin: Springer; 1992 a.

Weerda H. Kompendium plastisch-rekonstruktiver Eingriffe, 4. Aufl. Hamburg Norderstedt: Ethicon; 1992 b.

Weerda H. Fibrinkleber in der Ohrmuschelchirurgie. Tagungsbericht 29. Jahrestagung der DG für Plastische und Wiederherstellungschirurgie. Stuttgart: Thieme; Sonderdruck, 1993:17–19.

Weerda H. Die Ohrmuschelplastik. In: Ramanzadeh R, Hrsg. Alloplastische Verfahren und mikrochirurgische Maßnahmen. Reinbek: Einhorn; 1994 a:543–548.

Weerda H. Ear – the auricle. In: Soutar O, Tiwari R, eds. Excision and reconstruction in head and neck cancer. Edinburgh: Churchill Livingstone; 1994 b:215–226.

Weerda H. Hals-, Nasen-, Ohrenheilkunde. 2. Aufl. Stuttgart: Enke; 1994 c.

Weerda H. Partial and total reconstruction of the auricle. In: Schlag G, Ascher PW, Steinkogler FJ, Stammberger H, eds. Neurosurgery, Ophthalmic Surgery, ENT. Berlin: Springer; 1994 d.

Weerda H. Anomalien des äußeren Ohres. In: Naumann HH, Helms J, Herberhold C, Kastenbauer E (Hrsg). Otorhinolaryngologie in Klinik und Praxis. Band 1 Stuttgart New York: Thieme-Verlag; 1994 e: Ohr. 488–499.

Weerda H. Entzündungen des äußeren Ohres (Otitis externa). In: Naumann HH, Helms J, Herberhold C, Kastenbauer E, Hrsg. Otorhinolaryngologie in Klinik und Praxis. Band 1 Ohr. Stuttgart: Thieme; 1994 f:499–510.

Weerda H. Traumen und nicht entzündliche Prozesse. In: Naumann HH, Helms J, Herberhold C, Kastenbauer E, Hrsg. Otorhinolaryngologie in Klinik und Praxis. Band 1 Ohr. Stuttgart: Thieme; 1994 g:510–517.

Weerda H, Siegert R. Komplikationen der Ohrmuschel-Anlegeplastik und ihre Behandlung. Laryngo Rhino Otol. 1994 a;73:394–399.

Weerda H, Siegert R. Complications in otoplastic surgery and their treatment. Facial Plast Surg. 1994 b;10:287–297.

Weerda H. Gesichts- und Ohrmuschelverletzungen – Das Ich wieder herstellen. Karlsruhe: Braun Fachverlage, Therapiewoche. 1995;19:1103–1107.

Weerda H, Siegert R. Classification and Treatment of Auricular Malformations. In: Proceedings of the 1st International Round-Table Discussion on Auricular Reconstruction, Yokohama Japan; 1995 a.

Weerda H, Siegert R. Classification and Treatment of Auricular Malformations. Face. 1995 b;4:23–29.

Weerda H. Das frische Ohrmuscheltrauma. HNO. 1996 a;44:701–709.

Weerda H. Die Ohrmuschelrekonstruktion nach NAGATA – Vorteile und Nachteile gegenüber der BRENT-Technik. In: Berghaus A, Hrsg. Plastische und Wiederherstellungschirurgie. Reinbek: Einhorn; 1996 b.

Weerda H, Siegert R. Zugangswege zur plastischen Ohrmuschelrekonstruktion im Kindesalter. In: Schmelzle R, Hrsg. Plastische und Wiederherstellungschirurgie – Ein Jahrbuch. Bremen: UNI-MED; 1996.

Weerda H. Plastic surgery of the ear. In: Kerr AG, ed. Scott Brown's Otolaryngology, 6th ed. London: Heinemann- Butterworth; 1997 a:3/8/1–21.

Weerda H. Geschichte der Otoplastik. Laryngo Rhino Otol. 1997 b;76:715.

Weerda H, Siegert R. Die Komplikationen der Otoplastik und ihre Behandlung. Laryngo Rhino Otol. 1997;76:716.

Weerda H, Siegert R, Danter J. Auricular reconstruction for microtia: Nagata's technique in comparison to other methods. Eur Arch Otorhinolaryngol. 1997;254:54.

Weerda H. Discussion of personal technique in panel by Brent B. "Solving problems in autogenous auricular reconstruction". Presented at ear reconstruction '98. Choices for the Future. Chateau Lake Louise, Canada. 1998 a.

Weerda H. 3rd International Symposium on Auricular and Middle Ear Malformations, Ear Defects and their Reconstruction. FOCUS MUL. 1998 b;15:1.

Weerda H. Das Ohrmuscheltrauma – Kurzreferate der 32. Fortbildungsveranstaltung Hannover 1998. Köln: medio Druck & Logistik, 1998 c.

Weerda H. Epithetische Wiederherstellung im Gesicht. Dtsch Ärztebl. 1998 d;43:2711.

Weerda H, Siegert R. Classification of Auricular Malformations. Face. 1998 a;5:157–158.

Weerda H, Siegert R. Complications in otoplastic procedures. Face. 1998 b;1169–175.

Weerda H, Siegert R. First degree dysplasias: our surgical techniques. Face.1998 c;5:195–197.

Weerda H, Siegert R. Second degree dysplasias: our surgical techniques. Face. 1998 d;5:213–215.

Weerda H, Siegert R. Third degree dysplasias. our surgical techniques. Face. 1998 e;6:79–82.

Weerda H, Siegert R. Classification and treatment of acquired deformities. Face. 1998 f;6:79–82.

Weerda H, Siegert R . Auricular and Middle Ear Malformations, Ear Defects and their Reconstruction. The Hague/The Netherlands. Kugler Publications; 1998 g.

Weerda H, Siegert R. Third degree dysplasias: our surgical techniques. In: Weerda H, Siegert R, eds. Auricular and Middle Ear Malformations, Ear Defects and their Reconstruction. The Hague/ The Netherlands. Kugler Publications; 1998 h.

Weerda H, Siegert R. Complications after Otoplasty and their Treatment. Eur Arch Otorhinolaryngol. 1998 i;255:88.

Weerda H. Plastisch-rekonstruktive Chirurgie im Gesichtsbereich. Ein Kompendium für Problemlösungen. Stuttgart: Thieme; 1999 a.

Weerda H. Die subtotale und totale Ohrmuschelrekonstruktion. In: Krupp S, Hrsg. Plastische Chirurgie in Klinik und Praxis, Ecomed; 1999 b;Bd I/9.2:1–33.

Weerda H, Siegert R. Otoplastic Procedures and the Treatment of Complications. In: Bull, ed. Aesthetic Facial Surgery. Reinbek: Einhorn-Presse Verlag; 1999 a.

Weerda H, Siegert R. Rekonstruktion der Ohrmuschel: In: Kastenbauer ER, Tardy ME, Hrsg. Ästhetische und Plastische Chirurgie an Nase, Gesicht und Ohrmuschel. Stuttgart: Thieme, 1999 b.

Weerda H, Siegert R. Klassifikation und Behandlung der Ohrmuschelmißbildungen. Dt Ärztebl. 1999 c;96:A2216–A2218.

Weerda H, Gehrking E. Die (sonografisch kontrollierte) Feinnadelpunktionszytologie im Kopf-Halsbereich. HNO. 2000;48:419–420.

Weerda H. Reconstructive Facial Plastic Surgery. A Problem-Solving Manual. Stuttgart: Thieme; 2001.

Weerda H. Chirurgie der Ohrmuschel. Verletzungen, Defekte und Anomalien. Stuttgart: Thieme; 2004.

Weidner F, Tonak J. Das maligne Melanom der Haut. Erlangen: Perimed; ohne Jahresangabe.

Welling DB, Glasscock ME, Gantz BJ. Avulsion of the anomalous facial nerve at stapedectomy. Laryngoscope 1992; 102: 729–33.

Wellisz T. Reconstruction of the burned external ear with a Medpor porous polyethylene pivoting helix framework. Plast Reconstr Surg. 1993;91:811–818.

Welsh F. Otoplasty: excision of conchal floor cartilage. Aesthetic Plast Surg. 1980;4:87–93.

Wickstrom OW, Bromberg BE. Total ear reconstruction with allogenous costal cartilage and autogenous perichondrium. Acta Med Pl. 1980;21:87–92.

Wieland H. Einfache Operationstechnik zur Ohrmuschelkorrektur. Arch Otolaryngol. 1971;199:514–519.

Williams R, Havoonjian I, Isagholian K, Menaker G, Moy R. A clinical study of hair removal using the long-pulsed ruby laser. Dermatol Surg 1998;24: 837–842.

Wilmes E, Landthaler M, Schubert-Fritschle G. Therapie und Prognose maligner Melanome im Kopf-Hals-Bereich. Arch Oto Rhino Laryngol. 1988;Suppl II;185–186.

Wilmington D, Gray L, Jahrdoerfer R. Binaural processing after corrected unilateral conductive hearing loss. Hearing Research. 1994;74:99–114.

Wimmershoff MB, Hohenleutner U, Landthaler M. Isomorphic phenomenon: adverse effect after epilation with the long-pulsed ruby laser. Arch Dermatol 2000;136:1570–1571.

Wodak E. Über die Stellung und Form der menschlichen Ohrmuschel. Arch Klin Exp Ohren-Nasen-Kehlkopfheilk. 1967;188:331–336.

Wolfe MM. Protruding ears: The Psychological Effect and Plastic Correction. Med Record. 1936;144:306.

Wood-Smith D. Otoplasty. In: Rees T, Wood-Smith D, eds. Cosmetic facial surgery. Philadelphia: Saunders; 1973.

Woolford TJ, Morris DP, Saeed SR, Rothera MP. The implant- site split-skin graft technique for the bone- anchored hearing aid. Clin Otolaryngol. 1999;24:177–80.

Yamada A, Fukuda O, Soeda S. The evaluation of cleft earlobe. Plast Reconstr Surg. 1976;19:171.

Yanai A, Fukuda O, Nagata S, Tanaka H. A new method utilizing the bipedicle flap for reconstruction of the external auditory canal in microtia. Plast Reconstr Surg. 1985;76:464–468.

Yano K, Hata Y, Matsuka K, Ito O. Morphometric characteristics of cryptotia. Ann Plast Surg. 1994;33:178–183.

Yates JA, Patel PC, Millman B, Gibson WS. Isolated congenital internal auditory canal atresia with normal facial nerve function. Int J Pediatr Otorhinolaryngol. 1997;41:1–8.

Yeakley JW, Jahrsdoerfer RA. CT Evaluation of congenital aural atresia: What the radiologist and the surgeon need to know. J Comput Assist Tomogr. 1996; 20:724–731.

Yotsuyanagi T, Sawada Y, Tanaka I, Yokoi K et al. Postoperative management using a splint after reconstruction of microtia. In. Weerda H, Siegert R, eds. Auricular and Middle Ear Malformations, Ear Defects and their Reconstruction. The Hague/The Netherlands: Kugler Publication; 1998;39–43.

Yotsuyangi T. Earlobe reconstruction using a chondrocutaneous flaps. Plast Reconstr Surg. 1994;94:1075–1078.

Young F. Autogenous cartilage grafts, an experimental study. Surgery. 1941;10:7–10.

Young F. Correction of abnormaly prominent ears. Gynecol Obstet. 1944 a;78:541–550.

Young F. Cast and precast cartilage grafts. Surgery. 1944 b;15: 735–748.

Yousif N, Warren R, Matloub H, Sanger J. The lateral arm fascial free flap. In: Anatomy and Use in Reconstruction. Plast Reconstr Surg. 1990;86:1138–1145.

Zeifer B, Sabini P, Sonne J. Congenital absence of the oval window: radiologic diagnosis and associated anomalies. AJNR. 2000;21:322–327.

Zeis E. Die Literatur und Geschichte der plastischen Chirurgie. Leipzig: W Engelmann; 1838 a.

Zeis E. Von der Otoplastik oder Ohrbildung. In: Zeis E. Handbuch der plastischen Chirurgie. Berlin: G Reimer; 1838 b;IX Abteilung: 464–468.

Zeis E. Die Geschichte der Otoplastik. In: Zeis E. Die Literatur und Geschichte der plastischen Chirurgie. Leipzig: W Engelmann: 1838 (Reprinted by Amaldo Forini Bologna. 1963;270–275).

Zenner HP, Leysieffer H. Active electronic hearing implants for middle and inner ear hearing loss – a new era in ear surgery II: Current state of developments. HNO 1997;45:758–768.

Zenteno S. Auricular reduction. In: Proceedings of the Xth Congress of Internat Plast Reconstr Surgeon Confederation: Madrid; 1992.

Zubriczky von J. Verletzungen des menschlichen Gehörgangs. Monatsschr Ohrenheilk Laryngorhinol. 1935;69:208–218.

Zühlke D. Weiche, elastische Kunststoffe in der HNO-Heilkunde. Pract Oto-Rhino-Laryng. 1960;22:99–110.

Appendix 1: Examination Form For External Ear Patients

(adapted from one used by Burt Brent)

Name: ______________________ Age: ________ Date: ______________

Diagram of the deformity, measured length of the ear

Right ear Left ear

OPERATIVE PLAN

OP I: ______________________________

OP II: ______________________________

OP III: ______________________________

OP IV: ______________________________

Further operations: ______________________________

Family history, ear: ______________________________

Family history, general: ______________________________

____

Occupation: ______________________________

Childhood illnesses: ______________________________

______________________________ Previous surgery (general): ______________

Allergies: ______________________ Mental disorders: ______________

____

Nicotine, alcohol: ______________________________

Bleeding disorders: ______________________________

General condition: ______________________________

Hearing problems: ______________________________

____

Acute illnesses, infectious diseases: ______________________________

____

Chest findings: ______________________________

Audiological findings: ______________________________

____

____

CT-findings: ______________________________

____

____

Comments: ______________________________

____

____

____

MIDDLE EAR SURGERY

– Other previous operations (right side, left side, hospital, year, treatment records requested) –

____

____

____

____

____

____

Referring physician: ______________________________

OPERATION

Auricular reconstruction, stage one: ______________________________

Auricular reconstruction, stage two: ______________________________

Auricular reconstruction, stage three and further stages: ____________________

CONSENT

____

(Signature of the parents/guardian and/or patient)

Place, date: ______________________________

Patient Information for Informed Consent

Dear [Name of patient]

You have asked us to operate on your ear. This letter contains some information about what this procedure involves, and some advice you may find helpful.
Reconstruction of the ear proceeds in two or three stages. Each time you will have to stay in hospital for a few days (a maximum of 2 weeks).

Stage one:
In this operation, we take some cartilage from your ribs and use it to make a framework which will form the front surface of the ear. This framework is then transplanted beneath the skin near your ear. A small portion of the rib cartilage is saved under the skin of your chest, to be used later for further reconstructive stages.

Stage two:
About 2–3 months later, we free the cartilage framework from under the skin, and in the same operation we resurface the fold behind the ear with a skin graft taken from your head, chest, or buttock. Any rib cartilage that is left over is again placed beneath the skin of your chest, as it may be required for the next stage.

Stage three:
A further 2–3 months later, we will make fine adjustments to the contours of the ear or remove hairs.
Wound healing is then largely complete, but the skin over the cartilage framework is still very sensitive. We therefore recommend that you look after your new ear by protecting it against:

- Injury (contact sports)
- Mechanical stress (rubbing when washing, or from headwear)
- Exposure to damp heat (in the sauna)
- Exposure to too much sun
- Exposure to extreme cold

Do not wash your new ear until at least 2 weeks after the operation (and then very carefully). You should then regularly remove any sloughed-off skin, especially behind the ear. Scabs should be gradually dissolved with a moisturizing ointment or baby oil.
You should continue to wear a headband at night for three to four weeks to prevent any rubbing of the skin. You may not notice any soreness from this because it has a reduced level of sensation.
If the skin is subjected to excessive stress for any reason, and the whitish cartilage is exposed, cover it immediately with povidone-iodine (betadine) ointment and contact your specialist right away. It is important to cover the injured area with ointment as soon as possible, or it may dry out causing loss of the cartilage.

You should use a special dressing with steroid cream to cover the scar on your chest wall for about 4 weeks. This will result in a better scar. You can also treat the scar with a steroid cream for 2 weeks and with Contractubex gel for a further 4 weeks.

If you have any further questions, please contact us and we will do our best to answer them.

Appendix 2: Suture Materials

Manufactured by Ethicon, Inc. (see text for further suture materials)

Suture material	Strength	Needle	Thread length	Colour	Comments
Steel wire monofilament	5–0	ST-4 19.1 mm ▼sharp double armed	15 cm		For the buried suture of the supportive framework
	5–0	FS-2 19 mm ▼sharp	45 cm		Fixation of the cartilage block at the 2nd stage of Nagata's procedure
PDS II monofilament	4–0	PSL 30 mm ▼sharp	50 cm	Violet	Contouring of the helix
	5–0	PS-1-needle ▼sharp	45 cm	Violet	Contouring of the helix
	5–0	PS-3 16 mm ▼sharp	45 cm	Violet	Contouring of the helix
	5–0	P-3 13 mm, 3/8 ▼sharp	45 cm	Violet	Earlobe skin suture 1st stage
	6–0	P-1 Prime 11 mm, 3/8 ▼sharp	45 cm	Violet	Skin suture
	7–0	P-6, 8 mm ▼sharp	45 cm	Violet	Skin suture
VICRYL braided	4–0	ST-4 Black 19 mm double armed ● roundbodied	35 cm	Violet	For the cartilage supportive framework and subcutaneous suture
	4–0	P-3 13 mm, 3/8 ▼sharp	45 cm	Undyed	For the cartilage supportive framework and subcutaneous suture
	5–0	P-3 13 mm, 3/8 ▼sharp	45 cm	Undyed	Subcutaneous suture 1st stage
	6–0	P-1 11 mm, 3/8 ▼sharp	45 cm	Undyed	Subcutaneous suture 1st stage
PROLENE monofilament	2–0	PS-2 19 mm, 3/8 ▼sharp	45 cm	Blue	For conchal rotation
MERSILENE (polyester) braided	4–0	P-3 13 mm, 3/8 ▼sharp	45 cm	Undyed	Ear setback (pinnaplasty)
	3–0	FS-1 24 mm, 3/8 ▼sharp		Dyed or undyed	Conchal (caval) rotation
	2–0	FS-1 24 mm, 3/8 ▼sharp	45 cm	Dyed or undyed	Conchal (caval) rotation

Appendix 3: Self-help Groups

Auricular Dysplasias (Goldenhar Syndrome)

Goldenhar Family Support Group (UK)
Goldenhar Support Group
299 Burncross Road
Sheffield S35 1SA
United Kingdom
www.goldenhar.org.uk

Goldenhar Syndrome Support Network
(International Network)
9325 163 Street
Edmonton, Alberta
T5R 2P4 Canada
www.goldenharsyndrome.org

Facial Disfigurement

AboutFace USA
PO Box 158
South Beloit, IL 61080
USA
www.aboutfaceusa.org

Children's Craniofacial Association
134140 Coit Road
Dallas, TX 75240
USA
www.ccakids.com

Let's Face It (USA)
University of Michigan
School of Dentristy/Dentristry Library
1011 N. University
Ann Arbor, MI 48109-1078
www.dont.umich.edu/faceit/

Let's Face It (UK)
Christine Piff
72 Victoria Avenue
Westgate on Sea
Kent CT8 8BH
United Kingdom
www.lets-face-it.org.uk

Other Related Organizations

American Speech-Language-Hearing Association
10801 Rockville Pike
Rockville, MD 20852
USA
www.asha.org

Birth Defect Research for Children, Inc.
930 Woodcock Road
Orlando, FL 32803
USA
www.birthdefects.org

IBIS: International Birth Defects
Information Systems
www.ibis-birthdefects.org

Treacher Collins (Franceschetti) Syndrome

Treacher Collins Family Support Group
114 Vincent Road
Norwich NR1 4HH
United Kingdom
www.treachercollins.net

Index

A

B

C

D

E

Q

R

S

T

U

V

W

X

Y

Z